AJN / MOSBY

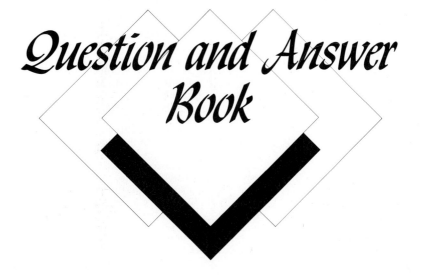

Question and Answer Book

For the NCLEX-RN Examination

Managing Editor

Rose Mary Carroll-Johnson, MN, RN. *Nurse Editor, Valencia, California*

Coordinators for this Edition

Judith K. Leavitt, MEd, RN. *Consultant, Ithaca, New York*

Paulette D. Rollant, MSN, RN, CCRN. *President, Multi-Resources, Inc., Grantville, Georgia*

Diane S. Smith, MSN, RN, CS, NP. *Psychiatric Nurse Practitioner, Grosse Pointe Center, Grosse Pointe Park, Michigan*

Francene M. Weatherby, PhD, RNC

Contributing Authors for this Edition

Deborah A. Ennis, MSN, RN, CCRN. *Associate Professor of Nursing, Harrisburg Area Community College, Harrisburg, Pennsylvania*

Peg Gray-Vickery, MS, RNC. *Doctoral Student, University at Buffalo School of Nursing, Buffalo, New York*

Marybeth Young, PhD, MSN, RNC. *Assistant Professor, Maternal-Child Nursing, Loyola University, Chicago, Illinois*

Contributing Authors for Previous Editions

Paula J. Albertson, BSN, RN
M. Regina Asaro, BSN, RN
Diane J. Baker, BSN, RN
Janis P. Bellack, PhD, MN, RN
Kay Bensing, MA, RN
Louise Bradford, RN, MSN
Nancy Jo Bush, MN, RN,
Geraldine C. Colombraro, MA, RN
Olivian DeSouza, MSN, RN
Gita L. Dhillon, CNM, MEd, RN
Deborah DiGiaro, MS, RN
Cynthia Dunsmore, MS, RN
Janice M. Dyehouse, MSN, RN
Doris S. Edwards, MS, RN
Lou Ann T. Emerson, MSN, RN
Linda Finke, MSN, RN
Silva Foxpuglisi, MS, RN
Julia B. George, PhD, RN
Jo Ann Gragnani, MS, MA, RN
Cindy Smith Greenberg, MS, RN, CPNP
Carol Seal Hildebrand, MSN, RN
Wendy B. Hollis, MN, RN
Carolyn Kay Jass, MS, RN
Ann L. Jessop, MSN, RN
Phyllis Walls Juett, MSN, RN
Elizabeth C. Kaiser, MSN, RN
Michele M. Kamradt, EdD, RN
Shari Wazney Keba, MSN, RN
Retha Vornholt Keenan, MSN, RN

Marie Trava King, MAN, RN
Deborah Koniak, EdD, RN
Beverly Kopala, MS, RN
Susan L. W. Krupnick, MSN, CCRN, CEN, CS, RN
Judith K. Leavitt, MEd, RN
Elizabeth J. Lipp, MS, RN
Mariann C. Lovell, MS, RN
Esther Matassarin-Jacobs, PhD, MSN, MEd, RN
Edwina A. McConnell, PhD, MS, RN
Michele Michael, MSN, RN
Mary Ann Niehaus, MSN, RN
B. Patricia Nix, MSN, RN
Mary Paquette, MN, RN
Joan Webster Reighley, MN, RN
Constance Ritzman, MSN, RN
Mary-Charles Santopietro, EdD, MS, EdM, RN
Victoria Schoolcraft, MSN, RN
Virginia Madden Shea, MS, RN
Brenda Hanson Smith, MSN, RNC
Janet Trigg, MSN, RN
Quilla D.B. Turner, PhD, MN, RN
Deborah L. Ulrich, MA, RN
Esther Coto Walloch, MN, RN
Gail D. Wegner, MS, RN
Elizabeth Elder Weiner, PhD, RN
Jean H. Woods, PhD, RNCS
Donna J. Woodside, EdD, RN
Nancy K. Worley, MSN, RN
Marybeth Young, PhD, MSN, RN

AJN/MOSBY

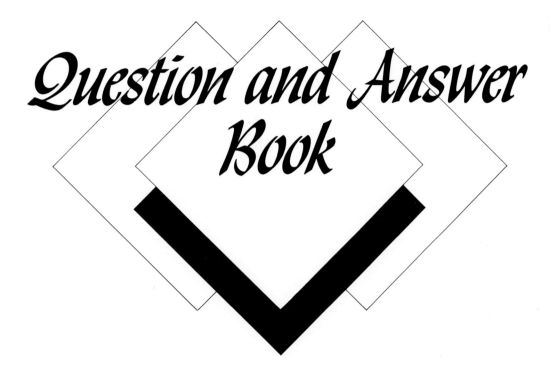

Question and Answer Book

For the NCLEX-RN Examination

THIRD EDITION

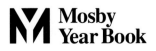

Mosby
Year Book

St. Louis   Baltimore   Boston   Chicago   London   Philadelphia   Sydney   Toronto

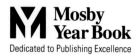

Mosby
Year Book
Dedicated to Publishing Excellence

Senior Editor: Nancy L. Coon
Managing editor: Susan R. Epstein
Project Manager: Karen Edwards
Production Editor: James Russell
Book and Cover Design: Gail Morey Hudson

THIRD EDITION

Accurate indications, adverse reactions, and dosage schedules for
drugs are provided in this book, but it is possible they may
change. The reader is urged to review the package information data
of the manufacturers of the medications mentioned.

First Edition 1984

Printed in the United States of America

Mosby–Year Book, Inc.
11830 Westline Industrial Drive
St. Louis, MO 63146

International Standard Book Number 0-8016-0015-4

GW/MV 9 8 7 6 5 4 3 2 1

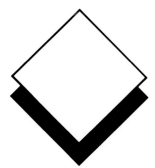

Introduction

Most registered nurses will remember in detail the experience of preparing for and taking the state licensing examination, or NCLEX-RN, as it has come to be called. When I took the exam in 1960-something, my friends and I took our textbooks, the *one* available review text, and a supply of suntan lotion, and retired to the beach to study (actually we crammed for a week). Yes, we all passed with flying colors, but how much more fortunate are the graduates of today. Not only is there a wide array of review books to choose from, but they come in many forms. In addition, the review courses are plentiful and affordable. Graduates can now pick the types of review and studying that complement their learning styles.

This volume completes a trio of offerings from the AJN Company and Mosby–Year Book. Here you will find a whole book of practice questions to use alone or in combination with the *AJN/Mosby Nursing Boards Review* text and the AJN/Mosby Nursing Boards Review course.

In this new third edition, Section 1 explains in detail the NCLEX-RN testing format and scoring methods. Strategies on how to read questions more carefully and select the correct answer are included to increase your test-wiseness. Techniques to help you reduce your stress on the day of the examination are also presented. Read this section first, and refer to it as often as necessary for reinforcement.

Sections 2 through 5 contain more than 1100 questions organized according to:

—Nursing Care of the Client with Psychosocial and Mental Health Problems
—Nursing Care of the Adult
—Nursing Care of the Childbearing Family
—Nursing Care of the Child.

The correct answers and rationales that explain all the possible answers follow each section. At the end of each rationale, you will be able to determine what section of the *AJN/Mosby Nursing Boards Review* contains the content and what aspect of the nursing process and client needs framework the question tests.

Section 6 contains two sample examinations for practice. The test items have been carefully mixed for content. Each examination includes four books of 95 questions each. When you feel ready, set aside time for each examination. The goal is to answer each book within 90 minutes (6 hours for each test). This period parallels the time you will be allowed on the NCLEX-RN.

In the appendix you will find each question categorized according to its nursing process and client need categories. This information can help you assess your knowledge and ability in each of these areas.

Develop a system for review that meets your needs. The table of contents for each section will help you locate questions that test specific health problems within that section. Based on your answers and your understanding of the answer rationales, you may decide you need to review content in a specific area using your textbooks or the *AJN/Mosby Nursing Boards Review*.

The test items in this book have been prepared by the national faculty who teach the AJN/Mosby Nursing Boards Review course. All are instructors, clinical specialists, or authors in the clinical specialty. They, along with all of us involved in the production of this book at the AJN Company and at Mosby–Year Book, wish you every success on the NCLEX-RN and in your career as a registered professional nurse.

Rose Mary Carroll-Johnson

Managing Editor

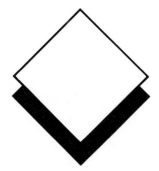

Contents

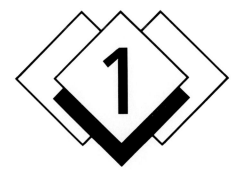

Preparing for the NCLEX-RN

Marybeth Young, PhD, MSN, RNC

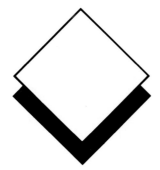

Preparing for the NCLEX-RN

PRETEST

1. Test items on the NCLEX-RN are based on case studies
   a. describing actual or potential health problems.
   b. emphasizing knowledge of physiology and safe, effective care.
   c. focusing on situations encountered by entry-level nurses.
   d. All of the above choices are correct.
2. The examination requires that the graduate nurse select
   a. one single, correct response.
   b. answers from "multiple-multiple" options.
3. Time allotted for each of the approximately 93 items in each section is
   a. 20 seconds.
   b. 30 seconds.
   c. 45 seconds.
   d. 60 seconds.
4. The integrated nursing exam contains about the same number of questions measuring applied knowledge of
   a. pediatric, maternity, and medical-surgical nursing.
   b. assessment, analysis, planning, implementation, and evaluation.
   c. acute illnesses and chronic health problems.
   d. risk factors and measures to promote health.
5. Which of the following test-taking hints is *not* useful in taking the licensure examination?
   a. Try to narrow the possible answers to two choices.
   b. Focus on key words such as *initially* or *least effective*.
   c. *Do not guess* if you are unsure of an answer.
   d. Be careful when erasing responses and changing them.

After completing the above pretest, you may find that you want more accurate information about the licensure examination ahead. Reading the following information may contribute to your success.

PREPARING FOR THE LICENSURE EXAM
Planning for Review: Unique Features of this Text.

You are preparing for professional entry at an exciting period of transition into the twenty-first century. The acute nursing shortage has increased recruitment among diverse ethnic groups, males, and those considering a career change. Clinical career ladders increasingly reward excellent practitioners. Research studies involve nurses at all levels and contribute to quality care. As acuity levels increase during very brief hospitalizations, nurses are challenged to collaborate in planning comprehensive home care. Health maintenance and health promotion are increasingly viewed as cost effective and a creative use of nursing expertise.

In order to practice safely in a changing health care system, you will need to use and refine clinical problem-solving skills. Thoughtful identification, analysis, and resolution of client problems have been part of your professional education and will continue through lifelong learning. This approach to client needs also may be applied as you prepare for the licensure examination, the NCLEX-RN. In this introductory section, suggestions are offered to help you successfully complete the test.

A summary of the exam format, suggested cognitive testing strategies, and approaches to reduce tension should help you develop an individualized plan for test preparation and review. Then you will be able to use the material in this text to organize your nursing knowledge and better understand the many aspects of safe practice.

KNOW THE TEST FORMAT

Just as the novice driver needs to know what to expect on the state driving test, each graduate nurse needs a clear idea of the professional licensure exam format. Knowing that you have some questions about the test itself or are unsure of your responses on the pretest, the following brief summary will provide answers.

Success on the national examination is required for entry into professional practice. The same multiple-choice test currently is administered throughout the United States twice each year. Computerized Adaptive Testing (CAT) currently is offered as a field test in selected sites across the nation. Eventually, this computer-interactive approach will eliminate some stress often experienced in a massive testing environment. If your state is involved in this testing approach or you participate in clinical simulation testing, information will be shared with you in advance. Until the test format changes in every state, which will take several years, the current paper-and-pencil test will be used to measure competence.

There are approximately 93 test items in each of 4 separate, integrated sections. (Some questions are "pilot items" and are not counted toward the pass/fail score. However, since these are not identified as such, respond to each item with equal attention.) Situations and questions represent a variety of client health problems and needs. One case study describing a plan for health promotion of a young family may be followed by another case study focusing on the safe care environment of an adolescent in an acute-care setting. Test items focus on critical requirements for competent practice rather than on separate specialty content, such as pediatric or surgical nursing.

The National Council of State Boards of Nursing organizes the licensure examination around a broad framework comprising the "Nursing Process" and "Categories of Human Needs." Each part of this plan is summarized briefly; implications for review are suggested.

Nursing Process

The nursing process provides organization for the test as it does for care planning in every clinical setting. Each nursing process phase is equally important in resolving health problems. This consistency is immediately evident to test takers who perceive this equal emphasis. These same graduates are quick to point out that the numbers of items testing maternity and psychiatric nursing are not equal; medical-surgical nursing is heavily emphasized. Table 1-1 suggests a possible test item focus for each phase of the nursing process.

Categories of Human Needs

Concepts that contribute to understanding human needs are another exam focus. Among these are basic human needs, the teaching-learning process, therapeutic communication, crisis intervention, and developmental theory. Knowledge of anatomy, physiology and pathophysiology, asepsis, nutrition, accountability, the group process, and mental health concepts is basic to the prac-

Table 1-1 Test item focus suggested by the nursing process

Phase	Possible item focus
Assessment	Identifying data base
	Selecting appropriate means to gather data
	Gathering information from client/family
	Noting significant observations/data
	Considering environmental factors
	Recognizing client/family strengths, limitations
Analysis	Prioritizing potential/actual problems
	Selecting an appropriate nursing diagnosis
	Interpreting meaning of test results
Planning	Setting measurable long/short-term goals
	Prioritizing goals
	Involving client/family in goal setting
	Examining/modifying existing plan
	Sharing plan with client/family/staff
Implementation	Carrying out nursing actions safely
	Understanding rationale for care
	Prioritizing care
	Assisting with self-care
	Calculating/administering medications safely
	Suggesting diet modifications
	Ensuring safety/comfort
	Preventing infection/injury
	Promoting mobility/independence
	Responding to emergencies
	Recording/sharing information
	Teaching to client's intellectual level
	Communicating appropriately with client/family/staff
	Supervising/delegating care
Evaluation	Comparing outcomes to goals
	Examining response to therapy
	Seeking more information
	Identifying learning outcomes
	Recognizing risks/problems of therapy
	Communicating outcomes to staff/family
	Reassessing/revising plan

tice of nursing and also is incorporated into many test items. The organization of client needs based on these concepts is identified by the National Council of State Boards of Nursing as "Categories of Human Needs" and is part of the test format. These four categories flow from the ANA Nursing Social Policy Statement and current research on job analysis for beginning practitioners. The greatest NCLEX-RN exam emphasis is on the categories of physiological integrity (42%-48%) and safe care environment (25%-31%). Health promotion and mainte-

Table 1-2   Categories of human needs

Categories	Nursing focus
Safe, effective care environment	Coordinating care Ensuring quality Setting goals Promoting safety Preparing client for treatments/procedures Implementing care
Physiological integrity	Promoting adaptation Identifying/reducing risks Fostering mobility Ensuring comfort Providing care
Psychosocial integrity	Promoting adaptation Facilitating coping
Health promotion/maintenance	Promoting growth and development Directing self-care Fostering support systems Prevention/early treatment of disease

Table 1-3   Test item focus suggested by categories of human needs

Human needs category	Possible test item focus
Safe, effective care environment	Understanding basic principles Using management skills Implementing protective measures Promoting safety Ensuring client/family rights Preventing spread of infection
Physiological integrity	Recognizing altered body function Using body mechanics Providing comfort measures Using equipment safely Understanding effects of immobility Recognizing untoward responses to therapy/medication/procedures Documenting emergency actions
Psychosocial integrity	Identifying mental health concepts Recognizing behavior changes Referring to resources Communicating appropriately
Health promotion/maintenance	Understanding family systems Teaching nutrition Promoting wellness Strengthening immune responses Recognizing adaptive changes to health alterations Considering cultural/religious impact on childbearing Supporting the dying/family

nance (12%-18%) and psychosocial integrity (9%-15%) are also incorporated (see Tables 1-2 and 1-3).

Some overlap is evident as you look at the nursing process framework and the categories of client needs. For example, the nursing process phase of planning addresses both physiological and psychosocial needs. However, if an individual has a severe deficit in fluid volume related to dehydration, emotional needs are attended to *after* setting a goal to resolve life-threatening physiological problems. Priority setting is critical to exam success, just as it is in clinical care giving.

Use your knowledge of the test format to help you identify and review concepts learned throughout your nursing education and to prepare thoughtfully for the examination. However, during the actual NCLEX-RN exam, do not attempt to identify whether safe, effective care or physiological integrity is tested in a particular item.

Applied knowledge, rather than mere recall of facts, is measured in most test questions. Detailed and sometimes lengthy case studies describe a client or family with emphasis on health needs, followed by several questions. In order to answer these, you will need to use knowledge gained from clinical experience and classroom learning to identify and resolve client problems. Expect to find test questions challenging and varying in difficulty. Application of knowledge may be subtle, such as selecting a toy appropriate for a hospitalized toddler in traction, or suggesting emergency treatment for a neighbor who splashes cleaning solution in her eyes. Remember that standards for care are based on general principles. Although environmental factors may affect client needs, priorities for safe care are based on those general principles.

HOW THE TEST IS SCORED

The exam grading method differs significantly from standardized achievement or aptitude tests. For example, instructions given before college placement exams urge students to avoid guessing. Directions given to you before the nursing licensure exam stress that guessing is not penalized. An educated guess may thus contribute to success. If you can narrow the four options to two possibilities, the probability is 50% for making a correct choice. Completing all questions becomes a critical goal because the grading process results in a pass/fail score based on the number of correct responses. Although individuals who fail the exam are informed of the approximate number of items missed, there is no numerical score.

There is no separate answer sheet, and responses are

marked by filling in circles at the left of each option. All stray pencil marks and underlining must be erased before turning in the test booklet so that the scanner does not pick them up during the grading process. A blank page is provided for mathematical calculations of medication doses and IV flow rates. This is also an ideal "scratch sheet" on which to note items you skip initially but plan to reexamine after completing the rest of the exam. This approach saves time and eliminates the need to scan the entire booklet to locate omitted responses.

Remember, the NCLEX-RN test plan has been developed to measure critical thinking and nursing competence. Knowing the framework of the exam should dispel some of your fears and help you to anticipate and prepare for the test. When the actual date arrives, do not think about the "test plan," but concentrate on the challenge of each case study and the related questions. Just as the driver attends the road test without wondering, "What is being tested now?" you need only address the problem-solving task.

WHERE SHOULD YOU BEGIN?

When you are familiar with this text and the test format, map out a personal plan for preparation and review. If independent study is planned, set realistic goals within the time available. Ideally, reviewing content over several months is preferable to "cramming" in a few weeks. Studying regularly, over time, helps to reinforce knowledge and improves your ability to apply that knowledge.

Begin your review plan by focusing on content that is less familiar to you or about which you feel insecure. Your results on standardized national tests, such as the AssessTest, could serve as a guide, or you may select several case studies and answer the questions that follow. After completing the test items, refer to the correct responses, rationale, and test format classification; then compare your problem-solving abilities to those of content experts. You may find it helpful to review the *AJN/Mosby Nursing Boards Review*, a nursing specialty or fundamentals text, or your class notes to resolve doubts or increase understanding. Look for patterns of test-taking difficulties as you review responses. Becoming aware of your strengths and weaknesses in test taking is an important phase of review and gives more meaningful feedback than counting correct and incorrect responses. By beginning with the greatest challenge and reinforcing understanding, your confidence is renewed as the date of the exam approaches.

COGNITIVE AND AFFECTIVE KEYS TO SUCCESS

There are three factors that are important in achieving success: *reading*, which affects both reviewing and test taking; *test wiseness*, which is defined as the ability to use a test situation to demonstrate learning; and the ability to *control tension* in a major examination, free-

Table 1-4   Cognitive strategies for success

Prepare	for safe practice
Plan a review	to broaden knowledge
Read carefully	for understanding
Identify key words	to focus attention
Narrow options	by critical thinking
Use an educated guess	not random choice
Set priorities	based on health risk
Trust decisions	avoid many erasures

ing the mind to concentrate on the written questions. Although these factors are interrelated, they are discussed separately. Suggestions and strategies are offered for use during your licensure exam experience (Table 1-4).

Cognitive Strategies to Promote Success

Reading with concentration is a learned skill that is critical for study, review, and successful examination performance. When preparing for the NCLEX-RN, select an environment that is well-lighted and suits your learning style. Avoid reading on a bed—its comfort may induce sleep rather than reinforce knowledge. Gather all materials in advance for the planned study session, including this review book, other appropriate texts, notes, and marker pens to highlight content needing subsequent review.

Skim the review text material, then read for understanding. Look up any unfamiliar terms. Make a note of further questions that come to mind as you review information. Use your knowledge of anatomy, physiology, and pathophysiology to visualize the impact of a specific health alteration. Review the disease process, preventive measures, restoration, and rehabilitation. Refresh your memory of procedures specifically used in treatment. Think about ways in which health might be improved.

While reading test items as practice or in a real situation, be especially observant of *key words*. Notice cues such as *age, risk factors,* and *coping mechanisms*. Clearly identify the question focus (e.g., the concerned parent, the ill child, or the caregiver). Use your knowledge of nursing to think through the question and consider possible responses even before reading all possible options.

Be sure to control the time you spend considering each situation and question. During each 90-minute test section you will not have the luxury of time to thoughtfully *reread* and reflect. For this reason, it is wise to omit the very complex problems that may take several minutes to resolve. Return to those challenges after completing the less difficult items.

Although you must read carefully to understand the questions, avoid reading into the words more than is actually stated. Assume that the health care agency described is ideal and well staffed. If you think that the client's needs would be met by a midnight snack of milk and crackers, do not qualify this with ". . . but it may be impossible to provide this at night."

During the exam, you have no resource for defining vocabulary. Use the sentence context to deduce the meaning of unfamiliar words. Refer to the case study for insight and clarification, and remember to apply your understanding of pathophysiology throughout the exam.

One word of caution about rereading questions as you complete a test section. Occasionally, a series of items describes a client's progress over several days of treatment. Do not alter care priorities for the day of admission based on results of later diagnostic tests.

The following examples give you an opportunity to apply several testing strategies to varied questions typical of the NCLEX-RN. Priority setting can be a challenge on a written test. One approach is to view each option as a true/false statement. This is especially helpful if several nursing implementations are correct but you are asked to select a *best* or *initial* action. Ask yourself, "Will the client's health or recovery be affected if one action is *not* carried out initially?"

Consider this test item:

Ms. Travis, a 44-year-old kindergarten teacher, was admitted last evening with a medical diagnosis of endocarditis. History includes a cholecystectomy 2 years ago and childhood rheumatic fever. Two days ago her dentist extracted an infected molar after an unsuccessful root canal procedure. Although she usually takes prophylactic penicillin before dental treatment, she forgot to do so. Present temperature is 103° F. IV ampicillin is ordered every 6 hours. She seems uncomfortable and very anxious, asking repeatedly if her son has arrived from a distant state.

1. During the initial assessment of Ms. Travis, the nurse notes that 600 ml of 5% dextrose in 0.225% normal saline has infused in 2 hours. Since the physician ordered 1000 ml in 10 hours, the *initial action* should be to
   - ☐ 1. notify the attending physician.
   - ☐ 2. assess respirations and breath sounds.
   - ☐ 3. recalculate the infusion rate.
   - ☐ 4. report the problem to the supervisor.

Note that the case study is very detailed. As you would do in a clinical setting, review the assessment data and filter out the information that has less impact on the client's present condition. Identify the actual and potential problems; then read the question and consider each option thoughtfully. As fluid volume is altered, physiological integrity clearly dictates priority assessments and *immediate* interventions.

In this example say to yourself, "The priority action is to notify the physician. True or False?"; then proceed to the other options. Although responses 1, 2, and 3 are appropriate, the *priority action* is to detect signs of fluid

volume excess related to very rapid infusion (option 2). Pulmonary edema could further complicate the client's condition. Option 4 is not an initial action, nor should the supervisor be notified until after consulting with the head nurse or unit manager.

2. After examining the client, the cardiologist orders the remaining 400 ml of IV fluids administered over 8 hours. The drop factor is 10/ml. The nurse would adjust the fluid rate to
   - ☐ 1. 4 drops per minute.
   - ☐ 2. 8 drops per minute.
   - ☐ 3. 12 drops per minute.
   - ☐ 4. 16 drops per minute.

Calculate the fluid rate using the standard equation. Be sure to label all values such as minutes and milliliters. The correct response for this question is option 2, 8 drops per minute. The client must be assessed very carefully during the next few hours. Lab data will be analyzed for further problems related to overhydration.

Other priority test items may focus on emergency nursing actions in varied health care settings. Problem solve thoughtfully and select an initial lifesaving action. Consider this item:

Mr. Kent had a bronchoscopic examination several hours ago. A topical anesthetic spray was used during the procedure. Since the physician ordered diet as tolerated and the client tolerated sips of water, he was given a general diet for lunch. As he begins to eat, his color turns gray; he appears to have difficulty breathing and then grasps his throat.

3. Select the correct priority action.
   - ☐ 1. Notify the anesthesiologist.
   - ☐ 2. Suction secretions from his oral pharynx.
   - ☐ 3. Perform a thrust maneuver.
   - ☐ 4. No action can be taken until further information is gathered.

The priority action is to ensure a patent airway, option 3. Further reflection may lead you to question if the client's swallowing and gag reflexes were assessed before the meal. In this example, as in many NCLEX-RN test items, one choice suggests the need for further information. Be very careful in selecting this response. Although it may be very helpful to have more assessment data, this case study provides sufficient data to direct quick and safe action.

Communication test items present a special challenge. As in actual practice, nonverbal cues and the environment affect the communication process. When reading case studies and questions focusing on nurse/client/family interactions, consider all information very carefully. Realize that a reference to an interaction or the presence of quotation marks does not automatically imply therapeutic use of self. Refer to Table 1-5 for suggested ways in which communication test items might vary with *nurse-client* interactions. Apply basic principles and be aware of possible communication blocks. Base choices on

Table 1-5   Focus of communications test items

Type of interaction	Approach
Interview	Asking purposeful questions
	Identifying risk factors
	Using appropriate vocabulary
	Listening to responses
	Maintaining confidentiality
Information giving	Describing tests/procedures
	Clarifying data
	Explaining treatment to client/ family
Teaching/ learning	Assessing health, learning needs
	Using developmentally appropriate terms
	Giving instructions to promote safety
	Demonstrating self-care
	Reinforcing group learning
	Observing a return demonstration
	Involving family in basic care
	Evaluating learning outcome
Therapeutic use of self	Establishing trust
	Identifying own communication skills
	Developing goal direction
	Listening actively
	Clarifying, reflecting
	Sharing observations
	Anticipating needs
	Reinforcing positive coping styles
	Supporting in loss
	Referring for help

sound rationale, rather than selecting a response that "sounds like" what you actually might say.

Consider the following case study and test items:

Ms. Fox, 57, visits the clinic for a Pap smear and describes occasional hot flashes and irregular menstrual periods. She plans to discuss estrogen replacement therapy with her gynecologist. In response to questions about life-style, she describes regular activity and rest patterns, and a well-balanced diet. A review of her history reveals that two sisters had breast cancer. When asked if she performs breast self-exams regularly, Ms. Fox appears upset. "I am so afraid of cancer! I'd rather not know if there is a problem! I could not cope with finding a mass."

4. Select an appropriate reply to the client:
   □ 1. "Fear is no reason to neglect your health."
   □ 2. "Your risk is very high because of family history."
   □ 3. "Tell me more about what you are feeling."
   □ 4. "You should not feel afraid; early detection is critical."

5. After further discussion, the client agrees to view videotapes on menopause and regular breast examination. Which of the following statements made by Ms. Fox indicates that further teaching is necessary?
   □ 1. "When my periods stop, I won't need to check my breasts."
   □ 2. "I understand that I should continue to take calcium."
   □ 3. "Even though my body is changing, I know I can get pregnant."
   □ 4. "If I take estrogen, I'll decrease fat intake and stop smoking."

Question 4 indicates an initial need for therapeutic communication. Although correct information should be conveyed, risk factors identified, and teaching emphasized, this client needs to express her feelings and concerns. Response 3 indicates the nurse's availability as a listener.

In question 5, the client verbalizes understanding of several elements of teaching and plans to take a more active role in health maintenance. All statements, except response 1, indicate learning has occurred. This lack of understanding about continuing breast self-exams even after menopause indicates a need for further teaching.

Some questions focusing on Human Needs Categories address potential problems within the environment. Consider the following test questions.

6. During a busy day in the outpatient clinic, the nurse suspects that a young child may have rubella. Of the following clients who were in contact with the child, which individual is at greatest risk?
   □ 1. John Norris, HIV positive, recovering from tuberculosis
   □ 2. Celia Moran, 8 months pregnant; rubella titer positive
   □ 3. Lori Ruiz, 1 month old; breastfeeding
   □ 4. Frances Long, chronic alcoholic with cirrhosis

7. As a nurse makes rounds on a pediatric unit, each of the following is observed. Which situation must be corrected immediately to ensure client well-being?
   □ 1. A school-aged amputee leaves his wheelchair at the bedside.
   □ 2. Several toddlers spread their toys on the playroom floor.
   □ 3. The stereo volume in the adolescent lounge is quite loud.
   □ 4. The newborn step-down ICU is 68° F.

Risk factors are very different in the above situations. In question 6, rubella exposure is particularly dangerous for any immunosuppressed client (option 1). Although insufficient information is given about the 1-month-old baby's nursing mother and there may be a risk to the client described in option 4, you are asked to identify the individual for whom exposure is *most dangerous*.

That client is John Norris. In assessing environmental conditions that may affect physiological functioning and safety, the very low nursery temperature (option 4) is a serious problem and may lead to cold stress. Examine the other options for potential safety problems. The child with a disability should have access to his wheelchair. Although toys should not be left in an area where they create a hazard, risk is minimal in the playroom. The loud music may subsequently affect hearing, but this is typical for adolescents. Since the case study does not mention that other clients are disturbed, there is no need for immediate action.

Some test items ask you to consider potential or actual problems identified in several clients and then decide on an appropriate action. Consider this item:

8. Each of the following assessments is documented by a night nurse on an adult surgical unit. Which observation should be reported *immediately* to the physician?
   □ 1. Jenny Bocci has a temperature of 100° F the night following surgery for a ruptured appendix.
   □ 2. Karen Rosen's knee is hot and swollen 2 days after cartilage repair.
   □ 3. William Clifford's dressing has purulent drainage shortly after the incision of an abscess.
   □ 4. George Henderson has blood-tinged urine 12 hours after a transurethral prostatectomy.

In reviewing the data, visualize the operative procedure and expected recovery. Identify problems that may delay healing. The physician should be notified immediately about the orthopedic client's postoperative condition. Option 2 indicates a serious problem that may lead to subsequent bone or systemic infection. All other observations are expected during convalescence for the surgical procedures described.

Affective Strategies for Success

It is difficult to separate cognitive and emotional factors in test performance. There are, however, distinctly separate ways to prepare for the mental and emotional challenges of the examination.

Long-range goal setting must include realistic life plans. Anticipate the time that study and review demand; avoid a major life change that increases tension. While a wedding date may be difficult to reschedule, consider delaying other emotionally charged events, such as a three-week hiking trip through Europe just before the exam.

Realistically evaluate your personal responses to test challenges. Look at past successes and ways you maintain energy and confidence under stress. How have you reacted to past major examinations? What physiological or psychological responses to stress are common for you? Many graduates report that tension headaches or gastrointestinal distress occur during the two days of testing. Some suggest that lapses of concentration are frequent

during a tiring day of problem solving. Expect that your thoughts may "drift" or that you may experience a "failure fantasy," as many other nurses have described. Expect some anger about a specific test item. You may feel that you could have written "better answers than those!"

In order to use your mind to its fullest and to demonstrate your competence as a nurse, you need to control the effects of anxiety. Several effective ways exist to reduce tension, including:

- relaxing and contracting muscles progressively from head to toe
- slow, deep breathing and deliberate calming
- guided imagery with focus on a peaceful scene
- meditation, prayer, positive thoughts
- focusing on a confident self

Select the method of stress reduction that has worked for you in the past, learn new approaches, and practice them during times of tension while studying. For example, to use imagery, see yourself in the setting that is most peaceful for you. Close your eyes and imagine the quiet, the scents, the scenery around you. Feel the warmth and energy. Relax and feel calm. Change the setting as you need to until it is the perfect relaxing pause. Recall these images during difficult moments in the exam when you need a brief recharge. You will feel your spirits lift and will experience clearer thinking.

Close to the test date, plan your travel to the exam site. If distance allows, visit the area in advance so that you know the best route and alternates. Consider seasonal problems that may affect travel time. It is critical to arrive at the testing site ahead of time, or you may be refused entry.

Anticipate that the massive test setting may be overwhelming. Plan ways that you can block out environmental distractions such as a noisy lobby, classmates who desire a last-minute review of content, or friends who wish to hold a lunch-hour postmortem on test items. Replace those stimuli with a walk during the noon break, a brief nap on the steps, or reminiscence about school experiences. This is one time in your professional life that *your* needs are a priority. Do what you must to remain calm and confident.

On the exam days, consider your own comfort and nutritional needs. Dress in nonconstricting and attractive clothing that helps you to feel good about yourself. It is wise to carry a jacket in anticipation of temperature changes within the testing room. Eat a high-protein breakfast, but avoid excessive caffeine and fluids so that repeated trips to the restroom can be avoided during the examination period. Carry fruit, a can of juice, and other quick-energy sources for breaks. This suggestion is especially helpful to prevent overwhelming fatigue during the final test section.

If you know that you often have a tension headache during a long day of concentration, carry a remedy with you. Prepare for other problems by bringing cough drops

Table 1-6   Keys to success on the NCLEX-RN

Know the Test Format
  An integrated exam
  Pass/fail score
  Single-response, multiple-choice items
  Based on measurement of safe nursing behaviors for
    common health problems
Review Concepts
  Growth and development
  Pharmacology and pathophysiology
  Effects of culture and nutrition on health
  The nursing process
  Categories of human needs
Where Should You Begin?
  Consider your strengths and your learning style
How Should You Prepare?
  Review course notes and texts
  Consider a review program
  Use human resources and support services
Strategies to Promote Success
  Begin with self-evaluation
  Sharpen test-taking skills
  Learn methods to reduce stress
  Be self-confident
Just Before the Exam
  Get a good night's rest
  Avoid late cramming
  Eat breakfast
During the NCLEX-RN
  Be precise in marking answer spaces
  Use time wisely
  Be "test wise"
  Keep emotions under control

Used with permission © 1982, 1988. Young, M., & Kopala, B.

or antacids. However, do not take medications that might cause drowsiness, since you need to remain alert and attentive during the 90-minute test periods.

Expect to encounter at least one unfamiliar health problem in the NCLEX-RN exam. Remain confident that you can use your knowledge of anatomy, physiology, pathophysiology, and nursing to solve the problem. Do not allow anger to destroy your concentration with thoughts such as "Why didn't we learn about that condition in school?" Rather, think to yourself, "I can try to answer these questions." Read cues that help you understand the nature of the health problem, or perhaps omit unfamiliar items and return to them later.

The keys to success are within you (see Table 1-6). Discover your strengths and potential by preparing thoroughly—mentally and emotionally. Study, review, practice test-taking strategies, and learn how to reduce personal tension. The rewards begin with your license to practice as a professional nurse. You are needed in the health care field of the 1990s, and you are welcomed as a caregiver and a colleague!

Answer Key for Pretest Questions on Page 3

1. d
2. a
3. d
4. b
5. c

REFERENCES

Kane, M., Kinsgsbury, C., Colton, D., & Estes, C. (1986). *A study of nursing practice, role delineation, and job analysis of entry-level performance for registered nurses.* Chicago: National Council of State Boards of Nursing, Inc.

National Council of State Boards of Nursing. (1987). *Test plan for the National Council licensure examination for registered nurses.* Chicago: National Council of State Boards of Nursing, Inc.

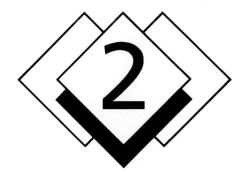

Nursing Care of the Client With Psychosocial and Mental Health Problems

Coordinator
Diane S. Smith, MSN, RN, CS, NP

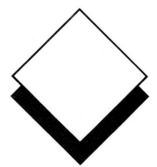

Questions

Joan Washington, RN, has been assigned as cofacilitator for a group of elderly residents in a local nursing home. The group of residents is composed of eight men age 70 to 85; the purpose of the group is to promote social interaction.

1. During the first meeting, Miss Washington introduces herself and asks each member to do the same. What information might be useful to the nurse at this time?
   - ☐ 1. The reasons for each resident's admission to the nursing home.
   - ☐ 2. A sociocultural history of each resident.
   - ☐ 3. The usual activity patterns of each resident.
   - ☐ 4. The interaction patterns in the group.

2. When Miss Washington asks the group what kinds of things they would like to focus on, the only responses she receives are comments such as, "You tell us; you're the leader," or, "Why do we need to come to this group anyway?" This behavior probably means
   - ☐ 1. Miss Washington has not explained the purpose of the group clearly enough.
   - ☐ 2. The residents are anxious (a typical response).
   - ☐ 3. The residents are angry about being in the group.
   - ☐ 4. An interpretation of these comments is not possible after only one meeting.

3. During one group meeting, Mr. Pankowski tells everyone of his apprehension about going to visit his daughter for a weekend. What would your best response be?
   - ☐ 1. "We wouldn't let you go if you weren't able."
   - ☐ 2. "Maybe others in the group have had similar feelings."
   - ☐ 3. "Have you ever had those feelings before?"
   - ☐ 4. "Mr. Abraham, tell Mr. Pankowski how you handled similar feelings."

4. Over a period of several weeks, Mr. Abels has monopolized most of the conversation in the group. How might the group facilitator best handle this?
   - ☐ 1. Take him aside and kindly tell him that others deserve a chance to talk, too.
   - ☐ 2. Ignore Mr. Abels' comments, and they will occur less often.
   - ☐ 3. Tactfully share your perception with the group and wonder aloud why they let it occur.
   - ☐ 4. Transfer Mr. Abels to another group.

Jane Thomas is a 57-year-old woman who was admitted to the psychiatric unit over the weekend. She says she is quite angry and thoroughly disgusted, even though she is smiling.

5. Which of the following best describes Mrs. Thomas' behavior?
   - ☐ 1. Suspicious.
   - ☐ 2. Demanding.
   - ☐ 3. Incongruent.
   - ☐ 4. Resistant.

6. What is the best response to this behavior?
   - ☐ 1. "Your smile does not seem to match what you are saying, Mrs. Thomas."
   - ☐ 2. "I wonder what you're really thinking, Mrs. Thomas."
   - ☐ 3. "Tell me more about your anger."
   - ☐ 4. "What were you thinking just now?"

7. Mrs. Thomas reflects on what the nurse has said and begins to think. After 1 minute, what would be an appropriate response for the nurse to make?
   - ☐ 1. Continue to allow her time to formulate her thoughts.
   - ☐ 2. Ask her, "Did I say something wrong?"
   - ☐ 3. Tell her, "I'm concerned about your silence, Mrs. Thomas."
   - ☐ 4. Tell her, "Just say the first thing that comes to mind, Mrs. Thomas."

8. Which of the following information would be most useful to discuss at today's client-care meeting?

☐ 1. Diagnosis.
☐ 2. Case history.
☐ 3. Psychological testing.
☐ 4. Approaches for present behavior.

9. Mrs. Thomas begins to become more reclusive and refuses to leave her room. What is the best nursing response when initiating contact with her?
☐ 1. "Come, let's go play some cards."
☐ 2. "Have I done something to frighten you?"
☐ 3. "I'll stay with you for awhile."
☐ 4. "What's on your mind?"

Ruby Sanchez comes to the mental health clinic and relates that since the death of her husband she feels really miserable. She states in a loud voice, "How could he do this to me? I just won't have it."

10. Which of the following stages of the grief reaction is Mrs. Sanchez most likely displaying at this time?
☐ 1. Denial.
☐ 2. Anger.
☐ 3. Bargaining.
☐ 4. Resolution.

11. Which of the following statements made by Mrs. Sanchez would be the most important in determining whether her response is normal or delayed or extended?
☐ 1. "My husband died 1 week ago."
☐ 2. "Most everything makes me cry."
☐ 3. "We were married for 42 years."
☐ 4. "We didn't have much in common in later years."

12. Based upon the data given by Mrs. Sanchez, which of the following would be the most appropriate statement of the nursing problem?
☐ 1. Prolonged grief reaction related to death of husband.
☐ 2. Anger related to loss of husband.
☐ 3. Denial of the loss.
☐ 4. Powerlessness over the situation.

13. What is the most therapeutic initial nursing approach to use in helping Mrs. Sanchez to deal with her feelings?
☐ 1. Help her to see the positive aspects of the relationship with her husband.
☐ 2. Describe the stages of the grieving process to her.
☐ 3. Support her expression of feelings she is experiencing now.
☐ 4. Tell her that in time she will feel better.

Della Quale is a 36-year-old married woman. She has two daughters, ages 7 and 9. She lives with her children and her husband, Dan, a 38-year-old construction foreman. Mrs. Quale has a history of cancer of the breast and had a radical mastectomy 6 years ago. Until 2 months ago, she was in excellent health. At that time, she began to complain of severe back pain and lost weight rapidly. Examination and surgery have revealed inoperable cancerous tumors on her spine, and she has been admitted to the oncology unit for palliative chemotherapy and radiation treatment. On admission, she is quiet and withdrawn, a thin, frail woman. She speaks only when spoken to and eats and drinks only when someone feeds her.

14. What is the nurse's highest priority in caring for the client at this time?
☐ 1. Help the client deal with her family's feelings of their impending loss.
☐ 2. Encourage verbal expression of the client's anger.
☐ 3. Ensure that the client receives adequate nutrition and hydration.
☐ 4. Allow the client to use any form of denial that she chooses.

15. Mrs. Quale continues to lose weight and refuses to move from her bed or to turn herself. This behavior may result in three of the following consequences. Which is *not* likely to occur?
☐ 1. Formation of decubitus ulcers.
☐ 2. Decreased staff interaction.
☐ 3. Anger and hostility from the nursing staff toward the client.
☐ 4. Contractures of the extremities.

16. Mrs. Quale refuses to see her children or to talk with them on the telephone. Such behavior may be understood as
☐ 1. The family needing to be more empathetic.
☐ 2. Moving through the grief process more quickly to resolution.
☐ 3. Psychological distancing resulting from the pain of separation and loss.
☐ 4. They are too young to know the difference.

17. One evening, the physician meets with Mrs. Quale and her husband to discuss her discharge and subsequent hospice care. Mrs. Quale is visibly distressed, and later that night she suffers an episode of respiratory arrest. Her medical condition is treated and stabilized, but she is visibly weakened and remains withdrawn. Which of the following nursing actions will *not* be therapeutic at this time?
☐ 1. Turning and positioning the client as needed.
☐ 2. Having the nurse consider her own feelings and beliefs about dying.
☐ 3. Sitting with the client quietly.
☐ 4. Encouraging her to feed and bathe herself to regain some autonomy.

18. When working with the dying client and the family, the nurse understands that three of the following are very likely to occur. Which one is *not*?
☐ 1. The family will respond to the dying member much as they have handled other major crisis situations.

☐ 2. The client will proceed through each of the stages of dying, regardless of outside help.

☐ 3. The family's greatest needs may be for competent physical care for the ill member and empathy for their situation.

☐ 4. Young children may see death as something experienced by others, but not themselves.

Mr. and Mrs. Carlson have learned recently that their 3-year-old daughter Jeannie has an untreatable malignant tumor.

19. Because Jeannie is 3 years old, the nurse can expect her to have which of the following views of death?

☐ 1. Someone bad will carry her away.

☐ 2. Death occurs, but it is not permanent.

☐ 3. Death and absence are the same.

☐ 4. Everyone must die.

20. Which of the following would probably *not* be effective in helping Jeannie express her reactions and feelings about her situation?

☐ 1. Provide her with dolls and puppets for symbolic play.

☐ 2. Provide paper and colors for her to draw with and have her describe her drawings.

☐ 3. Set up a regular time each day for her to talk about her feelings and concerns.

☐ 4. Read stories and talk about how the children in the stories feel.

Gail Miller is a 27-year-old woman admitted to the surgical unit of a general hospital following an accident in a small airplane. In the accident, her husband, the pilot, was killed. Mrs. Miller has a fractured left femur and some minor abrasions and contusions, but she is physiologically in stable condition. She has a 2-year-old son.

21. The day after admission, the nurse enters Mrs. Miller's room to find the shades drawn and Mrs. Miller in bed sobbing quietly. The most therapeutic response by the nurse would be

☐ 1. "It's a beautiful day outside. Let's get some sunshine in here."

☐ 2. "You seem distressed. What's upsetting you?"

☐ 3. "I'll come back when you are feeling better."

☐ 4. "It's not good for you to sit in here in the dark."

22. Mrs. Miller is exhibiting a normal response to grief. Which of the following would most likely be considered an *abnormal* grief response?

☐ 1. A period of preoccupation with the deceased person.

☐ 2. A period of emotional numbness.

☐ 3. Hoarding sleep medications.

☐ 4. Expressing angry feelings.

23. Which of the following would be most helpful as Mrs. Miller goes through the grief process?

☐ 1. Allow her long periods of solitary activity.

☐ 2. Schedule numerous activities for her in order to keep her mind occupied.

☐ 3. Arrange for a surprise visit from her son.

☐ 4. Allow her to work through the grief process at her own pace.

24. A week following Mrs. Miller's admission, her physician informs her that her admission tests reveal that she is pregnant. The nurse enters her room to find her crying hysterically. Which of the following would be most effective?

☐ 1. Tell her that you will return later when she has had a chance to gain control of herself.

☐ 2. Tell her that you will sit with her until she is ready to talk.

☐ 3. Administer a sedative immediately.

☐ 4. Ask her what the crying is about.

25. Two days after learning of her pregnancy, Mrs. Miller tells the nurse, "I'm going to have an abortion. I can't bear the thought of raising another child by myself." What is the best response?

☐ 1. "Well, it sounds as though you already have made a decision."

☐ 2. "You may be acting too hastily."

☐ 3. "Let's talk about it."

☐ 4. "You might be sorry in a year or two."

Ashley Carlisle, a newlywed, comes to the mental health clinic because of "nervousness." She relates to the nurse that "my stomach has butterflies a lot of the time. I haven't missed any work, but it's getting harder because I can't concentrate very long on anything."

26. What level of anxiety is Mrs. Carlisle most likely experiencing?

☐ 1. Mild.

☐ 2. Moderate.

☐ 3. Severe.

☐ 4. Panic.

27. Which of the following would be the best way to begin taking Mrs. Carlisle's nursing history?

☐ 1. "Tell me about your husband."

☐ 2. "What are you feeling now?"

☐ 3. "Have you ever felt this way before?"

☐ 4. "Does anyone else in your family ever get these feelings?"

Joan Taber calls out to the nurse's station every 10 minutes asking for something. She is a 67-year-old client who underwent a hip pinning 2 days before. The nursing staff is planning behavior modification techniques to deal with her persistent requests.

28. Which of the following is the first action for the nurse to take regarding Miss Taber's behavior?

☐ 1. Observe her behavior at regular intervals to obtain a baseline.

□ 2. Observe her ability to carry out her activities of daily living.

□ 3. Assess her need for pain medicine.

□ 4. Assess her reaction to the anesthetic.

29. An appropriate plan of nursing care for Miss Taber would be to

□ 1. Respond only when called by her.

□ 2. Administer pain medicine to her.

□ 3. Respond to her at consistent intervals even when she is not requesting something.

□ 4. Explain to her that the nurse has other clients to care for.

30. In behavior modification terms, the nursing action expressed above is undertaken because the nurse needs to

□ 1. Allay anxiety.

□ 2. Present reality.

□ 3. Respond to the client's need for safety.

□ 4. Avoid reinforcing demanding behavior.

31. Which of the following explains the major difference between normal anxiety and the syndrome associated with anxiety reactions?

□ 1. Normal anxiety is constant; an anxiety reaction is intermittent and rather short-lived.

□ 2. Normal anxiety is free floating; in an anxiety reaction, there is an impending sense of doom.

□ 3. An anxiety reaction is seldom controllable and usually must run its course.

□ 4. Normal anxiety is a fact of life and seldom becomes an anxiety reaction.

32. Miss Taber says to the nurse, "Dr. Wells has surely botched my case. I can't believe they'd let him continue to practice." The appropriate response of the nurse is

□ 1. "Dr. Wells is a fine doctor and one worthy of respect."

□ 2. "Dr. Wells has been sued before, and his practice is questionable."

□ 3. "You seem to have some concerns about Dr. Wells."

□ 4. "Dr. Wells usually provides good care."

Martin Oren is experiencing anxiety. He is married, has three children, and just lost his job as a coal miner. He comes into the hospital with severe indigestion and fears that he has a serious stomach disorder.

33. Signs and symptoms associated with anxiety are

□ 1. Complaints of apprehension, narrowed perception, stomach pains, and restlessness.

□ 2. Inability to get to sleep, early morning awakening, 10-pound weight loss, and lack of energy.

□ 3. Ideas of reference, grandiose delusions, hallucinations, and delusions.

□ 4. Spending or giving away large amounts of money.

34. If Mr. Oren goes into panic, the nurse would most likely note which of the following symptoms?

□ 1. Persecutory delusions, ideas of reference, and rhyming.

□ 2. Greatly reduced perception, extreme discomfort, and extreme agitation.

□ 3. Fugue state, amnesia, and multiple personalities.

□ 4. Extreme agitation, mood depression, and immobilization.

35. Nursing care during panic reaction would most likely include

□ 1. Allowing the client to express thoughts and feelings while calmly staying with him.

□ 2. Encouraging discussion of childhood events.

□ 3. Talking with the client about the future.

□ 4. Helping the client express and deal with anger.

36. Which of the following criteria should the nurse use to evaluate Mr. Oren's care?

□ 1. Coherence of thought processes and reality orientation.

□ 2. Absence of behavioral signs of nervousness and effective use of coping mechanisms.

□ 3. Cycle of mood swings.

□ 4. Self-reports of experiencing less fear.

John Luzinski, a 40-year-old married man, has demonstrated increased reluctance to leave his home over the past 3 months. He had been absent from his job frequently, and 1 month ago his employment was terminated. Since that time, he has not been outside his home. His wife informed their family physician, who arranged for him to be brought to the psychiatric hospital for evaluation.

37. From the information provided, Mr. Luzinski most likely displays symptoms of

□ 1. Acrophobia.

□ 2. Agoraphobia.

□ 3. Astraphobia.

□ 4. Claustrophobia.

38. The ego-defense mechanism being used by Mr. Luzinski is which of the following?

□ 1. Sublimation.

□ 2. Displacement.

□ 3. Substitution.

□ 4. Suppression.

39. What is the most effective technique in treating Mr. Luzinski's condition?

□ 1. Confrontation to determine if the fear is real.

□ 2. Immediate exposure to the situation he fears.

□ 3. Distraction each time he mentions the subject.

□ 4. Gradual desensitization by controlled exposure to the situation he fears.

40. To decrease the anxiety experienced when exposed to his situational phobia, Mr. Luzinski is started on a medication regimen. Which of the following would most likely be prescribed for him?

☐ 1. The antipsychotic fluphenazine (Prolixin), 2 mg TID PO.

☐ 2. The antipsychotic chlorpromazine (Thorazine), 25 mg BID PO.

☐ 3. The antimanic-depressive lithium carbonate, 300 mg TID/QID PO.

☐ 4. The anxiolytic diazepam (Valium), 2 mg TID PO.

41. Which of the following activities attended by Mr. Luzinski might indicate that he is experiencing less agoraphobia?

☐ 1. Milieu group in the dayroom.

☐ 2. Occupational therapy in the adjunctive-therapy room.

☐ 3. Recreational therapy on the outside volleyball court.

☐ 4. Sunday dinner in the hospital cafeteria.

Maria Morgan is a 16-year-old high school student brought to the psychiatric hospital by her mother. Since she was a small child, she has been preoccupied with excessive cleanliness, refusing to play in areas where she might soil her clothing, and bathing several times a day. Recently, she has begun to scrub her underarm areas so frequently that the skin is excoriated and bleeding. She states that she does not wish to offend anyone by her body odor. She is admitted with a diagnosis of obsessive-compulsive disorder.

42. The primary reason for Maria's symptoms is represented by which of the following?

☐ 1. A method of receiving attention.

☐ 2. A method of reducing anxiety.

☐ 3. A childhood value of staying clean.

☐ 4. A manipulative method of avoiding socialization.

43. Which ego-defense mechanisms are most prominently used in this disorder?

☐ 1. Introjection and projection.

☐ 2. Compensation and isolation.

☐ 3. Displacement and undoing.

☐ 4. Rationalization and repression.

44. What is the best rationale to explain Maria's type of disorder?

☐ 1. Anger is internalized and turned against the self.

☐ 2. Intellectualization fails as a defense mechanism.

☐ 3. Trust was never established in early significant relationships.

☐ 4. A distressing thought is cancelled out by some type of action.

45. Select the factors that are most important for the nurse to assess about Maria.

☐ 1. Actions, life events, unresolved conflicts, and activities of daily living.

☐ 2. Silly behavior, thought patterns, associations, and delusions.

☐ 3. Nervousness, vital signs, body language, and impending sense of doom.

☐ 4. Involvement of involuntary muscles, fears, attention level, and sleeping disorders.

46. When formulating the initial nursing care plan for Maria, which of the following should receive the highest priority?

☐ 1. Client will maintain her role in the family.

☐ 2. Client will eliminate her washing behavior.

☐ 3. Client will verbalize the underlying cause of her behavior.

☐ 4. Client will reestablish skin integrity.

47. Initially the nurse will most likely consider which of the following in planning care for Maria?

☐ 1. She will require strict limit setting in order to conform to the unit schedules.

☐ 2. She will need extra time to perform her rituals, so her anxiety will be manageable.

☐ 3. She will need to be isolated in order to feel less anxious about proximity to other clients.

☐ 4. She will need to be confronted about the senselessness of her behavior.

48. Which of the following is most important in planning nursing care for Maria?

☐ 1. Use constant reality orientation.

☐ 2. Set limits on washing behavior.

☐ 3. Administer diazepam (Valium), 5 mg as ordered.

☐ 4. Use assertiveness training.

49. Maria relates that she likes to watch TV, but is fearful of sitting on the chairs in the dayroom. What would be the most therapeutic intervention?

☐ 1. Sterilize one of the chairs in the dayroom and reserve it for Maria.

☐ 2. Move the TV into Maria's room.

☐ 3. Permit Maria to stand while watching TV.

☐ 4. Insist that she sit in the chair.

50. Three of the following interventions are appropriate. Which one is not?

☐ 1. Allow her to complete her ritual, once she has begun.

☐ 2. Allow her to make choices in her schedule.

☐ 3. Prevent her ritualistic behavior, once she has begun adjunctive therapy.

☐ 4. Provide protection from physical discomfort caused by her ritualistic behavior.

51. Which statement would be the most appropriate guideline when considering possible outcomes of Maria's care?

☐ 1. If given an antipsychotic medication, she will completely eliminate her symptoms.

☐ 2. If psychotherapy is used intensively, she will be able to deal with her repressed feelings and completely eliminate her symptoms.

☐ 3. If Maria is given sufficient opportunities to succeed in activities, her self-esteem will improve, and all her symptoms will be eliminated.

☐ 4. It is appropriate to develop methods to limit and confine symptoms, since these behaviors are very resistant to treatment.

52. Which of the following criteria would be used to evaluate Maria?

☐ 1. A reduction of washing behavior and resumption of daily activities.

☐ 2. Intact thought processes grounded in reality.

☐ 3. Able to go to school without fear.

☐ 4. Self-reports of decreased anxiety.

53. Which statement best demonstrates Maria's understanding of her problem?

☐ 1. "I suppose washing under my arms all the time is a crazy thing to do."

☐ 2. "I feel so clean when I get done washing, but it just doesn't last very long."

☐ 3. "I know I'm getting better, because I don't have as much body odor as I did in the beginning."

☐ 4. "I really don't think I have a problem. It's important to be clean if you want to have dates."

Tina Otis, 18 years old, is admitted to an inpatient psychiatric unit. She is 5 feet 7 inches tall and weighs 95 pounds. She attends a local university, where she is an excellent student. Although she appears weak, she exercises intensively, especially after meals. Her condition is diagnosed as anorexia nervosa. She has been dieting to lose weight and sees herself as needing to lose at least 25 more pounds to "get rid of my fat hips."

54. Three of the following conditions are frequently characteristic of the anorexic client. Which one is *not*?

☐ 1. Amenorrhea.

☐ 2. Delayed psychosexual development.

☐ 3. Covert dysfunctional family patterns.

☐ 4. Tachycardia.

55. Miss Otis exhibits much of the behavior considered typical of clients suffering from anorexia nervosa. Which of the following behaviors could be considered *atypical*?

☐ 1. Hoarding food.

☐ 2. Eating only low-calorie foods.

☐ 3. Napping frequently to conserve energy.

☐ 4. Strenuous exercising.

56. Which of the following has the highest priority in the treatment of this client?

☐ 1. Negotiate a behavioral contract with the client.

☐ 2. Teach her the basics of good nutrition.

☐ 3. Institute immediate measures to restore electrolyte and nutritional balance.

☐ 4. Observe her closely for 2 hours after each meal.

57. In setting up Miss Otis' treatment plan, three of the following would be appropriate. Which one would be *inappropriate*?

☐ 1. Provide opportunities for her to make her choices from an appropriate menu.

☐ 2. Provide positive reinforcement for each pound gained.

☐ 3. Encourage Miss Otis to be more independent.

☐ 4. Provide her with solitary time in her room after each meal.

58. When monitoring Miss Otis' eating patterns, it is essential for the nurse to recognize that she

☐ 1. Has an alteration in the functioning of the hypothalamus, which affects the appetite center.

☐ 2. Is unable to eat properly because of a physiological lack of appetite.

☐ 3. Represses and suppresses normal stomach hunger.

☐ 4. Is never aware of the sensation of hunger.

59. Miss Otis is started on a behavior modification program. She is encouraged to eat three well-balanced meals each day and to attempt to gain at least ½ pound each day. Each time she accomplishes this, she is allowed an additional privilege on the unit. This is an example of which of the following behavior modification techniques?

☐ 1. Avoidance of punishment.

☐ 2. Positive reinforcement.

☐ 3. Negative reinforcement.

☐ 4. Generalization.

60. Miss Otis continues to deny her problems and remains aloof from the staff and peers on the unit. Which of the following approaches would be the most effective?

☐ 1. Point out that she will be force-fed if she does not improve her eating habits.

☐ 2. Let her eat as little as she wishes, as she will not continue to lose weight after a plateau is reached.

☐ 3. Involve her in the preparation of her treatment plan, assisting in decisions concerning food, exercise, and hygiene.

☐ 4. Assign her a roommate who has good eating habits, so she will become more interested in good nutrition.

61. Which of the following is the most appropriate nursing response when Miss Otis describes her hips as fat?

☐ 1. "Actually you're too skinny; you don't look good that way."

☐ 2. "Look here in the mirror. Now, you can see your hips are not fat."

☐ 3. "I understand that your hips seem fat to you, but to others you appear very thin."

☐ 4. "It's difficult for me to understand how you can do this to yourself."

Horace Babcock is admitted to the mental health unit for evaluation. He has a 5-year history of numerous medical admissions for severe, intermittent headaches. Despite extensive diagnostic workups and tests that have revealed no organic basis for his symptoms,

he continues to believe he is ill. He holds a responsible job as an accountant, is married, and is the father of two young children.

62. Mr. Babcock's symptoms are most characteristic of which of the following diagnostic categories?
    ☐ 1. Hypochondriasis.
    ☐ 2. Psychosomatic illness.
    ☐ 3. Conversion disorder.
    ☐ 4. Malingering.

63. The day after admission, Mr. Babcock tells the nurse that he will be unable to participate in group therapy because his headaches have increased. What is the most therapeutic response from the nurse?
    ☐ 1. "Describe the pain to me."
    ☐ 2. "Go to your room and lie down. I'll call your doctor."
    ☐ 3. "You must go to group therapy. It's part of your treatment."
    ☐ 4. "Let's sit down and talk a bit about what group therapy involves."

64. Diazepam (Valium), 5 mg TID, is ordered for Mr. Babcock. This drug is primarily effective in treating which of the following?
    ☐ 1. Hallucinations.
    ☐ 2. Delusions.
    ☐ 3. Anxiety.
    ☐ 4. Mania.

65. Mr. Babcock is discharged with a prescription for diazepam (Valium), 5 mg TID. When teaching him how to use the medication at home, the nurse would *exclude* which of the following instructions?
    ☐ 1. "Do not combine medication with alcohol."
    ☐ 2. "If you need to take any other medication while taking this drug, consult with your physician first."
    ☐ 3. "Valium decreases muscular coordination and mental alertness, so use caution when driving."
    ☐ 4. "Drink at least eight glasses of water daily, since Valium will dehydrate you."

Tina Manchester, a 33-year-old widow and mother of four children, was visiting a neighbor when her house burned down. Her children were at home alone when the fire occurred. The two oldest children, age 10 and 8, were killed. The baby, Chrissie (2 months old), and Danny (4 years old) survived, but they were badly burned. Four months later, Tina is still waking at night with nightmares about the incident. She keeps remembering the sight of the firemen carrying her children out of the burning home. She cannot turn on a stove and see flames without becoming very anxious and scared. She visits a local mental health clinic and receives a diagnosis of post-traumatic stress disorder.

66. When describing the fire to the nurse at the clinic, Mrs. Manchester clearly leaves out part of the story. The best nursing response would be to

☐ 1. Ask several questions to help her remember what happened.
☐ 2. Allow her to tell as much of the story as she is comfortable relating.
☐ 3. Realize that she probably does not remember those parts of the story that are not painful.
☐ 4. Tell her that she must not hold back information if she wants to improve.

67. Mrs. Manchester says she feels very guilty about the children's deaths. She says, "I wish it had been me that died in the fire." Which of these responses is most appropriate for the nurse to make?
    ☐ 1. "Your feelings are normal for this type of accident, and we can talk more about them."
    ☐ 2. "Your feelings are different from most parents in this type of situation, so let's explore them further."
    ☐ 3. "Then who would take care of Chrissie and Danny?"
    ☐ 4. "Do you have a plan to kill yourself?"

68. One of the goals the nurse and Mrs. Manchester have agreed upon is that she will increase her involvement in out-of-the-home activities. Which of the following actions will probably be most effective in helping her achieve that goal?
    ☐ 1. Join a Parents Without Partners group.
    ☐ 2. Take a 1-week trip out of town.
    ☐ 3. Plan on taking the children to a film once a week.
    ☐ 4. Join a group of parents whose children died from accidental causes.

69. The mental health clinic has an emergency crisis intervention team to provide immediate care to prevent post-traumatic stress disorder. According to the Public Health Model, this is an example of
    ☐ 1. Primary prevention.
    ☐ 2. Secondary prevention.
    ☐ 3. Tertiary prevention.
    ☐ 4. Early diagnostic care.

Ada Cohen, age 60, is admitted to the hospital with symptoms of increasing forgetfulness, irritability, decreasing concentration, and feelings that others are out to get her. The medical diagnosis is Alzheimer's disease.

70. In view of the medical diagnosis, which of the following pieces of information would be most useful to obtain for immediate nursing care?
    ☐ 1. Family history concerning other members with similar disorders.
    ☐ 2. Her previous occupation, hobbies, and diversional activities.
    ☐ 3. Her past medical history.
    ☐ 4. Major stressors in her life.

71. Three of the following statements are true about this disease. Which one is *incorrect*?

☐ 1. There is degeneration of the cortex and atrophy of the cerebrum.

☐ 2. Death usually occurs 1 to 10 years following onset.

☐ 3. There is progressive deterioration of intellectual function and changes in personality and behavior.

☐ 4. The etiology of this disease is well-known and fairly uniform.

72. Memory loss for recent events is the most common symptom during the early stages of Alzheimer's disease. Of the following actions, which one will probably *not* help?

☐ 1. Answer questions repeatedly as needed using short, simple sentences.

☐ 2. Place a large calendar next to the client's bed.

☐ 3. Place the client's name in large letters outside of the door to her room.

☐ 4. Tell the client she is getting increasingly forgetful.

73. Mrs. Cohen has difficulty remembering where her room is on the unit. Which of the following would best help her to alleviate this problem?

☐ 1. Paint the door to her room light blue.

☐ 2. Assign her a buddy who will help her when she gets lost.

☐ 3. Put her picture and her name in large letters on the door to her room.

☐ 4. Assign her a room next to the nurses' station so the staff can assist her as necessary.

74. Mrs. Cohen's food intake is only marginally adequate, in part because of her inability to sit at the table and concentrate for the length of time necessary to eat the meal. Which approach would be most likely to ensure a nutritionally adequate intake?

☐ 1. Order a full liquid diet that will take her less time to eat.

☐ 2. Feed Mrs. Cohen.

☐ 3. Order six small, nutritionally balanced meals.

☐ 4. Offer small amounts of food whenever she appears ready to eat.

75. During a visit, Mr. Cohen asks to speak to the nurse. He tearfully tells her that his son and daughter are urging him to place Mrs. Cohen in a nursing home. Which of the following is the best response?

☐ 1. "Your wife will recover soon. Just give her time."

☐ 2. "Our social service department has a list of the best nursing homes in the area that you may want to consider."

☐ 3. "When you are finished visiting your wife, come up to the nursing station. I'll find a quiet place where we can talk."

☐ 4. "I'm sure you will be able to take care of your wife at home without that much difficulty."

Glenn Jones is a 33-year-old client admitted to the psychiatric unit with a diagnosis of major retarded depression. He has been hospitalized twice before with this diagnosis. He speaks negatively of himself and states that he has a history of recurrent depression. He has demonstrated no suicidal ideation and is not on "suicide status" at present, although he has been suicidal during previous hospitalizations. He is quiet and withdrawn and responds slowly to all stimuli.

76. Mr. Jones seems less lethargic today and agrees to participate in the occupational therapy program. To help make the session most successful for Mr. Jones, the nurse would do which one of the following?

☐ 1. Set up a large number of projects for Mr. Jones to choose from.

☐ 2. Introduce Mr. Jones to the other clients in occupational therapy.

☐ 3. Help to structure Mr. Jones' participation in occupational therapy to facilitate successful completion of one specific, small task.

☐ 4. Stay away from the client while he is in occupational therapy so that he is free to express himself.

77. Mr. Jones is to receive nortriptyline (Aventyl), 100 mg daily. Of the following side effects, which one is *not* expected with this medication?

☐ 1. Blurred vision.

☐ 2. Dry mouth.

☐ 3. Urinary retention or delayed urination.

☐ 4. Photophobia.

78. Which of the following behaviors or symptoms is Mr. Jones most likely to demonstrate?

☐ 1. Lack of cooperation with staff.

☐ 2. Flight of ideas.

☐ 3. Increased motor activity.

☐ 4. Pressured speech.

79. Which of the following nursing actions is considered nontherapeutic?

☐ 1. Identifying the aspects of cognitive changes that are important to the client.

☐ 2. Taking responsibility for the client's physical safety.

☐ 3. Refusing to acknowledge or discuss irrational demands.

☐ 4. Evaluating the effect of the antidepressant medication on the client.

Barney Chung, a 60-year-old widower, was brought by his son to the hospital after exhibiting increasingly withdrawn behavior over a period of 3 months. He had been living alone since coming to this country 12 years ago. He has been widowed 15 years, and he worked as a tailor until his retirement 3 years ago. He is now refusing to eat or bathe, must be escorted to

the bathroom, and does not respond verbally when addressed.

80. When orienting Mr. Chung to the unit, which of the following guidelines would be most appropriate?
    - ☐ 1. Ensure he meets everyone on the unit as soon as possible.
    - ☐ 2. Accompany him to his room and stay with him, giving concise information as needed.
    - ☐ 3. Accompany him to all activities, so he will be encouraged to participate.
    - ☐ 4. Assign him to a room with a talkative roommate, so he will not feel isolated.

81. In severe, major depression, which of the following defense mechanisms is most notable?
    - ☐ 1. Introjection.
    - ☐ 2. Projection.
    - ☐ 3. Suppression.
    - ☐ 4. Repression.

82. What is the most common cause of symptoms of depression that Mr. Chung exhibits?
    - ☐ 1. A hormonal imbalance.
    - ☐ 2. A problem with sexual identity.
    - ☐ 3. An unresolved parental conflict.
    - ☐ 4. A sense of real or imagined loss.

83. In planning activities for Mr. Chung during the initial stages of hospitalization, which of the following is most appropriate?
    - ☐ 1. Give him only one activity a day, so he will not become fatigued.
    - ☐ 2. Prepare a schedule of activities for him to follow each day.
    - ☐ 3. Let him choose what he wants to do each day.
    - ☐ 4. Wait until he indicates a willingness to participate before providing any activities.

84. During the first few days of his hospitalization, Mr. Chung comes to the dayroom when escorted but does not yet respond verbally. Which of the following statements would be most therapeutic?
    - ☐ 1. "I will sit with you, Mr. Chung. You may wish to talk later."
    - ☐ 2. "I will sit with you, Mr. Chung, so that you won't hurt yourself."
    - ☐ 3. "You won't get better if you don't talk to others, Mr. Chung."
    - ☐ 4. "I will sit with you, Mr. Chung. It's important for you to be comfortable in the dayroom."

85. Mr. Chung will be started on therapy with an antidepressant drug. The most appropriate choice would be which of the following?
    - ☐ 1. The tricyclic imipramine (Tofranil), 50 mg TID PO.
    - ☐ 2. The tricyclic amitriptyline (Elavil), 150 mg TID PO.
    - ☐ 3. The MAO inhibitor isocarboxazid (Marplan), 30 mg TID PO.
    - ☐ 4. The MAO inhibitor phenelzine sulfate (Nardil), 50 mg TID PO.

86. The possibility of suicide is a most important concern in the care of depressed clients. During which period is Mr. Chung most likely to attempt suicide?
    - ☐ 1. When he is mute and unlikely to tell anyone about it.
    - ☐ 2. When he is ready to go home.
    - ☐ 3. When his family goes on vacation.
    - ☐ 4. When he begins to demonstrate improvement.

87. The most important priority in caring for a client who is a high suicide risk is to
    - ☐ 1. Administer tranquilizers, so the client will be less suicidal.
    - ☐ 2. Monitor location and behavior constantly.
    - ☐ 3. Change the subject whenever suicide is mentioned, so ideation is less.
    - ☐ 4. Keep the client in isolation to prevent other clients from witnessing a possible attempt.

88. Mr. Chung has improved slowly. He consents to a series of electroconvulsive therapy treatments (ECT). Before the first treatment, he becomes anxious and states he does not wish to go to the treatment room. Which of the following is the most appropriate response?
    - ☐ 1. "You'll be asleep, Mr. Chung, and won't remember anything."
    - ☐ 2. "I'll call your doctor if you want, Mr. Chung, and let him know you have suddenly changed your mind about the treatment."
    - ☐ 3. "You don't have to go, Mr. Chung. You have the right to refuse any treatment. You seem anxious. Let's talk about it."
    - ☐ 4. "I'll go with you, Mr. Chung, and I'll be there throughout the treatment."

89. What are the most common side effects of ECT?
    - ☐ 1. Headache and dizziness.
    - ☐ 2. Nausea and vomiting.
    - ☐ 3. Confusion and memory loss.
    - ☐ 4. Diarrhea and gastrointestinal distress.

90. Which of the following medications is used in conjunction with ECT?
    - ☐ 1. Succinylcholine (Anectine) as a muscle relaxant.
    - ☐ 2. Methohexital (Brevital) as an anesthetic.
    - ☐ 3. Atropine sulfate as an anticholinergic.
    - ☐ 4. All of the above medications are used in conjunction with ECT.

91. Mr. Chung continues to improve and now attends group therapy daily. The most important benefit he would derive from this is
    - ☐ 1. Improved socialization skills.
    - ☐ 2. Improved reality orientation.

   ☐ 3. Greater insight into his problems through the concept of universality.

   ☐ 4. Greater insight and knowledge of self through feedback provided by group members.

Phyllis Rafferty's history reveals that she has had eight depressive episodes during the last 5 years and has been treated with antidepressants, antipsychotic medications, and psychotherapy during this time. During her current hospitalization, several consultations are held with psychiatrists who specialize in the treatment of depression. The decision is made, with the approval of the client and her daughter, to try electroconvulsive therapy (ECT).

92. One of the chief benefits of ECT is that it
   ☐ 1. Shortens the hospitalization period.
   ☐ 2. Often enables a client to be more accessible to psychotherapy.
   ☐ 3. Decreases the need for medication.
   ☐ 4. Enables the client to terminate psychiatric treatment.

93. Which of the following is *not* a nursing responsibility for ECT?
   ☐ 1. Remove dentures, hairpins, etc.
   ☐ 2. Administer medications, such as muscle relaxant, as ordered.
   ☐ 3. Prep the client as if she were going to OR.
   ☐ 4. Carry out the ECT treatment.

94. In order to deal effectively with the side effects that follow ECT, the first nursing action would be to do which of the following?
   ☐ 1. Reintegrate client into the therapeutic milieu.
   ☐ 2. Orient the client to place, time, and person.
   ☐ 3. Provide environmental stimulation as soon as treatment is completed for the day.
   ☐ 4. Initiate bed rest for client for remainder of the day.

Esther Bell has been admitted to a locked unit; her diagnosis is severe depression with history of insomnia and suicidal ideation. She is a 52-year-old divorced woman and is unemployed. She expresses feelings of hopelessness, anger at hospitalization, and self-deprecation. She reports having repeated thoughts of suicide and has a plan to "crash my car and die."

95. Upon completing the initial assessment, the nurse most accurately determines that Mrs. Bell's suicidal risk is at which level?
   ☐ 1. Low.
   ☐ 2. Medium.
   ☐ 3. High.
   ☐ 4. In remission.

96. Which of the following is *not* a high-risk group for suicidal behavior?
   ☐ 1. The elderly.
   ☐ 2. Adolescents.

   ☐ 3. Alcoholics and drug abusers.
   ☐ 4. A nonpsychiatric population in their 30s.

97. Mrs. Bell has treatment orders that include suicide precautions. Which of the following is *not* considered a suicide precaution?
   ☐ 1. Searching personal effects for toxic agents (drugs or alcohol).
   ☐ 2. Removing sharp instruments (razor blades, sewing equipment, glass bottles, and knives).
   ☐ 3. Removing clothes that could be made into straps (belts, stockings, and pantyhose).
   ☐ 4. Asking the client to focus on positive feelings.

98. The nurse knows that severe depression also may be classified as a
   ☐ 1. Somatoform disorder.
   ☐ 2. Affective disorder.
   ☐ 3. Anxiety disorder.
   ☐ 4. Personality disorder.

99. On what basis is the distinction made between severe and mild depression?
   ☐ 1. Somatic and motor activity.
   ☐ 2. Suicidal ideation.
   ☐ 3. Duration of symptoms.
   ☐ 4. Client's age at onset.

100. Mrs. Bell continues to be concerned about insomnia and wants to nap in the daytime. Which of the following short-term goals is *not* appropriate for this client?
   ☐ 1. Client will discuss feelings and concerns about sleep.
   ☐ 2. Client will state that she was able to get some sleep during the night.
   ☐ 3. Client will take several naps during the day.
   ☐ 4. Client will participate in exercise and activity in the daytime.

101. Nursing actions for the insomnia problem should include which of the following?
   ☐ 1. Ignore sleep patterns and complaints about insomnia.
   ☐ 2. Reassure the client that insomnia is not a serious problem.
   ☐ 3. Encourage short naps during the day.
   ☐ 4. Help the client to establish a bedtime routine to promote rest and sleep.

102. Mrs. Bell has been transferred to an open unit from the locked unit. Her physician has ordered imipramine (Tofranil). Tofranil is a(n)
   ☐ 1. Tricyclic antidepressant.
   ☐ 2. Phenothiazine.
   ☐ 3. MAO inhibitor.
   ☐ 4. Antianxiety agent.

103. The nurse teaches Mrs. Bell about Tofranil. Which statement is correct about this drug?
   ☐ 1. May take 2 to 4 weeks for an antidepressant effect.
   ☐ 2. May cause urinary frequency.

☐ 3. May cause increased salivation.

☐ 4. Should be taken intermittently when the client is severely depressed.

104. Which of the following would *not* be appropriate questions for the nurse to ask when assessing the depressed client?

☐ 1. "What are your expectations of yourself?"

☐ 2. "How do you cope with anger?"

☐ 3. "What kinds of things are pleasurable for you?"

☐ 4. "Don't you know that it is morally wrong to think of suicide?"

105. Which of the following would be the most appropriate goal for a nursing diagnosis of "ineffective individual coping related to feelings of hopelessness and anger"?

☐ 1. The client will deny feelings of hopelessness and anger.

☐ 2. The client will demonstrate cheerful affect.

☐ 3. The client will voice no complaints.

☐ 4. The client will share feelings with nurse and others.

106. Which of the following actions would be *least* effective in helping the client cope with painful feelings?

☐ 1. Focus on the positive aspects of life.

☐ 2. Encourage the client to share feelings.

☐ 3. Help the client to identify feelings.

☐ 4. Provide reality orientation, and encourage realistic expectations of self.

107. Mrs. Bell refuses to discuss discharge plans. She states she "can't go home alone, and no one wants to come live with me." Which of the following is the most appropriate action?

☐ 1. Accept her appraisal of the situation and encourage exploration of alternatives.

☐ 2. Call her family and work with them on plans for discharge.

☐ 3. Allow Mrs. Bell to discuss other topics of interest.

☐ 4. Insist that Mrs. Bell discuss discharge to her family home.

108. Mrs. Bell ruminates about her failures in relationships and work. Which of the following would be an *ineffective* intervention for rumination?

☐ 1. Introduce communication that expands her narrow frame of reference.

☐ 2. Tell her to stop ruminating about failure and to speak of positive goals.

☐ 3. Provide opportunities for activity and exercise.

☐ 4. Help the client reevaluate her strengths and weaknesses.

109. Mrs. Bell is angry with the nursing staff and her physician for continuing to discuss discharge planning. Three of the following nursing actions are appropriate to this situation. Which one is *not* appropriate?

☐ 1. Encourage client to verbalize feelings and concerns.

☐ 2. Use simple, direct explanations and open-ended questions.

☐ 3. Make plans with the client for physical activity and exercise.

☐ 4. Ignore angry outbursts; tell the client to remain calm.

Eunice King, a very neat and organized 42-year-old woman, is admitted to the intensive care unit. She is accompanied by her husband, who tells the nurse that he recently asked his wife for a divorce. He left the house yesterday to go on a 3-day business trip. Some of his meetings were cancelled, and he returned home today to find his wife unconscious. An empty bottle that had contained sleeping pills was on the bedside table.

110. In assessing the seriousness of Mrs. King's suicide attempt, which of the following facts is the most important?

☐ 1. She is unconscious.

☐ 2. She used a potentially lethal method.

☐ 3. She planned the attempt for a time when she thought no rescue was possible.

☐ 4. She did not leave a suicide note.

111. The following day, Mrs. King regains consciousness. She is in tears and tells the nurse, "I'm a failure at everything, as a woman, as a wife; and I've even failed at killing myself." When interpreting this statement, which of the following is *least* likely to be correct?

☐ 1. Mrs. King is depressed.

☐ 2. Mrs. King is remorseful about her suicide attempt, and therefore, it is unlikely that she will make a second attempt.

☐ 3. Mrs. King is feeling hopeless, and the potential for another suicide attempt is great.

☐ 4. Mrs. King is ambivalent about whether she wants to live or die.

112. A few days later, Mrs. King is transferred from the intensive care unit to the psychiatric unit. Which of the following nursing interventions has the highest priority?

☐ 1. Remove all potentially harmful items from the client's room.

☐ 2. Allow the client to express feelings of hopelessness and helplessness.

☐ 3. Note the client's capabilities and strengths in order to increase self-esteem.

☐ 4. Observe the client closely for suicidal ideation or gestures.

113. A week after admission, Mrs. King comes to breakfast in a new dress; her hair and makeup are immaculate; and she is quite cheerful. She tells the nurse that she is going to ask her physician for a

weekend pass. What does the nurse need to know regarding this abrupt change in behavior and affect?

☐ 1. Realize that the client is improving and discontinue suicide precautions.

☐ 2. Realize that her first weekend at home will be difficult, and offer anticipatory guidance.

☐ 3. Realize that a decrease in depression may be indicative of renewed suicide potential, and monitor the client carefully.

☐ 4. Realize that depressed clients often have mood swings, and no intervention is probably necessary.

114. The treatment team decides that one of the goals in treating Mrs. King is to increase her self-esteem. Which of the following is the most appropriate way of doing this in the early stages of treatment?

☐ 1. Suggest that she make her bed and keep her room in order.

☐ 2. Introduce her to another client who is an excellent chess player and suggest that he teach her to play.

☐ 3. Suggest that she lead the evening sing-along.

☐ 4. Since she is an excellent cook, suggest that she start a cooking class for the other clients.

115. Another treatment goal for Mrs. King is reducing dependency. Which of the following is an *inappropriate* way to reduce dependency needs in a client?

☐ 1. Provide only the help needed.

☐ 2. Encourage the client to solve her own problems.

☐ 3. Frequently rotate the staff caring for the client.

☐ 4. Encourage participation in unit activities.

Dorothy Pinsky, a 49-year-old homemaker, was recently admitted to the psychiatric unit because of anxiety and suicidal behavior. Her adult life has always been centered on her family and home. Her two oldest children are married and live in nearby towns; her two youngest children are away at college. She had expressed feelings of hopelessness and somatic complaints before hospitalization.

116. Mrs. Pinsky presents the typical symptoms of which of the following?

☐ 1. Paranoid schizophrenia.

☐ 2. Manic-depressive reaction, manic phase.

☐ 3. Psychotic depression.

☐ 4. Substance abuse.

117. Which of the following is the most important nursing action at this time?

☐ 1. Monitor her food intake.

☐ 2. Institute suicide precautions.

☐ 3. Encourage her interest in her family.

☐ 4. Reassure her that her physical complaints are unwarranted.

118. Mrs. Pinsky is indeed a potential suicide victim. She is most likely to commit suicide

☐ 1. Immediately after admission.

☐ 2. At the point of her deepest depression.

☐ 3. When the depression begins to lift.

☐ 4. Just before discharge.

119. Mrs. Pinsky's psychiatrist is thinking of changing her medicine to a monoamine oxidase (MAO) inhibitor. Of the following characteristics, which one should the nurse be most aware of?

☐ 1. They are short acting.

☐ 2. They cause tachycardia.

☐ 3. They cause an increase in appetite.

☐ 4. They potentiate the effects of other drugs.

120. Mrs. Pinsky will begin electroconvulsive therapy (ECT) today. She tells the nurse that she is very afraid. The best response is

☐ 1. "Don't be afraid, your doctor has had 18 years of experience in giving ECT."

☐ 2. "It's not good for you to worry so much."

☐ 3. "You do seem frightened; I will stay with you. Let's talk about it."

☐ 4. "Most people say the same thing; so you are not alone."

Sixty-two-year-old Rose Magrone is admitted to the psychiatric unit with a diagnosis of agitated depression.

121. Which of the following behaviors would the nurse *not* expect to observe with this diagnosis?

☐ 1. Extreme restlessness.

☐ 2. Pacing.

☐ 3. Handwringing.

☐ 4. Sleeping 10 to 12 hours a day.

122. The physician orders amitriptyline (Elavil) 25 mg TID, for Mrs. Magrone. Which classification of psychotropic drugs includes amitriptyline (Elavil)?

☐ 1. Tricyclic antidepressants.

☐ 2. Monoamine oxidase inhibitors.

☐ 3. Phenothiazines

☐ 4. Antihistamines

123. A few days after starting the medication, Mrs. Magrone complains of a dry mouth, constipation, and blurred vision. These symptoms are characteristic of the action of this drug on which of the following body systems?

☐ 1. Cardiovascular.

☐ 2. Endocrine.

☐ 3. Autonomic nervous.

☐ 4. Respiratory.

124. Mrs. Magrone takes her medication as ordered. Three days later, she still exhibits signs of agitation, anxiety, and restlessness. What is the most likely explanation for this?

☐ 1. She is not actually taking the medication.

☐ 2. She is not responding to the medication.

3. Symptomatic relief is not usually achieved until 2 to 4 weeks after therapy is started.

4. The dosage is too small to be effective.

125. Mrs. Magrone refuses to take the next scheduled dose of her medication, because she finds the side effects too annoying. Which of the following is the most effective nursing action?

1. Tell Mrs. Magrone that skipping one dose is not important.

2. Explain to her that the side effects might diminish in a few days.

3. Ask her to discuss the side effects with her physician.

4. Advise her that she will probably have to get electroconvulsive therapy if she fails to take her medication.

Sarah Perkins, age 35, is admitted to the hospital because of increasing feelings of extreme worthlessness and sinfulness, disinterest in eating and personal hygiene, weight loss, and problems with sleep. These problems began shortly after Mrs. Perkins learned that her husband was having an affair with her best friend. A diagnosis of major depression with psychotic features is made.

126. During the initial interview, Mrs. Perkins states, "I really can't blame him. He's such a fine person, and I'm such a terrible wife." How might the nurse best respond?

1. "Everyone has good qualities, Mrs. Perkins. I'm sure you do too."

2. "Tell me why you think you're so terrible?"

3. "You're not feeling very good about yourself right now. Let's talk about it."

4. "You'll feel better about yourself after a few days in the hospital."

127. Mrs. Perkins' response to this situation most likely may be viewed as

1. Normal, because of the severity of the precipitating stress.

2. A reaction to what she perceives as a severe blow to her security.

3. The result of a maturational crisis.

4. Transitory and likely to be self-limiting.

128. The nurse notes that Mrs. Perkins is having difficulty making decisions. Which approach would be most therapeutic?

1. Firmly, but kindly, indicate that she is expected to make decisions.

2. Explain how important decision making is to her recovery.

3. Provide an opportunity for her to make small decisions when she appears ready to do so.

4. Do not ask her to make decisions.

129. Mrs. Perkins stays in her room most of the time and is not interested in any activities or persons on the unit. Which action by the nurse would be most therapeutic?

1. Allow her the time alone that she requires.

2. Require her to attend at least one activity per day.

3. Spend short, frequent periods of time with her.

4. Explain that becoming more active will help her feel better.

130. Mrs. Perkins is to receive a series of electroconvulsive therapy (ECT) treatments. Which of the following understandings about this procedure is most important when providing care to the client?

1. The preparation for this is basically the same as for any procedure in which a general anesthetic is used.

2. ECT is not very effective in the treatment of endogenous or melancholic depressions, so Mrs. Perkins should not get her hopes up.

3. ECT is highly controversial and is used only as a last resort.

4. ECT has no short-term side effects.

131. Before her first treatment, Mrs. Perkins is quite anxious. Which action by the nurse would be most therapeutic?

1. Administer diazepam (Valium), 10 mg IM.

2. Encourage her to sit quietly in her room and breathe deeply.

3. Take her to the dayroom for a cup of coffee.

4. Remain with her and discuss topics she introduces.

132. What nursing action would be most appropriate for Mrs. Perkins following ECT?

1. Remain quietly with her until the confusion subsides.

2. Ask her to remain in bed until the physician arrives.

3. Assess her orientation to time, place, and person by frequent assessment.

4. Call her by name and reorient her to the unit as soon as possible.

133. One day while talking with the nurse, Mrs. Perkins states, "I guess I haven't been thinking very clearly. I'm beginning to think that there may be other ways of dealing with the things that have been happening in my life." This statement best indicates which phase of the nurse-client relationship?

1. Initiating.

2. Working.

3. Terminating.

4. Orienting.

Muriel Moskovitz, a 42-year-old homemaker, is admitted to the psychiatric unit with a diagnosis of psychotic depression.

134. The nurse's first priority is to

1. Establish reality orientation.

☐ 2. Ensure client safety.

☐ 3. Promote self-esteem.

☐ 4. Improve cognitive perceptions.

135. While interviewing Mrs. Moskovitz, the nurse asks what led to her coming to the hospital. Mrs. Moskovitz said, "I'm wicked and it's God's wrath." The most appropriate therapeutic response by the nurse would be which of the following?

☐ 1. "You are not wicked, Mrs. Moskovitz."

☐ 2. "What do you mean by that?"

☐ 3. "Why is God punishing you?"

☐ 4. "We'll talk about this later."

136. Mrs. Moskovitz's physician prescribes a course of electroconvulsive treatments for the client. She asks the nurse what is going to happen to her. Which of the following is the most appropriate explanation to give her?

☐ 1. "You will have a small seizure that will help you to forget what is bothering you."

☐ 2. "Electrodes will be placed on your temples, and a light electrical shock will be delivered to your brain."

☐ 3. "The anesthesiologist will put you to sleep, and you will not even be aware of what is happening."

☐ 4. "You will be given something to help you relax, and you will not feel the actual shock."

137. After Mrs. Moskovitz's first electroconvulsive treatment, the nurse stays with her and the physician leaves. After initially regaining consciousness, Mrs. Moskovitz seems to go to sleep. What would the nurse do?

☐ 1. Try to wake her.

☐ 2. Let her sleep.

☐ 3. Summon the physician.

☐ 4. Administer a prescribed stimulant.

138. Mrs. Moskovitz is slow about getting herself dressed and ready for breakfast. What should the nurse do?

☐ 1. Permit her to take as much time as she wishes.

☐ 2. Tell her she will not get breakfast if she arrives late.

☐ 3. Serve her breakfast in her room.

☐ 4. Help her to get dressed and get to breakfast.

139. Mrs. Moskovitz says to the nurse, "I'm really not worth all the time it takes for you to help me." What is the best response for the nurse to make?

☐ 1. "Even though you feel that way, I am here to help you. I think it is worthwhile."

☐ 2. "You should not think of yourself that way."

☐ 3. "I don't have anything else I have to do right now."

☐ 4. "Soon you will be able to start doing more for yourself, so it won't take so much of my time."

140. After 3 weeks of treatment, Mrs. Moskovitz begins to take more responsibility for herself and expresses an interest in getting ready for discharge. What should the nurse do?

☐ 1. Assess Mrs. Moskovitz's current level of self-esteem.

☐ 2. Institute suicide precautions.

☐ 3. Encourage her to become more involved with the activities on the ward.

☐ 4. Discuss with her her denial of the long-term effects of her depression.

141. Mrs. Moscovitz tells the nurse, "I feel guilty, now that my children are grown, because I didn't do more for them when they were little." Which is the most therapeutic response for the nurse to make?

☐ 1. "What have your children done to make you feel that way?"

☐ 2. "Parents often feel guilty about things that have to do with their children."

☐ 3. "You probably did the best you could for them."

☐ 4. "What other feelings do you have toward your children besides guilt?"

142. The day before her discharge, Mrs. Moscovitz is late for her last interview with the nurse. When the nurse mentions the late arrival, Mrs. Moscovitz blurts out, "Don't nag me! I'm an adult." What is the best response for the nurse to make?

☐ 1. "You seem angry when it seems as though someone's nagging you."

☐ 2. "You're not acting as we would expect an adult to act."

☐ 3. "It must be hard for you to think of leaving the hospital."

☐ 4. "Being on time is part of being responsible for yourself."

Marilyn Brooks has been brought to the hospital by her husband, who states she has become increasingly agitated and overactive during the past 2 weeks. She did not sleep last night. Upon admission, Mrs. Brooks refuses to sit down and continues to move about rapidly, speaking in a loud, tense voice.

143. The medical-biological model of psychiatric illness is based on three of the following assumptions. Which assumption is *not* a tenet of this model?

☐ 1. A client suffering from emotional disturbances has an illness or defect.

☐ 2. The illness has characteristic symptoms or syndromes.

☐ 3. Mental illnesses are properly within the charge of the physician.

☐ 4. Psychiatric illness stems from social and environmental conditions.

144. The manic behavior displayed by Mrs. Brooks is best explained by which of the following statements?

☐ 1. Repression is used to avoid inner feelings of loneliness and poor self-esteem.

2. Suppression is used to avoid inner feelings of dependency and inadequacy.
3. Displacement is used to shift inner feelings to the environment.
4. Denial is used to avoid inner feelings of depression.

145. Which of the following would be the best initial response to Mrs. Brooks?
   1. "I'm glad to see you have so much energy today, Mrs. Brooks."
   2. "I need you to help me pass the breakfast trays, Mrs. Brooks."
   3. "Let me introduce you to another new client, Mrs. Brooks."
   4. "I will go with you to your room, Mrs. Brooks."

146. When managing Mrs. Brooks' behavior on the unit, which of the following actions would *not* be helpful?
   1. Suggest activities that require her attention for long periods of time.
   2. Attempt to minimize environmental stimuli.
   3. Encourage her to complete short projects in occupational therapy.
   4. Use distracting techniques when necessary to channel her attention appropriately.

147. The physician orders lithium therapy. The therapeutic blood level is maintained between which of the following?
   1. 0.5 to 1.2-1.5 mEq/L
   2. 1.0 to 1.5 mEq/L
   3. 0.5 to 1.5 mg/ml
   4. 1.0 to 1.5 mg/ml

148. As part of a teaching plan on lithium carbonate, clients are instructed to have lithium levels determined every 1 to 3 months. Which statement best describes the reason for this?
   1. Lithium carbonate can produce potassium depletion.
   2. Triglyceride levels can increase as the lithium level increases.
   3. Lithium carbonate in large quantities produces sedation.
   4. There is a very narrow margin of safety between the therapeutic level and toxic level of lithium carbonate.

149. Which of the following symptoms would Mrs. Brooks most likely exhibit if she developed mild lithium toxicity?
   1. Urinary retention, increased appetite, and abdominal distension.
   2. Dry mouth, decreased appetite, and constipation.
   3. Macular rash, fever, and hematuria.
   4. Diarrhea, muscle weakness, and polydipsia.

150. As his wife begins to improve, Mr. Brooks states he wishes her to return home and asks what he can do to help his wife after discharge. Which of the following would be the most appropriate information to give Mr. Brooks?
   1. Get someone to stay with her, since she probably will not be stable enough to be left alone.
   2. While his wife receives lithium therapy, it is necessary to have her blood lithium levels monitored regularly.
   3. Manic-depressive illness is hereditary, so they should never have any children.
   4. Ensure that she has a prescription for tranquilizers, so that she can start taking them if her symptoms of mania recur.

151. Mrs. Brooks receives instructions about lithium before discharge. Learning has most probably occurred when she notifies the outpatient clinic that she has experienced which of the following?
   1. Vomiting and diarrhea for 48 hours.
   2. Swollen lymph nodes.
   3. Dry mouth.
   4. Symptoms of an upper respiratory tract infection.

John Peters, a 60-year-old investment analyst, was admitted to the psychiatric unit with a diagnosis of manic-depressive disorder, manic phase, and alcohol abuse. His wife left him a week ago. Two days ago, he was counseled by his work supervisor for telling several clients to sell all their stocks immediately and not to ask questions.

152. In obtaining a family history, which of the following would the nurse most expect to find?
   1. A high incidence of childhood illnesses.
   2. Alcohol or drug abuse as a young adult.
   3. Parents were divorced when he was a child.
   4. One parent is described as having been "very happy" or "very down."

153. A diagnostic category, affective disorders, includes extremes in mood and affect. Of the following, which is *not* characteristic of a manic-depressive disorder?
   1. Vegetative behavior.
   2. Hypomanic behavior.
   3. Thought disorder.
   4. Clang associations.

154. Which of the following is *not* characteristic of manic-depressive clients in a manic phase?
   1. High risk for violence.
   2. Attempt to boss the staff around.
   3. Denial of feelings of depression and sadness.
   4. Hypersomnolence.

155. Upon Mr. Peters' admission, his son said to the nursing staff, "You had better do your job right and calm him down." Which of the following responses would be most helpful at this time?

☐ 1. "You must really be fed up. I've never seen anyone this maniacal."

☐ 2. "You must be very worn out dealing with your father's behavior. It will be very helpful to both of you that you brought him to the hospital."

☐ 3. "I can appreciate your embarrassment. He is really high, isn't he?"

☐ 4. "You must wonder why your father is acting aggressively in order to gain attention."

156. Despite evidence to the contrary, Mr. Peters tells the nurse to, "Go get your money. The banks have failed. Only I know this." In assessing Mr. Peters' behavior, what do his remarks most likely indicate?

☐ 1. Short attention span.

☐ 2. Irritability.

☐ 3. Thought disorder.

☐ 4. Overtalkativeness.

157. The psychiatrist orders lithium carbonate, 300 mg QID PO, for Mr. Peters. The laboratory results indicate a serum lithium level of 1.5 mEq/L. The client does not exhibit or complain of any side effects. Which nursing action is most appropriate?

☐ 1. Suggest that the psychiatrist repeat the test.

☐ 2. Withhold the next dose of lithium and notify the psychiatrist.

☐ 3. Administer the next dose of lithium.

☐ 4. Observe Mr. Peters' degree of pressured speech.

158. For clients taking lithium, it is critical that the nurse observe the client's food intake. Lithium toxicity is most likely to occur if the client has insufficient intake of which of the following?

☐ 1. Fat and carbohydrates.

☐ 2. Potassium and iron.

☐ 3. Sodium and fluids.

☐ 4. Protein

159. The nursing history is a vital component of the nursing process. Which of the following, obtained through the history, is most likely to contraindicate treatment of a client with lithium?

☐ 1. Kidney damage.

☐ 2. High suicide risk.

☐ 3. High level of physical activity.

☐ 4. Hyperthyroidism.

160. In order to provide Mr. Peters with the most therapeutic environment during his hospitalization, which of the following would be most important for the nurse to keep in mind?

☐ 1. Assign him to a semiprivate room with another client who has a similar problem.

☐ 2. Assign him to a private room.

☐ 3. Realize that the presence or absence of a roommate is not particularly important for him.

☐ 4. Place him in the seclusion-quiet room and in restraints as soon as possible after admission.

161. In order to intervene effectively when Mr. Peters is talking rapidly and indicating a flight of ideas, the nursing staff would consistently remind him to do which of the following?

☐ 1. Verbalize how he feels about his work as an investment analyst and his behavior.

☐ 2. Tell himself that his verbalizations are a flight of ideas, which is indicative of his depression.

☐ 3. Speak more slowly, so that he can be understood better.

☐ 4. Describe as many details of his problems as possible.

162. To help reduce the overt aggression demonstrated by Mr. Peters, the nursing staff would use three of the following measures. Which measure would *not* be indicated?

☐ 1. Participation in competitive games.

☐ 2. Physical exercise.

☐ 3. Reduction in environmental stimuli.

☐ 4. Encouraging the client to discuss feelings associated with angry behavior.

163. In planning for Mr. Peters' discharge and future functioning, it is important for his son to be aware of his father's need for health education. Client education would most likely include which of the following aspects?

☐ 1. Recognize behaviors that indicate increased excitement such as irritability, agitation, and verbal and motor hyperactivity.

☐ 2. Teach the son to make most major decisions for his father.

☐ 3. Encourage the father to handle business matters quickly and aggressively.

☐ 4. Teach father and son all possible drug toxicities.

164. In evaluating Mr. Peters' readiness for discharge, the client should demonstrate three of the following. Which would *not* be indicative of readiness for discharge?

☐ 1. Self-care.

☐ 2. Stating requests appropriately and negotiating power with staff and other clients.

☐ 3. Frequent expressions of anger and hostility.

☐ 4. A decrease in manipulative or acting-out behaviors.

165. The psychiatric-mental health nurse who assesses psychiatric clients in the emergency room encounters Mr. Peters 6 months after discharge. He is hyperverbal, rude, hostile, and insulting to the emergency room staff. When conducting the initial nursing assessment, the most important question to ask early in the interview is

☐ 1. "What happened when you returned to work?"

☐ 2. "Are you and your wife still separated?"

☐ 3. "Have you stopped taking your lithium?"

☐ 4. "What makes it difficult for you to talk about your problem?"

William White is a 42-year-old salesman of boats and outdoor equipment for water recreation. He has a history of mood swings. His wife finally persuaded him to admit himself to the hospital following his latest episode of extremely unusual behavior. She reported that he's excited because he is the top salesperson in the company, but added that many of the sales were initiated by her husband's having put his own money down as deposits. When the final contracts are due, she said, he will become very depressed because he won't be able to get his money back in order to pay his own bills.

166. When assessing Mr. White's behavior, the nurse will most likely note which one of the following behaviors?
☐ 1. Withdrawal from reality.
☐ 2. Overactivity.
☐ 3. Delusions of persecution.
☐ 4. Hallucinations

167. During the first few days on the unit, Mr. White comes up to the nurse several times and says, "You're an asshole." How would the nurse best deal with this inappropriate language?
☐ 1. Reflect that he seems to be upset about something.
☐ 2. Interpret the defense to Mr. White as projection.
☐ 3. Tell him that kind of language will not be tolerated.
☐ 4. Seclude him until his speech is less offensive.

168. Mr. White may fail to eat because he
☐ 1. Feels he does not deserve to eat.
☐ 2. Feels the food is poisoned.
☐ 3. Is too busy.
☐ 4. Does not like hospital food.

169. After 1 week on the unit, Mr. White has lost 10 pounds. Which of the following will be most likely to prevent further weight loss?
☐ 1. Increase the size of his portions at each meal.
☐ 2. Remain with him at meals to ensure that he eats everything.
☐ 3. Restrict between-meal snacks, so that he will be more hungry at mealtime.
☐ 4. Provide between-meal, nutritious foods that Mr. White can eat in a short time.

170. Mr. White refuses to eat, stating that he has too much to do. Which of the following is the best nursing response?
☐ 1. "Come and eat at the table."
☐ 2. "Here is a sandwich for you to eat."
☐ 3. "You will be able to work later."
☐ 4. "What are you doing that takes so much of your time?"

171. Mr. White is scheduled for occupational therapy (OT). The chief aim of OT for Mr. White is to
☐ 1. Teach social skills for group living.
☐ 2. Stimulate interest in the environment.
☐ 3. Provide a constructive outlet for excessive energy.
☐ 4. Provide an environment where confrontation and reality testing are maximized.

Monica Wendall is a 17-year-old mother of an 8-month-old son. The nurse is discussing the baby's progress with Mrs. Wendall during a regularly scheduled visit to the well-baby clinic. Mrs. Wendall expresses her frustration over her baby's recent illness and reveals her fear of harming the baby and her feelings of wanting to throw the baby to the floor.

172. When assessing the mother's potential for child abuse, which factor from the mother's history would be most important to know?
☐ 1. Whether the mother has completed high school.
☐ 2. The mother's age at menarche.
☐ 3. Whether the mother, as a child, was physically abused by her parents.
☐ 4. The socioeconomic status of the mother's family of origin.

173. When assessing the mother's current potential for child abuse, which factor is the most important to determine?
☐ 1. Is the mother currently pregnant?
☐ 2. Has the mother actually harmed the baby?
☐ 3. Did the mother want the baby at the time of birth?
☐ 4. Has the mother cared for small children before, such as baby-sitting or caring for younger siblings?

174. In planning for this family's care, the nurse would do best to consider which of the following facts about teenage mothers?
☐ 1. They often have unrealistic expectations about the love and caring they will receive from the baby.
☐ 2. They often have realistic expectations of the baby's patterns of growth and development.
☐ 3. They often have adequate knowledge about the child care, nutrition, and health needs of the baby.
☐ 4. They usually have excellent role models for parenting from their own parents.

175. Based on the current information and client needs, which of the following clinic-sponsored programs would be the most appropriate initial referral for Mrs. Wendall?
☐ 1. The birth control clinic.
☐ 2. The nutritional counseling program.

☐ 3. Early childhood development and parenting classes.

☐ 4. Classes in first aid and cardiopulmonary resuscitation.

Roberta Lane is a 42-year-old, married mother of four children ages 23, 21, 17, and 9. Mrs. Lane appears at the medical clinic this morning with a bandaged nose and a black eye. As the nurse enters the examining room, Mrs. Lane laughs, points to her face and says, "See this! My husband did this. I was in the emergency room 4 hours the other night getting patched up. He really did a good job on me this time." With that comment, Mrs. Lane becomes sad and stares at the floor.

176. Which of the following approaches is most appropriate when responding to Mrs. Lane's comment?

☐ 1. Respect Mrs. Lane's need to deny the problem and do not probe further into the issue.

☐ 2. Comment that if Mrs. Lane is not going to put a stop to this situation there is not much the nurse can do to help.

☐ 3. Acknowledge Mrs. Lane's sadness and ask directly about the circumstances surrounding this current battering incident.

☐ 4. Refer Mrs. Lane for psychotherapy.

177. The nurse's attitudes toward women who remain in a relationship in which multiple battering incidents have occurred often influence the ability to be helpful to these women. Which of the following feelings are most commonly experienced by the nurse?

☐ 1. Apathy and ignoring behavior.

☐ 2. Frustration and disappointment.

☐ 3. Guilt and shame.

☐ 4. Denial and repression.

178. Which of the following attitudes, if conveyed by health care professionals, inhibits self-disclosure by the battered women?

☐ 1. Indifference to the seriousness of the situation.

☐ 2. Concern over the detail of the situation.

☐ 3. Interest in previous medical records to determine the history of the battering incidences.

☐ 4. Feeling that the victim brought the battering on herself.

179. When planning her care, which of the following is most important for Mrs. Lane?

☐ 1. The phone numbers of the local crisis hot line and the local battered-women's shelter.

☐ 2. Referral to a psychotherapist.

☐ 3. Referral to assertiveness training classes for women.

☐ 4. No referral will be needed unless the battering occurs again or is witnessed by an adult.

Thomas Benson, a 14-year-old boy, is admitted to an inpatient psychiatric unit with the diagnosis of con- duct disorder. **He has been running away from home, taking illegal drugs, skipping classes, and now he has been arrested for shoplifting. His family is very discouraged and does not feel he can be controlled at home.**

180. The nurse assigned to Tom can expect him to behave in which of the following ways the first few days on the unit?

☐ 1. Exhibit depressed and withdrawn behavior.

☐ 2. Express a desire to spend most of the time alone.

☐ 3. Tease and bait the staff.

☐ 4. Display good interpersonal skills.

181. This behavior is primarily Tom's way of

☐ 1. Avoiding or expressing feelings of anger or depression.

☐ 2. Attempting to make friends.

☐ 3. Behaving like a normal teenager.

☐ 4. Denying his lack of social and intellectual abilities.

182. The most appropriate initial goal of nursing care will be which of the following?

☐ 1. Client will sit and talk with a primary nurse for 30 minutes daily.

☐ 2. Client will verbalize his understanding of why his family feels frustrated with him.

☐ 3. Client will decrease acting-out behavior.

☐ 4. Client will increase contact with other clients.

183. The most appropriate action for Tom's early treatment would be to

☐ 1. Have the client's friends visit daily.

☐ 2. Have the client discuss with the nurse why his family is upset with him.

☐ 3. Set firm and definite limits on his acting-out behavior.

☐ 4. Allow the client to use abusive language until he is able to regain some control.

Susan Porter has been hospitalized in an alcohol-rehabilitation unit for 3 weeks. She was given a pass, but has returned to the psychiatric unit in an agitated state. She spits on the primary nurse, then kicks her and tries to choke her. Despite efforts to encourage verbalization, Miss Porter continues to try to be physically abusive. Using a team approach, the staff members place Miss Porter in 4-point (all extremities) leather restraints and reassure her that they will help her regain control of herself.

184. Miss Porter's history indicates that during her drinking bouts, she has periods of amnesia and blackouts; when she withdraws from drinking she has delirium tremens. Given this history, the multidisciplinary health team assigned to this client would best conclude that her alcoholism is in which stage?

☐ 1. Early.

☐ 2. Middle.

☐ 3. Late or chronic.

☐ 4. Recovered.

185. When dealing with a potentially violent client, staff would use three of the following alternatives to restraints and seclusion. Which one would be *inappropriate*?

☐ 1. Identify the anxiety (e.g., say, "It seems as though you feel very bad. Tell me what is going on.").

☐ 2. Encourage the client to verbalize instead of act out (e.g., "What happened while you were out on pass that made you so angry?").

☐ 3. Sit close to client and provide reassurance (e.g., say "Let me give you some kind words.").

☐ 4. Tell the client she is getting out of control and will have to be restrained if she refuses to take the prescribed medication.

186. If staff members have sufficient time to prepare themselves to restrain a client, they should do all of the following. If it is vital to restrain the client quickly, which component can be done following the restraint procedure?

☐ 1. Obtain a physician's order for restraints.

☐ 2. Remove their own glasses, ties, earrings, pens, and any other articles that the client can seize in order to hurt them.

☐ 3. Distract the client with a blanket or sheet.

☐ 4. Have four staff members available in order to avoid client and staff injury.

187. During the time that Miss Porter is in restraints, she experiences vivid hallucinations and persecutory delusions. She continues to be agitated and combative for several hours. Blood is drawn for drug screening. The most likely substance used by Miss Porter while on pass is

☐ 1. Barbiturates.

☐ 2. Opiates.

☐ 3. Diazepam (Valium).

☐ 4. Phencyclidine (PCP).

188. Three of the following behaviors indicate that the goals regarding the use of physical restraints have been met. Which one does *not*?

☐ 1. The client tolerates physical restraints.

☐ 2. The client verbalizes angry feelings and calms down considerably.

☐ 3. The client does not demonstrate aggressive behavior such as abusive language.

☐ 4. The client promises to quiet herself.

Lydia Smith, a 26-year-old nurse, was leaving the hospital at midnight at the end of her shift when she was sexually assaulted in the parking lot of the hospital. After the assault, Mrs. Smith went to the emergency room for treatment.

189. The initial treatment of a rape victim can significantly affect the psychological impact the assault will have on the victim. The first information elicited from Mrs. Smith should be which of the following?

☐ 1. The marital state of the victim.

☐ 2. The victim's perception of what occurred.

☐ 3. Whether or not the rapist was known to her.

☐ 4. How she feels about having an abortion if she becomes pregnant.

190. Rape is generally considered to be an act of

☐ 1. Aggression.

☐ 2. Bestiality.

☐ 3. Exposure.

☐ 4. Sexual passion.

191. Mrs. Smith called her husband to come to the hospital. Which of the following statements is most often true about the reactions of significant others?

☐ 1. They are usually very supportive and helpful to the victim.

☐ 2. They are usually apathetic, because they do not empathize with the victim.

☐ 3. They may require time and professional assistance for resolution of this crisis.

☐ 4. They may derive positive experiences by providing emotional support for the victim.

192. Mrs. Smith may not have a true emotional crisis as a result of the assault. Which factor will contribute most to decreasing the severity of the trauma?

☐ 1. Support from counseling.

☐ 2. Support from her nursing colleagues.

☐ 3. Support from the hospital administration.

☐ 4. Support from her husband and the effectiveness of her coping mechanisms.

Sarah Long, a 35-year-old electrician, is brought by the police to the emergency room. The officer tells the triage nurse that Miss Long called the police to report a man had broken into her apartment and raped her. The nurse notes Miss Long has several bruises and lacerations on her face and is very quiet; she gives only her name.

193. What is the first action that the nurse should implement with Miss Long?

☐ 1. Obtain a specimen of semen for documentation for the future court case.

☐ 2. Suture lacerations and clean all wounds.

☐ 3. Call Miss Long's family.

☐ 4. Reassure Miss Long that she is safe and will not be harmed further.

194. In planning care for Miss Long, the nurse's first actions should be oriented toward

☐ 1. Controlling symptoms.

☐ 2. The diagnosis.

☐ 3. The behavior.

☐ 4. Her intellectual capacity.

195. The nurse has established a rapport with Miss Long. Which of the following would *not* be helpful during the early stages of crisis intervention?
    □ 1. Encourage her to identify the frightening events.
    □ 2. Help her to understand the crisis.
    □ 3. Assess her thoughts of suicide.
    □ 4. Identify her resources and support systems.

196. The use of crisis intervention is based on several important assumptions. Which of the following is *not* characteristic of the crisis model?
    □ 1. Interventions focus on immediate, concrete problems rather than on many aspects of the client's life.
    □ 2. Interventions are consistent with the client's culture and life-style.
    □ 3. Interventions include the client's significant others.
    □ 4. Interventions will be initiated by the nurse and not by the client.

Nicholas Bonono is a 43-year-old married man who is chronically suspicious and lacks trust in people. In the past few months, he has become convinced his brother is attempting to steal his property. Although he is still functioning in his position as an accountant, his family, marital, and social relationships have deteriorated. He is admitted to the hospital with a diagnosis of paranoid disorder.

197. Mr. Bonono demonstrates which of the following?
    □ 1. Persecutory hallucinations.
    □ 2. Persecutory delusions.
    □ 3. Persecutory illusions.
    □ 4. Persecutory phobias.

198. Which of the following ego-defense mechanisms are most prominently used by Mr. Bonono?
    □ 1. Denial and projection.
    □ 2. Denial and repression.
    □ 3. Displacement and projection.
    □ 4. Displacement and repression.

199. Since Mr. Bonono is mistrustful of others, which nursing action would be most appropriate?
    □ 1. Have him attend many activities, so he will meet as many clients and personnel as soon as possible.
    □ 2. Be very cheerful at all times, so he will sense positive feelings from the nursing staff.
    □ 3. Be consistent with personnel and schedules, so that structure is provided for his daily activities.
    □ 4. Use touch appropriately to reinforce reality.

200. Mr. Bonono is started on a regimen of chlorpromazine (Thorazine), 50 mg TID PO. What is the primary reason for the use of psychotropic drugs?
    □ 1. To keep clients sedated and easier to manage.
    □ 2. To alleviate symptoms, so that additional therapies may be more effective for clients.
    □ 3. To assist clients in gaining insight into their problems.

    □ 4. To improve the self-esteem of clients.

201. The clients on the unit are going on a picnic in the park. What information should Mr. Bonono be given regarding the side effects of his medication before he leaves?
    □ 1. Wear a hat and a long-sleeved shirt.
    □ 2. Report constipation and fatigue.
    □ 3. Report dry mouth and a stuffy nose.
    □ 4. Watch for signs of jaundice.

202. Mr. Bonono says to the nurse, "I really have been intolerant of others all these years." Which response by the nurse is preferable?
    □ 1. "Why do you say that, Mr. Bonono?"
    □ 2. "With whom have you been intolerant, Mr. Bonono?"
    □ 3. "Tell me about it, Mr. Bonono."
    □ 4. "What would you do differently now, Mr. Bonono?"

Rodman Dooley is a 45-year-old man whose wife has accompanied him to the hospital. Mrs. Dooley states that her husband has recently become very suspicious of their neighbors and has almost engaged in physical conflicts with one man on two occasions. He has accused other persons of trying to spy on him when they are merely going about their own business. In the interview, Mrs. Dooley states that this behavior began a few weeks after Mr. Dooley was on an airplane that was hijacked to another country. The admissions officer decides to admit Mr. Dooley for observation.

203. What is the nurse's first priority in working with Mr. Dooley?
    □ 1. Help him to establish a trusting relationship.
    □ 2. Make him aware that stress precipitated his behavior.
    □ 3. Improve his self-esteem.
    □ 4. Improve his social functioning.

204. Mr. Dooley states that he consented to being admitted only to please his wife and that there is really nothing wrong with him. What is the best nursing response?
    □ 1. "Why would she want you here if you didn't need help?"
    □ 2. "You have been creating some problems for her."
    □ 3. "The only way you will get help is if you admit you need it."
    □ 4. "What has been going on in your life lately?"

205. The nurse assigned to meet with Mr. Dooley is delayed 30 minutes by an emergency. Which of the following is the best action to take?
    □ 1. Acknowledge the lateness, but do not dwell on it.
    □ 2. Explain the reason for the delay.
    □ 3. Make another appointment with the client.
    □ 4. Apologize for being late.

206. Two nurses are discussing Mr. Dooley's progress when the client unexpectedly walks around the corner and overhears his name. He says, "What were you saying about me?" Which is the best response for the nurse to make?
- ☐ 1. "We were discussing your progress."
- ☐ 2. "We often talk about clients."
- ☐ 3. "It would be better if we didn't talk about it."
- ☐ 4. "Does it bother you that we talk about you?"

207. Which of the following best indicates that Mr. Dooley is developing a trusting relationship with a nurse?
- ☐ 1. He recounts his delusions with the nurse.
- ☐ 2. The nurse can explain the reasons for his delusions.
- ☐ 3. He can describe his feelings to the nurse.
- ☐ 4. The nurse feels more at ease with him.

Sheila Dumas appears to be in her early twenties. She was found curled up in a corner of a bus station. When she was asked her name all she would say was "good baby." The police brought her to the psychiatric unit. Miss Dumas' guardian is an aunt who has been responsible for her since her parents were killed when Miss Dumas was 10. The aunt reports that Miss Dumas has had similar episodes in the past. Her condition has been managed with medication, and she has not had a psychotic episode in more than 2 years. The current episode occurred when Miss Dumas refused to continue taking her medication.

208. Which of the following areas should the nurse gather data about first?
- ☐ 1. The client's perception of reality.
- ☐ 2. The client's physical condition.
- ☐ 3. The observations of the client made by others in the bus station.
- ☐ 4. The client's speech patterns.

209. Whenever the nurse tries to talk with Miss Dumas, the client responds with baby talk or gibberish. How would the nurse react?
- ☐ 1. Correct her speech.
- ☐ 2. Discontinue efforts to communicate with her.
- ☐ 3. Give simple, explicit directions to her.
- ☐ 4. Request a consultation with a speech therapist for her.

210. The physician prescribes haloperidol (Haldol), 6 mg IM q30min for three doses. Which of the following would the nurse do before each dose?
- ☐ 1. Draw a blood specimen.
- ☐ 2. Do a neurological check.
- ☐ 3. Offer her fluids.
- ☐ 4. Take her blood pressure.

211. After the third dose of the medication, Miss Dumas is still talking baby talk and appears to be hallucinating. What would the nurse do?
- ☐ 1. Call the physician for further orders.
- ☐ 2. Administer another dose of the medication.
- ☐ 3. Record the results of the medication.
- ☐ 4. Observe the client for an hour.

212. After the client is past the acute hallucinatory period, the physician orders 4 mg of haloperidol (Haldol) qid. Which of the following is the best explanation for the nurse to give the client about the side effects of the drug?
- ☐ 1. "This medication may make you feel a little light-headed, especially in the morning, but it will help your symptoms."
- ☐ 2. "You will probably experience considerable drowsiness with this drug, but it will help you function better."
- ☐ 3. "This medication has no major side effects, and it will help you to tell what is real from what you may be imagining."
- ☐ 4. "You will be able to stop using this drug before very long, because it will get rid of your disordered thinking."

213. Miss Dumas appears to be listening to something. The nurse hears nothing. What is the most appropriate nursing response?
- ☐ 1. Give her an additional dose of her antipsychotic medication.
- ☐ 2. Ignore the behavior.
- ☐ 3. Contact her physician and request a seclusion order.
- ☐ 4. Talk with her about what she is experiencing.

214. Miss Dumas says to the nurse, "My mama says I shouldn't talk to you." Which of the following is the most appropriate response?
- ☐ 1. "Your mother has been dead for over 10 years."
- ☐ 2. "When did she say that?"
- ☐ 3. "I think you don't want to talk to me."
- ☐ 4. "I understand that belief is very real to you. It would be helpful for us to talk about it."

215. Which of the following is the best way to get Miss Dumas to participate in recreational activity?
- ☐ 1. Ask her what sports she enjoys, and find ways for her to join other clients in these activities.
- ☐ 2. Assign a staff member to play catch with her.
- ☐ 3. Give her a list of available choices, and have her select her preference.
- ☐ 4. Give her time to develop an interest, and initiate activity.

216. To what extent would the nurse encourage the involvement of Miss Dumas' aunt in her therapy?
- ☐ 1. Not at all, since Miss Dumas is an adult.
- ☐ 2. Only as much as Miss Dumas requests.
- ☐ 3. As much as the aunt can participate.
- ☐ 4. The aunt should be encouraged to enter therapy herself.

Several weeks after her wedding, Jane O'Grady was brought to the hospital by her husband. He reported she had disrobed in the supermarket and had urinated on the floor while singing the "Battle Hymn of the Re-

public." Her husband emphasized that this was very unusual behavior, since she has always been reserved, rather shy, and religious. Mrs. O'Grady called the nurse "Holy Mary" and said she finally was in a place where "there are lots of saints." She also whispered that God talks to her through the television.

217. Mrs. O'Grady's present behavior and events that possibly led to her hospitalization are discussed at a team conference. Which of the following nursing actions should be given the highest priority?
   □ 1. Concentrate on helping her relate to her husband.
   □ 2. Concentrate on helping her relate to a few staff members.
   □ 3. Concentrate on having her improve her grooming and appearance.
   □ 4. Concentrate on getting her involved in social activities on the unit.

218. As the nurse approaches her, she says, "I don't want to talk." What is the best nursing response?
   □ 1. "You don't want to talk?"
   □ 2. "Why don't you want to talk to me?"
   □ 3. "There is no need to talk with me."
   □ 4. "I'll sit with you for awhile."

219. A nursing student and Mrs. O'Grady pass by a room where other nursing students and clients are involved in a grooming and makeup session. The nursing student explains, "These sessions are on Tuesday and Thursday afternoons. The women learn how to apply makeup." What is the rationale for this nursing student's remark?
   □ 1. Impress the other clients and the instructor.
   □ 2. Encourage the success of the nurse-client relationship.
   □ 3. Orient the client to reality.
   □ 4. Persuade the client to join the group.

220. Mrs. O'Grady yells for the nurse. As the nurse arrives and enters her room, she says, "Do you see? There! God is appearing." Which of the following is the best nursing response?
   □ 1. "No, I don't see Him, but I understand He is real to you."
   □ 2. "He is not there. You must be imagining things."
   □ 3. "Show me where God appears to you."
   □ 4. "God is appearing?"

221. The nurse's response when Mrs. O'Grady asks for confirmation of her hallucination is based on which one of the following?
   □ 1. Agree that the client perceives the hallucination in order to avoid increasing the client's anxiety.
   □ 2. Tell the client to reexamine her feelings.
   □ 3. Give an honest reply with the focus on what the client believes to be real.
   □ 4. Tell the client that she is imagining things.

222. Mrs. O'Grady's anxiety has increased since her admission 3 days ago. Which behavior is Mrs. O'Grady most likely to demonstrate?
   □ 1. Receptive to psychotherapy.
   □ 2. Shows insight about the causes of her illness.
   □ 3. Less able to focus her attention on the reality of the situation.
   □ 4. Less inclined to talk with her husband.

Chi Wu is admitted to the hospital because of increasing withdrawal. He moves very slowly and is largely uncommunicative. His medical diagnosis is schizophrenia, catatonic type.

223. The best initial goal is which of the following?
   □ 1. Client will establish a trusting relationship with the nurse.
   □ 2. Client will increase his social skills.
   □ 3. Client will increase his level of communication.
   □ 4. Client will be oriented to reality.

224. The nurse on the unit begins to establish a relationship with Mr. Wu. Which of the following would be most effective in establishing communication at this time?
   □ 1. Sit quietly with Mr. Wu.
   □ 2. Talk about current world problems.
   □ 3. Ask about the problems Mr. Wu is experiencing now.
   □ 4. Tell Mr. Wu about all of the activities on the unit.

225. Mr. Wu becomes more communicative. The nurse plans to include him in activities that will provide opportunities for socialization. Which of the following would be most appropriate?
   □ 1. Square dancing in the gym.
   □ 2. Learning to play chess.
   □ 3. Picnicking on the hospital grounds.
   □ 4. Playing video games.

226. After a week of therapy with chlorpromazine (Thorazine), the nurse notices that Mr. Wu walks with a shuffling gait. What action should be taken by the nurse?
   □ 1. Take his blood pressure before the next dose.
   □ 2. Withhold the drug until the symptom disappears.
   □ 3. Suggest a neurological consultation.
   □ 4. Obtain an order for an antiparkinsonian drug.

227. After the nurse has discussed an upcoming 3-week vacation, Mr. Wu stops coming to their scheduled meetings and begins spending more time alone in his room. What best explains his response?
   □ 1. He feels threatened by the closeness of their relationship.
   □ 2. He is having a cyclical exacerbation of his illness.
   □ 3. He is responding to the impending loss.

☐ 4. He does not feel the need for the relationship anymore.

Arthur Maling has been admitted to the substance-abuse unit. He is 51 years old and has a history of increasing alcohol ingestion over the last 35 years. He currently drinks 1½ quarts of whiskey daily. He is married, but his wife has moved out of their home because of his drinking problem.

228. Which of these would most likely be included in Mr. Maling's admission orders?
☐ 1. High-protein diet, vitamins C and B-complex, chlordiazepoxide (Librium)
☐ 2. High-fat diet, vitamins B-complex and E, chlorpromazine (Thorazine)
☐ 3. Liquid diet, vitamins A and E, meperidine (Demerol)
☐ 4. Liquid diet, vitamins C and B-complex, phenytoin (Dilantin)

229. Prolonged use of alcohol may result in neuronal damage to the central nervous system. This may result in Korsakoff's organic syndrome (severe memory loss and confabulation). What is the physiological cause of this condition?
☐ 1. Encephalomalacia.
☐ 2. Destruction of brain tissue and often a marked deficiency of vitamin B[1] (thiamin).
☐ 3. Convulsions during withdrawal.
☐ 4. Dystonic reactions.

230. That evening, Mr. Maling begins to show signs of alcohol withdrawal. The first symptoms are
☐ 1. Hypotension, bradycardia, and decreased salivation.
☐ 2. Fever, dehydration, and convulsions.
☐ 3. Tremors, nervousness, and diaphoresis.
☐ 4. Vomiting, diarrhea, and incontinence.

231. If Mr. Maling experiences hallucinations during withdrawal, which would be the best nursing practice?
☐ 1. A quiet room and prn medication.
☐ 2. Bed rest, soft music, and fluids.
☐ 3. Hot tea every 2 hours, blood pressure check every 30 minutes, and restraints.
☐ 4. Ice cream every 2 hours, blood pressure check every 15 minutes, and restraints.

232. Mrs. Maling comes to see her husband. After the visit, she asks the nurse about Al-Anon. Which is the best response?
☐ 1. "Al-Anon is a support group for families of alcoholics. How do you feel about joining?"
☐ 2. "Al-Anon is a support group for families of alcoholics. Do you feel you need this, since you haven't been living with your husband?"
☐ 3. "Al-Anon is a support group for families of alcoholics. I'm sure you'd get a lot of help from joining."

☐ 4. "Al-Anon is a support group for families of alcoholics. Everyone who has a spouse who abuses alcohol should join."

233. The chances of an alcoholic becoming permanently sober are variable. Which factor is most necessary for Mr. Maling to be successful?
☐ 1. Willingness to atone for past behavior.
☐ 2. Recognition of the problem and motivation to change.
☐ 3. Support from his family and from his employer.
☐ 4. Membership in Alcoholics Anonymous.

234. Mr. Maling starts taking disulfiram (Antabuse). He will continue to take this after discharge. Which drugs should he be clearly instructed *not* to take?
☐ 1. Aspirin and acetaminophen (Tylenol).
☐ 2. Most cough medicines.
☐ 3. Heart and blood pressure medications.
☐ 4. Antacids and laxatives.

235. Mr. Maling starts attending Alcoholics Anonymous (AA) meetings in the hospital before discharge. Which statement about Alcoholics Anonymous is most correct?
☐ 1. It is a therapy group in which membership is recommended after discharge from a substance-abuse program.
☐ 2. It is a self-help group in which members acknowledge their illness and share experiences concerning abuse and control of alcohol intake.
☐ 3. It is a self-help group led by professionals who have achieved sobriety.
☐ 4. It is a therapy group that discourages relationships outside the organization.

236. Eight months after discharge, Mr. Maling returns to visit. He attends AA regularly, his wife has returned to him and attends Al-Anon regularly, and he remains on the disulfiram (Antabuse) regimen. Which is the best description of Mr. Maling?
☐ 1. A cured alcoholic.
☐ 2. A former alcoholic.
☐ 3. A recovering alcoholic.
☐ 4. A recovered alcoholic.

Bert Trysdale is a 19-year-old who was admitted at 4:35 AM to the orthopedic unit from surgery. He had fractured the shaft of his right femur in a motorcycle accident. The surgeon did an open reduction and inserted an intramedullary nail. Mr. Trysdale is in traction, and a unit of whole blood is hanging. He has been sleeping, and his vital signs are stable.

237. When the nurse enters the room to hang the container with the IV fluid to follow the unit of blood, Mr. Trysdale is awake and alert. He says, "How about a pint of rye instead?" Which of the following is the most therapeutic response?
☐ 1. "We don't have any of that in the hospital."
☐ 2. "It's a little early in the day for that, isn't it?"

☐ 3. "It sounds as though you feel you could use a drink."

☐ 4. "Sorry, but liquor is not allowed in the hospital."

238. The nurse enters the room later to find Mr. Trysdale trying to undo his traction. How would the nurse respond?

☐ 1. "The traction must be left in place, or more damage will be done to your leg. What is bothering you about it?"

☐ 2. "You're in an awfully big hurry to get up. What made you try to undo your traction?"

☐ 3. "If you aren't comfortable, maybe I can get you some sedation."

☐ 4. "The traction is necessary to immobilize your leg, so that it can heal. You must leave it alone."

239. The nursing assessment notes on the evening shift say that Mr. Trysdale seems anxious, has tremors, is perspiring, and has requested something for nausea. When the nurse gives Mr. Trysdale his IM medication for nausea, he says, "Is that gonna put me out?" How would the nurse respond?

☐ 1. "Do you want to be put out?"

☐ 2. "This is only for your nausea."

☐ 3. "Are you used to taking drugs?"

☐ 4. "You seem to be having a difficult time."

240. Mr. Trysdale continues to complain of generalized discomfort. He is visibly more anxious by the end of the evening shift and has not been able to fall asleep. He has not taken anything by mouth all day, even though he received a general soft diet at dinner time. The nurse suspects Mr. Trysdale may be going through drug or alcohol withdrawal. What would the nurse do first?

☐ 1. Call Mr. Trysdale's physician, and discuss the symptoms.

☐ 2. Observe Mr. Trysdale closely for further symptoms.

☐ 3. Arrange to transfer Mr. Trysdale to the detoxification unit.

☐ 4. Administer the sedative prescribed for Mr. Trysdale.

241. Mr. Trysdale begins screaming at 2:40 AM. When the nurse enters the room, he is trying to get out of bed and is crying out, "They're all over the bed! Get me outta this bed!" How should the nurse respond initially?

☐ 1. Gesture as if to brush off whatever Mr. Trysdale thinks he sees.

☐ 2. Reassure Mr. Trysdale that there is nothing in his bed. Talk calmly, stay with him, and orient him to his surroundings.

☐ 3. Speak in a calm voice until Mr. Trysdale has settled down; then get help to restrain him.

☐ 4. Administer a dose of the tranquilizer that the physician ordered.

242. After initially calming down, Mr. Trysdale becomes agitated again. He says, "What's happening to me? Why are you keeping me here?" Which of the following is the best response?

☐ 1. "We are trying to help you, but you must try to get control of yourself."

☐ 2. "When was the last time you took drugs or had a drink? You seem to be going through substance withdrawal."

☐ 3. "I think you are having withdrawal symptoms. We are going to take care of you and help you through this."

☐ 4. "You must be quiet and not disturb the other clients. We are keeping you here because you are sick."

243. Which of the following supportive nursing measures is appropriate while Mr. Trysdale is acutely agitated?

☐ 1. Encourage ambulation for him every hour.

☐ 2. Offer fluids every 2 hours.

☐ 3. Provide distractions, such as television.

☐ 4. Give mild, natural stimulants, such as coffee or tea.

244. After 3 days, Mr. Trysdale seems to be through the most dangerous stage of withdrawal. He has told the nurse that he has been a heavy drinker ever since he entered high school. He has never gone through withdrawal before, he says, and the experience has scared him enough that he wants to give up drinking. Which of the following goals has the highest priority for the client?

☐ 1. Client will admit to a drinking problem.

☐ 2. Client will give up the use of alcohol permanently.

☐ 3. Client will join Alcoholics Anonymous or similar self-help group and attend meetings.

☐ 4. Client will accept the support of others to give up drinking.

245. After being hospitalized for 2 weeks, Mr. Trysdale has learned crutch walking and is ready for discharge. The evening before he is to be discharged, the nurse enters his room and finds him drinking a can of beer. How should the nurse respond?

☐ 1. "It really must be difficult for you to give up drinking when you've been doing it for a long time."

☐ 2. "It is so disappointing to see that you are not willing to change your habits."

☐ 3. "After all the work you've done, how can you throw it away like this?"

☐ 4. "Are you testing me to see how I'll react?"

246. The day that Mr. Trysdale is discharged, he says to the nurse who has worked with him the most, "Even though I slipped up last night, I know I'm gonna be able to quit for good." How should the nurse respond?

1. "No matter how much you want to quit, it's going to be tough. Why not ask for help when you need it?"
2. "I'm proud that you are getting back on track. We all slip sometimes."
3. "You haven't really committed yourself to giving up drinking. You're not going to get better until you do."
4. "Don't make promises you're not ready to keep. You're the only one you hurt when you act like you did last night."

Roy Clements, a 26-year-old man, is admitted to the hospital in an acute psychotic state. He crawls around the unit on his hands and knees, making barking sounds. He came in accompanied by several friends, who revealed that the client took an unknown amount of lysergic acid diethylamide (LSD).

247. LSD belongs to which of the following classifications of drugs?
    1. Opiates.
    2. Barbiturates.
    3. Hallucinogens.
    4. Stimulants.

248. Which of the following is *not* characteristic of LSD?
    1. Physical addiction.
    2. Psychological dependence.
    3. Acute panic states.
    4. Heightened sensory perceptions.

249. Drug-dependent clients respond best to
    1. Psychoanalysis.
    2. Behavior modification.
    3. Family therapy.
    4. Group therapy led by former drug abusers.

250. Immediately after admission to the unit, Mr. Clements' psychotic behavior worsens. He tears at his clothes and hair, attempts to smash the television set in the dayroom with a chair, and threatens to attack another client. The best immediate nursing action is to
    1. Turn off the TV to reduce stimulation.
    2. Place the client in seclusion.
    3. Ask the physician for a stat order for sedation.
    4. Restrain the client in a chair in the dayroom.

251. Of the following reasons for the use of seclusion, which one is *not* valid?
    1. To reduce environmental stimulation.
    2. To prevent a client from hurting himself.
    3. To prevent a client from hurting others.
    4. To reduce the need for constant observation.

252. Mr. Clements sees red spiders crawling on his bed. Which of the following is the appropriate nursing response?
    1. "Come on, Mr. Clements, you're putting me on."
    2. Swat at the red spiders as if to kill them in Mr. Clements' presence.
    3. "I understand you believe you see the red spiders, Mr. Clements. I am not seeing any."
    4. Logically explain that red spiders are not present in his bed.

253. Later, Mr. Clements states that he is the king of Siam, and as one of his subjects, the nurse should bow in his presence. Select the most appropriate nursing response.
    1. Bow and pay respect to Mr. Clements.
    2. "Being a king might make a person feel very powerful."
    3. "If you're the king of Siam, I am Queen Jezebel."
    4. Place him in seclusion until he is able to control himself.

254. Select the medication that best helps control hallucinations and delusions.
    1. Haloperidol (Haldol)
    2. Isocarboxazid (Marplan)
    3. Diazepam (Valium)
    4. Imipramine (Tofranil)

References

American Journal of Nursing Company. (1992). *AJN/Mosby nursing boards review* (8th ed.). St. Louis: Mosby–Year Book.

American Psychiatric Association. (1987). *Diagnostic and statistical manual of mental disorders* (3rd ed. revised). Washington, DC: Author.

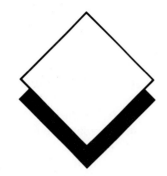

Correct Answers

1. no. 4	**40.** no. 4	**79.** no. 3	**118.** no. 3
2. no. 2	**41.** no. 3	**80.** no. 2	**119.** no. 4
3. no. 2	**42.** no. 2	**81.** no. 1	**120.** no. 3
4. no. 3	**43.** no. 3	**82.** no. 4	**121.** no. 4
5. no. 3	**44.** no. 4	**83.** no. 2	**122.** no. 1
6. no. 1	**45.** no. 1	**84.** no. 1	**123.** no. 3
7. no. 1	**46.** no. 4	**85.** no. 1	**124.** no. 3
8. no. 4	**47.** no. 2	**86.** no. 4	**125.** no. 2
9. no. 3	**48.** no. 2	**87.** no. 2	**126.** no. 3
10. no. 2	**49.** no. 3	**88.** no. 3	**127.** no. 2
11. no. 1	**50.** no. 3	**89.** no. 3	**128.** no. 3
12. no. 2	**51.** no. 4	**90.** no. 4	**129.** no. 3
13. no. 3	**52.** no. 1	**91.** no. 4	**130.** no. 1
14. no. 3	**53.** no. 1	**92.** no. 2	**131.** no. 4
15. no. 2	**54.** no. 4	**93.** no. 4	**132.** no. 4
16. no. 3	**55.** no. 3	**94.** no. 2	**133.** no. 2
17. no. 4	**56.** no. 3	**95.** no. 3	**134.** no. 2
18. no. 2	**57.** no. 4	**96.** no. 4	**135.** no. 2
19. no. 3	**58.** no. 3	**97.** no. 4	**136.** no. 4
20. no. 3	**59.** no. 2	**98.** no. 2	**137.** no. 2
21. no. 2	**60.** no. 3	**99.** no. 1	**138.** no. 4
22. no. 3	**61.** no. 3	**100.** no. 3	**139.** no. 1
23. no. 4	**62.** no. 1	**101.** no. 4	**140.** no. 1
24. no. 4	**63.** no. 4	**102.** no. 1	**141.** no. 4
25. no. 3	**64.** no. 3	**103.** no. 1	**142.** no. 1
26. no. 2	**65.** no. 4	**104.** no. 4	**143.** no. 4
27. no. 2	**66.** no. 2	**105.** no. 4	**144.** no. 4
28. no. 1	**67.** no. 1	**106.** no. 1	**145.** no. 4
29. no. 3	**68.** no. 4	**107.** no. 1	**146.** no. 1
30. no. 4	**69.** no. 2	**108.** no. 2	**147.** no. 1
31. no. 2	**70.** no. 2	**109.** no. 4	**148.** no. 4
32. no. 3	**71.** no. 4	**110.** no. 3	**149.** no. 4
33. no. 1	**72.** no. 4	**111.** no. 2	**150.** no. 2
34. no. 2	**73.** no. 3	**112.** no. 1	**151.** no. 1
35. no. 1	**74.** no. 3	**113.** no. 3	**152.** no. 4
36. no. 2	**75.** no. 3	**114.** no. 1	**153.** no. 4
37. no. 2	**76.** no. 3	**115.** no. 3	**154.** no. 4
38. no. 2	**77.** no. 4	**116.** no. 3	**155.** no. 2
39. no. 4	**78.** no. 1	**117.** no. 2	**156.** no. 3

157. no. 3	**182.** no. 3	**207.** no. 3	**231.** no. 1
158. no. 3	**183.** no. 3	**208.** no. 2	**232.** no. 1
159. no. 1	**184.** no. 3	**209.** no. 3	**233.** no. 2
160. no. 2	**185.** no. 3	**210.** no. 4	**234.** no. 2
161. no. 3	**186.** no. 1	**211.** no. 1	**235.** no. 2
162. no. 1	**187.** no. 4	**212.** no. 1	**236.** no. 3
163. no. 1	**188.** no. 4	**213.** no. 4	**237.** no. 3
164. no. 3	**189.** no. 2	**214.** no. 4	**238.** no. 1
165. no. 3	**190.** no. 1	**215.** no. 2	**239.** no. 4
166. no. 2	**191.** no. 3	**216.** no. 3	**240.** no. 1
167. no. 1	**192.** no. 4	**217.** no. 2	**241.** no. 2
168. no. 3	**193.** no. 4	**218.** no. 4	**242.** no. 3
169. no. 4	**194.** no. 3	**219.** no. 3	**243.** no. 2
170. no. 2	**195.** no. 2	**220.** no. 1	**244.** no. 4
171. no. 3	**196.** no. 4	**221.** no. 3	**245.** no. 1
172. no. 3	**197.** no. 2	**222.** no. 3	**246.** no. 1
173. no. 2	**198.** no. 1	**223.** no. 1	**247.** no. 3
174. no. 1	**199.** no. 3	**224.** no. 1	**248.** no. 1
175. no. 3	**200.** no. 2	**225.** no. 3	**249.** no. 4
176. no. 3	**201.** no. 1	**226.** no. 4	**250.** no. 2
177. no. 2	**202.** no. 4	**227.** no. 3	**251.** no. 4
178. no. 4	**203.** no. 1	**228.** no. 1	**252.** no. 3
179. no. 1	**204.** no. 4	**229.** no. 2	**253.** no. 2
180. no. 3	**205.** no. 2	**230.** no. 3	**254.** no. 1
181. no. 1	**206.** no. 1		

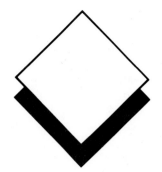

Correct Answers with Rationales

KEY TO ABBREVIATIONS
Section of the Review Book

P = Psychosocial and Mental Health Problems
  T = Therapeutic Use of Self
  L = Loss and Death and Dying
  A = Anxious Behavior
  C = Confused Behavior
  E = Elated-Depressive Behavior
  SM = Socially Maladaptive Behavior
  SS = Suspicious Behavior
  W = Withdrawn Behavior
  SU = Substance Use Disorders

Nursing Process Category

AS = Assessment
AN = Analysis
PL = Plan
IM = Implementation
EV = Evaluation

Client Need Category

E = Safe, Effective Care Environment
PS = Physiological Integrity
PC = Psychosocial Integrity
H = Health Promotion and Maintenance

1. no. 4. The present interaction pattern allows the nurse to work in the here-and-now and not proceed based on preconceived ideas. Present interaction includes not only verbal aspects (who talks to whom), but also nonverbal ones (e.g., facial expressions, body movements, seating patterns). Options no. 1, no. 2, and no. 3 will be important later, once the group is established. P/T, IM, E

2. no. 2. The residents are anxious, and their response is not unusual. This is the establishing phase of the group. While the nurse may not have clearly explained the purpose of the group, a characteristic of this stage is anxiety related to uncertainty over what will actually occur in the group. The members may express anger; however, it is usually a manifestation of anxiety at the beginning of a new experience. P/T, AN, E

3. no. 2. The purpose of the group is interaction. Option no. 2 will permit discussion and possible problem solving by the entire group. Option no. 4 singles out one resident, in effect, closing the others out of the interaction. Option no. 1 is negation and false reassurance and cuts off further exploration. Option no. 3 keeps the focus on an individual rather than encouraging group interaction. Look for open-ended questions and statements. P/T, IM, PC

4. no. 3. Commenting on your perceptions will allow the group to discuss their feelings and has the potential for serving as a learning situation. Monopolizing the conversation is a group issue and needs to be addressed in the group, not on an individual basis. What are the dynamics occurring that allow only one person to talk? Ignoring the behavior does not help Mr. Abels to learn how to be with other people appropriately. If transferred to another group, Mr. Abels might repeat the behavior, and it will give a message to other group members that exclusion can occur as a result of the decision of the facilitator alone. P/T, IM, E

5. no. 3. The client's verbal and nonverbal communications do not correspond. If she is angry and disgusted, she should not be smiling. Her words and behavior are incongruent. Mrs. Thomas is not demonstrating suspicious (fear of harm from

others), demanding (unnecessary and insistent requests), or resistive (unwilling to cooperate) behavior. P/T, AN, PC

6. no. 1. The best way to deal with incongruence is to point out the inconsistency observed between verbal and nonverbal communication to the client. Options no. 2, no. 3, and no. 4 do not address the incongruent behavior and are not as helpful to the client. P/T, IM, PC

7. no. 1. After the nurse has confronted her with the inconsistency, allow her some time to think about what was said before expecting her to respond. Rather than show concern, as in option no. 3, the nurse might do better to simply wonder why the client is silent. Option no. 2 reflects a lack of understanding about giving feedback and the need to provide the client time to reflect before responding. The suggestion of free association (no. 4) seems inappropriate at this time. P/T, IM, PC

8. no. 4. The health care team can begin a plan of care based on initial assessment of the incongruent behavior. Part of the plan of care will include approaches or possible interventions for specific behaviors displayed by the client. It is most likely that options no. 2 and no. 3 have not been completed or even initiated yet. The diagnosis is provisional at this time and is based on the client's needs and behavior. The focus of no. 1 is on the behavior. P/T, PL, E

9. no. 3. Clients who become more withdrawn are frequently regarded as needing human contact. This can best be done through a one-to-one relationship, beginning at the client's level. The nurse offers physical presence and avoids probing questions and does not demand options or premature participation. Options no. 2 and no. 4 reflect a lack of understanding of withdrawn behavior. P/L, AN, PC

10. no. 2. From the data presented, both affect and words indicate anger. "I'm sure he's really OK" would indicate denial. Bargaining would be suggested by "I would never argue with him again if he could come back." Depression would be demonstrated by crying, immobility, and inability to sleep and eat, or sleeping and eating too much. Resolution would be shown by statements that acknowledge the death and view the deceased realistically. P/L, AN, PC

11. no. 1. This option provides information about the duration of the response. A commonly seen grief reaction usually resolves in 6 to 12 months and is usually resolved in 12 months. Options no. 2, no. 3, and no. 4 may be normal grief reaction statements, but they do not help to discern between normal and dysfunctional grief. P/L, AS, H

12. no. 2. The overt problem being expressed at this time is anger. From the data provided, the anger seems to be associated with the very recent death of her husband and how the loss is being experienced by her. P/L, AN, H

13. no. 3. The intensity and admixture of feelings during the initial grieving process may leave the client confused, sad, anxious, or guilty. Talking about feelings (ventilation) aids in their recognition and resolution. Recounting the positive aspects of her husband occurs in the resolution stage. Educating the client to the normal grief process is important once the overwhelming feelings are explored. Option no. 4 is premature and might be experienced as negation and false reassurance, leaving the client feeling isolated and misunderstood. P/L, IM, H

14. no. 3. The client's basic physical needs must be met first. It might be more beneficial to help the family deal with their feelings and help the overwhelmed client verbally express any of the feelings she is experiencing. P/L, PL, PC

15. no. 2. By her "helpless" nonparticipation, she has increased the chance of more staff interaction and assistance. Decubitus ulcers may result from immobility and associated stasis of blood flow. Nurses may feel anger toward client because Mrs. Quale is not demonstrating "good client" behavior. Contractures in an already debilitated client are more likely with immobility. P/L, AN, PS

16. no. 3. The children may reject their mother as a defense against their perceived rejection by her. Since it may be too painful for Mrs. Quale to deal with her children, the separation keeps her from increasing her awareness of how they are actually feeling. The client may be afraid that her changed body image would repel her children and further decrease her self-esteem. She uses denial to protect herself from the changes and to fully experience her impending losses, thus prolonging the grief process. P/L, AN, H

17. no. 4. The client may be unable to achieve this physically or mentally. Nursing care measures in option no. 1 are necessary. The nurse who explores her own feelings usually gains greater awareness and self-control; thus she is able to focus more on the client's need rather than her own needs. The presence of the nurse may be comforting and demonstrates acceptance of the client. P/L, IM, PS

18. no. 2. A client may or may not experience each of the stages of dying, in order or not. People are usually consistent in their reactions to major crises. It is very important for the nurse to remember the needs of the family. A child's level of cognitive development will determine the response to death. P/L, AS, H

19. no. 3. To a 3-year-old, death is the same as going away for awhile. Children ages 6-9 personify death (someone bad carries them away). Children ages 5-6 believe death is reversible. Children ages 9-10 recognize that everyone must die. P/L, AS, H

20. no. 3. Children generally do not express their emotions or concerns in a verbal, direct manner as an adult does, especially to strangers such as the hospital staff. They are able to express their concerns better through stories, drawings, or other forms of play as indicated in options no. 1, no. 2, and no. 4. Through these media, children may state directly how they feel, or their emotions may be inferred through observation. P/L, IM, PC

21. no. 2. This approach is direct. It allows the client to talk about her feelings using broad statements. Options no. 1, no. 3, and no. 4 avoid dealing directly with Mrs. Miller's sorrow and grief. This may foster the client's repressing her grief and developing a delayed grief reaction. P/L, IM, PC

22. no. 3. Suicidal thoughts are fairly common in reactive depression, but hoarding sleep medications may indicate actual planning of a suicide attempt, which is an abnormal grief response. Options no. 1, no. 2, and no. 4 are common manifestations of a normal grief reaction. P/L, AS, H

23. no. 4. Although it is appropriate to offer support during the crisis period of a grief reaction, it is also important to allow the client to move through the process at her own pace. Mrs. Miller's depression is an expected stage of normal grief, and she should be allowed to experience her sorrow. Too little or too much introspection may be counterproductive. A "surprise" visit from her son would not be part of a collaborative care plan. P/L, IM, PC

24. no. 4. This is the only option that affords the client broad openings for ventilation of affect. P/L, IM, PC

25. no. 3. This answer indicates the absence of a value judgment by the nurse, while encouraging the option of discussing the decision. Option no. 1 is a premature closure of the subject. Options no. 2 and no. 4 are judgmental statements and may elicit a defensive response to the decision rather than encouraging further consideration. All three (nos. 1, 2, and 4) discourage further discussion of her feelings. P/L, IM, H

26. no. 2. In moderate anxiety, the person's ability to perceive and concentrate is decreased. Physical discomforts increase, and overall level of functioning decreases. This client is still functioning and able to focus on work with effort, but her discomfort is increasing. At this point, the anxiety is moderate. Without intervention, it is likely to become severe, whereby the person's perceptual field is greatly reduced, sense of time is distorted, and all behavior

is aimed at getting relief. During mild anxiety, the person is alert, and the perceptual field is increased. When in a panic, the person's emotional tone is associated with awe, dread, and terror. P/A, AN, PC

27. no. 2. This helps the client identify and express the feelings she is experiencing at the time. It provides the nurse with more data to help the client recognize her anxiety and begin to relate her behavior to the feelings she is experiencing. It is best in the beginning of assessment to focus on the here-and-now and start with a general perspective rather than being directive or asking about past experiences. P/A, IM, PC

28. no. 1. In order to establish an effective behavior-modification program, baseline data must first be collected about the behavior (e.g., frequency, amount, and time). Although options no. 2 and no. 3 are important because activities of daily living and pain contribute to the behavior, they themselves do not provide a complete picture of client behavior. Any reaction to the anesthetic already would have occurred. P/A, AS, PS

29. no. 3. The client is probably afraid that she will be left alone. Responding to the client at consistent intervals when she is not calling for something will reduce the calling behavior and, one hopes, increase her confidence that she will be attended to. Her underlying fear can be dealt with by checking on her consistently and frequently. Option no. 1 promotes the client's frequent requests. Pain may not be the only reason she is uncomfortable. Option no. 4 only makes the client feel guilty and does not address the underlying problem of her fear of being alone. P/A, IM, E

30. no. 4. If demanding behavior is reinforced, it will be repeated. To change undesired behavior, reinforce more appropriate behavior. Options no. 1 through no. 3 address possible underlying dynamics for the behavior, but are not considered essential for behavior change and are not as helpful for changing the behavior. P/A, PL, E

31. no. 2. During an anxiety reaction, the client thinks that something bad will happen; with normal anxiety there is no such underlying feeling. Both have the same physiological and psychological manifestations. Normal anxiety is not constant; there can be a wide range of levels from mild to severe. An anxiety reaction can be controlled with proper interventions to reduce the level of distress. Normal anxiety could become an anxiety reaction if stress renders normal coping mechanisms inadequate. P/A, AS, PC

32. no. 3. The techniques used in option no. 3 are reflection and restatement. Option no. 1 defends the doctor, no. 2 agrees with the client, and no. 4

is reassurance, all of which are nontherapeutic statements because they do not allow further exploration of the client's concerns and feelings. P/A, IM, PC

33. no. 1. These are the physiological and psychological manifestations of anxiety. Characteristics of depression are listed in option no. 2, no. 3 describes thought disorders related to psychosis, and no. 4 is also characteristic of mania and depression. P/A, AS, PC

34. no. 2. The person in panic is severely agitated, which shows in verbal and nonverbal behavior. Option no. 1 lists symptoms of psychotic behaviors; option no. 3 indicates a dissociative state. Option no. 4 is only partially correct; mood depression is not usually characteristic of a panic reaction. P/A, AS, PC

35. no. 1. Stay calm and help the client mobilize thoughts and feelings. Option no. 2 deals with the immediate solution. Option no. 3 is a cognitive skill that a person in panic may not be able to use until he has calmed down. Clients in a panic state are usually experiencing fear, dread, and terror. P/A, IM, PC

36. no. 2. The nurse must assess the psychological and physiological indicators of anxiety as well as the client's effective use of coping mechanisms. Incoherent thought processes, mood swings, or lack of reality orientation have not been the problem. Although self-reporting is important, a more comprehensive evaluation is in order. P/A, EV, PC

37. no. 2. This is an increasingly recognized phobia. Literally "fear of the marketplace," agoraphobia is displayed by those who specifically fear being in a public place from which they feel they may not be able to escape. The "scope or territory" of what is considered the safety and security of home varies. Acrophobia is the fear of heights; astraphobia is the fear or dread of thunder and lightning; claustrophobia is the fear of closed places. P/A, AN, PC

38. no. 2. In a phobic disorder, the anxiety is displaced from the original source and then transferred, resulting in a phobia. Sublimation is a higher-order ego defense that involves the positive rechanneling of drives to a socially acceptable modality. Substitution involves replacing the original unacceptable wish, drive, emotion, or goal with one that is more acceptable. Suppression occurs when the client chooses not to think about something. P/A, AS, PC

39. no. 4. The most common behavior modification technique used to treat phobic disorders is gradual desensitization. Under controlled conditions, the client is slowly exposed to the object or situation feared. Confrontation is useful only when the client

has the ability to hear the information and the readiness to work on the problem. Premature confrontation might result in panic or regression. Immediate exposure could create even greater anxiety. Distraction will not enable the client to overcome his fear and resume functioning. P/A, PL, PC

40. no. 4. Agoraphobia is classified as occurring with or without panic attacks. However, anxiety is experienced with exposure to the feared object or situation, and an anxiolytic may be prescribed at the beginning of desensitization. Fluphenazine and chlorpromazine are indicated for the treatment of psychosis. Lithium carbonate is an antimanic-depressive medication. P/A, IM, PS

41. no. 3. Since agoraphobia is fear of the outside, his presence on the volleyball court might be indicative of his increased ability to leave the hospital building. Milieu group, occupational therapy, and Sunday dinner are held on the unit in general and, although they are important elements of the treatment program, the client is still in a closed environment. P/A, EV, PC

42. no. 2. The ritualistic behavior demonstrated by the client with an obsessive-compulsive disorder is considered a symbolic attempt to control anxiety. Obsessive-compulsive behaviors may secondarily result in attention, but the behavior is an attempt to handle an anxiety-provoking situation. An obsessive-compulsive disorder reveals an uncontrollable thought and impulse pattern, and it may result in isolation. It may originate from a feeling of anxious dread and is persistently impelling, not manipulative. P/A, AN, PC

43. no. 3. Displacement of the ego-dystonic idea into an unrelated and senseless activity temporarily lowers the anxiety of the individual. By carrying out the act, the client attempts to undo the uncontrollable impulse. In introjection, a psychic representation of a loved or hated object is taken into one's ego system. In projection, a person attributes to another ideas, thoughts, feelings, and impulses that are a part of his or her inner perceptions, but are unacceptable. Compensation is a conscious or unconscious defense mechanism by which a person tries to make up for an imagined or real deficiency that is physical, psychological, or both. Isolation involves setting apart an idea from the feeling tone. Rationalization is an unconscious defense mechanism in which an irrational behavior, motive, or feeling is made to appear reasonable. Repression is an unconscious defense mechanism by which a person removes from consciousness those ideas, impulses, and affects that are unacceptable. P/A, AN, PC

44. no. 4. The obsessive-compulsive disorder is characterized by obsessive thoughts that are cancelled

out by symbolic acts or rituals to reduce anxiety. Although the behavior may be self-destructive, it is an attempt to control irrational thinking and feared impulses. This behavior does not involve an attempt to explain or justify it cognitively (intellectualization). P/A, AN, PC

45. no. 1. Obsessive-compulsive clients are assessed for the ritualistic behavior, possible sources of conflict in life situations, the degree to which the ritual or repetitive behavior interferes with activities of daily living, and potential unresolved conflicts. Assessment of thought patterns, associations, and delusions would be important if the nurse believed the client to be psychotic. Options no. 3 and no. 4 must, always be assessed, but in determining whether or not the client has an obsessive-compulsive disorder, the nurse must first determine the client's specific daily actions. P/A, AS, PC

46. no. 4. It is necessary to reestablish and maintain physiological integrity while working on the long-range goal of decreasing the washing behavior. If this is not focused on initially, infection could result. Option no. 1 is a higher level of functioning. Once the client has stabilized physically (or concurrently), it is helpful to begin working on the problem behavior. Expression of feeling is important, but understanding the causes may not be the equivalent of changing the behavior. Determining the "why" may or may not be a useful short-term goal. P/A, PL, E

47. no. 2. Plan sufficient time for her to perform necessary rituals early in her treatment; to prohibit or strictly limit this behavior would induce extreme anxiety, as would strict limit setting. Confrontation of irrationality may induce further defense of it. This particular compulsion seems to be accompanied by near-delusional thoughts of offending others. P/A, PL, E

48. no. 2. In dealing with ritualistic behavior, the nurse must help the client by setting limits on the destructive, repetitive behavior. Allow the client to carry out the behavior to some degree, but not to the point of injury. The client also should be presented with reality in a matter-of-fact manner. Her primary problem does not seem to involve assertive behavior. Medication may be ordered to help the client with uncontrollable anxiety. P/A, PL, PC

49. no. 3. This allows some participation in a unit activity as tolerated by the client. Option no. 1 would be an overreaction by the nurse and is inappropriate. Moving the TV does not address the problem, encourages isolation, and elicits a reaction from others in the unit. Option no. 4 would likely result in the client becoming more anxious. P/A, IM, PC

50. no. 3. Providing Maria with a schedule will slowly help limit her ritualistic behaviors, but it should not be expected to prevent them altogether. The remaining actions would all be helpful. P/A, IM, PC

51. no. 4. Although new medications to treat this disorder may be approved soon, these behaviors are known to be very resistant to treatment. Nursing care plans can aim at modifying or limiting ritualistic behaviors rather than attempting to eliminate them altogether. The obsessive-compulsive disorder is not a psychosis. Options no. 2 and no. 3 may be true, but initially the behavior must be controlled because of the physical threat. P/A, EV, PC

52. no. 1. To evaluate nursing care for the obsessive-compulsive client, first look for a decrease in the ritualistic behavior and resumption of activities of daily living, such as personal care. Thought process regarding her obsessive beliefs and self-reports of reduced anxiety will also need to be evaluated. P/A, EV, PC

53. no. 1. Obsessive-compulsive clients usually recognize the behavior is senseless and receive no pleasure from the activity. Anxiety and tension are only temporarily reduced. Option no. 2 indicates some beginning insight. Options no. 3 and no. 4 indicate no insight on the part of the client. P/A, AS, H

54. no. 4. Bradycardia (not tachycardia) is characteristic with weight loss. Amenorrhea is a common finding. Delayed psychosexual development related to earlier unresolved issues of separation and individualization is frequently seen. There may be a family pattern reflecting a facade of happiness and harmony, which covers underlying conflict and dysfunction among the family members. P/A, AS, PC

55. no. 3. These clients are not concerned with conserving energy; rather they typically exercise frequently in order to expend the number of calories equal to the amount they estimate are consumed. Options no. 1, no. 2, and no. 4 are all commonly manifested behaviors in clients experiencing anorexia nervosa who demonstrate an intense interest in food and the relentless pursuit of perceived thinness. P/A, AS, PC

56. no. 3. These clients are often in life-threatening electrolyte and nutritional imbalance. Death rates of up to 20%-30% among diagnosed cases have been cited in the literature. Options no. 1, no. 2, and no. 4 are all important to implement after physiological integrity is established. P/A, IM, PS

57. no. 4. It is important to keep an anorexic client within view of the staff for at least 1 hour after

meals to discourage induction of vomiting. Options no. 1 and no. 3 promote some positive control and independence, which the client needs instead of starving herself to gain control. Providing support and reinforcement allays anxiety and increases compliance. P/A, IM, E

58. no. 3. Althought much is still unknown about this disorder, the anorexic denies, suppresses, and represses stomach hunger. Thus, she may ignore feelings of hunger. Hypothalamic and physiological functions may be normal. P/A, AN, PC

59. no. 2. A desired response is followed by a desired or positive consequence. Option no. 1 is the presentation of an aversive stimulus immediately following an undesired response. Option no. 3 occurs when the removal of a stimulus strengthens the tendency to behave in a certain way. Option no. 4 is the process of transferring learning from one situation to other similar situations. P/A, IM, PC

60. no. 3. Involvement in preparation and management of the treatment plan will help the client gain control and mastery and practice self-responsibility. Threats create a power struggle that reenacts old, familiar, and pathological family patterns. Option no. 2 can be life threatening, since about 15% of anorexic clients die from starvation. Option no. 4 is not helpful because the core issue is control and distorted self-image, not good eating habits. Indeed, the client may be very knowledgeable about nutrition. P/A, IM, PC

61. no. 3. Clients with anorexia nervosa see themselves as overweight regardless of how thin they are. Even when they look in the mirror, they see themselves as fat. The most appropriate nursing response is to tell them how the nurse sees their size in a factual way without judgments or statements that may decrease their self-esteem. P/A, IM, PC

62. no. 1. Hypochondriasis is an exaggerated concern with one's physical health although no organic pathological condition (psychosomatic illness) and no subjective loss of function (conversion disorder) exists. Other dissociative reactions are a mechanism for minimizing or avoiding anxiety by keeping parts of the individual's experience out of conscious awareness (e.g., amnesia, fugue state, multiple personality). He is not malingering, because he holds a responsible job despite his complaints. P/A, AN, PC

63. no. 4. These clients tend to react with increased anxiety and symptoms to new and different situations. Clear and concise explanations of treatments and procedures help to allay the anxiety. The focus for intervention should not be the symptom (i.e., pain) but the precipitating event (i.e., group interaction). Option no. 2 fosters avoidance of the pos-

sible stressor(s) and encourages reliance on others to relieve the symptom (pain). Option no. 3 avoids any interaction by exerting authoritative control and sets up a possible power struggle. P/A, IM, PC

64. no. 3. Hallucinations, delusions, and mania would be treated with antipsychotic medication, not diazepam. P/A, IM, H

65. no. 4. The first three options are true for diazepam (Valium). Valium and alcohol are both CNS depressants; the combination could severely depress the CNS. Valium can cause possible interactions/toxicity when taken with other medications. P/A, IM, PS

66. no. 2. As Mrs. Manchester deals with her feelings of guilt, anger, and fear, she will begin to remember the rest of the painful event. Allow her time to remember without probing. Asking questions might help the client recall additional details of the story, but it might also increase her anxiety and contribute to a sense of being overwhelmed by the situation. It is common for clients experiencing post-traumatic stress disorder to have lapses in memory regarding details that are too painful to remember. Telling the client that she is withholding information may only add to her sense of frustration, anxiety, and guilt. P/A, IM, PC

67. no. 1. For those with post-traumatic stress disorder, the pain of surviving and the accompanying guilt often lead to their wish that they, too, had died. For many survivors, the situation can compound their guilt if they feel they should have been at the scene of the trauma or were there but survived when others did not. The client's feelings are those normally expressed in this type of situation. Option no. 3 does not convey a sense of acceptance of the feelings and only adds more guilt. It is always important for the nurse to assess risk of suicide; however, option no. 4 is not sensitive to the client's feelings of guilt at that moment. P/A, IM, PC

68. no. 4. Support groups of people who have suffered similarly can be very helpful in teaching clients how to deal with the situation. They can also provide a forum where the client can express feelings shared by others in an accepting atmosphere. It might be helpful for the client to join Parents Without Partners after the crisis period in order to develop a support network for the future. An out-of-town trip might add to her sense of guilt about having left her children alone when the accident occurred. While planning weekly outings with her children might be helpful, the activities chosen should be more appropriate for their age group. P/A, IM, H

69. no. 2. Crisis intervention, a form of secondary prevention, seeks to prevent psychiatric disorders through early intervention in order to allow the client to regain equilibrium. Primary prevention seeks to prevent psychiatric disorders through community education and special programs targeting high-risk groups. Tertiary prevention is aimed at reducing the long-term impact resulting from psychiatric disorders and includes rehabilitation programs. Early diagnostic care is only *one* component of secondary prevention. P/A, PL, H

70. no. 2. Knowledge of past occupations, hobbies, etc., will help keep interactions based upon reality. Present medical conditions and past methods of coping with stress are more immediately useful in planning nursing care than are prior medical history and stressors. Family history would be important later in assessing previous episodes of this disorder and how they were handled. P/C, AS, PC

71. no. 4. The etiology of Alzheimer's disease is currently unknown. Blood tests confirming the disorder are under investigation. Currently, it can only be truly diagnosed by an autopsy. Options no. 1, no. 2, and no. 3 are true of Alzheimer's disease because decreased immunity or a virus attacks the tissue of the cerebral cortex, causing progressive deterioration of intellectual functioning and behavior. P/C, AN, PC

72. no. 4. Realization that memory loss is occurring often causes anxiety and depression in these clients. The first three options will help the client remain oriented to time, person, and place and maintain self-esteem for as long as possible. P/C, IM, PC

73. no. 3. Her picture and name on the door draw upon long-term memory, which is more likely to remain intact. Mrs. Cohen would have a difficult time remembering the light-blue door because of short-term memory loss. Assigning her a buddy or placing her close to the nurses' station will reinforce her feelings of dependency and loss of control. P/C, IM, E

74. no. 3. Serving smaller amounts of food at more frequent intervals will increase the probability of an adequate intake, as well as preserve the dignity of the client. A full liquid diet would not be palatable and would decrease her appetite. Feeding Mrs. Cohen would decrease her self-worth because of being forced to be in an unnecessarily dependent position. Serving food whenever Mrs. Cohen is ready could lead to an unbalanced diet; it is difficult to monitor the type of food and amount eaten. P/C, IM, PS

75. no. 3. This response indicates a willingness to offer support and to allow Mr. Cohen to ventilate his feelings at a difficult time. Alzheimer's disease is a degenerating illness, and she will progressively worsen. Option no. 2 is poorly timed. Mr. Cohen has not come to terms with this alternative solution.

No. 4 reflects denial on the nurse's part. Alzheimer's disease clients require demanding around-the-clock care, which may be too difficult for an elderly person. P/C, IM, H

76. no. 3. The client with major depression has low self-esteem, feelings of worthlessness, and very little physical energy. A structured, positive experience will help to increase self-esteem. Setting up too many tasks will overwhelm him. Introducing Mr. Jones to other people will make him feel more self-conscious. Staying away will reinforce the withdrawal and low self-esteem. Having him express himself freely is inappropriate in occupational therapy. P/E, IM, H

77. no. 4. Options no. 1, no. 2, and no. 3 are all side effects of nortriptyline, a tricyclic antidepressant. Major tranquilizers most often have this side effect. P/E, AN, PS

78. no. 1. The depressed client is likely to demonstrate anger, withdrawal, or hostility at times. The other options are seen in mania. P/E, AS, PC

79. no. 3. Refusal may be seen as rejection of the client. Focus on the client's needs. It is important to find out which changes the client wants to make. Depressed clients are more likely to make suicidal attempts. The nurse monitors the blood levels of the antidepressant because they have a critical therapeutic window effect, meaning that at a certain range in the blood they are most effective. P/E, IM, E

80. no. 2. The severely depressed client can best understand simple information, given slowly and directly. The presence of the nurse will be comforting to him in new surroundings. Introducing him to everyone and asking him to perform too many activities will be overwhelming. Placing him next to a talkative client would be a mismatch that would exaggerate Mr. Chung's quietness. P/E, IM, E

81. no. 1. The depressed client may have hostile, angry, and primitive internal introjections. Projection is a defense mechanism used in character disorders and by paranoid individuals. Suppression and repression are common defense mechanisms used in neurotic disorders. P/E, AS, PC

82. no. 4. The perception that something or someone meaningful has been lost is the most important contributing factor in depression. Hormonal imbalance is related to postpartum depression. Sexual identity problems are related to either adolescent adjustment problems or homosexuality. Character disorders such as sociopathy, where problems with authority figures exist, result from unresolved parental conflict. P/E, AN, PC

83. no. 2. A regular schedule provides structure and removes the burden of making decisions from the depressed client. Giving him only one activity a

day will reinforce his feelings of inadequacy and withdrawal. A depressed client's thinking processes are too slowed to allow him to choose activities or take the initiative in participating. He is in the hospital for the structure he could not provide for himself. P/E, IM, E

84. no. 1. Nonverbal communication may be necessary with a severely depressed client. The presence of the nurse indicates to him that he is regarded as a worthwhile person. Option no. 2 assumes that he is self-destructive. At this point, Mr. Chung lacks the energy to hurt himself. Option no. 3 is a judgmental response. The nurse needs to accept his discomfort and not place demands on Mr. Chung when he does not feel comfortable around others. P/E, IM, PC

85. no. 1. A tricyclic antidepressant is used first, because there are fewer restrictions with this class of drugs. The dosage for imipramine may initially be lower and increased gradually. Amitriptyline has sedative side effects, and the dose stated is too high for initial administration. The MAO inhibitors, isocarboxazid and phenelzine sulfate, are generally contraindicated in the elderly and would be used only if the tricyclic antidepressants did not work. P/E, IM, PS

86. no. 4. When depression is severe, the client has insufficient energy to plan and execute a suicide attempt. When improvement begins, the risk of suicide is the greatest. If he is ready to go home, he is not suicidal. When his family goes on vacation, he might feel more depressed because he is being left behind, but would not necessarily become suicidal. P/E, AN, E

87. no. 2. Keeping the suicidal client under constant, close observation is mandatory protection from self-inflicted harm. Tranquilizers are contraindicated while taking antidepressants and will not eliminate the suicidal ideation. Suicidal feelings should be talked about and worked through until the internalized feelings of hostility are resolved. Other clients could be helpful in monitoring a suicidal client's behavior by lending support and increasing concern regarding the client's whereabouts. P/E, PL, E

88. no. 3. The nurse is demonstrating a positive attitude toward the client, reality orientation, and respect for the client's participation in his treatment. The nurse offers self and an opportunity to clarify and ventilate concerns. Mr. Chung demonstrates anxiety about the unknown, and option no. 1 does not address the unknown aspects of the ECT procedure and negates his anxiety. It is true that Mr. Chung does not have to go, but at his age of 60 years, ECT might be safer than MAO inhibitors in helping him overcome his depression. P/E, IM, E

89. no. 3. The most common ECT side effects are confusion and memory loss for recent events. It is reassuring to the client to know that this is a temporary condition. Headaches and dizziness are common side effects of MAO inhibitors. Nausea and vomiting are common side effects of many drugs. Diarrhea and gastrointestinal distress are common side effects of lithium carbonate. P/E, AS, PS

90. no. 4. All of these drugs may be used for the safest and most effective administration of ECT. ECT causes seizures, so a muscle relaxant is given to prevent fractures. An anesthetic is used to reduce sensations of the seizure. Atropine sulfate is used to decrease secretions and to relax smooth muscles. P/E, IM, PS

91. no. 4. Group members provide feedback for each other through a variety of responses and reactions. This improves insight and self-knowledge. Group therapy's aim is not to increase socialization skills, because the focus is to work on one's own problems. Improved reality orientation is done through the use of calendars, clocks, and name tags. Universality, or the feeling that other people have the same problem, does provide comfort that one is not alone, but does not provide insight into the nature of depression. P/E, EV, H

92. no. 2. Currently, the most frequent use of electroconvulsive therapy (ECT) is to treat severe depression that has not responded to medication or psychotherapy. Following ECT, the client often becomes more accessible to psychotherapy. A shortened hospital stay is a benefit of ECT, but not the chief benefit. After the client has had some psychotherapy, the length of hospitalization may be shortened, but follow-up care is usually required. ECT does not necessarily lessen the need for medication. P/E, PL, PC

93. no. 4. Ordinarily, hospital policies and procedures require that the physician administer the shock to the client. Some of the nurse's responsibilities during ECT are cited in options no. 1 through no. 3. P/E, IM, E

94. no. 2. Immediately following ECT, the client is given the same nursing care as that of any unconscious client. The client will experience drowsiness and confusion upon awakening. Orienting the client will decrease anxiety or fears. There is no reason for the client to remain in bed after vital signs have stabilized. Resumption of normal activity on the unit by the client soon after treatment places ECT in its proper perspective as one of a number of therapeutic modalities. P/E, IM, PS

95. no. 3. Mrs. Bell exhibits behaviors or symptoms that are considered at high risk for suicide: severe depression, history of suicidal ideation, hopeless-

ness, anger at hospitalization, and a suicidal plan. Her age, sex, and divorced and unemployed status also place her at high risk. P/E, AN, PC

96. no. 4. The elderly, adolescents, alcoholics, and drug abusers are statistically high-risk groups for suicidal behavior; people in their 30s are not. P/E, AS, PC

97. no. 4. Suicidal clients often have problems talking about painful feelings; they need encouragement to express their feelings and concerns about suicide and hopelessness. Options no. 1, no. 2, and no. 3 are the responsibilities of a nurse when caring for a client with high risk of suicide. P/E, IM, E

98. no. 2. The DSM-III-R classifies depression as an affective disorder. Somatoform disorders are conditions characterized by complaints of physical distress. Anxiety disorders are conditions characterized by feelings of fear and symptoms such as palpitations, tachycardia, and tremors. Personality disorders are conditions characterized by longstanding problems with relationships and acting out behaviors. P/E, AN, PC

99. no. 1. A mild depression is primarily affective in nature (sadness, dejection, discouragement), while severe depression includes severe affective signs as well as a decrease in activity, thought patterns, communication, and socialization, and an increase in somatic symptoms and vegetative signs. Suicidal ideation can be associated with any level of depression. Duration of symptoms and age do not indicate severity, and mild depression can be lengthy. P/E, AS, E

100. no. 3. Napping in the daytime encourages increased withdrawal from social activity and also prevents the client from being tired enough to sleep through the night. Encouraging discussion of feelings and concerns will reduce anxiety associated with lack of sleep. Option no. 2 will engage client in participating in self-care. Option no. 4 provides structure and normalization of routine for the client. P/E, PL, E

101. no. 4. Helping the client establish bedtime routines to promote rest and sleep will be a learning situation to practice in the hospital and to use at home; success builds hope and self-esteem. It would not be therapeutic to ignore sleep patterns and complaints because that discounts a client's concerns. Reassurance is rarely therapeutic. Option no. 3 would defeat the goal of normalization of sleep patterns. P/E, IM, PS

102. no. 1. Tofranil is a tricyclic antidepressant. P/E, IM, PS

103. no. 1. Tofranil causes urinary retention rather than urinary frequency. It may produce dry mouth, not increased salivation. Tofranil cannot be taken on an as-needed basis since it requires a blood con-

centration to be effective, which takes 2-4 weeks to establish itself. P/E, IM, H

104. no. 4. This option is a closed-ended, judgmental question and is not appropriate. The remaining options all help the nurse to establish a useful data base. P/E, AS, PC

105. no. 4. Denying feelings and complaints would not be helpful. Sharing painful feelings is vital in learning to cope with them. P/E, PL, E

106. no. 1. Focusing on the positive aspects of life has merit but is the least effective of the four actions given to meet the stated goal. Options no. 2 and no. 3 are basic to the nurse-client relationship no matter what the client problems may be. They are considered to be effective in helping clients to cope. Option no. 4 is an effective method of providing alternatives, which assists in coping and decision-making. P/E, IM, PC

107. no. 1. This action allows Mrs. Bell to maintain control and self-direction in her life and yet focus on concerns of discharge. Options no. 2 and no. 4 work against the nurse-client relationship and undermine the client's control over her life. Option no. 3 fosters denial of the problem areas of her life and does not accomplish therapeutic goals. P/E, IM, H

108. no. 2. Rumination can be mild to severe. It can be found in obsessive, depressive, and psychotic disorders. Telling a client to stop does little good. Introducing communication that expands her narrow frame of reference will enhance interaction and redirect her thinking. Providing opportunities for activity and exercise will provide structure, redirection, and broaden the use of energy for clients who ruminate. Option no. 4 enhances self-awareness and self-esteem. P/E, IM, PC

109. no. 4. Angry outbursts are a positive behavior for depressed clients and should never be ignored. Options no. 1, no. 2, and no. 3 are all appropriate communication techniques and strategies for working with all clients. P/E, IM, H

110. no. 3. Most individuals who are intent on suicide still wish very much to be rescued. The fact that Mrs. King tried to eliminate the possibility of rescue indicates the seriousness of the attempt and should alert the staff to the possibility of another attempt. A client may be unconscious as a result of a suicide gesture that was not intended to be serious. Many clients who are not serious use a potentially lethal method and kill themselves accidentally. Not leaving a suicide note may indicate nonintent; however, it may also indicate impulsive and serious intent. P/E, AS, PC

111. no. 2. The client's response does not indicate remorsefulness about the suicide attempt, but disappointment at her ineffectiveness in carrying it out successfully. She is depressed and feeling hopeless, so the potential for another suicide attempt is great. As with most suicidal people, she is probably ambivalent about whether she wants to live or die. P/E, AN, E

112. no. 1. Although all the options are appropriate, the first priority is to protect the client from suicidal gestures. Options no. 2 and no. 3 are correct actions; however, they are not the highest priority when dealing with a high-potential suicide risk. Option no. 4 is of a higher priority and would be implemented as soon as the safety needs addressed in option no. 1 were accomplished. P/E, IM, E

113. no. 3. Any change in behavior may mean that the client has worked out a suicide plan. The apparent lifting of her depression may mean that Mrs. King now has the energy to carry out her plan. While any client's first weekend at home is stressful, for this client and her history, a weekend pass at this time is contraindicated, premature, and potentially dangerous. Depressed clients may have mood swings; however, the abruptness of this client's change and her request for a weekend pass must be explored and considered cautiously. P/E, AN, PC

114. no. 1. In treating low self-esteem, it is important to begin by giving clients minimal tasks that they can accomplish without failure. All the other suggestions contain the possibility of failure or are too stressful when the client is feeling helpless, or both. P/E, IM, H

115. no. 3. These clients need the security of being allowed to build a trusting relationship with a staff member. Dependence on the staff can more appropriately be dealt with by firm limit setting and encouragement to be more independent. Providing only the help needed and encouraging problem-solving would foster independence on the part of the client. Option no. 4 is an early attempt to reduce dependent behavior. P/E, IM, PC

116. no. 3. Anxiousness, hopelessness, somatic complaints, depressions, suicidal behavior, and a sense of loss are symptoms of involutional states classified as psychotic depression. Middle age, a life centered on family and home, and children leaving the "nest" are other clues. Paranoid schizophrenia is characterized by a concrete and pervasive delusional system that is generally persecutory. No data are presented to suggest a history of mood swings, manic behavior, or substance abuse. P/E, AN, PC

117. no. 2. This client has already attempted suicide. Observation and protective measures should be instituted immediately. Although food intake is a concern with clients expressing depression, it is not the most important nursing action listed. Data sug-

gest that this client has already exhibited a high involvement with her family. The nursing intervention strategies would best address diversifying her interests at this time. Reassurance is rarely therapeutic. Based on the data presented, it would be presumptive to indicate that physical complaints are unwarranted. P/E, IM, E

118. no. 3. During times of deepest depression, the client lacks the energy to plan and carry out a suicide attempt. When depression lessens, the client has energy to act on self-destructive thoughts and impulses. P/E, AS, PC

119. no. 4. Serious drug interactions occur when MAO inhibitors are given in combination with tricyclic antidepressants, narcotics, alcohol, anticholinergics, antidiabetic agents, barbiturates, reserpine, sympathomimetics, and dibenzepin derivatives. Option no. 1 is incorrect, since these drugs are slower to act than other antidepressants. While tachycardia may sometimes occur, the most common side effect of MAO inhibitors is hypertensive crisis. MAO inhibitors do not increase appetite; in fact, they may cause nausea and vomiting. Specific, important dietary restrictions are required when taking them. Client warnings and instructions must be provided, preferably in writing. P/E, AS, PS

120. no. 3. This comment by the nurse acknowledges the client's fear. Staying with the client also tends to allay anxiety. To tell the client who expresses fear to not be afraid discourages expression of the feelings. Options no. 2 and no. 4 are incorrect because they minimize the importance of these feelings. P/E, IM, E

121. no. 4. Their agitation causes these clients to be hyperactive, and they usually have difficulty getting sufficient sleep. Agitated depression is characterized by psychomotor restlessness, pacing, and handwringing. P/E, AS, PC

122. no. 1. Amitriptyline (Elavil) is a tricyclic antidepressant. Although the monoamine oxidase inhibitors (MAOI) are also antidepressants, the MAOI mode of action is distinctly different from the tricyclic antidepressants. Phenothiazines are antipsychotic medications. Antihistamines have sedative effects and may combat the side effects of the antipsychotic medications. P/E, AN, PS

123. no. 3. Dry mouth, constipation, and blurred vision are anticholinergic responses, indicative of side effects upon the autonomic nervous system. Cardiovascular and endocrine system side effects such as dysrhythmias and impotence can occur with amitriptyline (Elavil) but are not mentioned in this question. Respiratory system reactions are uncommon. P/E, AN, PS

124. no. 3. This is a major reason for noncompliance with tricyclic antidepressants. Symptomatic relief

does not usually occur until after 2 to 4 weeks of therapy, and clients often become noncompliant unless instructed about this time lag. Three days is an insufficient time to judge clinical effectiveness. Twenty-five milligrams TID is a therapeutic dose of amitriptyline (Elavil). P/E, AN, PS

125. no. 2. The side effects of tricyclic antidepressant medications are most apparent during initiation of treatment and diminish as therapy progresses. Drug therapy requires regularity of administration for effectiveness. Although the client may discuss the side effects with her physician, it also is appropriate for the nurse to discuss them. It is nontherapeutic to threaten clients with electroconvulsive therapy. P/E, IM, H

126. no. 3. This indicates to the client that her distress was heard and permits exploration of feelings she is experiencing now. The second option asks for an explanation that the client is probably unable to give. The first option may make the client feel the nurse is minimizing or unaware of her feelings. The client with a major depression will not feel better about herself within a few days. P/E, IM, PC

127. no. 2. One theory regarding the etiology of major depressive episodes is that symptoms reflect the individual's response to a severe threat to security (a loss). The loss may be real or imagined and is perceived by an individual, such as Mrs. Perkins, as a threat to her very being. A psychotic depression is not a normal response regardless of the severity of the precipitating stress. The incident described is a situational, not maturational, crisis. Major depressions may last for a long time and require hospitalization. P/E, AN, PC

128. no. 3. Focusing on making small decisions such as "Do you want to wear the blue blouse or red blouse?" is a first step in building self-esteem. The client may be unable to make decisions at this time and will need assistance. Explaining the importance of decision making is premature and likely to make her feel worse. Making all decisions for her will keep the client regressed and dependent. P/E, IM, H

129. no. 3. Short, frequent contacts, as tolerated, will assist in establishing the nurse-client relationship. Once this is accomplished, the client can be encouraged to participate in activities on the unit. Depressed clients need human contact. Aloneness will cause further alterations in the client's thought processes. However, she may be unable to attend activities yet. Explanations about the therapeutic value of activities are not a motivator for the depressed person. P/E, IM, PC

130. no. 1. The preparation is basically the same as for any procedure in which a general anesthetic is used,

since electroconvulsive therapy (ECT) produces a loss of consciousness. Include all measures (e.g., NPO, removal of dentures) necessary to preserve the safety of the client. There is continuing controversy about the use of ECT, and many myths about it persist. Clients who have not responded to adequate trials of antidepressant medication may experience a reduction of symptoms following ECT. Short-term side effects of ECT are confusion, transient memory loss, and headache. P/E, AN, E

131. no. 4. The human contact provided by remaining with the client and conversing with her at her level of readiness will help to lighten the anxiety she is feeling. Valium and deep breathing lessen anxiety, but more important is the client's need to express her fears and to be given proper reassurance by the nurse. Mrs. Perkins must not eat or drink because an anesthetic will be administered. P/E, IM, E

132. no. 4. Prompt reorientation lessens the anxiety generated by the confusion. Some degree of confusion may persist during the day; however, observations by staff can take place in the day-room. The client will remain in bed or on a stretcher until she is oriented, her vital signs stabilize, and she can safely join ward activities. There are no data to indicate the need for a physician. P/E, IM, PS

133. no. 2. The working phase is characterized by the client's confronting problems and learning alternative methods of coping and problem solving. The initiating phase also may be called the orienting phase. In the terminating phase, the client and nurse summarize and evaluate the work of the relationship and express feelings and thoughts about termination. P/E, AN, E

134. no. 2. The first priority with any depressed client is to ensure safety because of a high risk of suicide. Promoting self-esteem, reducing cognitive distortion, and presenting reality consistently to the client are very important, but safety is the highest priority. P/E, PL, E

135. no. 2. Encourage the client to express feelings in a realistic manner. Do not accept irrational statements. Do not argue with her, imply her beliefs are true, or dismiss her. The client will become more tenacious in holding on to this delusion if the nurse tries to argue her out of it. Option no. 3 implies that the client's delusion is true. Option no. 4 evades the issue and dismisses the client's concern. P/E, IM, PC

136. no. 4. Before electroconvulsive therapy, give the client accurate information in a way that does not increase anxiety. Options no. 1, no. 2, and no. 3 are accurate but raise the client's anxiety by failing to provide any reassurance. P/E, IM, E

137. no. 2. It is normal for the client to fall asleep, and she does not need to be disturbed. There is no

reason to wake the client, give a stimulant, or call the physician. P/E, IM, E

138. no. 4. Assist the client in doing activities of daily living until she is able to do them on her own. Depressed clients have psychomotor retardation and need help in mobilizing themselves. It may be beyond Mrs. Moskovitz's control to be punctual every day. ECT clients should be integrated into the unit routines and milieu as soon as possible to obtain maximum benefit. P/E, IM, PS

139. no. 1. Acknowledge the client's feelings without implying that they are true or shared by the nurse. The depressed client cannot alter her way of thinking at this point in treatment. Mrs. Moskovitz may feel devalued and unimportant by options no. 3 and no. 4. P/E, IM, PC

140. no. 1. When a client shows a change in behavior, the nurse should assess the behavior to understand the nature of the change and how to respond. Such a change might imply suicidal intent, but this cannot be determined without further questioning. There is insufficient data to warrant suicide precautions, increased participation in ward activities, or to suggest denial of her depression. P/E, IM, PC

141. no. 4. Expressions of guilt often conceal unexpressed resentment and anger. The client needs to have the opportunity to identify and verbalize such feelings. Option no. 1 focuses on the children rather than the client. Options no. 2 and no. 3 make a universal conclusion about parenting and give false reassurance. P/E, IM, PC

142. no. 1. Using reflection helps to identify feelings and gives the client the opportunity to express them directly. Options no. 2 and no. 4 may be perceived by Mrs. Moskovitz as punitive or as reprimands. The nurse should first help the client identify and deal with her feelings before focusing on dealing with separation and the transition. P/E, IM, PC

143. no. 4. The first three options are all correct. A pure medical-biological model does not address social and environmental conditions. However, some physicians may consider that these conditions have some influence on the illness. The medical-biological model assumes mental illnesses are disease entities. A disease can be classified, diagnosed, and labeled, and is within the purview of the physician. P/E, AN, PC

144. no. 4. Manic behavior in manic-depressive illness (bipolar disorder) is the result of denial of underlying depression. The client copes with these feelings by demonstrating excessive activity. The other defense mechanisms listed, such as repression, suppression, and displacement, may also be used; but no. 4 is most characteristic of manic-depression. P/E, AN, PC

145. no. 4. The presence of the nurse may facilitate client adjustment to new surroundings and personnel. A decrease in environmental stimulation is necessary for its calming effect. The overactivity of Mrs. Brooks should not be rewarded, because these clients are prone to self-injury and burnout. Involving the client in activities and introducing her to new people will increase her psychomotor activity. P/E, IM, PC

146. no. 1. A short attention span is characteristic of manic behavior, and she would be unable to manage activities requiring extended concentration. Decreasing stimulation, channeling energy, and using distraction techniques are calming and therapeutic for manic clients. P/E, IM, PC

147. no. 1. The therapeutic blood-level range of lithium is 0.5 to 1.2-1.5 mEq/L. Lithium levels are not measured in mg/ml, but rather in mEq/L. P/E, AS, PS

148. no. 4. The therapeutic level and toxic level of lithium are so close that blood levels must be monitored carefully. The therapeutic level is 0.5 to 1.2-1.5 mEq/L. Above 1.5 mEq/L, significant side effects occur. The toxicity level is 2.0 to 3.0 mEq/L. Options no. 1, no. 2, and no. 3 are not the reasons for determining lithium levels. P/E, AN, PS

149. no. 4. These are symptoms of mild lithium toxicity. Options no. 1, no. 2, and no. 3 are not characteristic of lithium toxicity. P/E, AS, PS

150. no. 2. Once the therapeutic blood level is achieved, it should be monitored at least monthly for outpatients. The prognosis for manic-depressive episode is good, so Mrs. Brooks probably does not need anyone to stay with her. Genetic research studies suggest there is a dominant X-linked factor present for the transmission of manic-depressive illness. This factor is thought to occur in families in which one or more members have had manic as well as depressive episodes. However, the couple decides whether or not to have children. Tranquilizers are not indicated. P/E, IM, H

151. no. 1. Vomiting and diarrhea may be signs of lithium toxicity or may be due to other causes. Loss of fluid will increase the concentration of medicine in the blood and may produce toxicity. Dryness of the mouth, although a side effect of lithium, is not serious. Swollen lymph nodes and upper respiratory symptoms would be associated with a health problem (e.g., infection) rather than with lithium toxicity. P/E, EV, H

152. no. 4. There is thought to be a genetic component to manic-depressive illness. Manic-depressive illness is a biochemical imbalance and is not related to childhood illnesses. There is no relationship to the abuse of alcohol during adolescence and the onset of manic-depressive illness in adulthood.

Having parents divorce during one's childhood might contribute to an unresolved grief reaction leading to chronic depression. However, this past history is usually not the cause of manic excitement. P/E, AS, PC

153. no. 4. Clang associations occur in schizophrenia, not in manic-depressive disorders. Vegetative behavior is seen during the depressive phase of manic-depressive illness. Hypomanic behavior is seen during the acute manic phase of manic-depressive illness. A thought disorder is present during mania and depression and usually consists of morbid self-blame. P/E, AS, PC

154. no. 4. The mania seen in such clients is thought to be an attempt to ward off an underlying depression. These clients characteristically sleep very little during a manic episode. The other options describe manifestations of hyperactivity, confused thinking, aggressiveness, and poor judgment that are characteristic of manic behavior. P/E, AS, PC

155. no. 2. Providing empathy and indicating to the son that his actions will help his father are indicated. It would not be beneficial to the son to hear that his father is worse than anyone else the staff has dealt with or implying that he is not capable of caring for his father. Interpreting the father's behavior will not help at this point. Option no. 3 assumes that the son is embarrassed by his father's illness. P/E, IM, H

156. no. 3. Although Mr. Peters may be overly talkative, and irritable and may have a short attention span, his remark specifically typifies the delusion of grandeur that is a disorder of thought. P/E, AN, PC

157. no. 3. Administer the upcoming dose, since the normal serum-level range is 0.5 to 1.2-1.5 mEq/L. The nurse would ask for the test to be repeated or withhold the next dose if the client showed signs of toxicity. If pressured speech were still present, the nurse would record the observation and inform the physician. P/E, IM, PS

158. no. 3. With insufficient sodium, lithium is retained and the client becomes toxic. The body needs sodium in order to excrete lithium. Insufficient fat and carbohydrates will lead to weight reduction, and eventually the dosage may need to be readjusted; but these foods are not critical to the proper absorption and elimination of lithium. Potassium is necessary when taking diuretics, and iron is important when anemia exists. Proteins are critical when damaged tissue is present. P/E, AN, PS

159. no. 1. Kidney damage does occur in association with lithium treatment in some clients. If the client already has a problem of this type, it is more appropriate to try other medication before using lithium. Lithium may be helpful in controlling suicidal urges when the client is coming out of the depres-

sion. Physically active clients should be advised to watch fluid and sodium intake. Lithium is known to decrease the amount of circulating thyroid hormones. P/E, AS, PS

160. no. 2. Manic clients are very disruptive, usually hyperirritable, and often very hostile to other clients. Mr. Peters may or may not need restraints or seclusion on admission, but throughout his hospitalization, he needs an atmosphere of decreased stimuli, which is best achieved in a private room. In addition, client rights necessitate as unrestrictive an atmosphere as possible. Therefore, seclusion and restraints are not used unless absolutely necessary. P/E, IM, E

161. no. 3. Having the client speak more slowly may help him to focus and identify some of his difficulties. Having him verbalize his feelings will only increase his anger and his mania. Insight into the nature of his illness will not be absorbed because he is not able to hear too many details at this point. Therefore, he needs to have support rather than insight. P/E, IM, PC

162. no. 1. Competitive games are stimulating and escalate aggression; therefore, physical exercise of a noncompetitive nature is the more constructive way to aid the client to discharge aggressive and angry feelings. Reduction of stimuli and ventilation of feelings are also therapeutic interventions for the client during the manic phase. P/E, IM, E

163. no. 1. Recognizing signs and symptoms of escalating, excited behavior will enable the client and his son to seek early treatment of a recurrent episode of mania. By making most major decisions, the son would increase his father's feelings of worthlessness. Option no. 2 has been the client's pattern anyway, especially during a hypomanic state; he needs to learn assertive behavior. Teaching the family about possible side effects of lithium is important, but if the client can recognize symptomatology of hypomanic behavior, he can inform the doctor that the medication can be increased. P/E, PL, H

164. no. 3. This kind of behavior is apt to be seen on admission, not discharge. In order for a client to be deemed ready for discharge, he must be able to perform activities of daily living. Options no. 2 and no. 3 indicate that he has changed his behavioral pattern of aggressiveness to one of assertiveness, and that the client believes in himself and feels worthy of asking for his needs directly. P/E, EV, PS

165. no. 3. Although at some point options no. 1, no. 2, and no. 4 must be assessed, the most important initial determination is the degree of compliance with the medication regimen. P/E, AS, PC

166. no. 2. Overactivity in motor behavior, speech, and thought patterns is characteristic of manic-depressive, manic-phase clients. Mr. White is not psychotic. He does have distortions of reality, but no associative looseness, delusions, hallucinations, or inappropriate affect. P/E, AS, PC

167. no. 1. Thought processes of the hypomanic client move rapidly. Focusing on inappropriate language only prolongs it. Mr. White is unable to grasp the meaning of his behavior at this time or to control it even when threatened or ordered to stop. Seclusion is a drastic measure for abusive language and not helpful in reducing its occurrence. P/E, IM, PC

168. no. 3. Hyperactivity is a behavior seen in the manic client. Option no. 1 indicates a psychotic depression with guilty delusions. Option no. 2 would be typical behavior of a paranoid schizophrenic and no. 4 is a possibility but is unlikely. If he were not hyperactive, he would experience his hunger and request other food. P/E, AN, PS

169. no. 4. It is unrealistic to expect Mr. White to sit and eat large quantities of food. Providing nutritious snack foods will increase his overall intake. Keeping him company may only intensify his feelings of dependency, causing him to be angry and more hyperactive. P/E, IM, PS

170. no. 2. High-calorie finger foods and drinks can be consumed easily while standing or moving. He is not able to sit long enough to eat and will become irritated at the suggestion of putting off his work. Option no. 4 will put him on the defensive and not facilitate his eating. P/E, IM, E

171. no. 3. Large motor skills such as painting, drawing, and rug making on a loom provide for appropriate discharge of energy and tension. Occupational therapy is designed to teach people hobbies so they have other resources for relaxing; it is not the place to teach social skills, nor is it the appropriate environment for reality testing and confrontation. P/E, PL, H

172. no. 3. One important determinant of abuse by parents is whether they were abused as children. Child abuse can be a learned behavior. Education, age of menarche, and socioeconomic status are not of themselves indicators of potential or actual child abuse. P/SM, AS, E

173. no. 2. One important factor in the current situation is to determine if the abuse has already occurred. If this has happened, then more protective measures are necessary. This is the most important fact to determine when planning care. Being pregnant, not wanting her baby at the time of birth, and previous experience in caring for children do not indicate potential or actual child abuse. P/SM, AS, E

174. no. 1. Most teenage pregnancies result because the teenager thinks her unmet needs for love and affection can be provided by a baby. These expectations are unrealistic and lead to anger, frustration, and possible abuse, when the mother realizes the child cannot fulfill her needs. Teenagers often have a lack of knowledge about patterns of growth and development, child care, nutrition, and health needs of a baby. The pregnant teenager may not have an excellent role model for parenting from her own parents. P/SM, PL, E

175. no. 3. The most helpful initial interventions are to support the mother in the process of learning about realistic growth and development of the child and to teach her appropriate child-care and parenting skills. The information given does not address whether contraception, nutritional counseling, first aid, or cardiopulmonary resuscitation are referral needs. P/SM, IM, H

176. no. 3. The most appropriate response is to acknowledge Mrs. Lane's feelings and then explore the incident directly. By acknowledging the sadness, the nurse shows respect for her feelings and empathizes with Mrs. Lane's pain. By exploring the issue directly, the nurse conveys concern and caring and reduces Mrs. Lane's embarrassment and shame over the incident. It is important that the nurse indicate that it is acceptable to talk about this problem. Talking directly about the problem conveys confidence and a sense of control. Mrs. Lane has acknowledged, not denied, that she has a problem. Option no. 2 fails to address the client's feelings and will increase her shame and low self-esteem. Assessment about battering is an appropriate role and responsibility of nurses. A referral for psychotherapy can be made at a later point if the client wishes. P/SM, IM, PC

177. no. 2. The most common feelings experienced by the nurse are those of frustration and disappointment that the woman continues to remain in the destructive situation. These feelings influence the nurse's ability to remain nonjudgmental and objective. If the nurse is not aware of these feelings, it is easy to give up or avoid engaging the client in problem solving and exploration of alternate methods of dealing with the situation. It is unlikely that a nurse would experience apathy or ignore the behavior. Guilt, shame, denial, and repression are feelings that usually occur in battered women, rather than being a response of the nurse. P/SM, AN, E

178. no. 4. Blaming the victim is a most common response to victims of battering. When this attitude is conveyed, the victim becomes reluctant to share the details of her experience or to discuss her feelings or engage in problem solving. This attitude

often leaves the victim feeling helpless and powerless. Although indifference in the nurse is nontherapeutic, blaming the victim is a more powerful deterrent to self-disclosure by battered women. Some degree of concern over the detail of the situation may promote self-disclosure by the battered woman. Inquiring into the client's history should not affect self-disclosure. P/SM, AN, E

179. no. 1. The most important information to provide is the numbers of the crisis center and the battered-women's shelter, so the victim has resources available to her if the incident occurs again or if the battered woman needs support to help her come to a decision about the situation. Assertiveness training classes and psychotherapy are usually beneficial; however, the most important and highest priority referrals are no. 1. It is neither professional nor ethical to withhold information needed by the client. Battering recurs and needs no witnesses for proof. P/SM, IM, H

180. no. 3. Teasing is a way of testing the ability of staff to handle acting-out behavior. If staff members are consistent and can control his behavior, the client will learn trust. He will need to know, also, that staff members understand his underlying fears. If these two components are present, the adolescent will be in a climate conducive to helping him learn new behavior patterns. The client's pattern of behavior is acting out and will continue until firm limits are set. None of the information indicates that he will want to be alone much of the time. Good interpersonal skills require more self-control than Thomas' behavior demonstrates. P/SM, AS, PC

181. no. 1. The acting-out behavior can provide a diversion from the overwhelming fears the adolescent experiences. It can also be a way of channeling feelings or a way of asking adults for help. Conduct disorders, however, are not a normal part of adolescence. The data do not indicate that the client perceives problems in social or intellectual functioning. P/SM, AN, PC

182. no. 3. The adolescent will first need to decrease his acting-out behavior. He will then be ready to move on to other treatment goals. Acting out also pushes staff and peers away, so he will be unable to interact effectively with others until he can control his behavior. Acting-out behavior is an indication of anxiety. Initially, Tom would not be able to tolerate sitting and talking for 30 minutes daily. The client is very self-involved at this point and may not be able to empathize or be aware of his family's feelings. P/SM, PL, E

183. no. 3. Limit setting is the method staff can use to provide the necessary control over acting-out behavior. Visits from friends could be disruptive.

Such a visit could be used as a reward for showing self-control. The therapy should focus on the client at this time rather than his family because he may not understand nor want to know why his family is upset with him. Limit-setting should extend to control of abusive language. P/SM, IM, PC

184. no. 3. Delirium tremens is characteristic of the late stage of alcoholism. In the early stage, insomnia and tremors occur. In the middle stage, blackouts, amnesia, and physical changes such as chronic gastritis and fatty infiltration of the liver occur. A recovering alcoholic is not drinking and may be able to reduce some of the health problems that occurred as a consequence of alcohol ingestion. P/SM, PL, PS

185. no. 3. Options no. 1, no. 2, and no. 4 are appropriate interventions. Identifying feelings, encouraging expression, and setting limits are therapeutic. Sitting close to the client would be avoided, since many potentially violent clients perceive closeness as an invasion of their territory and as a controlling maneuver on the part of staff. In response, the client is even more likely to assault the person who comes close. P/SM, IM, E

186. no. 1. Unless options no. 2 through no. 4 are carried out, the staff or the client may be at greater risk of injury. Rarely would a physician refuse to write this order after the fact. Such an order also can be included as part of an institution's protocol for care of the potentially violent client. Tossing a sheet or blanket over a potentially violent client is another technique often included in standard protocols for control of potentially or actually violent behavior. P/SM, IM, E

187. no. 4. Clients who have ingested barbiturates, opiates, or diazepam (Valium) would have developed a general depressant-withdrawal syndrome. PCP ingestion is associated with vivid hallucinations and persecutory delusions. P/SM, AN, PS

188. no. 4. The behaviors listed in options no. 1 through no. 3 indicate that the client is regaining control. The behavior in no. 4 is more likely a way to manipulate staff. In short, the client is promising to behave in an unlikely way, considering her history of alcohol abuse. P/SM, EV, E

189. no. 2. Determination of the victim's perception of the rape is of value initially. Marital status and identity of rapist may be contributory, but they are not the most important information. To inquire about abortion is premature unless client indicates a wish to talk about this possibility. P/SM, AS, PC

190. no. 1. Rape is not considered a crime of passion, but rather one of violent aggression. Bestiality refers to sexual relations with an animal. Exposing one's sexual organs when socially inappropriate is

called exhibitionism. Venting anger and hostility and exercising power and control motivate the rapist, rather than sexual passion. P/SM, AN, PC

191. no. 3. It is very often a crisis for the significant other as well as for the victim. It is difficult for the significant other to perceive the victim as unchanged. Although option no. 4 is a possibility, no. 3 is more likely. P/SM, AN, H

192. no. 4. This will have the most significant effect in decreasing the trauma. Some victims develop posttraumatic stress disorder following a severe trauma like rape. Counseling and support from nursing colleagues and hospital administrators who are aware of Mrs. Smith's plight are also important. P/SM, IM, H

193. no. 4. The client who has been raped is very anxious and fears being harmed. Being touched is very likely to be anxiety producing. First, establish rapport, then assess the level of anxiety. Attention to lacerations, wounds, and obtaining a semen specimen can be done later in the visit. The decision to notify a family member can be made later in conjunction with the client. P/SM, IM, E

194. no. 3. Miss Long is in crisis, and she is experiencing many changes. Nursing actions that focus on behavior deal with immediate needs. The symptoms will abate as her anxiety decreases. Her diagnosis and intellectual capacity have implications for care, but actions that address her presenting behaviors are most important initially. P/SM, PL, E

195. no. 2. During the early stages of crisis intervention, the client will be unable to clearly understand the crisis situation; the understanding will come later. If frightening events are identified, Miss Long will be able to regain some feelings of control. Talking relieves anxiety for many people. A rape victim feels much shame and repulsion for what has happened to her body. Sometimes, the victim may feel the rape was her fault and suicidal thoughts may follow. Support systems and resource identification are necessary components of crisis intervention. P/SM, IM, PC

196. no. 4. Crisis theory is founded on the assumption that all plans will be developed in collaboration with the client. The underlying philosophy is that people have the resources to help themselves. The growth-and-development philosophy that is part of crisis theory is undermined when clients are not involved in their own decision making. The client's self-esteem will be lowered and she can feel devalued if decisions are made for her. Options no. 1, no. 2, and no. 3 describe important and necessary aspects of crisis intervention. P/SM, IM, PC

197. no. 2. He has symptoms of a persecutory delusional system. The idea that his brother is attempting to steal his property is almost certainly a false belief, a misunderstanding of reality. A hallucination is an imagined sensory perception that occurs without an external stimulus. An illusion is a misinterpretation of a sensory stimulus of a real experience. A phobia is a persistent, irrational, obsessive, intense fear of a situation or an object that results in increased tension and anxiety. P/SS, AN, PC

198. no. 1. Denial and projection are most common in paranoia. In denial, a person treats obvious reality factors as though they do not exist because these factors are intolerable to the conscious mind. In projection, a person attributes his or her own unacceptable emotions and qualities to others. Repression is the involuntary, unconscious forgetting of unacceptable or painful impulses, thoughts, feelings, or acts. Displacement refers to the transferring of unacceptable feelings aroused by an object or situation to a more acceptable substitute. P/SS, AN, PC

199. no. 3. As the client becomes more socially adapted, delusions are used less. Structuring activities will assist in decreasing delusions. Ability for group participation comes slowly, if at all. Cheerful behavior on the part of others increases the suspiciousness of the paranoid client. These clients tend to misinterpret the touch, experiencing it as control, anger, or invasion of their territory or person. P/SS, IM, PC

200. no. 2. Psychotropic drugs are used to lessen symptoms (e.g., paranoia, delusions, anxiety, and psychomotor excitement) so that clients can benefit more from milieu therapy and psychotherapy. Initially, psychotropic drugs may sedate a client. However, sedation is not the intention. Psychotropic medications do not, of themselves, assist clients in gaining insights. They only contribute indirectly to improved self-esteem by enabling the client to benefit from therapy. P/SS, AN, PS

201. no. 1. Although the symptoms listed may all be side effects of chlorpromazine, protection from photosensitivity is most appropriate because the picnic is outdoors. Constipation, dry mouth, and stuffy nose occur because of the anticholinergic effect of chlorpromazine (Thorazine). Fatigue is usually transient and relieved as dosage is adjusted and individualized for each client. Cholestatic jaundice is a rare side effect that is usually benign, self-limiting, and reversible. Jaundice is not caused by exposure to light. P/SS, IM, PS

202. no. 4. His statement demonstrates insight into past behavior. This response will help him to work on patterns of more acceptable behavior. The nurse's response also gives him the opportunity to tell her

about the people and situations in which he thinks he was tolerant. Generally, it is better to avoid "why" questions since many clients feel as if they are being put on the spot or do not know why. It is more therapeutic to focus on ways to change behavior rather than a particular person. The approach in option no. 3 is too broad and unfocused. Mr. Bonono needs help in learning ways to make his behavior more acceptable to others. P/SS, IM, PC

203. no. 1. The first priority in working with a suspicious client is to establish a trusting relationship so that other goals can be accomplished. The reality of the situation cannot be dealt with and insight cannot be achieved until a trusting relationship is established. Mr. Dooley's self-esteem should improve at a later point in his treatment. Mr. Dooley's social functioning also should improve as a result of improved self-esteem and as the client discontinues behaviors that disrupt his social relationships. P/SS, PL, E

204. no. 4. Ask questions that encourage the client to explore his situation and come to his own realization of his problems. Option no. 1 would be too confronting and threatening to the client. If his anxiety is kept within reasonable control, he will be better able to explore his difficulties. In no. 2, the nurse sides with the wife, which the client may experience as accusatory. Option no. 3 is likely to cause the client to hold more firmly to his delusions. P/SS, IM, PC

205. no. 2. An explanation for the lateness is most important. Establishing trust requires giving accurate information about what is happening in the client's environment. This avoids the problem of the client drawing conclusions that support a misinterpretation of events. If the nurse merely acknowledges lateness, the client's suspiciousness may lead him to conclude the nurse does not want to see him. The nurse will not be viewed as a reliable person if the appointment is cancelled after the delay. An apology rather than an explanation could be misinterpreted. P/SS, IM, PC

206. no. 1. Communications with clients should always be honest. This is even more important with suspicious clients, so as not to contribute to the suspicious delusions. Options no. 2, no. 3, and no. 4 may raise the client's anxiety needlessly, reinforce his delusional system, and increase his suspicions of others. P/SS, IM, PC

207. no. 3. When a suspicious client is willing to share feelings with a nurse, this is evidence that a trusting relationship is being formed. His delusions are an indication of anxiety and increase with greater anxiety. Trust with the nurse is not related to an explanation of the client's delusions by the nurse.

Although desirable, the nurse's feeling at ease does not necessarily indicate that Mr. Dooley is developing a trusting relationship with the nurse. P/SS, EV, H

208. no. 2. The highest priority in assessment of a psychotic client is to evaluate physical well-being. Such a client may be suffering from an illness or fluid and/or electrolyte imbalances. She also may have physical injuries either self-inflicted or from an assault. Her perception of reality is also important to assess potential safety risks and reality testing and to begin to set goals and plan the client's care. Observations at the bus station may or may not provide some useful information. Speech patterns may provide useful information, yet no. 2 has the highest priority. P/W, AS, PS

209. no. 3. Establishing a therapeutic relationship with psychotic clients requires communicating, even when they seem out of touch with reality. Make directions and expectations as clear and unambiguous as possible. The client is regressed, and baby talk or gibberish is part of her regression. It would not be therapeutic or effective to deal with her speech problem at this time. Therapeutic verbal and nonverbal communication by a professional person is a critical need of this client. Therapeutic communication and medication, not a speech therapist, will help the client. P/W, IM, PC

210. no. 4. The most common side effect of antipsychotic drugs is hypotension. Monitoring the blood pressure is necessary to ensure that appropriate measures can be taken if blood pressure falls below safe levels. Lying and standing blood pressures should be taken to test for orthostatic hypotension before each dose. A blood specimen and neurological checks are not necessary before administering each dose of medication. Observation of parkinsonian side effects is important throughout hospitalization but is not necessary before each of these three doses. Fluids do not need to be offered. P/W, AS, PS

211. no. 1. Control of psychotic symptoms may require as many as 10 doses of the medication within a matter of 5 to 6 hours. If the client is not experiencing any untoward side effects, further doses probably will be ordered by the physician. A nurse cannot administer any more haloperidol without a physician's order or a protocol. The nurse must always record the results of the medication. The point of this question is the nurse's next action. It is not necessary to observe the client for an hour but rather to assess intermittently and to ensure that the client is safe. P/W, IM, PS

212. no. 1. Mild hypotension may be present with haloperidol and may cause light-headedness when the client arises. This symptom usually disappears after

2 to 3 weeks. The drug controls psychotic symptoms. It is unlikely that the client will experience considerable drowsiness. Option no. 3 is inaccurate; the medication does have some major side effects, and the second part of the remark could be misunderstood by the client. The client will need medication for an extended time; the current psychotic episode was precipitated when she discontinued her medication. P/W, IM, E

213. no. 4. The nurse must make an assessment before assuming a client is hallucinating. A client should not be medicated before the nursing assessment and nursing diagnosis. The nurse must not jump to conclusions. It is not helpful to the client for the nurse to ignore the behavior; assessment is necessary. If hallucinating, the client may become worse if secluded, unless someone stays with her. P/W, IM, PC

214. no. 4. Acknowledge that hallucinations are real to the client, but encourage her to communicate with staff present in the unit. Although option no. 1 does present reality, it is not therapeutic to the client at this time. Option no. 2 does not address a relevant issue and does not provide the client with the direction she needs (i.e., to talk with the nurse). In option no. 3, the nurse makes an assumption but has no data on which to base her conclusion. P/W, IM, PC

215. no. 2. A psychotic client may be unable to make choices or engage in activities with other clients without support. Assigning a staff member gives the client an opportunity to build a relationship. The client may not yet be able to describe what sports she enjoys, make choices, engage in activities with others, or develop an interest and initiate activity. P/W, IM, E

216. no. 3. Involving the aunt will enable the nurse to assess the aunt's ability to promote continued progress for the client. The nurse needs to assess the client's support system. The nurse needs to be more actively involved in the decision-making process because Miss Dumas may not be able to determine or make her needs known at this time. The nurse has not yet assessed the extent to which the aunt is helpful to Miss Dumas. There is no data on which to base the conclusion in option no. 4. P/W, PL, H

217. no. 2. Building a one-to-one relationship with the schizophrenic client is very important, since this is a problem for her. A relationship with one staff member can lead to relationships with others if the client is able to increase trust. Usually it is not feasible for the client to work with one staff person for a 24-hour day, but the client should be assigned to as few staff members as possible. The new marriage and accompanying life-style changes may

have precipitated this crisis and psychological decompensation. An assessment of the relationship would be necessary before concentrating on helping her relate to her husband. Options no. 3 and no. 4 are important aspects of care, but can only be successful after the client develops a trusting relationship with the nursing staff. P/W, PL, E

218. no. 4. Perseverance and patience are essential when working with a schizophrenic client. The nurse must continue to demonstrate interest and sincerity until the client feels able to trust the nurse in increasing ways. The other options demand more verbalization and changes in behavior that are not appropriate at this time. P/W, IM, PC

219. no. 3. The schizophrenic client's mistrust and inability to interpret reality accurately inhibit the ability to make sense of what is happening. Here the nurse is orienting the client to the environment. Immediate involvement in unit activities may be too stimulating or demanding at this time and may cause the client's anxiety to escalate unnecessarily. P/W, IM, PC

220. no. 1. The nurse should cast doubt on the client's perceptions, while at the same time not denying the validity of the perceptions to the client. Attempts to reason with the client or argue about, challenge, or reinforce the ideas only serve to entrench them more firmly. P/W, IM, PC

221. no. 3. As above. Options no. 1, no. 2, and no. 4 could precipitate an increase in the client's level of anxiety. P/W, AN, PC

222. no. 3. Anxiety is one of the most crucial elements in the development of schizophrenia. As anxiety decreases, clients become more reality oriented and more approachable, and their behavior becomes more appropriate. Insight and receptivity to psychotherapy are usually not seen when there is an increase in anxiety. Option no. 4 may be true; however, she probably would initially exhibit an attention or memory deficit. P/W, AS, PC

223. no. 1. Establishing a trusting relationship will decrease the client's anxiety and make it possible for the nurse to work toward other goals, such as increasing communication and improving social skills. P/W, PL, E

224. no. 1. Sitting quietly will promote interpersonal contact without pressuring the client to communicate beyond his level of readiness. Options no. 2, no. 3, and no. 4 will probably result in further retreat from socialization because the client is frightened about the level of interaction the nurse is attempting. P/W, IM, PC

225. no. 3. A picnic on the hospital grounds provides the opportunity for interaction with other clients and staff in a noncompetitive, nondemanding setting. Options no. 1, no. 2, and no. 4 are either

physically demanding or require a high level of perceptual and cognitive awareness and may result in failure, further inhibiting socialization. P/W, IM, E

226. no. 4. Parkinsonian side effects are common with phenothiazine drugs. Unless severe, their presence is not an indication to stop the drug. Option no. 1 would be an excellent intervention if the client were experiencing orthostatic hypotension, another side effect of thorazine. Option no. 2 will not assist the client who is experiencing extrapyramidal effects of the antipsychotic agent. A neurological consultation would only be indicated if there were additional focal symptoms and if an antiparkinson agent did not alleviate the extrapyramidal symptoms. P/ W, IM, PS

227. no. 3. People tend to respond to current or anticipated losses as they have responded to losses in the past. Schizophrenic clients have difficulty dealing with closeness; however, a relationship has been established, and there is an impending absence of the client's primary nurse, which the client internalizes as loss and abandonment. Schizophrenia does not have a pattern of cyclic exacerbation as in manic-depressive illness; this client is responding to a well-defined, precipitating event. He apparently does feel he needs the relationship and is subsequently withdrawing from the nurse to get ready for the perceived loss of the relationship. P/ W, AN, PC

228. no. 1. A diet with extra protein and C and B vitamins is indicated to compensate for the poor nutritional state present in many substance abusers. The addition of chlordiazepoxide will decrease anxiety and assist in detoxification. Cirrhosis of the liver, a common side effect of chronic alcoholism, necessitates a low-fat diet. Vitamin E, a fat-soluble vitamin, is stored in the body and may not be depleted. Chlorpromazine (Thorazine) is contraindicated in withdrawal states from alcohol. Although fluids are important to counteract dehydration, emphasis should be on high protein intake to build up the depleted nutritional state. Meperidine (Demerol) is an analgesic and is contraindicated with impaired hepatic function. Although phenytoin (Dilantin) is an important consideration to eliminate the possibility of seizures (as are fluids to counteract dehydration) chlordiazepoxide (Librium) is the first drug of choice to reduce initial symptoms of anxiety in the acute phase. P/SU, IM, PS

229. no. 2. Poor dietary habits of many substance abusers cause marked deficiency in thiamin. This results in symptoms of Korsakoff's syndrome. Encephalomalacia, convulsions, and dystonia are consequences of impaired CNS functioning, not the causative factors of Korsakoff's syndrome. P/SU, AN, PS

230. no. 3. These symptoms are accompanied by nausea and increased pulse rate and blood pressure. Alcohol withdrawal results in psychomotor agitation. The symptoms in option no. 1 are a result of autonomic nervous system depression. Option no. 2 lists manifestations of alcohol withdrawal, but they are not the first symptoms observed. The symptoms in option no. 4 would not be a direct result of alcohol withdrawal, but may occur as a secondary consequence (e.g., from seizures). P/SU, AS, PS

231. no. 1. Provide an environment with minimal stimulation. Remaining with the client provides reassurance and decreases anxiety. Although bed rest and fluids, excluding caffeine products, are indicated, soft music is an environmental stimulus and would, therefore, be contraindicated. Caffeine, a stimulant found in tea, and high fat content, found in ice cream, are contraindicated in alcohol withdrawal. Restraints are only necessary if client is a safety threat to himself or others. Use of restraints should be avoided, as they tend to agitate and confuse the disoriented client. Vital signs need to be monitored as necessary, but the nurse needs to minimize intrusions to maintain a quiet and calm environment. P/SU, IM, PS

232. no. 1. The nurse gives information but leaves the opportunity for Mrs. Maling to ventilate her feelings and decide for herself. Option no. 2 implies that only the alcoholic is affected by the disease, whereas it is insidious to the family system. Although many find Al-Anon helpful, participation is not mandatory and should be an individual consideration. P/SU, IM, H

233. no. 2. The client must acknowledge the illness and be motivated to change his pattern of living. Atonement for past behavior is not nearly as important as motivation for change of future behavior. A strong support system is helpful in facilitating recovery; however, recovery is self-dependent. P/ SU, EV, H

234. no. 2. Most cough medicines contain varying amounts of alcohol and would cause him to become ill if he were to combine them with disulfiram. Aspirin, acetaminophen, antacids, and laxatives are over-the-counter drugs that do not contain alcohol and, therefore, would not cause adverse effects. Heart and blood pressure medications, which are also prescribed by the physician, may be medically indicated. Individuals taking disulfiram (Antabuse) must learn to read product labels to ascertain if alcohol is an ingredient. P/SU, IM, PS

235. no. 2. Alcoholics Anonymous is run entirely by alcoholics who have achieved or are attempting to

achieve sobriety. It is not group therapy, nor is it led by professionals. It does not discourage relationships, but instead recognizes the need for support. P/SU, AN, H

236. no. 3. A client who achieves sobriety after alcohol abuse is considered a recovering alcoholic. Alcoholism is not curable but can be controlled. Options no. 2 and no. 4 imply a resolved disease state, whereas the potential for active alcoholism remains throughout the client's life. P/SU, AN, PC

237. no. 3. Encourage the client to talk about feelings, using techniques such as reflection. Avoid judgmental responses, such as no. 2, that close off communication. Neither option no. 1 nor no. 4 allows exploration of Mr. Trysdale's feelings on drinking. P/SU, IM, PC

238. no. 1. Clear explanations about treatment are appropriate. The nurse would then assess the client's status. Option no. 2 sounds judgmental. Sedation may not be indicated. While it is good to provide explanations to a client, no. 4 does not allow the nurse to explore the reason why Mr. Trysdale undid his traction. P/SU, IM, PS

239. no. 4. Reflection encourages the client to describe how he is feeling, so the nurse can assess, analyze, and plan care appropriately. Option no. 1 is a closed question and does not encourage exploration of the client's feelings. Option no. 2 does not allow the nurse to explore with the client what he is experiencing and, therefore, does not provide the nurse with the necessary information to make a complete assessment. In option no. 3, the nurse is making an assumption that could make the client feel judged and prevent further exploration. P/SU, IM, PC

240. no. 1. Collaborate with the physician in order to plan appropriately. Adequate assessment has been obtained by the nurse over the course of a shift. Option no. 3 is not a nursing decision. The physician will make this decision based on the diagnosis. If the client's condition has changed, the sedative may be medically contraindicated. The physician should be alerted to any dramatic changes in client status. P/SU, IM, PS

241. no. 2. Point out reality to persons who are having hallucinations from substance withdrawal. Reassure and orient them frequently. Option no. 1 serves to reinforce his hallucinations. A physician's order is required to apply restraints, and reassurance may be all that is needed as an initial nursing action. Nursing measures to calm and orient Mr. Trysdale should be done first. If the behavior continues, the administration of the prescribed tranquilizer may be necessary later. P/SU, IM, E

242. no. 3. Persons in withdrawal need reassurance that they will be taken care of and will not be left alone. The client is unable to control himself at this time, and it is an inappropriate time to question him about his drinking habits. P/SU, IM, PC

243. no. 2. The highest priority is to prevent dehydration, but caffeine drinks would increase agitation. This client has a physical problem that makes ambulation impossible. Keep the environment as quiet and distraction free as possible. P/SU, IM, PS

244. no. 4. The client has already admitted he has a problem. The most realistic and highest priority goal for him is to accept the help of others. Options no. 2 and no. 3 are long-term goals, not the first or immediate concern. P/SU, PL, H

245. no. 1. Handle lapses nonjudgmentally and in a way that encourages the client to use the help of others to find new ways of coping. Option no. 2 is a judgment statement. The fact that Mr. Trysdale is drinking does not imply that he is unwilling to change. The client needs to be reassured that it is difficult, rather than chastised for his lapse. The focus should be on the client's needs and behaviors. He must assume responsibility and motivation for his recovery. P/SU, IM, PC

246. no. 1. Identify the difficulties associated with trying to stop alcohol intake, so that the client does not continue to fall back on superficiality and denial. Continue to encourage the client to seek help from others. Option no. 2 supports the client's denial of the difficulty involved with abstaining from alcohol. Value judgments and threats are contraindicated and deny Mr. Trysdale the necessary support he needs at this time. P/SU, IM, H

247. no. 3. Hallucinogens cause an individual to lose contact with reality and hallucinate. Opiates are a class of drug that contain or are derived from opium. Barbiturates are a group of powerful sedative drugs that bring about relaxation and sleep. Stimulants are a class of drug whose major effect is to provide energy and alertness. P/SU, AN, PS

248. no. 1. There is no evidence that LSD is physically addicting. Heightened sensory perception can lead to an acute panic state. P/SU, AN, PC

249. no. 4. No treatment modality has been very effective with drug abusers, and the relapse rate is about 90%. Treatment by former addicts has had the best results, because these persons, through their own experiences, are familiar with the behaviors of the drug abuser. The aim of psychoanalysis is to restructure the personality. Behavior modification uses learning principles to improve behavior and has not proven to be very effective in treating drug dependence. Family therapy does not focus on the

drug abuser, but instead treats family roles and attitudes. P/SU, AN, PC

250. no. 2. One of the effects of LSD is heightened sensory perceptions, which can be very frightening to the client and cause an acute panic state in which the client can hurt himself and others. Seclusion will help to reduce environmental stimulation and protect both this client and others. Turning off the television and restraining the client are not sufficient. Client safety and dignity must be maintained. An order for sedation can be obtained later. P/SU, IM, PS

251. no. 4. Clients should be observed constantly when in seclusion, and seclusion should be used only when it is the most effective therapy for the client at that time. The client needs a quiet and calm environment to counteract heightened sensory perception. The use of seclusion to protect the client from harming self or others is legitimate, since safety is always an utmost concern. P/SU, PL, PC

252. no. 3. The nurse must help the client sort out what is real and what is not by giving reality-based feed-

back. Option no. 1 belittles the client's feelings and is condescending. Option no. 2 does not help the client determine what is real and what is hallucination. Discussing the hallucination, as suggested in option no. 4, will give it credence and increase the likelihood of recurrence. What the nurse discusses with a client reinforces it in the client's mind. P/SU, IM, PC

253. no. 2. Mr. Clements is having a delusion. Delusions are created in the mind to make up for or meet an underlying need. Option no. 2 responds to the possible need underlying this client's delusion. Options no. 1 and no. 3 foster his grandiose and aberrant thinking and do not orient him to reality. The presence of visual hallucinations does not necessitate the use of seclusion. P/SU, IM, PC

254. no. 1. Haloperidol is a major tranquilizer, the purpose of which is to treat psychosis or thought disorders. Diazepam is an antianxiety drug. Imipramine (Tofranil) and isocarboxazid (Marplan) are antidepressants. P/SU, AN, PC

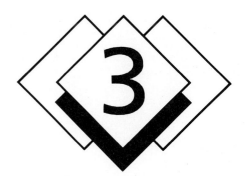

Nursing Care of the Adult

Coordinator

Paulette D. Rollant, MSN, RN, CCRN

Contributors

Deborah A. Ennis, MSN, RN, CCRN
Peg Gray-Vickery, MS, RNC

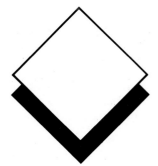

Questions

A nurse comes upon an auto accident and discovers a young man lying beside the road. He has a carotid pulse but does not seem to be breathing.

1. Which action would be *incorrect*?
   - ☐ 1. Clear the mouth.
   - ☐ 2. Hyperextend the neck.
   - ☐ 3. Perform a chin-lift maneuver.
   - ☐ 4. Inhale deeply and smoothly deliver several rapid breaths.

2. If the victim had oral injuries, the nurse would deliver mouth-to-nose resuscitation. Which of the following would be correct for mouth-to-nose resuscitation but *not* correct for mouth-to-mouth?
   - ☐ 1. More force is required.
   - ☐ 2. The victim's mouth is closed during inspiration.
   - ☐ 3. The victim's mouth is open during expiration.
   - ☐ 4. The victim's neck is extended.

3. An Ambu-bag is available. If it is used with one hand, how many milliliters of air can be delivered?
   - ☐ 1. 1000.
   - ☐ 2. 800.
   - ☐ 3. 600.
   - ☐ 4. 400.

4. The victim has a blood pressure of 60/0 mm Hg and a pulse of 140. Following adequate ventilation, the first treatment priority is
   - ☐ 1. Sodium bicarbonate.
   - ☐ 2. Range of motion.
   - ☐ 3. Turn, cough, and deep-breathe.
   - ☐ 4. Fluid infusion.

5. The victim is admitted to the emergency room with chest injuries. Which piece of assessment data would be the most helpful to the physician in assessing blood loss and deciding what action to take?
   - ☐ 1. What was the cause of the injury.
   - ☐ 2. History of mentation since the accident.
   - ☐ 3. Time of injury.
   - ☐ 4. Sex of the victim.

6. A thoracentesis is performed, but no fluid or air is found. Blood is administered IV, but the client's vital signs do not improve. A central venous pressure line is inserted, and the initial reading is 20 cm. The nurse notes distension of the jugular vein. The most likely cause of these findings is
   - ☐ 1. Spontaneous pneumothorax.
   - ☐ 2. Ruptured diaphragm.
   - ☐ 3. Hemothorax.
   - ☐ 4. Pericardial tamponade.

Carl Bates, a 75-year-old man, underwent abdominal surgery for a bowel obstruction. In the immediate postoperative period, he developed signs and symptoms of hypovolemic shock.

7. Below what systolic blood pressure level is perfusion to the vital organs markedly compromised in a usually normotensive client?
   - ☐ 1. 100 mm Hg.
   - ☐ 2. 90 mm Hg.
   - ☐ 3. 80 mm Hg.
   - ☐ 4. 70 mm Hg.

8. Blood levels of angiotensin and renin are increased during shock. What clinical findings would the nurse assess for as a result of these blood levels?
   - ☐ 1. Peripheral vasoconstriction.
   - ☐ 2. Peripheral vasodilatation.
   - ☐ 3. Increased respiratory rate.
   - ☐ 4. Decreased respiratory rate.

9. Why is dopamine frequently used to treat shock?
   - ☐ 1. It is a powerful vasodilator.
   - ☐ 2. It has no untoward side effects.
   - ☐ 3. Cardiac function is not affected.
   - ☐ 4. Kidney perfusion is maintained.

10. What is the best parameter for adequate fluid replacement in a client who is in shock?
    - ☐ 1. Systolic blood pressure above 100 mm Hg.
    - ☐ 2. Systolic blood pressure above 90 mm Hg.

☐ 3. Urine output of 30 ml/hr.
☐ 4. Urine output of 20 ml/hr.

11. A fluid challenge is begun with Mr. Bates. Which assessment will give the best indication of client response to this treatment?
☐ 1. CVP readings and hourly urine outputs.
☐ 2. Blood pressure and apical rate checks.
☐ 3. Lung sounds and arterial blood gases.
☐ 4. Electrolytes, BUN, and creatinine results.

12. Why are adrenergic agents particularly useful in treating hypotension and controlling superficial bleeding?
☐ 1. They cause dilatation of peripheral vessels.
☐ 2. They cause constriction of peripheral vessels.
☐ 3. They decrease the cardiac output.
☐ 4. They block the effects of acetylcholine.

13. Adrenergic drugs, such as epinephrine (Adrenalin), are given in emergency situations for what primary reason?
☐ 1. To increase cardiac output by increasing the rate and strength of myocardial contraction.
☐ 2. To increase tone and motility of the gastrointestinal tract.
☐ 3. To prevent spasm and constriction of peripheral vessels.
☐ 4. To prevent cardiac dysrhythmias.

14. The most serious side effect of the adrenergic drugs that the nurse monitors for is
☐ 1. Dilated pupils.
☐ 2. Headache.
☐ 3. Cardiac dysrhythmias.
☐ 4. Nervousness.

15. Mr. Bates' arterial blood gas results are: pH 7.30, PO_2 58, PCO_2 34, HCO_3 19. What acid-base imbalance would these results most likely indicate?
☐ 1. Metabolic acidosis.
☐ 2. Metabolic alkalosis.
☐ 3. Respiratory acidosis.
☐ 4. Respiratory alkalosis.

16. Why are acid-base imbalances life threatening?
☐ 1. Enzyme activity is inhibited.
☐ 2. Increased catecholamines cause cardiac stimulation.
☐ 3. Increased metabolites depress nerve activity.
☐ 4. Increased enzyme activity causes a hypermetabolic state.

17. Mr. Bates' first line of defense when his body is attempting to compensate for his acid-base problem would be which of the following?
☐ 1. Hormonal activity.
☐ 2. Increased alveolar CO_2.
☐ 3. Retention of bicarbonate by the kidneys.
☐ 4. Blood-buffering systems.

Ted Fontaine has done well in surgery and returns to his unit after a cholecystectomy. During the night, the nurse discovers his incisional area has become hard and elevated, his blood pressure is 80/60, and his pulse is 124. Blood studies show his hematocrit and hemoglobin are both low, his platelet count is 100,000/mm³, and his prothrombin time is prolonged. Whole blood is administered, but Mr. Fontaine does not improve. The nursing history reveals Mr. Fontaine took prednisone for a year before admission.

18. Information is obtained from clients regarding previous use of corticosteroids to help identify
☐ 1. Secondary adrenocortical insufficiency.
☐ 2. Addison's disease.
☐ 3. Primary adrenocortical insufficiency.
☐ 4. Azotemia.

19. Mr. Fontaine is most likely exhibiting signs of
☐ 1. Acute tubular necrosis.
☐ 2. Azotemia.
☐ 3. Disseminated intravascular coagulation (DIC).
☐ 4. Waterhouse-Friderichsen syndrome.

20. Drug therapy for Mr. Fontaine will probably include
☐ 1. Tranquilizers.
☐ 2. Vitamins.
☐ 3. Adrenocorticosteroids.
☐ 4. Adrenocorticosteroids and pressor agents.

21. Additionally, Mr. Fontaine will most likely need which of the following treatments?
☐ 1. Heparin and packed red blood cells (PRBC).
☐ 2. Whole blood.
☐ 3. Peritoneal dialysis.
☐ 4. Antibiotics.

22. If not successfully treated, Mr. Fontaine's condition could result in
☐ 1. Addisonian crisis.
☐ 2. Renal failure.
☐ 3. Hemophilia.
☐ 4. Neutropenia.

23. Mr. Fontaine's fever climbs to 104.6° F (40.3° C). His physician orders hypothermia equipment and asks the nurse to maintain his body temperature at 99.6° F (37.5° C). At what body temperature would the nurse discontinue the hypothermia treatment?
☐ 1. 97.6° F (36.4° C)
☐ 2. 98.6° F (37° C)
☐ 3. 99.6° F (37.5° C)
☐ 4. 100.6° F (38.1° C)

Sinja Mung, a 55-year-old Korean, is employed as a cook in a local restaurant. He awakens one night with crushing substernal chest pain, diaphoresis, and nausea. His wife calls the paramedics, and Mr. Mung is taken to the closest emergency room. He has the classic signs of myocardial infarction.

24. Mr. Mung arrives in the emergency room, still in pain; he is quickly assessed by the nurse and the physician. The best initial nursing action is to

☐ 1. Start an IV.

☐ 2. Give the pain medication as ordered by the physician.

☐ 3. Prepare him for immediate transfer to the coronary care unit.

☐ 4. Get a complete history from his wife.

25. The pain experienced by Mr. Mung is probably a result of

☐ 1. Vasoconstriction because of arterial spasms.

☐ 2. Myocardial ischemia.

☐ 3. Fear of death.

☐ 4. Irritation of nerve endings in the cardiac plexus.

26. Which area of the heart most frequently suffers the most damage in a myocardial infarction?

☐ 1. Conduction system.

☐ 2. Heart valves.

☐ 3. Left ventricle.

☐ 4. Right ventricle.

27. Which of the following also would be included in the admission process?

☐ 1. Contact client's place of employment.

☐ 2. Ensure that someone stays with significant others.

☐ 3. Keep family and significant others informed of progress and status.

☐ 4. Secure information about client's medical insurance status.

28. When the nurse talks to Mr. Mung's wife, she reports that he had experienced some angina for months before admission but had not sought medical attention. What is the probable reason for his neglect?

☐ 1. He has a high threshold for pain.

☐ 2. He lacks knowledge about health maintenance.

☐ 3. He denied the significance of the pain.

☐ 4. He was afraid it would be interpreted as psychosomatic.

29. Mr. Mung experiences a cardiac arrest. What would be the first nursing action in this situation?

☐ 1. Call the physician on duty.

☐ 2. Establish an airway.

☐ 3. Start closed-chest massage.

☐ 4. Give a bolus of sodium bicarbonate.

30. What initial nursing assessment would best indicate that Mr. Mung has been resuscitated?

☐ 1. Skin warm and dry.

☐ 2. Pupils equal and react to light.

☐ 3. Palpable carotid pulse.

☐ 4. Positive Babinski reflex.

31. Mr. Mung was transferred to the coronary care unit after an ECG indicated a posterior-wall infarction. Upon arriving at the unit, he complained of chest pain. In assessing the pain, which of the following is *not* characteristic of the pain of an acute myocardial infarction?

☐ 1. Intense and crushing.

☐ 2. Relieved by nitroglycerin.

☐ 3. May radiate to one or both arms, neck, or jaw.

☐ 4. Is of long duration and not relieved by rest.

32. What is the narcotic of choice in this situation?

☐ 1. Morphine sulfate.

☐ 2. Meperidine (Demerol).

☐ 3. Codeine sulfate.

☐ 4. Hydromorphone chloride (Dilaudid).

33. Upon his admission to the coronary care unit, oxygen was ordered. The primary purpose of oxygen administration in this situation is to

☐ 1. Relieve dyspnea.

☐ 2. Relieve cyanosis.

☐ 3. Increase oxygen concentration in the myocardium.

☐ 4. Supersaturate the red blood cells.

34. The most dangerous period for a client following a myocardial infarction is

☐ 1. The first 24 to 48 hours.

☐ 2. The first 72 to 96 hours.

☐ 3. 4 to 10 days after myocardial infarction.

☐ 4. From onset of symptoms until treatment begins.

35. What is the most lethal complication in the period after myocardial infarction?

☐ 1. Cardiogenic shock.

☐ 2. Ventricular dysrhythmias.

☐ 3. Pulmonary embolus.

☐ 4. Cardiac tamponade.

36. Which fact is accurate about cardiogenic shock?

☐ 1. It is easily treated with drugs.

☐ 2. It can be prevented with close monitoring.

☐ 3. The mortality rate is very high.

☐ 4. It is difficult to identify high-risk clients.

37. Cardiac-enzyme studies are helpful in diagnosing a myocardial infarction. These studies are most indicative of

☐ 1. Cardiac ischemia.

☐ 2. Location of the myocardial infarction.

☐ 3. Cardiac necrosis.

☐ 4. Size of the infarct.

38. Which drug is a first choice to reduce premature ventricular contractions?

☐ 1. Procainamide (Pronestyl).

☐ 2. Phenytoin (Dilantin).

☐ 3. Lidocaine (Xylocaine).

☐ 4. Digoxin (Lanoxin).

39. Which of the following is a more common side effect of this drug?

☐ 1. Tachycardia.

☐ 2. Decreased respirations.

☐ 3. Seizures.

☐ 4. Sedation.

40. Valsalva's maneuver can result in bradycardia, which can be very dangerous for the myocardial infarction client. Which nursing action will prevent Valsalva's maneuver?

☐ 1. Administer oral laxatives prn.

☐ 2. Teach the client to hold his breath when changing position.

☐ 3. Service liquids at room temperature.

☐ 4. Encourage the client to deep-breathe frequently.

41. Mrs. Mung tells the nurse she is afraid her husband is going to die. Anticipatory grieving is important for her to experience at this time. Which of the following nursing actions would probably *hinder* her experiencing anticipatory grieving?

☐ 1. Have her participate in her husband's care when possible.

☐ 2. Let her express her fears about the possibility of his dying.

☐ 3. Give her frequent reports about her husband's condition.

☐ 4. Tell her that the nurses are very competent.

42. Mr. Mung, now considerably improved, wants to talk about his sexual activity after he has been discharged from the hospital. What would be the nurse's initial approach?

☐ 1. Give him some written materials and then answer questions.

☐ 2. Plan a teaching session with Mr. Mung and his wife.

☐ 3. Answer his questions accurately and directly.

☐ 4. Provide enough time and privacy so that he can express his concerns fully.

43. Mr. Mung is to be discharged on a low-cholesterol diet. Which of the following foods is lowest in cholesterol?

☐ 1. Liver.

☐ 2. Tuna fish.

☐ 3. Shellfish.

☐ 4. Rice.

44. Which of the following would *not* contribute to Mr. Mung's risk of another myocardial infarction?

☐ 1. His brother had a myocardial infarction 2 years ago.

☐ 2. He has diabetes.

☐ 3. He smokes a pack of cigarettes daily.

☐ 4. He takes four aspirins daily.

45. Mr. Mung lives in a two-story house but has bathrooms upstairs and downstairs. Which of the following is the most correct teaching for him with regard to activity after discharge?

☐ 1. "Do what you feel like."

☐ 2. "Do not do any walking except to the bathroom from bed. Take your meals in the bedroom."

☐ 3. "Walk around in the house; do not walk up or down steps until you have seen the doctor."

☐ 4. "Do all the walking you wish inside and outside. You can climb stairs inside the house."

Henry Duboff, a 50-year-old white man, awakens in the middle of the night with severe dyspnea, bilateral basilar rales, and expectoration of frothy, blood-tinged sputum. He is brought to the hospital in congestive heart failure complicated by pulmonary edema.

46. Dyspnea is a characteristic sign of congestive heart failure. This is primarily the result of

☐ 1. Accumulation of serous fluid in alveolar spaces.

☐ 2. Obstruction of bronchi by mucoid secretions.

☐ 3. Compression of lung tissue by a dilated heart.

☐ 4. Restriction of respiratory movement by ascites.

47. In congestive heart failure, edema develops primarily because

☐ 1. Diffusion is inhibited.

☐ 2. The capillary bed dilates.

☐ 3. Venous pressure increases.

☐ 4. Osmotic pressure increases.

48. Edema caused by cardiac failure tends to be

☐ 1. Painful.

☐ 2. Dependent.

☐ 3. Periorbital.

☐ 4. Nonpitting.

49. Left-sided congestive heart failure is most often associated with which sign or symptom?

☐ 1. Dyspnea.

☐ 2. Distended neck veins.

☐ 3. Hepatomegaly.

☐ 4. Pedal edema.

50. Force of cardiac contraction (systole) is *decreased* by excess of which of the following?

☐ 1. Calcium ions.

☐ 2. Chloride ions.

☐ 3. Potassium ions.

☐ 4. Sodium ions.

51. Respirations of the client with congestive heart failure are usually

☐ 1. Rapid and shallow.

☐ 2. Deep and stertorous.

☐ 3. Rapid and wheezing.

☐ 4. Cheyne-Stokes.

52. What is the optimal bed position for the client with congestive heart failure?

☐ 1. Position of comfort, to relax the client.

☐ 2. Semirecumbent, to ease dyspnea and metabolic demands on the heart.

☐ 3. Upright, to decrease danger of pulmonary edema.

☐ 4. Flat, to decrease edema formation in the extremities.

53. Why are IV drugs more effective in a client with congestive heart failure than IM or oral administration?

☐ 1. Altered circulation slows the action of IM and ingested drugs.

☐ 2. Altered circulation speeds the action of IM and ingested drugs.

☐ 3. An enlarged heart needs a stronger dose.

☐ 4. There is no difference between IV, IM, and PO drug absorption in clients with congestive heart failure.

54. The nurse's main concern when caring for the client receiving both digitalis and furosemide (Lasix) is to

☐ 1. Take central venous pressure readings.

☐ 2. Observe for decreased edema.

☐ 3. Observe for signs and symptoms of hypokalemia.

☐ 4. Force fluids.

55. How do rotating tourniquets relieve the symptoms of acute pulmonary edema?

☐ 1. Cause vasoconstriction.

☐ 2. Cause vasodilatation.

☐ 3. Decrease the amount of circulating blood.

☐ 4. Increase the amount of circulating blood.

56. When tourniquets are applied to extremities to relieve the symptoms of pulmonary edema, one tourniquet is rotated, in order, every

☐ 1. 5 minutes.

☐ 2. 15 minutes.

☐ 3. 30 minutes.

☐ 4. 60 minutes.

57. Mr. Duboff is restricted to a 2000-mg sodium diet. He is instructed to not salt his food and to avoid

☐ 1. Whole milk.

☐ 2. Canned tuna.

☐ 3. Plain nuts.

☐ 4. Eggs.

58. Mr. Duboff is counseled regarding his potassium intake while he is receiving diuretics. Which of the following foods have very low levels of potassium?

☐ 1. Meats and milk.

☐ 2. Citrus fruits.

☐ 3. Potatoes.

☐ 4. Cereals and breads.

Rosalind Avery is being admitted with a diagnosis of thrombophlebitis.

59. Which of the following signs and symptoms would the nurse most expect to find when assessing Mrs. Avery?

☐ 1. A negative Homans' sign.

☐ 2. Pallor of the legs.

☐ 3. Shiny, atrophic skin on the legs.

☐ 4. Unilateral leg swelling.

60. Which of the following actions is most appropriate for Mrs. Avery?

☐ 1. Apply warm, dry packs to the involved site.

☐ 2. Elevate her legs 45°.

☐ 3. Maintain her on bed rest for 10 to 14 days.

☐ 4. Provide range-of-motion to both legs at least twice every shift.

61. Mrs. Avery starts receiving heparin sodium. Which of the following rationales for heparin therapy is most correct?

☐ 1. It dissolves existing thrombi.

☐ 2. It inactivates thrombin that forms.

☐ 3. It inactivates thrombin that forms and dissolves existing thrombi.

☐ 4. It interferes with vitamin K absorption.

62. Which of the following lab tests needs to be monitored while Mrs. Avery is being given heparin?

☐ 1. Bleeding time.

☐ 2. Partial thromboplastin time (PTT).

☐ 3. Prothrombin consumption test (PCT).

☐ 4. Prothrombin time (PT).

63. Which of the following would *not* be a sign or symptom of overdosage of heparin?

☐ 1. Rectal bleeding.

☐ 2. Positive Homans' sign.

☐ 3. Smoky, dark urine.

☐ 4. Epistaxis.

64. Which of the following drugs blocks the action of heparin?

☐ 1. AquaMEPHYTON.

☐ 2. Atropine sulfate.

☐ 3. Protamine sulfate.

☐ 4. Vitamin K.

65. Mrs. Avery is to take warfarin sodium (Coumadin) at home. Which of the following would be included in her discharge instruction?

☐ 1. Keep a vial of vitamin A available at all times.

☐ 2. Report any blood in stools or urine to her doctor.

☐ 3. Take aspirin for headaches.

☐ 4. Use a firm toothbrush.

Shara Ahmed was admitted to the hospital with chest pain and shortness of breath. She stated that she was treated for thrombophlebitis of the left thigh 3 months ago and is not taking any medicines for it. Her admitting diagnosis is possible pulmonary embolism. Her arterial blood gases on admission were: pH 7.52, Pco_2 27, HCO_3 22, ba: excess 0, Po_2 53, O_2 saturation 91%.

66. The above values suggest that on admission Mrs. Ahmed was exhibiting

☐ 1. Respiratory alkalosis.

☐ 2. Respiratory acidosis.

☐ 3. Metabolic alkalosis.

☐ 4. Metabolic acidosis.

67. By examining her arterial blood gases (ABGs), the nurse knows that Mrs. Ahmed is most probably

☐ 1. Breathing slowly and shallowly.

☐ 2. Breathing rapidly and deeply.

☐ 3. Restless and in obvious oxygen hunger.

☐ 4. Comatose.

68. Which of the following would be the most serious symptom for Mrs. Ahmed?

☐ 1. Resonance over the chest on percussion.

☐ 2. Expirations 1-2 times longer than inspirations.
☐ 3. Central cyanosis.
☐ 4. Peripheral cyanosis.

69. What is the normal ratio of P_{CO_2} to HCO_3?
☐ 1. 1:10.
☐ 2. 1:20.
☐ 3. 10:1.
☐ 4. 20:1.

Gordon McLaughlin has a history of chronic obstructive pulmonary disease, but presents with edema of the legs and feet, distended neck veins, and a large, palpable liver.

70. What is Mr. McLaughlin most likely suffering from?
☐ 1. Atelectasis.
☐ 2. Pulmonary embolus.
☐ 3. Cor pulmonale.
☐ 4. Pleurisy.

71. As the nurse enters Mr. McLaughlin's room, his oxygen is running at 6 L/min, his color is pink, and his respirations are 9/min. What is the best initial action?
☐ 1. Take his vital signs.
☐ 2. Call the physician.
☐ 3. Lower the oxygen rate.
☐ 4. Put the client in Fowler's position.

72. What is the primary purpose of instructing Mr. McLaughlin to use pursed-lip breathing?
☐ 1. Prolonged exhalation helps prevent air trapping.
☐ 2. This trains the diaphragm to aid inspiration.
☐ 3. It improves the delivery of oral and nasal inhaler medications.
☐ 4. It facilitates the movement of thick mucus.

73. Percussion is ordered for Mr. McLaughlin to facilitate the movement of thick mucus out of the lungs. In which of the following situations would percussion be *contraindicated*?
☐ 1. Hemoptysis.
☐ 2. Pneumonia.
☐ 3. Cystic fibrosis.
☐ 4. Atelectasis.

74. What would the nurse expect Mr. McLaughlin's potassium level to be?
☐ 1. Normal.
☐ 2. Elevated.
☐ 3. Low.
☐ 4. Unrelated to the pH.

Mike Pierce, a 45-year-old steel-mill worker, is admitted through the emergency room with complaints of stabbing chest pain that becomes worse with coughing, chills, diaphoresis, and rust-colored sputum. He states it came on suddenly.

75. What is the most probable diagnosis associated with these symptoms?

☐ 1. Angina.
☐ 2. Congestive heart failure.
☐ 3. Pneumonia.
☐ 4. Pulmonary edema.

76. What is very likely the causative factor of this diagnosis?
☐ 1. Chemical irritant.
☐ 2. Coronary artery disease.
☐ 3. Fluid overload.
☐ 4. Pneumococci.

77. Mr. Pierce's diagnosis is pneumonia of the right lower lobe. What would the nurse expect to find on physical assessment?
☐ 1. Bradycardia.
☐ 2. Shallow respirations.
☐ 3. Diminished breath sounds on the left.
☐ 4. Pericardial rub.

78. A chest x-ray confirms consolidation in right lower lobe. When percussing this area, what sound would the nurse most expect to hear?
☐ 1. Tympany.
☐ 2. Resonance.
☐ 3. Dullness.
☐ 4. Hyperresonance.

79. While inspecting Mr. Pierce's thorax, the nurse observes that the client is splinting. What is this?
☐ 1. Client exhales with pursed lips.
☐ 2. Client holds his chest rigid.
☐ 3. Client uses neck and shoulder muscles to exhale.
☐ 4. Client flares the nares on inspiration.

80. Which of the following would be included in a nursing plan for Mr. Pierce?
☐ 1. Cough and deep-breathe TID to minimize chest discomfort.
☐ 2. Give intermittent, positive-pressure breathing treatments without percussion to minimize chest discomfort.
☐ 3. Give 3 to 4 L of fluid a day.
☐ 4. Avoid analgesics to keep from suppressing respirations.

81. What is the major advantage of the Venturi mask ordered for Mr. Pierce?
☐ 1. It can be used while the client eats.
☐ 2. Precise high or low flow rates of oxygen can be delivered.
☐ 3. Humidification of oxygen is unnecessary.
☐ 4. It administers oxygen in concentrations of 95% to 100%.

82. Gentamicin (Garamycin), 60 mg PO q8h, is ordered for Mr. Pierce. Which of the following would the nurse monitor most closely when this drug is given?
☐ 1. BUN and serum creatinine.
☐ 2. Hemoglobin and hematocrit.
☐ 3. SGOT and SGPT.
☐ 4. PT and PTT.

83. Atelectasis develops in Mr. Pierce's right lower lobe. What is this?
    - ☐ 1. Edematous fluid in the alveoli.
    - ☐ 2. Residual consolidation.
    - ☐ 3. Purulent exudate in the pleura.
    - ☐ 4. Collapsed, airless alveoli.

84. When suctioning mucus from Mr. Pierce's lungs, which of the following nursing actions would *not* be appropriate?
    - ☐ 1. Lubricate the catheter tip.
    - ☐ 2. Use sterile technique.
    - ☐ 3. Suction 40 to 60 seconds at one time.
    - ☐ 4. Hyperoxygenate the client.

Horace Brown is skin tested for tuberculosis using PPD.

85. Which of the following types of organism causes tuberculosis?
    - ☐ 1. Bacterium.
    - ☐ 2. Fungus.
    - ☐ 3. Virus.
    - ☐ 4. Spore.

86. When the visiting nurse reads Mr. Brown's skin test, it is positive. Which of the following indicates a positive tuberculin test?
    - ☐ 1. Induration is 15 mm or larger.
    - ☐ 2. Induration is 5 to 9 mm.
    - ☐ 3. Induration is 0 to 4 mm.
    - ☐ 4. Induration is 10 mm or larger.

87. A positive reaction to PPD indicates that
    - ☐ 1. The client has active tuberculosis.
    - ☐ 2. The client has been exposed to *Mycobacterium tuberculosis.*
    - ☐ 3. The client will never have tuberculosis.
    - ☐ 4. The client has never been infected with *Mycobacterium tuberculosis.*

88. The health team meets and reviews Mr. Brown's history. Because of the positive skin test and a history of pulmonary disease, the physician prescribes oral rifampin (Rimactane) and isoniazid (INH) for at least 9 months. When informing Mr. Brown of this decision, the nurse knows that the purpose of this choice of treatment is to
    - ☐ 1. Cause less irritation to the gastrointestinal tract.
    - ☐ 2. Destroy resistant organisms and promote proper blood levels of the drugs.
    - ☐ 3. Gain a more rapid systemic effect.
    - ☐ 4. Delay resistance and increase the tuberculostatic effect.

89. Which of these occurrences in Mr. Brown would probably be indicative of an untoward effect of isoniazid (INH)?
    - ☐ 1. Purpura.
    - ☐ 2. Peripheral neuritis.
    - ☐ 3. Hyperuricemia.
    - ☐ 4. Optic neuritis.

90. To prevent the untoward effect of isoniazid (INH), another drug is added to Mr. Brown's chemotherapy. Which drug is this likely to be?
    - ☐ 1. Vitamin B_{12}.
    - ☐ 2. Vitamin B_1 (thiamin).
    - ☐ 3. Vitamin C (ascorbic acid).
    - ☐ 4. Vitamin B_6 (pyridoxine).

91. Mr. Brown is taught that a fairly common side effect of the drug rifampin (Rimactane) is
    - ☐ 1. Reddish-orange color of urine, sputum, and saliva.
    - ☐ 2. Ectopic dermatitis.
    - ☐ 3. Eighth cranial nerve damage.
    - ☐ 4. Vestibular dysfunction.

92. Mrs. Brown is skin tested for tuberculosis and has a negative result. However, because of her husband's newly diagnosed tuberculosis, the physician recommends chemotherapy for her. What is the drug of choice for preventive therapy of tuberculosis?
    - ☐ 1. Streptomycin.
    - ☐ 2. Paraaminosalicylic acid (PAS).
    - ☐ 3. Isoniazid (INH).
    - ☐ 4. Ethambutol (Myambutol).

93. Before starting on preventive drug therapy for tuberculosis, Mrs. Brown will probably receive
    - ☐ 1. Serum creatinine and BUN.
    - ☐ 2. SGOT and SGPT.
    - ☐ 3. Dexamethasone suppression test.
    - ☐ 4. Serum cortisol level.

94. Mr. Brown also received a skin test for histoplasmosis. Histoplasmosis is often mistaken for
    - ☐ 1. Lung cancer.
    - ☐ 2. Pneumonia.
    - ☐ 3. Tuberculosis.
    - ☐ 4. Bronchitis.

95. The drug of choice in the treatment of histoplasmosis is
    - ☐ 1. Isoniazid (INH).
    - ☐ 2. Amphotericin B.
    - ☐ 3. Paraaminosalicylic acid (PAS).
    - ☐ 4. Streptomycin.

Steven Nelson undergoes a left thoracotomy and a partial pneumonectomy. Chest tubes are inserted, and one-bottle water-seal drainage is instituted in the operating room.

96. Postoperatively, Mr. Nelson is placed in Fowler's position on either his right side or back in order to
    - ☐ 1. Reduce incisional pain.
    - ☐ 2. Facilitate ventilation of the left lung.
    - ☐ 3. Equalize pressure in the pleural space.
    - ☐ 4. Promote drainage by gravity.

97. Which of the following would be considered most normal within the first 24 hours postoperatively with one-bottle water-seal drainage?

☐ 1. No fluctuation in the water-seal tube.

☐ 2. Intermittent, slight bubbling from the water-seal tube.

☐ 3. Bright-red bloody drainage.

☐ 4. Orders to maintain suction at 30 cm H_2O.

98. Water-seal chest drainage involves attaching the chest tube to a

☐ 1. Bottle at a level above the bed.

☐ 2. Tube that is submerged under water.

☐ 3. Tube that is open to the air.

☐ 4. Drainage bottle.

99. Fluid oscillating in the tubing in the water-seal bottle indicates

☐ 1. The equipment is working well.

☐ 2. The chest tube is clogged.

☐ 3. The end of the tube is not under water.

☐ 4. Air has leaked into the chest cavity.

Miguel Orlando, a 50-year-old construction worker, is admitted to the unit with a tentative diagnosis of cancer of the lung.

100. Which of the following symptoms is a common, presenting symptom of bronchogenic carcinoma?

☐ 1. Dyspnea on exertion.

☐ 2. Foamy, blood-tinged sputum.

☐ 3. Wheezing sound on inspiration.

☐ 4. Cough or change in a chronic cough.

101. Several diagnostic tests have been ordered. Bronchoscopy and bronchial washings have been scheduled. When teaching Mr. Orlando what to expect postoperatively, what would be the nurse's highest priority?

☐ 1. Food and fluids will be withheld for at least 2 hours.

☐ 2. Warm saline gargles will be done q2h.

☐ 3. Coughing and deep-breathing exercises will be done q2h.

☐ 4. Only ice chips and cold liquids will be allowed for 2 hours.

102. Mr. Orlando has a left upper lobectomy. Which action by the nurse would best facilitate effective coughing and deep-breathing postoperatively?

☐ 1. Encourage him to take a day at a time and do his best to cough and deep-breathe.

☐ 2. Give him a back rub in order to relax him before coughing and deep-breathing.

☐ 3. Administer pain medication 20 minutes before coughing and deep-breathing.

☐ 4. Position him for postural drainage with cupping and vibration 10 minutes before coughing and deep-breathing.

103. What is the purpose of the long glass tube that is immersed 3 cm below the water level in Mr. Orlando's water-seal bottle?

☐ 1. To humidify the air leaving the pleural space.

☐ 2. To allow the drainage to mix with sterile water.

☐ 3. To monitor the respirations by visualizing the fluctuations.

☐ 4. To prevent atmospheric air from entering the chest tube.

104. Continuous bubbling in the water-seal bottle is observed during morning rounds. Which of the following factors best accounts for this phenomenon?

☐ 1. The system is functioning adequately.

☐ 2. There is an air leak in the system.

☐ 3. The lung has reexpanded.

☐ 4. The suction pressure is low.

105. Mr. Orlando's vital signs have been stable, and he has been alert and oriented. Today, however, he has had several periods of confusion. His physician orders arterial blood gases. The respiratory therapist draws the blood but asks the nurse to apply pressure to the area, so that she can leave and take the specimen to the lab. How long does the nurse apply pressure to the area?

☐ 1. 2 minutes.

☐ 2. 5 minutes.

☐ 3. 8 minutes.

☐ 4. 10 minutes.

106. The arterial blood gas values are pH 7.5, P_{CO_2} 33.5, P_{O_2} 45.7, oxygen saturation 86.7%. Which value is within normal limits?

☐ 1. Oxygen saturation.

☐ 2. P_{O_2}.

☐ 3. P_{CO_2}.

☐ 4. None of these values is normal.

107. At the end of the hour, Mr. Orlando's arterial blood gases are pH 7.45, P_{CO_2} 34.7, P_{O_2} 71.8, oxygen saturation 95.6%. The nurse will most likely expect Mr. Orlando to be

☐ 1. Combative.

☐ 2. Less confused.

☐ 3. More confused.

☐ 4. About the same.

John Baker, age 50, has experienced bouts of retrosternal burning and pain for 6 months. His condition has recently been diagnosed as esophagitis related to reflux of gastric contents into the esophagus with resultant mucosal injury.

108. When documenting Mr. Baker's health history, the nurse would most likely expect him to report that his symptoms are worse

☐ 1. When he is active and busy.

☐ 2. While lying down.

☐ 3. While sitting.

☐ 4. When he is upset and under stress.

109. In assessing the client's dietary habits, the nurse finds that he has increased symptoms with foods that are associated with lowered esophageal-sphincter pressure. What are those foods?

☐ 1. Poultry and yogurt.

☐ 2. Fruits and vegetables.

☐ 3. Fatty foods and chocolate.

☐ 4. High-fiber foods and vanilla.

110. Esophageal problems associated with reflux may necessitate a change in life-style such as which of the following?

☐ 1. Increase the amount of exercise.

☐ 2. Discontinue smoking and alcohol.

☐ 3. Increase body weight.

☐ 4. Raise the foot of the bed to sleep.

111. Cancer of the esophagus occurs more commonly in men over age 50 and is associated with esophageal obstructions. Which of the following statements guides the nurse's approach to client education?

☐ 1. Histologically, the cells are very malignant.

☐ 2. Symptoms develop late, and lymphatic spread occurs early.

☐ 3. Ulceration and hemorrhage occur.

☐ 4. Malnutrition and aspiration are present.

112. How can gastric regurgitation best be reduced?

☐ 1. Eat small, frequent meals; avoid overeating.

☐ 2. Have a small evening meal, followed by a bedtime snack.

☐ 3. Belch frequently.

☐ 4. Swallow air.

Vernon Crabtree, 47 years old, is admitted with a diagnosis of possible gastric ulcer.

113. Mr. Crabtree undergoes gastric endoscopy. When may food and fluids be given following this examination?

☐ 1. Upon the client's request.

☐ 2. When the gag reflex returns.

☐ 3. Within 30 minutes after the test.

☐ 4. As soon as the client returns to the ward.

114. The physician orders guaiac tests of all stools to determine the presence of

☐ 1. Hydrochloric acid.

☐ 2. Undigested food.

☐ 3. Occult blood.

☐ 4. Inflammatory cells.

115. Unlike Mr. Crabtree, the client with a duodenal ulcer is most likely to complain of pain

☐ 1. During a meal.

☐ 2. 15 minutes after eating.

☐ 3. 1 to 4 hours after meals.

☐ 4. About 30 minutes after eating.

116. When Mr. Crabtree requests a cigarette, the best response of the nurse would be which of the following?

☐ 1. One cigarette a day is all that is permitted.

☐ 2. Nicotine increases gastric acid and stomach activity.

☐ 3. Nicotine decreases gastric acid and lessens stomach activity.

☐ 4. Cigars are less harmful than cigarettes.

117. Mr. Crabtree is advised by his physician not to drink coffee. The nurse explains that coffee

☐ 1. Increases mental stress.

☐ 2. Stimulates gastric secretions.

☐ 3. Increases smooth muscle tone.

☐ 4. Elevates systolic blood pressure.

118. Mr. Crabtree does not respond to medical treatment for his peptic ulcer. He is advised to have a subtotal gastrectomy. In preparing for client teaching, the nurse knows this procedure involves removal of what?

☐ 1. Cardiac sphincter and upper half of the stomach.

☐ 2. Pyloric region of the stomach and duodenum.

☐ 3. Entire stomach and associated lymph nodes.

☐ 4. Lower one-half to two-thirds of the stomach.

119. In anticipation of clarifying information for client education, the nurse knows that vagotomy is done as part of the surgical treatment for peptic ulcers in order to

☐ 1. Decrease secretion of hydrochloric acid.

☐ 2. Improve the tone of the gastrointestinal muscles.

☐ 3. Increase blood supply to the jejunum.

☐ 4. Prevent the transmission of pain impulses.

120. Which of the following facts best explains why the duodenum is not removed during a subtotal gastrectomy?

☐ 1. The head of the pancreas is adherent to the duodenal wall.

☐ 2. The common bile duct empties into the duodenal lumen.

☐ 3. The wall of the jejunum contains no intestinal villi.

☐ 4. The jejunum receives its blood supply through the duodenum.

121. During Mr. Crabtree's immediate postoperative care, why must the nurse be particularly conscientious to encourage him to cough and deep-breathe at regular intervals?

☐ 1. Marked changes in intrathoracic pressure will stimulate gastric drainage.

☐ 2. The high abdominal incision will lead to shallow breathing to avoid pain.

☐ 3. The phrenic nerve will have been permanently damaged during the surgical procedure.

☐ 4. Deep-breathing will prevent postoperative vomiting and intestinal distension.

122. Mr. Crabtree has a nasogastric tube. It will be removed when there is

☐ 1. Inflammation of the pharyngeal mucosa.

☐ 2. Absence of bile in gastric drainage.

☐ 3. Return of bowel sounds to normal.

☐ 4. Passage of numerous liquid stools.

123. Mr. Crabtree is told about the dumping syndrome. The nurse explains to him that it is

☐ 1. The body's absorption of toxins produced by liquefaction of dead tissue.

   □ 2. Formation of an ulcer at the margin of the gastrojejunal anastomosis.

   □ 3. Obstruction of venous flow from the stomach into the portal system.

   □ 4. Rapid emptying of food and fluid from the stomach into the jejunum.

124. When administering Mr. Crabtree's medication, the nurse knows that aluminum hydroxide gel (Amphogel) is preferred to sodium bicarbonate in treating hyperacidity because, unlike sodium bicarbonate, aluminum hydroxide gel

   □ 1. Is not absorbed from the bowel.

   □ 2. Does not predispose to constipation.

   □ 3. Dissolves rapidly in all body fluids.

   □ 4. Has no effect on phosphorus excretion.

125. Which of the following statements by Mr. Crabtree about the diet protocol for the treatment of dumping syndrome would indicate a need for additional teaching?

   □ 1. "I plan to eat a diet low in carbohydrates and high in protein and fat."

   □ 2. "I plan to eat a diet high in carbohydrates and low in protein and fat."

   □ 3. "I will eat slowly and avoid drinking fluids during meals."

   □ 4. "I will try to assume a recumbent position after meals for 30 minutes to 1 hour to enhance digestion and relieve symptoms."

126. Mr. Crabtree asks the nurse how he would know if he has dumping syndrome. The nurse would include which of the following clinical symptoms when discussing dumping syndrome?

   □ 1. Explosive diarrhea, loss of appetite, nausea, and vomiting.

   □ 2. Explosive diarrhea, nausea, vomiting, and borborygmi.

   □ 3. Flushing, dizziness, diaphoresis, and hypertension.

   □ 4. Flushing, dizziness, headache, and hypertension.

127. When Mr. Crabtree is started on propantheline bromide (Pro-Banthine), the nurse monitors for the primary dose-limiting side effect of

   □ 1. Dry mouth.

   □ 2. Hiccoughs.

   □ 3. Visual blurring.

   □ 4. Urinary retention.

Don Sharp, a 17-year-old college student, is stricken with periumbilical pain while playing baseball. Because the pain increases rapidly in intensity during the next few hours, his fraternity brothers take him to the dispensary. The nurse puts Don to bed and calls the physician. The physician makes a diagnosis of acute appendicitis and orders that Don be admitted to the university hospital immediately for an emergency appendectomy.

128. Don asks why this happened today. The nurse responds with the knowledge that the most common precipitating cause of acute appendicitis is which of the following?

   □ 1. Chemical irritation by digestive juices.

   □ 2. Mechanical obstruction of the lumen of the appendix.

   □ 3. Mechanical irritation of overlying pelvic viscera.

   □ 4. Ischemic damage from mesenteric thrombosis.

129. Peritonitis resulting from rupture of an inflamed appendix is primarily the result of

   □ 1. Chemical irritation by digestive juices.

   □ 2. Bacterial contamination by intestinal organisms.

   □ 3. Mechanical pressure exerted by the distended bowel.

   □ 4. Ischemic damage from mesenteric thrombosis.

130. In order to promote capillary proliferation and formation of scar tissue, Don may be given a supplementary dose of which vitamin?

   □ 1. E.

   □ 2. B_1.

   □ 3. C.

   □ 4. D.

Tina Cortez is admitted to the hospital because of nausea and abdominal pain after having eaten a fatty meal. Her condition was diagnosed as cholelithiasis (gallstones). A cholecystectomy with common bile duct exploration is performed.

131. Mrs. Cortez has arrived in the postanesthesia room. She is semiconscious. Her vital signs are within normal limits. Which of the following nursing actions would be *inappropriate*?

   □ 1. Apply a warm blanket to her body.

   □ 2. Place her in semi-Fowler's position.

   □ 3. Attach her T-tube to gravity drainage.

   □ 4. Set up low, intermittent suction for her nasogastric tube.

132. Mrs. Cortez had an uneventful stay in the postanesthesia room and has returned to her room. She complains of abdominal pain. Her physician has ordered meperidine (Demerol), 50 to 100 mg q3h, prn for pain. Which of the following is an *inappropriate* criterion when deciding how much to administer?

   □ 1. Mrs. Cortez's vital signs.

   □ 2. Anesthetics and drugs used during surgery.

   □ 3. The amount of discomfort Mrs. Cortez is exhibiting.

   □ 4. The time and amount of any previous doses of Demerol.

133. When planning Mrs. Cortez's care for the next 24 hours, the nurse should select which of the following as the primary goal?
    □ 1. To prevent respiratory complications.
    □ 2. To assess level of consciousness.
    □ 3. To maintain range of joint motion.
    □ 4. To promote normal bowel function.

134. Which of the following would be most indicative of complications during the first 24 hours postoperatively?
    □ 1. Serous drainage on the surgical dressing.
    □ 2. Golden-colored fluid draining from the T-tube.
    □ 3. Urinary output of 20 ml/hr.
    □ 4. Body temperature of 99.8° F (37.6° C).

135. Mrs. Cortez, like many people who require a cholecystectomy, is obese. Because of her obesity, she would be most closely observed for which of the following complications?
    □ 1. Clay-colored, fatty stools.
    □ 2. Inadequate blood clotting.
    □ 3. Cardiac irregularities.
    □ 4. Delayed wound healing.

136. The nurse knows that Mrs. Cortez needs further discharge teaching if she states which of the following?
    □ 1. "I will not climb stairs for a month."
    □ 2. "I will make a follow-up appointment with my surgeon."
    □ 3. "Eating fatty foods may cause me some discomfort for awhile."
    □ 4. "Redness or swelling in the incision must be reported to my surgeon immediately."

Joan Belzer, a 45-year-old obese stockbroker and mother of three, is admitted with a diagnosis of possible cholecystitis.

137. Which of the following signs and symptoms are most likely to be included in the initial assessment of Mrs. Belzer?
    □ 1. Abdominal pain, usually in the left upper quadrant.
    □ 2. Dyspepsia following carbohydrate ingestion.
    □ 3. Fullness and eructation following protein ingestion.
    □ 4. Nausea and vomiting.

138. Mrs. Belzer is having severe pain. The physician has ordered morphine sulfate, 10 mg IM every 3 to 4 hours prn for severe pain or 6 mg IM every 3 to 4 hours prn for moderate pain. What would the nurse do?
    □ 1. Ask her if she is allergic to morphine.
    □ 2. Give 6 mg of morphine sulfate IM.
    □ 3. Give 10 mg of morphine sulfate IM.
    □ 4. Verify the order with the physician who wrote it.

139. Since Mrs. Belzer is scheduled for a cholecystogram, which of the following questions is best to ask her?
    □ 1. Are you on a low-sodium diet?
    □ 2. Have you ever had a barium study?
    □ 3. Have you ever had a nasogastric tube inserted?
    □ 4. Are you allergic to any drugs?

140. Two days later, Mrs. Belzer has a cholecystectomy and is now ready to return to her room from the recovery room. Mrs. Belzer has an IV of 5% dextrose in 0.45% normal saline infusing at 100 ml/hr, a T-tube connected to gravity drainage, and a nasogastric tube connected to low intermittent suction. What does the T-tube indicate?
    □ 1. Stones were removed from the cystic bile duct.
    □ 2. Stones were removed from the gallbladder.
    □ 3. The common bile duct was explored.
    □ 4. The cystic duct was removed.

141. During the first 2 hours postoperatively, Mrs. Belzer's nasogastric tube drains greenish liquid; then the drainage suddenly stops. What is the first action to take?
    □ 1. Irrigate it as ordered with distilled water.
    □ 2. Irrigate it as ordered with normal saline.
    □ 3. Notify her physician.
    □ 4. Reposition it.

142. Mrs. Belzer asks the nurse how long it will be before she can have something to eat. The nurse replies
    □ 1. "Are you hungry already?"
    □ 2. "Since you are slightly overweight, now would be a good time for you to begin reducing."
    □ 3. "The doctor makes that decision."
    □ 4. "Usually clients start clear liquids after active bowel sounds return and the stomach tube is removed."

143. On Mrs. Belzer's second postoperative day, the T-tube drains 30 ml during the morning shift the nurse is working. What is the best action?
    □ 1. Irrigate the T-tube with 50 ml normal saline.
    □ 2. Irrigate the T-tube with 50 ml distilled water.
    □ 3. Nothing; this is normal.
    □ 4. Notify the physician.

144. Mrs. Belzer asks when the T-tube will be removed. What would be best to tell her?
    □ 1. Usually 3 to 4 days after surgery.
    □ 2. Usually 6 to 8 days after surgery, and following an x-ray of the cystic duct.
    □ 3. Usually 10 to 12 days after surgery, and following a T-tube cholangiogram.
    □ 4. When the drainage exceeds 500 ml/day.

Joseph Morris, a 40-year-old man, is admitted to the hospital with severe left midepigastric pain and nausea and vomiting. This is his second admission for acute pancreatitis.

145. In assessing Mr. Morris, the nurse knows that common causes of pancreatitis are
    □ 1. Alcohol abuse and congestive heart failure.
    □ 2. Alcohol abuse and biliary tract disease.
    □ 3. Epileptic seizures and pancreatic fibrosis.
    □ 4. Pancreatic fibrosis and chronic obstructive pulmonary disease.

146. Which of the following is an exocrine function of the pancreas?
    □ 1. Secrete insulin and glucagon.
    □ 2. Secrete digestive enzymes.
    □ 3. Promote glucose uptake by the liver.
    □ 4. Facilitate glucose transport into the cells.

147. What is the initial treatment plan for acute pancreatitis?
    □ 1. Keep the gastrointestinal tract at rest to prevent pancreatic stimulation.
    □ 2. Provide adequate nutrition to enhance healing.
    □ 3. Prevent secondary complications such as peritonitis.
    □ 4. Maintain adequate fluid and electrolyte balance.

148. Which of the following drugs may best be used in conjunction with analgesics to decrease the pain of pancreatitis?
    □ 1. Magnesium hydroxide (Maalox).
    □ 2. Prochlorperazine (Compazine).
    □ 3. Propantheline bromide (Pro-Banthine).
    □ 4. Pancreatin (Viokase).

149. Which diagnostic test best measures the response to treatment in the client with pancreatitis?
    □ 1. Serum amylase.
    □ 2. Abdominal CAT scan.
    □ 3. Serum aspartate aminotransferase (AST).
    □ 4. Erythrocyte sedimentation rate (ESR).

Carol Hansen, age 19, is admitted to the hospital with a diagnosis of infectious hepatitis.

150. Initially, what laboratory test shows elevated values in viral hepatitis?
    □ 1. Serum ammonia.
    □ 2. Serum bilirubin.
    □ 3. Prothrombin time.
    □ 4. Serum transaminase.

151. Which of the following goals would be given highest priority during the initial hospitalization?
    □ 1. Prevent decubitus ulcers.
    □ 2. Limit physical activity.
    □ 3. Eliminate emotional stress.
    □ 4. Promote activity and diversion.

152. Which of the following diets most probably will be prescribed for Miss Hansen?
    □ 1. High fat.
    □ 2. Low sodium.
    □ 3. High calorie.
    □ 4. Low carbohydrate.

Albert Gates is a 48-year-old transient, unskilled laborer who has a 33-year history of alcohol abuse and a 12-year history of cirrhosis. He is admitted with the complaint of hematemesis and rectal bleeding. While in the emergency room, he has a bright-red emesis of approximately 400 ml, which is positive for blood. His admission diagnosis is bleeding esophageal varices with ascites. His blood pressure is 100/50 mm Hg, pulse 112, respirations 24, temperature 99° F (37.2° C) rectally. His breath smells of alcohol and he reports having drunk whiskey within the past 3 hours. He has an IV of 5% dextrose and water running at 125 ml/hr.

153. Which of the following is an *incorrect* statement about cirrhosis?
    □ 1. It is a chronic disease resulting in inflammation, degeneration, and necrosis of the liver.
    □ 2. It causes obstruction of the venous and sinusoidal channels of the liver.
    □ 3. It is frequently caused by alcohol abuse.
    □ 4. It causes decreased resistance to blood flow through the liver.

154. Mr. Gates' initial care plan would include which of the following?
    □ 1. Elicit an alcohol consumption history.
    □ 2. Obtain a social service referral.
    □ 3. Secure a visit from an Alcoholics Anonymous representative.
    □ 4. Plan for a psychiatric evaluation.

155. Which of these actions would the nurse be prepared to institute for the client who is experiencing delirium tremens?
    □ 1. Provide a dark, quiet room; restraints; and side rails.
    □ 2. Arrange a room away from the nurse's station and keep the TV on continuously.
    □ 3. Keep the client's room door closed and a bright light on in the room.
    □ 4. Provide a room with lighting that decreases shadows, and have someone in constant attendance.

156. Which of the following would most likely be observed during an assessment of Mr. Gates?
    □ 1. Spider angiomas, palmar erythema, headache, and lower abdominal pain.
    □ 2. Peripheral edema, right upper quadrant pain, hemorrhoids, and decreased urine output.
    □ 3. Hepatomegaly, decreased peripheral pulses, cool extremities, and intermittent claudication.
    □ 4. Dyspnea, pruritus, inspiratory stridor, and intermittent jaundice.

157. Which of the following laboratory results would *not* be expected with the diagnosis of cirrhosis?
    □ 1. Decreased serum folic acid and albumin.
    □ 2. Decreased platelets and increased bilirubin.
    □ 3. Decreased prothrombin time and leukocytes.
    □ 4. Elevated SGPT, SGOT, and LDH.

158. The most important pathological factor contributing to the formation of esophageal varices that the nurse needs to consider when planning care for Mr. Gates is

☐ 1. Increased platelet count.

☐ 2. Portal hypertension.

☐ 3. Increased pulmonary artery pressure.

☐ 4. Renal failure.

159. In assessing Mr. Gates, the nurse knows that portal hypertension usually does *not* cause

☐ 1. Esophageal varices.

☐ 2. Pulmonary edema.

☐ 3. Ascites.

☐ 4. Hemorrhoids.

160. Mr. Gates continues to bleed from the esophaeal varices. Before the insertion of a Sengstaken-Blakemore tube, what will the nurse need to do?

☐ 1. Check each balloon for leaks, and label all tube ports.

☐ 2. Clamp the lumen of the nasogastric tube.

☐ 3. Insert ice water into the gastric balloon.

☐ 4. Insert mercury into the esophageal balloon.

161. The nurse needs to make additional preparations before inserting the Sengstaken-Blakemore tube. Which of the following would be *inappropriate* before insertion?

☐ 1. Place the client in a high-Fowler's position.

☐ 2. Administer a neomycin enema.

☐ 3. Instruct the client about the procedure.

☐ 4. Lubricate the tube with water-soluble lubricant.

162. The tube has been inserted, and the balloons have been inflated. An *incorrect* action would be which of the following?

☐ 1. Insert a nasogastric tube above the esophageal balloon and connect it to intermittent suction.

☐ 2. Tape the tube to provide some traction and decrease movement.

☐ 3. Place the client in a supine position.

☐ 4. Tape a scissors to the bedside to be used to cut the tube in the event of severe respiratory distress.

163. Complications resulting from the use of Sengstaken-Blakemore tube can occur. For the nurse caring for Mr. Gates, the priority complication to monitor for would be

☐ 1. Ulceration of the esophagus and gastric mucosa.

☐ 2. Esophageal perforation.

☐ 3. Upward dislodgment of the gastric balloon.

☐ 4. Downward dislodgment of the esophageal balloon.

164. If Mr. Gates' bleeding is not controlled by the Sengstaken-Blakemore tube, the nurse would be prepared to administer which of the following?

☐ 1. Hydralazine (Apresoline).

☐ 2. Vasopressin (Pitressin).

☐ 3. Meprobamate (Miltown).

☐ 4. Diazepam (Valium).

165. In caring for Mr. Gates with the Sengstaken-Blakemore tube in place, which of the following actions is *inappropriate*?

☐ 1. Monitor intake and output carefully.

☐ 2. Give frequent oral hygiene.

☐ 3. Maintain bed rest.

☐ 4. Sedate client.

166. Several days later, the Sengstaken-Blakemore tube is gradually deflated and removed because Mr. Gates' bleeding has subsided. When teaching Mr. Gates about prevention of esophageal bleeding, what would he be instructed to do?

☐ 1. Eat a well-balanced, high-calorie, moderate high-protein, low-fat, low-sodium diet.

☐ 2. Eat a low-protein, high-carbohydrate diet.

☐ 3. It is OK to maintain alcohol intake if diet is balanced.

☐ 4. Eat a general diet with no restrictions.

Mr. Gates was discharged. Four months later, he is readmitted in a comatose state.

167. Knowing Mr. Gates' history, what condition would the nurse most likely suspect?

☐ 1. Brain tumor.

☐ 2. Hepatic encephalopathy.

☐ 3. Respiratory failure.

☐ 4. Parkinson's disease.

168. While caring for Mr. Gates, the nurse must consider that the most important pathophysiological factor contributing to his current state is which of the following?

☐ 1. Increased prothrombin time.

☐ 2. Portal hypertension.

☐ 3. Increased serum ammonia levels.

☐ 4. Increased serum bilirubin.

169. Mr. Gates' urine output falls below 20 ml/hr, and a central venous pressure (CVP) line is placed in his subclavian vein. What initial nursing intervention would be done after inserting, calibrating, and zeroing the line?

☐ 1. Check vital signs.

☐ 2. Check CVP reading.

☐ 3. Check his intake for the last 12 hours.

☐ 4. Measure output for 1 more hour.

170. Which of the following is an unlikely assessment for clients with a diagnosis of hepatic encephalopathy?

☐ 1. Asterixis.

☐ 2. Decreased level of consciousness.

☐ 3. Muscle twitching.

☐ 4. Exophthalmos.

171. Which of the following would the nurse be prepared to administer to Mr. Gates?

☐ 1. Neomycin and lactulose (Cephulac) enema.
☐ 2. Protein tube feeding.
☐ 3. Phenobarbital (Luminal).
☐ 4. Phenytoin sodium (Dilantin).

172. What is the therapeutic effect of the treatment in question 171?
☐ 1. To decrease muscular twitching.
☐ 2. To induce sedation.
☐ 3. To provide nutrition that promotes healing.
☐ 4. To prevent formation of ammonia.

173. In planning care for Mr. Gates, which of the following statements best describes the necessary dietary alterations?
☐ 1. High carbohydrate, protein, and fat.
☐ 2. Low protein and low fat.
☐ 3. Low carbohydrate and fat.
☐ 4. High fiber.

174. Mr. Gates' condition improves. In planning discharge health teaching, which of the following is *inappropriate* for the nurse to include?
☐ 1. The need for a balance between activity and rest.
☐ 2. How to avoid constipation.
☐ 3. What kinds of foods to avoid.
☐ 4. The need to drink 3 to 4 L of water each day.

James Yamamoto, age 45, is an unemployed carpenter who drinks heavily. He has been hospitalized on four occasions for acute alcoholism. He was admitted to the hospital after having vomited a large quantity of bright-red blood and smaller quantities of coffee-ground emesis.

175. On admission, which one of the following clinical manifestations of the client's pathological liver condition *cannot* be observed by the nurse?
☐ 1. Ascites.
☐ 2. Mild jaundice.
☐ 3. Purpuric spots on his arms and legs.
☐ 4. Esophageal varices.

176. Following are the most probable causes of Mr. Yamamoto's cirrhosis. Which has the most important implications for long-term nursing care plans?
☐ 1. Obstruction of major bile ducts.
☐ 2. Chronic ingestion of alcoholic beverages.
☐ 3. Long-term nutritional inadequacy.
☐ 4. Viral inflammation of liver cells.

177. Immediately following Mr. Yamamoto's admission to the hospital, which of the following would be provided in order to make him more comfortable?
☐ 1. Vigorous backrub.
☐ 2. Scrupulous mouth care.
☐ 3. Complete tub bath.
☐ 4. Shave and haircut.

178. The nurse anticipates that the client will experience nausea and vomiting. Which of the following an-

tiemetics would be the best to administer for the nausea and vomiting?
☐ 1. Prochlorperazine maleate (Compazine).
☐ 2. Hydroxyzine pamoate (Vistaril).
☐ 3. Hydroxyzine hydrochloride (Atarax).
☐ 4. Dimenhydrinate (Dramamine).

179. Accurate observation of Mr. Yamamoto's jaundice should be recorded, as which of the following might likely be expected to develop?
☐ 1. Hiccoughs.
☐ 2. Pruritus.
☐ 3. Anuria.
☐ 4. Diarrhea.

180. Why would Mr. Yamamoto be weighed daily?
☐ 1. To allow correction of a nutritional deficiency.
☐ 2. To monitor accumulation of edema and ascites.
☐ 3. To assess breakdown of tissue protein.
☐ 4. To monitor enlargement of the liver and spleen.

181. Because of his chronically poor physiological state, assessments and nursing actions would *not* be directed toward preventing which of the following?
☐ 1. Pneumonia.
☐ 2. Decubitus ulcers.
☐ 3. Cystitis.
☐ 4. Gynecomastia.

Larry Pearson, 38 years old, is admitted with complaints of headache, hyperhydrosis (excessive sweating), and lethargy. After extensive diagnostic tests, acromegaly is diagnosed.

182. In anticipating care of Mr. Pearson after his transsphenoid microsurgery for a small tumor, the priority nursing assessment postoperatively is to check for cerebrospinal fluid drainage from
☐ 1. The dressing anterior to the right ear.
☐ 2. The incision in the mouth between the upper gum and lip.
☐ 3. The nasal packing in the right nostril.
☐ 4. The occipital dressing.

Sara Garcia, a 19-year-old woman, is admitted to the hospital with a diagnosis of possible pituitary tumor. She has been having headaches and galactorrhea.

183. Overproduction of which of the following pituitary hormones can cause galactorrhea?
☐ 1. Follicle-stimulating hormone (FSH).
☐ 2. Estrogen.
☐ 3. Progesterone.
☐ 4. Prolactin.

184. Which of the following diagnostic tests would provide the *least* helpful information in diagnosing a pituitary tumor?
☐ 1. Hormonal assays.
☐ 2. CT scan.

☐ 3. Visual fields.

☐ 4. Serum calcium.

185. A hypophysectomy is planned for Miss Garcia. What would be the most important nursing action in the immediate postoperative period?

☐ 1. Instruct her to cough and deep-breathe.

☐ 2. Assess urinary output hourly.

☐ 3. Keep her in a supine position.

☐ 4. Perform nasotracheal suctioning frequently.

186. What long-term problem may result from having had a hypophysectomy?

☐ 1. Hypopituitarism.

☐ 2. Acromegaly.

☐ 3. Cushing's disease.

☐ 4. Diabetes mellitus.

187. Before Miss Garcia leaves the hospital, she confides to you that she is worried that she will never be able to have children. What information relative to her case is most correct?

☐ 1. The surgery has had no effect on her reproductive hormones.

☐ 2. Her sexual libido may be decreased, but not her ability to conceive.

☐ 3. A decrease in gonadal hormones is common, but replacements can be given.

☐ 4. The ovaries can function independently without the pituitary hormones.

Rose Schiller had a subtotal thyroidectomy today for removal of a nodule and is to return from the recovery room soon.

188. Which of the following questions is most important to ask Mrs. Schiller postoperatively?

☐ 1. Do you feel uncomfortable?

☐ 2. Do you have any tingling of your toes, fingers, or around your mouth?

☐ 3. Do your arms or legs seem heavier than usual?

☐ 4. Please tell me your name and where you are?

189. Which of the following positions would Mrs. Schiller be placed in when she returns from the recovery room?

☐ 1. High-Fowler's with the neck supported.

☐ 2. Left lateral recumbent with the upper part of the back supported.

☐ 3. Semi-Fowler's with the neck supported.

☐ 4. Supine with sandbags at the head.

190. Postoperatively, the nurse continues to assess for signs and symptoms of hypocalcemia. Which of the following are most indicative of incipient tetany?

☐ 1. Abdominal cramping and convulsions.

☐ 2. Dyspnea and cyanosis.

☐ 3. Positive Chvostek's and Trousseau's signs.

☐ 4. Muscular flaccidity and hypotension.

191. Which of the following pieces of equipment would be kept on hand for Mrs. Schiller?

☐ 1. An arterial line.

☐ 2. A nerve stimulator.

☐ 3. A tracheostomy set.

☐ 4. Rotating tourniquets.

192. Which of the following drugs would be readily available for Mrs. Schiller?

☐ 1. Calcitonin.

☐ 2. Calcium gluconate.

☐ 3. Calcium chloride.

☐ 4. Saturated solution of potassium iodine (SSKI).

193. Which of the following nursing actions is *inpropriate* for the postoperative thyroidectomy client?

☐ 1. Encourage minimal vocalization after surgery.

☐ 2. Support the head with at least two or three pillows.

☐ 3. Check the back of the neck for drainage.

☐ 4. Provide oral fluids as tolerated.

The nurse is preparing a care plan for Julia Canon, a 28-year-old, newly diagnosed diabetic.

194. What nursing action is vital to implementing this care plan for Miss Canon?

☐ 1. Determine if she is a ketosis-prone or a ketosis-resistant diabetic.

☐ 2. Assess her knowledge of the disease process.

☐ 3. Ask if her family has a history of diabetes.

☐ 4. Instruct Miss Canon that her life-style will never be the same.

195. Which of the following is true regarding diabetes?

☐ 1. Diabetes is an acute disorder that responds only to insulin treatment.

☐ 2. Diabetes is a curable illness.

☐ 3. Diabetes is characterized by an abnormality of carbohydrate metabolism.

☐ 4. Diabetes is not a significant cause of death in the United States.

196. The nurse's understanding of diabetes suggests that Miss Canon's symptom of polyuria is most likely caused by what physiological change?

☐ 1. Glucose, acting as a hypertonic agent, draws water from the extracellular fluid into the renal tubules.

☐ 2. Increased insulin levels promote a diuretic effect.

☐ 3. Electrolyte changes lead to the retention of sodium and potassium.

☐ 4. Microvascular changes alter the effectiveness of the kidneys.

197. The nursing care plan includes teaching Miss Canon how to prepare and give herself insulin injections. What is the most important reason for instructing her to rotate injection sites?

☐ 1. Lipodystrophy can result and is extremely painful and unsightly.

☐ 2. Poor rotation technique can cause superficial hemorrhaging.

☐ 3. Lipodystrophic areas can result, causing erratic insulin absorption rates from these areas.

☐ 4. Injection sites can never be reused.

198. Regular insulin is ordered for Miss Canon. The first dose is administered at 7:30 AM. The nurse would monitor Miss Canon for a hypoglycemic reaction at what time?

☐ 1. After breakfast.

☐ 2. After lunch.

☐ 3. After dinner.

☐ 4. After bedtime.

199. Which of the following are symptoms of hypoglycemia that the nurse would teach Miss Canon before discharge?

☐ 1. Polydipsia and polyuria.

☐ 2. Elevated urine glucose.

☐ 3. Rapid, deep respirations.

☐ 4. Rapid, shallow respirations.

200. Miss Canon is now prepared for discharge. She is concerned about continuing her aerobics program. What would the nurse suggest to her?

☐ 1. Aerobic exercise is too strenuous for diabetics.

☐ 2. An exercise program is an important part of diabetic management, when balanced with insulin and diet.

☐ 3. She should limit her activities to brisk walking.

☐ 4. Exercise increases the risk of diabetic complications (e.g., peripheral neuropathy).

Olga Schumacher, a 65-year-old woman, is admitted with the diagnosis of hyperglycemic, hyperosmolar, nonketotic coma. Her blood glucose level is 1000 mg/dl.

201. Characteristic findings of diabetes do *not* include

☐ 1. Polyuria caused by the excessive amounts of glucose in the urine.

☐ 2. Polyphagia caused by starvation at the cellular level.

☐ 3. Polydipsia caused by polyuria.

☐ 4. Weight gain caused by excessive appetite.

202. Which terms would best describe the most likely condition of Mrs. Schumacher's skin on admission?

☐ 1. Warm, flushed, and dry.

☐ 2. Cool and clammy.

☐ 3. Cool and dry.

☐ 4. Warm, pale, and clammy.

203. The highest priority of care when Mrs. Schumacher is admitted is to

☐ 1. Force fluids orally to 4 L or more per 24 hours as ordered.

☐ 2. Administer large doses of regular insulin as ordered.

☐ 3. Administer 2 to 3 L IV fluids in first 1 to 2 hours as ordered.

☐ 4. Administer large doses of NPH or Lente insulin as ordered.

204. When Mrs. Schumacher regains consciousness, she is told she has diabetes. She replies, "I might as well be dead. I'll never be able to lead a normal life again." The best response to this is

☐ 1. "After I teach you everything you need to know, you'll find out you're wrong."

☐ 2. "Don't worry. Everything will be fine."

☐ 3. "The doctor gave you some medicine that will take care of everything."

☐ 4. "You will have to do some things differently to control this disease, but you can still lead a normal life."

Martha Carter, 65 years old, has had diabetes for 10 years. The diabetes has been controlled by diet and tolbutamide (Orinase). Recently, she has complained of discomfort in her left leg.

205. The classic sign/symptom of arterial insufficiency of the lower extremities is which of the following?

☐ 1. Intermittent claudication.

☐ 2. Peripheral parasthesias.

☐ 3. Shiny, atrophic skin over the tibia.

☐ 4. Pain on dorsiflexion of the foot.

206. Promoting arterial blood flow to Mrs. Carter's feet is a nursing goal. Which nursing action would best achieve this?

☐ 1. Encourage her to dorsiflex her toes frequently.

☐ 2. Keep her feet covered with socks at all times.

☐ 3. Apply external heat to the feet.

☐ 4. Massage the feet briskly TID.

207. Mrs. Carter is scheduled for a left femoral-popliteal bypass graft. The day before surgery, she says to you, "I know this is only the beginning; soon they'll take my leg." Which response is most appropriate now?

☐ 1. "Many persons who have had this surgery have not needed an amputation."

☐ 2. "That may be a possibility some day, but don't worry about it now."

☐ 3. "I see this is worrying you. What would losing your leg mean to you?"

☐ 4. "There have been vast improvements in vascular surgery."

208. During Mrs. Carter's first few postoperative days, her diabetes can be best controlled by

☐ 1. Restarting her oral agent as soon as possible.

☐ 2. Administering an intermediate insulin daily.

☐ 3. Ensuring she eats all the food on her trays.

☐ 4. Administering short-acting insulin based on q4h blood glucose.

209. When the nurse goes into Mrs. Carter's room to give her morning care, she is very irritable and tells the nurse to get out of her room. What is the best initial action?

☐ 1. Assess her for other signs of hypoglycemia.

☐ 2. Ask her if she would like you to come back later.

☐ 3. Allow her to express her anger and stay with her.

☐ 4. Recognize that she may be confused and orient her to her surroundings.

210. While Mrs. Carter is in the hospital, the nurse reviews a diabetic diet with her. Which fact is most accurate?

☐ 1. Recent research indicates fats should be eliminated.

☐ 2. Dietetic fruits may be eaten as free foods.

☐ 3. A regular meal pattern need not be followed since she is not taking insulin.

☐ 4. Complex carbohydrates such as breads and cereals should be included in her diet.

211. Mrs. Carter is to be discharged soon. Which of the following would be *inappropriate* to include in her teaching plan?

☐ 1. Change position hourly to increase circulation.

☐ 2. Inspect feet and legs daily for any changes.

☐ 3. Keep legs elevated on two pillows while sleeping.

☐ 4. Keep the incision clean and dry.

Maria Adams, age 70, has been diagnosed with Addison's disease.

212. While completing the nursing history, the nurse anticipates that Mrs. Adams would most likely complain of

☐ 1. Weakness, decreased skin pigmentation, and weight gain.

☐ 2. Weakness, increased skin pigmentation, and weight loss.

☐ 3. Weakness, pallor, and weight loss.

☐ 4. Insomnia, weight loss, and nervousness.

213. Which action would be most appropriate when administering care to Mrs. Adams?

☐ 1. Encourage exercise.

☐ 2. Protect her from exertion.

☐ 3. Provide a variety of diversional activities.

☐ 4. Permit as much activity as she desires.

214. Which of the following nursing actions for the client with Addison's disease would be *inappropriate*?

☐ 1. Observe for fluid and electrolyte imbalances.

☐ 2. Administer varying amounts of cortisol as ordered.

☐ 3. Administer aldosterone as ordered.

☐ 4. Watch for symptoms of hypertension and tachycardia.

215. Which symptoms would alert the nurse to a deterioration in Mrs. Adams' condition (i.e., addisonian crisis)?

☐ 1. Increased blood pressure, polyuria, and pulmonary edema.

☐ 2. Increased blood pressure and oliguria.

☐ 3. Decreased blood pressure and urine output of 10 ml/hr.

☐ 4. Decreased blood pressure and urine output of 10 ml/hr.

216. Mrs. Adams will be treated with replacement glucocorticoid, cortisone, and fludrocortisone acetate (Florinef). In developing the teaching plan, the nurse identifies which of the following as *inappropriate* to include?

☐ 1. The different types and actions of medications.

☐ 2. The need to wear or carry medical alert identification of condition and medications.

☐ 3. The use of hydrocortisone IM in an emergency.

☐ 4. The need for a life-style change, even with the use of replacement medications.

Jack Thomas, a 56-year-old personnel director, is admitted for a cystoscopy. While admitting him, you learn that he has a urinary tract infection, smokes half a pack of cigarettes a day, and had a hernia repaired 20 years ago. He takes chlorothiazide (Diuril) for high blood pressure and follows a mild sodium-restricted diet.

217. Which of the following factors most increases the risk of Mr. Thomas' developing septic shock postoperatively?

☐ 1. Cystoscopy in the presence of a urinary tract infection.

☐ 2. High blood pressure.

☐ 3. Sodium-restricted diet.

☐ 4. Smoking.

218. While the nurse is preparing Mr. Thomas for the procedure, he says, "I think I'm going to die." What is an appropriate nursing response?

☐ 1. "Don't worry, your doctor is one of the best."

☐ 2. "This procedure has a very low mortality rate."

☐ 3. "What ever gave you that idea?"

☐ 4. "You think you're going to die?"

219. Mr. Thomas returns from the recovery room at 9 AM alert and oriented, with an IV infusing. His pulse is 80, blood pressure is 120/80, respirations are 20, and all are within normal range. At 10 AM and at 11 AM, his vital signs are stable. At noon, however, his pulse rate is 84, blood pressure is 110/74, and respirations are 24. What nursing action is most appropriate?

☐ 1. Increase the IV rate.
☐ 2. Notify his physician.
☐ 3. Take his vital signs again in 15 minutes.
☐ 4. Take his vital signs again in an hour.

220. Which of the following is an *early* sign of septic shock?
☐ 1. Cool, clammy skin.
☐ 2. Hypotension.
☐ 3. Increased urinary output.
☐ 4. Restlessness.

221. The nurse shows Mr. Thomas a list of foods and asks him to select any items included in his diet. His selection of which item probably indicates that he understands his dietary restrictions?
☐ 1. Beef broth.
☐ 2. Cheese.
☐ 3. Dried apricots.
☐ 4. Peanut butter.

222. Before Mr. Thomas is discharged, the nurse evaluates the effects of teaching. Which of the following statements best indicates that Mr. Thomas understands hypertension and his treatment?
☐ 1. "I only add a little salt while preparing my food, and I salt my food lightly at the table."
☐ 2. "I have blurred vision once in a while, but high blood pressure doesn't cause that."
☐ 3. "I know smoking increases my blood pressure and that I should stop, but it's very hard to do."
☐ 4. "I take my blood pressure pill whenever I get a severe headache."

During her hospitalization for a cataract extraction, Martha Cook acquires a urinary tract infection.

223. Besides instructing Mrs. Cook on how, when, and why she should take her antibiotics, the nurse knows that the most important thing Mrs. Cook needs to learn to clear the infection is which of the following?
☐ 1. To drink up to 3 L of fluid each day.
☐ 2. How to cleanse her perineum after voiding.
☐ 3. To limit fluids to increase the bacteriostatic activity of the urine.
☐ 4. To acidify the urine by drinking cranberry juice.

224. Because her urinary tract infection is still present several weeks after hospital discharge and following several courses of antibiotic therapy, she is scheduled for an intravenous pyelogram (IVP). If Mrs. Cook experiences any of the following reactions after injection of the contrast material for IVP, which one would have to be reported immediately?
☐ 1. Feeling of warmth.
☐ 2. Flushing of the face.
☐ 3. Salty taste in the mouth.
☐ 4. Urticaria.

225. The IVP reveals that Mrs. Cook has a renal calculus. She is believed to have a small stone that will pass spontaneously. To increase the chance of her passing the stone, the nurse would force fluids and do which of the following?
☐ 1. Teach her to strain all urine.
☐ 2. Have her ambulate.
☐ 3. Keep her on bed rest.
☐ 4. Give medications to relax her.

226. Which factor predisposes the development of renal calculi?
☐ 1. Bed rest for a client with multiple myeloma.
☐ 2. Use of a tilt table for a client who has a spinal cord injury.
☐ 3. Forcing fluids in a client on bed rest.
☐ 4. Decreasing calcium in the diet of a client with Paget's disease.

Randolph Parker, a 64-year-old carpenter, has a diagnosis of bladder cancer.

227. A risk factor of bladder carcinoma is
☐ 1. Cigarette smoking.
☐ 2. Family history.
☐ 3. Low-bulk diet.
☐ 4. Stress.

228. What is the most common clinical finding in carcinoma of the bladder?
☐ 1. Abdominal pain.
☐ 2. Gross, painless hematuria.
☐ 3. Palpable tumor.
☐ 4. Melena.

229. Mr. Parker is scheduled for a cystectomy with the creation of an ileal conduit in the morning. He is wringing his hands and pacing the floor when the nurse enters his room. What is the best approach?
☐ 1. "Good evening, Mr. Parker. Wasn't it a pleasant day, today?"
☐ 2. "Mr. Parker, you must be so worried, I'll leave you alone with your thoughts."
☐ 3. "Mr. Parker, you'll wear out the hospital floors and yourself at this rate."
☐ 4. "Mr. Parker, you appear anxious to me. How are you feeling about tomorrow's surgery?"

230. In addition to emotional support, range-of-motion (ROM) exercise is another nursing action that would be included in the nursing care plan for Mr. Parker. Why?
☐ 1. Ambulation will be restricted for 1 week postoperatively.
☐ 2. There is an increased risk of thrombophlebitis following pelvic surgery.
☐ 3. Cystectomies are extremely painful and limit the client's ability to move.
☐ 4. ROM helps to make the client feel he is involved in his care.

231. After surgery, Mr. Parker has a nasogastric tube in place but continues to complain of nausea. Which action would the nurse take?
- ☐ 1. Call the physician immediately.
- ☐ 2. Administer the prescribed antiemetic.
- ☐ 3. Irrigate the tube to check for patency.
- ☐ 4. Reposition the client.

232. Why is a nasogastric tube inserted postoperatively for Mr. Parker?
- ☐ 1. To administer tube feedings.
- ☐ 2. To test gastric secretions for bacteria.
- ☐ 3. To reduce the risk of paralytic ileus.
- ☐ 4. To increase the abdominal girth.

233. What color should Mr. Parker's urinary stoma be?
- ☐ 1. Brown.
- ☐ 2. Dark-red.
- ☐ 3. Light-brown.
- ☐ 4. Pink to red.

234. Mr. Parker's postoperative vital signs are a blood pressure of 80/40 mm Hg, a pulse of 140, and respirations of 32. Suspecting shock, which of the following orders would the nurse question?
- ☐ 1. Put the client in modified Trendelenburg's position.
- ☐ 2. Administer oxygen at 100%.
- ☐ 3. Monitor urine output qh.
- ☐ 4. Administer morphine 10 mg IM q3-4h.

Gwen Harris is admitted to the unit with a diagnosis of acute renal failure. This is her first hospitalization for this disease. She is awake, alert, oriented, and complaining of severe back pain and abdominal cramps. Her vital signs are blood pressure 170/100 mm Hg, pulse 110, respirations 30, and oral temperature 100.4° F (38° C). Her electrolytes are sodium 120 mEq/L, potassium 7 mEq/L; her urinary output for the first 8 hours is 50 ml.

235. Mrs. Harris is displaying signs of which electrolyte imbalance?
- ☐ 1. Hyponatremia.
- ☐ 2. Hyperkalemia.
- ☐ 3. Hyperphosphatemia.
- ☐ 4. Hypercalcemia.

236. The normal medical management of Mrs. Harris' sodium imbalance is most likely to be
- ☐ 1. Fluid restriction.
- ☐ 2. Fluid replacement.
- ☐ 3. Whole blood replacement.
- ☐ 4. Sodium replacement.

237. When taking Mrs. Harris' blood pressure, you observe the presence of Trousseau's sign. This is an indication of
- ☐ 1. Hyponatremia.
- ☐ 2. Hyperkalemia.
- ☐ 3. Hypocalcemia.
- ☐ 4. Anemia.

238. Which of the following are the most appropriate nursing actions for Mrs. Harris?
- ☐ 1. Intake and output, daily weight, and routine cardiopulmonary assessment.
- ☐ 2. Intake and output, up ad lib, and restrict fluids.
- ☐ 3. Daily weight, force fluids, and daily measurement of dependent edema.
- ☐ 4. Daily weight, up ad lib, and restrict fluids.

239. Mrs. Harris' urinary output suddenly increases to 150 ml/hr. The nurse assesses that she has entered the second phase of acute renal failure. Nursing actions throughout this phase include observation for signs and symptoms of
- ☐ 1. Hypervolemia, hypokalemia, and hypernatremia.
- ☐ 2. Hypervolemia, hyperkalemia, and hypernatremia.
- ☐ 3. Hypovolemia, hypokalemia, and hyponatremia.
- ☐ 4. Hypovolemia, hypokalemia, and hypernatremia.

Stanley Kleszewski is admitted to the hospital in acute renal failure. His symptoms include oliguria, lethargy, and elevated blood urea nitrogen (BUN).

240. Which statement best explains the elevation in his BUN?
- ☐ 1. Increased protein metabolism.
- ☐ 2. Hemolysis of red blood cells.
- ☐ 3. Damage to the kidney cells.
- ☐ 4. Decreased protein metabolism.

241. A low-protein diet is ordered for Mr. Kleszewski. What is the rationale the nurse would give the client for this type of diet?
- ☐ 1. Minimize protein breakdown.
- ☐ 2. Reduce the metabolic rate.
- ☐ 3. Decrease sodium intoxication.
- ☐ 4. Minimize the development of edema.

242. The nurse's aide assists with Mr. Kleszewski's care. Which assignment to the aide would be the nurse's priority to check?
- ☐ 1. Obtaining his vital signs.
- ☐ 2. Recording his intake and output.
- ☐ 3. Monitoring the amount of food he consumes.
- ☐ 4. Checking his bowel movements.

Wilmont Brown is admitted to the unit with the diagnosis of chronic renal failure.

243. Assessing the laboratory findings, which of the following results would you most likely expect to find on Mr. Brown?
- ☐ 1. BUN 10 to 30 mg/dl, potassium 4.0 mEq/L, creatinine 0.5 to 1.5 mg/dl.
- ☐ 2. Decreased serum calcium, blood pH 7.2, potassium 6.5 mEq/L.

3. BUN 15 mg/dl, increased serum calcium, creatinine 1.0 mg/dl.

4. BUN 35 to 40 mg/dl, potassium 3.5 mEq/L, pH 7.35, decreased serum calcium.

244. A likely cause of Mr. Brown's decreased serum calcium is
    1. Poor nutritional intake of calcium.
    2. Poor vitamin D intake.
    3. Elevated serum phosphorus.
    4. Elevated serum potassium.

245. Mr. Brown starts having Kussmaul's respirations. Which of the following statements best describes the rationale for this occurrence?
    1. The kidneys cannot excrete the hydrogen ion or reabsorb bicarbonate.
    2. The kidneys cannot excrete the bicarbonate ion or reabsorb the hydrogen ion.
    3. The kidneys are unable to excrete the potassium ion, resulting in acidosis.
    4. The kidneys are unable to excrete sodium and phosphorus, resulting in alkalosis.

246. Laboratory studies on Mr. Brown reveal hyperkalemia, the most serious electrolyte problem associated with renal failure. Hyperkalemia occurs for all but one of the following reasons. Which explanation is *not* accurate?
    1. Hyperkalemia results from failure of the excretory ability of the kidneys.
    2. Hyperkalemia results from the breakdown of the cellular protein that releases potassium.
    3. Hyperkalemia results from acidosis, which causes the shift of potassium from the intracellular to the extracellular space.
    4. Hyperkalemia results from decreased serum calcium because these electrolytes are inversely related.

247. Which of the following drugs would be *ineffective* in lowering Mr. Brown's serum potassium level?
    1. Glucose and insulin.
    2. Polystyrene sulfonate (Kayexalate).
    3. Calcium gluconate.
    4. Aluminum hydroxide.

248. Peritoneal dialysis is considered as a possible means of treatment for Mr. Brown. Which of the following is the main *disadvantage* of peritoneal dialysis?
    1. Vascular access is required.
    2. The possibility of contracting hepatitis is great.
    3. It is a slow method of treatment.
    4. Fluid and electrolyte exchange is gradual.

249. The most common and severe complication that requires assessment during peritoneal dialysis is
    1. Respiratory distress.
    2. Peritonitis.
    3. Hemorrhage.
    4. Abdominal pain.

250. The physicians decide against peritoneal dialysis for Mr. Brown. Treatment with hemodialysis is ordered and an external shunt is created. Which of the following nursing actions would be of highest priority with regard to the external shunt?
    1. Heparinize it daily.
    2. Avoid taking blood pressure measurements or blood samples from the affected arm.
    3. Change the Silastic tube daily.
    4. Instruct the client not to use the affected arm.

251. During the hemodialysis procedure, Mr. Brown complains of nausea, vomits, and is disoriented. Which of the following would be the first nursing action?
    1. Slow the rate of dialysis.
    2. Administer protamine zinc.
    3. Reassure the client; anxiety frequently accompanies the procedure.
    4. Place the client in Trendelenburg's position.

Fredrick Rasmussen is a 69-year-old retired salesman. He is admitted with a diagnosis of urinary retention. His physician immediately inserts a Foley catheter. While being admitted, Mr. Rasmussen tells the nurse that he is going to have his prostate "shaved," because it is enlarged.

252. Which of the following parameters would be monitored throughout Mr. Rasmussen's preoperative period?
    1. Fluid intake.
    2. Intake and output.
    3. Urinary output.
    4. Urinary pH.

253. Mr. Rasmussen is scheduled for a transurethral resection of the prostate (TURP) tomorrow. During preoperative teaching, he asks where his incision will be. What is the most appropriate response?
    1. "The incision is made in the abdomen."
    2. "The incision is made in the lower abdomen."
    3. "The incision is made in the perineum between the scrotum and the rectum."
    4. "There is no incision. The doctor inserts an instrument through the urethra, the opening in the penis."

254. When Mr. Rasmussen returns from the recovery room, he has an IV infusing at 100 ml/hr, a three-way Foley catheter in place, and constant bladder irrigation. What would the nurse do first when increased blood in the urine is detected?
    1. Increase the speed of the irrigation.
    2. Release the traction on the Foley.
    3. Irrigate the catheter manually.
    4. Notify the physician.

255. Mr. Rasmussen complains of pain and bladder spasms. Which of the following nursing actions is

most appropriate after determining that the drainage system is patent?

☐ 1. Administer narcotics plus anticholinergic drugs, as ordered.
☐ 2. Help him to a sitz bath.
☐ 3. Decrease the speed of the irrigation.
☐ 4. Decrease the traction on the Foley.

256. Nursing strategies can help prevent which of the following complications associated with a transurethral resection of the prostate (TURP)?

☐ 1. Epididymitis.
☐ 2. Incontinence.
☐ 3. Osteitis pubis.
☐ 4. Thrombophlebitis.

257. Which of the following would be included in the discharge teaching for Mr. Rasmussen?

☐ 1. "Avoid straining at stools."
☐ 2. "Avoid heavy lifting for approximately 2 weeks after surgery."
☐ 3. "Drive your car whenever you are ready to do so."
☐ 4. "Refrain from sexual intercourse for 12 weeks."

258. Which of the following statements indicates that Mr. Rasmussen understands his discharge instruction?

☐ 1. "I know my urine may be slightly pink-tinged."
☐ 2. "I know my urine should be clear all the time."
☐ 3. "I know my urine should be clear most of the time."
☐ 4. "I'll let my doctor know if I have any urinary dribbling."

John Halston, a retired bank manager, is admitted for evaluation of an enlarged prostate.

259. Which of the following is a common early symptom of prostate hypertrophy?

☐ 1. Difficulty urinating.
☐ 2. Impotence.
☐ 3. Urinary infection.
☐ 4. Hematuria.

260. The physician wants to examine Mr. Halston's prostate gland. What equipment will be necessary for the exam?

☐ 1. A Foley catheter.
☐ 2. Lubricant and gloves.
☐ 3. Urethral dilators.
☐ 4. A rectal tube.

261. Mr. Halston is scheduled to have an IV pyelogram (IVP) and cystoscopy. What nursing measure is essential to prepare him for the IVP?

☐ 1. Force fluids before the exam.
☐ 2. Insert a Foley catheter.
☐ 3. Administer cleansing enemas.
☐ 4. Administer iopanoic acid (Telepaque) tablets the evening before.

262. Mr. Halston undergoes a transurethral resection of the prostate (TURP) under spinal anesthesia. He returns to his room with continuous bladder irrigation (CBI). Which of these statements best explains the reason for the CBI?

☐ 1. To decrease bladder atony.
☐ 2. To remove blood clots from the bladder.
☐ 3. To maintain patency of the urethral catheter.
☐ 4. To dilute the concentrated urine.

263. The nursing assistant reports to the nurse that Mr. Halston is confused. "He keeps saying he has to urinate, but he has a catheter in place." Which of the following responses would be most appropriate for the nurse to make?

☐ 1. "His catheter is probably plugged. I'll irrigate it shortly."
☐ 2. "He may be confused. What else did he say or do?"
☐ 3. "That may be a sign of internal bleeding."
☐ 4. "The urge to urinate is usually caused by the catheter. He may also have bladder spasms."

264. Which of the following symptoms can be expected temporarily when Mr. Halston's Foley catheter is removed?

☐ 1. Urgency.
☐ 2. Dribbling.
☐ 3. Urinary retention.
☐ 4. Decreased urinary output.

Rennie Lacona, age 78, is admitted to the hospital with the diagnosis of benign prostatic hypertrophy (BPH). He is scheduled for a transurethral resection of the prostate (TURP).

265. When planning for Mr. Lacona's care, which of the following is *not* important to consider when evaluating his ability to withstand surgery?

☐ 1. Age.
☐ 2. Nutritional status.
☐ 3. Race.
☐ 4. Function of the involved area.

266. It would be *inappropriate* to include which of the following points in preoperative teaching?

☐ 1. TURP is the most common operation for BPH.
☐ 2. An explanation of the purpose and function of a 2-way irrigation system.
☐ 3. Expectation of bloody urine, which will clear as healing takes place.
☐ 4. He will be pain free.

267. If a client has had a perineal prostatectomy, which of the following is the most appropriate during the postoperative period?

☐ 1. Take rectal temperatures, not only to determine body temperature, but also to note the adequacy of perineal circulation.

☐ 2. A Foley catheter with a 30-ml inflation bag is used to promote hemostasis.

☐ 3. For comfort, have the client sit on a semiinflated air ring.

☐ 4. Have the client sit on a hard surface to support the perineal incision.

268. Which of the following is *inappropriate* to include in the nursing plan in the immediate postoperative period?

☐ 1. Monitor for signs and symptoms of shock (e.g., vital signs, level of consciousness).

☐ 2. Monitor for hemorrhage.

☐ 3. Observe patency of the catheter, color of the drainage.

☐ 4. Assess sexual potency.

269. Which of the following daily nursing actions would be *inappropriate* to include?

☐ 1. Position the catheter to drain freely.

☐ 2. Encourage adequate amount of fluids unless contraindicated by preexisting problems.

☐ 3. Ambulate the client.

☐ 4. Measure I&O.

270. Which one of the following is the most common complication following a prostatectomy that has implications for nursing assessment and intervention?

☐ 1. Urinary tract infection.

☐ 2. Cardiac arrest.

☐ 3. Pneumonia.

☐ 4. Thrombophlebitis.

271. When doing discharge planning for Mr. Lacona, what would be the high priority?

☐ 1. Diet.

☐ 2. Fluid restriction.

☐ 3. Bladder training.

☐ 4. Resumption of sexual relations.

Heidi Papps is a 25-year-old woman who has been experiencing intermittent bouts of diarrhea for the past 2 years. This condition has become increasingly worse for the past 2 months. She is seeking medical attention, because her self-medication program is no longer working. Miss Papps is admitted to the hospital for diagnostic testing.

272. Which of the following is the most appropriate when preparing a client for a proctosigmoidoscopy?

☐ 1. On the morning of the examination administer enemas until the returns are clear.

☐ 2. Maintain the client NPO for 24 hours preceding the examination.

☐ 3. Give a strong cathartic on both the evening before and the morning of the examination.

☐ 4. Give sitz baths three times daily for 3 days preceding the examination.

273. What position is best for a client during a proctoscopic examination?

☐ 1. Prone.

☐ 2. Right Sims'.

☐ 3. Lithotomy.

☐ 4. Knee-chest.

274. Which nursing response is the most appropriate when preparing a client for a proctosigmoidoscopy?

☐ 1. "You need have no anxiety concerning this procedure. You will experience no pain or discomfort."

☐ 2. "You will experience a feeling of pressure and the desire to move your bowels during the brief time that the scope is in place."

☐ 3. "You can reduce your discomfort during the procedure to a minimum by bearing down as the proctoscope is introduced."

☐ 4. "You will experience no discomfort during the procedure, because a topical anesthetic will be applied to the anus."

275. The physician wants a stool sample to check for amoebae. What is the correct procedure for obtaining a stool specimen for examination for amoebae?

☐ 1. Deliver the specimen immediately to the laboratory while still warm and fresh.

☐ 2. Mix the specimen with chlorinated lime solution before taking it to the laboratory.

☐ 3. Refrigerate the specimen until it is picked up by a laboratory technician.

☐ 4. Store the specimen in a warm water bath until time for delivery to the laboratory.

276. The tests confirm Miss Papps has ulcerative colitis. Which of the following is most characteristic of the stools in ulcerative colitis?

☐ 1. Diarrhea with blood and mucus.

☐ 2. Clay-colored with blood and mucus.

☐ 3. Gray and foamy.

☐ 4. Semisolid, green with blood and mucus.

277. Miss Papps' prothrombin time is considerably lowered. This most likely indicates

☐ 1. Decreased absorption of vitamin K.

☐ 2. Decreased absorption of vitamin C.

☐ 3. Decreased absorption of protein and potassium.

☐ 4. Decreased absorption of sodium, potassium, chloride, and fats.

278. Opiates and anticholinergic drugs are ordered for Miss Papps during her initial hospitalization, primarily to decrease

☐ 1. Acute intestinal hypermotility and spasms.

☐ 2. Gastric secretions.

☐ 3. Irritability and nervousness.

☐ 4. Pain.

279. Miss Papps does not respond to therapy. A colectomy and ileostomy are proposed. This surgery involves which of the following?

☐ 1. Removal of the rectum with a portion of the colon brought through the abdominal wall.

□ 2. Removal of the colon with a portion of the ileum brought through the abdominal wall.

□ 3. Removal of the ileum with a portion of the colon brought through the abdominal wall.

□ 4. A "pull-through" procedure.

280. Which of the following is *not* anticipated after this type of surgery?

□ 1. Weight gain.

□ 2. Liquid stool.

□ 3. Reestablishment of a regular bowel pattern.

□ 4. Irritation of the skin around the stoma.

Abel Hawkins, a 47-year-old computer programmer, is admitted with a suspected small-bowel obstruction. He is 5 feet 7 inches tall and weighs 210 pounds. An IV of 5% dextrose in 0.45% saline with 20 mEq KCl is to infuse at 150 ml/hr. A nasogastric tube is inserted and connected to continuous, medium suction; it immediately begins to drain large amounts of gastric drainage.

281. While taking a nursing history from Mr. Hawkins, the nurse would particularly monitor for an indication of a predisposition to bowel malignancy. Which disease of the bowel does *not* indicate such a predisposition?

□ 1. Hemorrhoids.

□ 2. Colitis.

□ 3. Amebiasis.

□ 4. Polyps.

282. When examining Mr. Hawkins' abdomen, which technique is performed last?

□ 1. Auscultation.

□ 2. Inspection.

□ 3. Palpation.

□ 4. Percussion.

283. Which of the following factors is most consistent with a small-bowel obstruction?

□ 1. Diarrhea with blood and mucus.

□ 2. Increased flatus.

□ 3. Malnutrition.

□ 4. Projectile vomiting.

284. What is the major problem for Mr. Hawkins if the intestinal blood supply is *not* compromised?

□ 1. Alteration in body image.

□ 2. Decreased tissue perfusion.

□ 3. Fluid and electrolyte deficiency.

□ 4. Pain.

285. Mr. Hawkins has a Miller-Abbott tube inserted in an effort to relieve the bowel obstruction. Which of the following is contraindicated?

□ 1. Position the client on his right side until the tube passes the pyloric sphincter.

□ 2. Tape the client's tube securely to the nose.

□ 3. Connect the tube to suction.

□ 4. Give mouth and nose care after any manipulation.

286. If Mr. Hawkins needed emergency surgery, thus precluding thorough preoperative teaching, which of the following would be the most important for the nurse to review with Mr. Hawkins?

□ 1. Deep-breathing exercises.

□ 2. Painless movement from side to side.

□ 3. Relaxation techniques.

□ 4. Use of an IPPB machine.

Orville Kaufman, a 54-year-old business executive, was admitted for severe abdominal pain, nausea, and vomiting. His abdomen was rigid and tender to the touch; there were no bowel sounds, and his temperature was 101° F (38.3° C) rectally. Mr. Kaufman has a 4-year history of diverticulitis for which he has been treated medically. On admission, he needed emergency surgery for a ruptured diverticulum. It is now 3 days after surgery, and he has a transverse colostomy.

287. Based upon the location of the colostomy, the nurse would most likely expect that Mr. Kaufman's normal stool consistency would be

□ 1. Liquid.

□ 2. Semiformed.

□ 3. Well formed.

□ 4. Hard and solid.

288. When teaching Mr. Kaufman how to irrigate his colostomy, which of the following points is *incorrect* to include?

□ 1. Use a catheter with a shield or cone.

□ 2. Hang the irrigation reservoir about 18 to 24 inches above the stoma.

□ 3. Irrigate twice a day until regulated, then decrease to once a day.

□ 4. Clear all air from the tubing before irrigation.

289. Skin care around the stoma is critical. In performing Mr. Kaufman's skin care, which of the following is *contraindicated?*

□ 1. Observe for any excoriated areas.

□ 2. Use karaya paste and rings around the stoma.

□ 3. Apply mineral oil to the area for moisture.

□ 4. Clean the area daily with soap and water before applying the bag.

290. Regulation of Mr. Kaufman's colostomy will be most enhanced if he

□ 1. Eats balanced meals at regular intervals.

□ 2. Irrigates after lunch each day.

□ 3. Restricts exercise to walking only.

□ 4. Eats fruit at all three meals.

291. When helping Mr. Kaufman to accept his colostomy, which of the following actions is *inappropriate?*

□ 1. Encourage him to look at the stoma.

□ 2. Emphasize his positive attributes.

□ 3. Involve the family in his care.

□ 4. Have him do his own irrigations right from the start.

The surgeon informs Jeff Oakes that he has cancer of the rectum and advises that he undergo surgery for the removal of the rectum and formation of a permanent colostomy.

292. A gastric suction tube was inserted before Mr. Oakes was sent to surgery, in order to
  □ 1. Facilitate administration of high caloric, nutritious liquids immediately after completion of the procedure.
  □ 2. Prevent accumulation of gas and fluid in the stomach both during and following surgical action.
  □ 3. Provide a reliable means of detecting gastrointestinal hemorrhage during the operative procedure.
  □ 4. Serve as a stimulus to restore normal peristaltic movement following recovery from anesthesia.

293. What is the primary purpose of inserting an indwelling Foley catheter before taking Mr. Oakes to the operating room?
  □ 1. To facilitate distension of the bladder with saline during surgery.
  □ 2. To provide a ready check for renal function throughout surgery.
  □ 3. To reduce the possibility of bladder injury during the procedure.
  □ 4. To prevent contamination of the operative field resulting from incontinence.

294. Sections of colon both above and below the site of tumor were removed in order to prevent
  □ 1. Direct extension and metastatic spread of the tumor.
  □ 2. Postoperative paralysis and distension of the bowel.
  □ 3. Accidental loosening of bowel sutures postoperatively.
  □ 4. Pressure injury to the perineal suture line.

295. When considering whether Mr. Oakes will receive tube feedings postoperatively, the nurse remembers tube feedings are designed to provide adequate nutrition for all of the following clients *except*
  □ 1. Those who have difficulty in swallowing.
  □ 2. Those who are comatose.
  □ 3. Those who do not have a functioning gastrointestinal tract.
  □ 4. Those who are anorexic.

296. How would the nurse prepare Mr. Oakes for the first irrigation of his colostomy?
  □ 1. Explain that the procedure will be short and painless.
  □ 2. Give him a pamphlet to read that outlines the procedure.
  □ 3. Talk with his spouse.
  □ 4. Show him pictures, and have him talk to a person with a well-regulated colostomy.

297. Which of the following would be best suited for irrigation of Mr. Oakes' colostomy?
  □ 1. 10% saline solution.
  □ 2. Mild soap solution.
  □ 3. Warm tap water.
  □ 4. Dilute hydrogen peroxide.

298. Which of the following is the most likely to promote success when Mr. Oakes is irrigating his colostomy?
  □ 1. Size of the stoma.
  □ 2. Excitement.
  □ 3. Hunger.
  □ 4. Relaxation.

Alan Simms, a 56-year-old accountant, is admitted to the hospital with a tentative diagnosis of cancer of the colon.

299. The symptoms of colon cancer vary depending on where in the colon the lesion is located. Which would *not* be a classic symptom of colon cancer?
  □ 1. Change in bowel habits.
  □ 2. Excessive flatus.
  □ 3. Pain on the right side.
  □ 4. Anorexia and nausea.

300. Which of the following diagnostic tests will confirm the diagnosis of colon cancer most conclusively?
  □ 1. Carcinoembryonic antigen (CEA).
  □ 2. Barium enema.
  □ 3. Biopsy of the lesion.
  □ 4. Stool examination.

301. Mr. Simms is found to have a lesion of the distal sigmoid colon and rectum. An abdominoperineal resection is planned. A bowel preparation is begun. After Mr. Simms has received three doses of neomycin, he complains of frequent stools. What would the nursing action be?
  □ 1. See if there is an order for antidiarrheal medication.
  □ 2. Explain to Mr. Simms that this is the desired result.
  □ 3. Ask Mr. Simms to record his stools.
  □ 4. Withhold the laxative that was ordered as part of the prep.

302. Mr. Simms and his wife have been taught about the nature of the surgery. The nurse asks Mr. Simms to repeat what he has learned. Which of the statements most indicates the need for follow-up by the nurse?
  □ 1. "Maybe my colostomy won't have to be permanent."
  □ 2. "My perineal wound may not be healed when I go home."
  □ 3. "I will be able to have normal bowel movements from my colostomy."
  □ 4. "I will have three incisions."

303. Mr. Simms recovers from surgery. He is scheduled to return to the hospital in a month for a course of chemotherapy. Before leaving, he says to you, "I'm not sure I want to come back. Maybe I'll just take my chances." What would be the best response?
   □ 1. "It is your decision, and you should do what you feel is right."
   □ 2. "What concerns you the most about coming back?"
   □ 3. "Have you discussed this with your wife and doctor?"
   □ 4. "The survival rate with adjuvant chemotherapy is quite high."

304. Mr. Simms is to be started on a regimen of 5-fluorouracil (5-FU). During the time that he is receiving this drug, it is most important to
   □ 1. Force fluids to maintain a good output.
   □ 2. Practice good asepsis to prevent him from getting an infection.
   □ 3. Give frequent mouth care with lemon swabs.
   □ 4. Monitor his blood pressure during drug administration.

Aretha Gamble, a 65-year-old retired teacher, is admitted for tests. Her major complaints include crampy, lower left abdominal pain and frequent, bloody stools with mucus.

305. Which of the following diagnoses is likely to manifest the above signs and symptoms?
   □ 1. Appendicitis.
   □ 2. Cholecystitis.
   □ 3. Diverticulitis.
   □ 4. Pancreatitis.

306. When assessing Mrs. Gamble, the nurse would observe for
   □ 1. Jaundice and clay-colored stools.
   □ 2. Rigid, tender abdomen and absence of bowel sounds.
   □ 3. Nausea, vomiting, and pruritus.
   □ 4. Dyspnea and chest pain.

307. Which of the following diagnostic examinations is most likely to be ordered for Mrs. Gamble?
   □ 1. Lower gastrointestinal series, barium enema, and colonoscopy.
   □ 2. Upper gastrointestinal series, and gastric analysis.
   □ 3. Cholecystogram and abdominal CT scan.
   □ 4. Schilling test and sigmoidoscopy.

308. Mrs. Gamble receives a diagnosis of diverticulitis. Before her discharge, which of the following would be *inappropriate* to include in a teaching session?
   □ 1. Practice stress-management techniques.
   □ 2. Eat a high-residue diet.

   □ 3. Take psyllium hydrophilic mucilloid (Metamucil).
   □ 4. Eat foods that are highly refined.

Peggy Swan, a 52-year-old woman, is admitted to the emergency room in an unconscious state. She is accompanied by a friend. Mrs. Swan passed out while shopping. The nurse notes that she is exhibiting Biot's respirations, her color is fair, blood pressure is 120/80, temperature is 99.6° F (37.5° C) rectally, and there are no cuts or bruises. Her pupils react sluggishly to light and are unequal. The friend informs the nurse that Mrs. Swan has a history of hypertension and complained of a headache while they were shopping.

309. What action would the nurse do first?
   □ 1. Prepare a lumbar puncture setup.
   □ 2. Insert a Levin tube.
   □ 3. Start an IV after taking a blood sample to check her glucose level.
   □ 4. Send her to x-ray for a chest film.

310. Routine procedure for an unconscious client who has just been admitted would include
   □ 1. Vital signs q15min until stable.
   □ 2. Lumbar puncture.
   □ 3. Emergency tracheostomy.
   □ 4. Nasogastric tube insertion, flexing client's neck to close the epiglottis.

311. Unequal pupillary light reflexes in the unconscious client are *not* likely to be a symptom of
   □ 1. Ketoacidosis.
   □ 2. Brain contusion.
   □ 3. Epidural hematoma.
   □ 4. Brain tumor.

312. Biot's respirations can be best described as
   □ 1. Shallow, then increasingly deep, in a pattern, with periods of apnea.
   □ 2. Extremely slow and fairly regular.
   □ 3. Several short breaths followed by irregular periods of apnea.
   □ 4. Rapid and deep.

313. Mrs. Swan now is displaying decerebrate posturing in response to pressure on the trapezius muscle. Decerebrate posturing is exhibited by which of the following?
   □ 1. Extension of lower and upper extremities.
   □ 2. Extension of lower and flexion of upper extremities.
   □ 3. Flexion of lower and upper extremities.
   □ 4. Flexion of lower extremities and extension of upper extremities.

314. The most likely cause of Mrs. Swan's condition is
   □ 1. Meningitis.
   □ 2. Intracranial hematoma.
   □ 3. Diabetic ketoacidosis.
   □ 4. Cerebral concussion.

315. Mrs. Swan is scheduled for a craniotomy. What is the most important aspect of her preoperative care?
    ☐ 1. Notify her relatives.
    ☐ 2. Assess and establish a neurological baseline.
    ☐ 3. Obtain a complete history and physical.
    ☐ 4. Find out where the lesion is located.

316. What will be most important to include in Mrs. Swan's postoperative nursing?
    ☐ 1. Maintenance of adequate respiratory function.
    ☐ 2. Frequent pupil and neurological checks.
    ☐ 3. Dressing checks q8h.
    ☐ 4. Vital signs q4h.

317. Mrs. Swan's breathing is assisted by a respirator, and she requires suctioning. She has been lying on her right side for 2 hours. The nurse would follow which of the following procedures?
    ☐ 1. Turn her to her other side, then suction her.
    ☐ 2. Suction her, then turn her.
    ☐ 3. Turn her to her back, then suction her.
    ☐ 4. Just suction her; position does not affect the procedure.

318. Which of the following is the most correct statement?
    ☐ 1. If an endotracheal tube is to be left in for an extended time, a tracheostomy is usually performed.
    ☐ 2. An IPPB machine may be used for ventilation in cardiopulmonary resuscitation.
    ☐ 3. Stroking the trachea helps inhibit coughing.
    ☐ 4. Postural drainage should be performed immediately following meals.

319. Which of the following steps would be *inappropriate* when suctioning a client?
    ☐ 1. Use a sterile catheter.
    ☐ 2. Instruct the client to cough before inserting the catheter into the trachea.
    ☐ 3. Instill 1 to 3 ml sterile normal saline into the trachea, if secretions are thick.
    ☐ 4. Suction the trachea after suctioning the mouth.

320. Which of the following is most correct about cuffed tracheostomy tubes?
    ☐ 1. Deflate the cuff before suctioning.
    ☐ 2. Suction the pharynx before the cuff is deflated.
    ☐ 3. A hissing sound is desirable.
    ☐ 4. Sterile normal saline is used to inflate the cuff.

321. Complications of tracheostomy tubes include all the following *except*
    ☐ 1. Tracheal stenosis.
    ☐ 2. Tracheoesophageal fistula.
    ☐ 3. Pulmonary infections.
    ☐ 4. Xerostomia.

322. If the client "fights" the respirator, which of the following actions would *not* be appropriate?
    ☐ 1. Remove the respirator, ventilate with an Ambu-bag, and then reinstate the respirator.
    ☐ 2. Check the respiratory rate and air flow.

    ☐ 3. Give morphine sulfate or muscle relaxants as ordered.
    ☐ 4. Restrain the client.

323. Which group of drugs does *not* cause respiratory depression?
    ☐ 1. Sedatives.
    ☐ 2. Tranquilizers.
    ☐ 3. Antiinflammatories.
    ☐ 4. Narcotics.

During the first 8 hours following a head injury, Jack Water, age 25, excretes 3000 ml urine; his fluid intake has been 800 ml, and no diuretics have been given.

324. The above clinical signs are probably indicative of
    ☐ 1. Cerebral edema.
    ☐ 2. Diabetes insipidus.
    ☐ 3. Cerebral contusion.
    ☐ 4. Cerebral concussion.

325. The affected area of Mr. Water's brain is probably the
    ☐ 1. Anterior pituitary lobe.
    ☐ 2. Cerebral cortex.
    ☐ 3. Posterior pituitary lobe.
    ☐ 4. Thalamus.

326. Although not immediately life threatening, the condition from which Mr. Water is suffering, if not treated, will lead to
    ☐ 1. Increased intracranial pressure.
    ☐ 2. Hypovolemia and electrolyte imbalance.
    ☐ 3. Cerebral infection.
    ☐ 4. Retrograde amnesia.

327. What would you expect the specific gravity of Mr. Water's urine to be?
    ☐ 1. Low.
    ☐ 2. High.
    ☐ 3. Normal.
    ☐ 4. Variable.

Elizabeth Allen, 88 years old, is admitted to the hospital with the diagnosis of a head injury. She fell and hit her head after suffering a transient ischemic attack (TIA).

328. The admitting nurse, after completing her assessment, notes all of the following. Which one is *not* commonly found in clients who have suffered a TIA?
    ☐ 1. Paresthesias.
    ☐ 2. Vertigo.
    ☐ 3. Tachycardia.
    ☐ 4. Disorientation.

329. In planning care, the nurse knows that noninvasive diagnostic tests may be ordered to evaluate the TIAs. Which one of the following is considered an invasive test?

□ 1. Electroencephalogram.
□ 2. CT scan.
□ 3. Echoencephalogram.
□ 4. Arteriogram.

330. Three days after Mrs. Allen's admission, the nurse assesses a change in her behavior. She is easily distracted and unable to concentrate. Her recent memory is failing. She is more confused, combative, and abusive. This behavior most likely stems from an injury or defect in which lobe of the brain?
□ 1. Temporal.
□ 2. Frontal.
□ 3. Occipital.
□ 4. Parietal.

331. What would be the best nursing approach for Mrs. Allen at this time?
□ 1. Devise a reorientation program.
□ 2. Request a psychiatric consultation.
□ 3. Decrease the environmental stimuli.
□ 4. Assign someone to stay with her, and implement safety precautions.

Emma Brandt, 59 years old, is eating dinner when she suddenly is unable to lift her fork or speak clearly. Her husband rushes her to the hospital, where the examining physician finds her to be unconscious and diagnoses her condition as a cerebrovascular accident (CVA).

332. While caring for Mrs. Brandt during her unconscious, acute stage, the nurse routinely assesses her status. Which is the most important assessment the nurse would make?
□ 1. Patency of airway and adequacy of respirations.
□ 2. Pupillary reflexes.
□ 3. Level of awareness.
□ 4. Response to sensory stimulation, such as a pinprick on a lower extremity.

333. On admission, Mrs. Brandt's vital signs were temperature 99.4° F (37.4° C), pulse 97, respirations 27, blood pressure 260/140 mm Hg. Based on these assessments, what is the most probable cause of the CVA?
□ 1. Obesity.
□ 2. Kidney disease.
□ 3. Hypertension.
□ 4. Hypercholesterolemia.

334. Which of the following best represent assessment priorities during Mrs. Brandt's admission process?
□ 1. Religion, marital status, insurance.
□ 2. Level of consciousness, vital signs, motor function.
□ 3. Medical and social history.
□ 4. Vital capacity of the lungs.

335. When preparing a bed and equipment for Mrs. Brandt's use, which one of the following is most important to include?

□ 1. Footboard.
□ 2. Suction machine.
□ 3. Bed-linen cradle.
□ 4. Sandbags and trochanter rolls.

336. Why should Mrs. Brandt receive frequent mouth care?
□ 1. She will experience severe thirst during the time that she is unable to take liquids orally.
□ 2. Her oral mucosa will become dried and cracked because of mouth breathing during coma.
□ 3. Her mouth may contain dried blood from having bitten her tongue or lips during a seizure.
□ 4. Tactile stimulation of the tongue and buccal mucosa will facilitate the return of consciousness.

337. While Mrs. Brandt is hospitalized, the nurse is concerned with preventing the complications of prolonged bed rest. Mrs. Brandt already has a reddened area over the sacrum and coccyx. The nurse knows that the most important action to prevent a decubitus ulcer is to
□ 1. Keep the skin area clean, dry, and free from urine, feces, and perspiration.
□ 2. Place an alternating-air-pressure or water mattress on the bed.
□ 3. Massage the reddened area with lotion or oil to stimulate circulation.
□ 4. Turn and reposition the client at least q2h; avoid positioning her on the affected side if possible.

338. Which of the following is the most correct statement about positioning the stroke client?
□ 1. Flexor muscles are generally stronger than extensors.
□ 2. Extensor muscles are generally stronger than flexors.
□ 3. The fingers should be flexed tightly.
□ 4. The footboard should be flush with the mattress.

Two days after Mrs. Brandt's admission, she has a steady rise in her temperature accompanied by a slow pulse and labile respirations.

339. What do these symptoms most likely suggest?
□ 1. Absorption of the clot in the damaged area of the brain.
□ 2. Injury to the vital centers in the brainstem.
□ 3. Development of hypostatic pneumonia.
□ 4. Bacterial infection of the central nervous system.

340. A lumbar puncture is ordered for Mrs. Brandt. During the procedure, in order to maintain the client in the proper position, the nurse would
□ 1. Discourage distracting conversation among personnel.
□ 2. Restrain the client's arms in a folded position over her chest.
□ 3. Prevent plantar flexion of both the feet and toes.

☐ 4. Hold the client on her side and keep the uppermost shoulder from falling forward.

341. After reviewing the lab results of the spinal fluid, the nurse notes the following. Which result is *abnormal?*
   ☐ 1. Color clear.
   ☐ 2. Glucose 60 mg/dl.
   ☐ 3. Red blood cell count 40/mm³.
   ☐ 4. White blood cell count 2/mm³.

342. As Mrs. Brandt's condition improves and she regains consciousness, her behavior becomes erratic. She frequently swears at the nurse who provides her daily care and cries without apparent cause. Mr. Brandt is very upset about his wife's unpredictable and often unpleasant behavior. What would the nurse explain to Mr. Brandt?
   ☐ 1. She is probably suffering from emotional lability characteristic of clients with CVA.
   ☐ 2. She is reacting to medications such as hydrochlorothiazide, which frequently cause behavior changes.
   ☐ 3. She seems to be hostile and angry because of her illness; to avoid upsetting her, it is wisest for the family not to visit so frequently.
   ☐ 4. She is in need of long-term psychiatric therapy.

A 35-year-old man is admitted to the emergency room with a possible spinal injury following an auto accident. The client, Joseph Reed, is conscious. He is unable to move his legs or his arms on command.

343. When transferring a client with a possible spinal cord injury, what is the most important consideration for the nurse to remember?
   ☐ 1. Support the lower extremities, since they are likely to be weak or paralyzed.
   ☐ 2. Explain what you are about to do, so the client can assist you.
   ☐ 3. Support the back with additional pillows to prevent further spinal trauma.
   ☐ 4. Immobilize the head, neck, and back to prevent further spinal trauma.

344. Which of the following would occur if Mr. Reed has spinal shock?
   ☐ 1. Spastic paralysis.
   ☐ 2. Hypertension.
   ☐ 3. Diaphoresis below the level of the injury.
   ☐ 4. Urinary retention.

345. Mr. Reed has complete destruction of the spinal cord at C3-4. Select the most important action for a nurse caring for this kind of client in the acute stage following injury.
   ☐ 1. Turn and position at least q2h.
   ☐ 2. Immobilize the head and neck.

☐ 3. Maintain a patent airway and adequate ventilation.
   ☐ 4. Monitor renal output.

346. Immediately after his injury, Mr. Reed's bladder will
   ☐ 1. Be spastic.
   ☐ 2. Be atonic.
   ☐ 3. Empty with slightest stimulus.
   ☐ 4. Be normal.

347. Which one of the following statements is correct concerning the relationship between the branches of the autonomic nervous system?
   ☐ 1. The parasympathetic branch excites all systems, and the sympathetic inhibits all systems.
   ☐ 2. The parasympathetic branch excites most systems except the gastrointestinal tract and urinary bladder, and the sympathetic has the opposite effect.
   ☐ 3. The sympathetic branch stimulates most systems but inhibits the gastrointestinal tract and urinary bladder; the parasympathetic branch inhibits most systems but stimulates the gastrointestinal tract and urinary bladder.
   ☐ 4. There is no relationship between the two branches.

348. What is characteristic of a reflex arc?
   ☐ 1. Always includes a sensory and motor neuron.
   ☐ 2. Always terminates in a muscle or gland.
   ☐ 3. Always has its center in the brain or spinal cord.
   ☐ 4. All the above are characteristic of a reflex arc.

349. When would the nurse expect Mr. Reed to exhibit mass reflex activity?
   ☐ 1. Immediately.
   ☐ 2. Within 24 hours.
   ☐ 3. In a few months.
   ☐ 4. Never.

350. A bowel and bladder routine is to be established for Mr. Reed. He has had a Foley catheter, and it is being clamped for intervals to increase bladder capacity. The plan is to use an external catheter and to teach him to stimulate voiding by stimulating his thigh. After the catheter has been clamped for 1 hour, Mr. Reed complains of a headache, is sweating, and has an elevated blood pressure. The most probable cause of these signs and symptoms is
   ☐ 1. Hyperreflexia of parasympathetic system.
   ☐ 2. Hyperreflexia of sympathetic system.
   ☐ 3. Hyperreflexia of sensory system.
   ☐ 4. Septicemia resulting from lack of flushing of bacteria from the bladder.

351. The most probable stimulus for this episode is
   ☐ 1. Bowel distension.
   ☐ 2. Stimulation of urinary sphincter by Foley catheter.

☐ 3. Bladder distension.

☐ 4. Fear.

352. Mr. Reed is progressing well with rehabilitation. He says that the dietitian has cautioned him about the amount of milk he drinks and told him that this could contribute to his problems with kidney stones. He says he is drinking no more than he did before the accident and wonders why it would be a problem now. The nurse's response would include which of the following facts?

☐ 1. He probably is drinking more milk than before and just does not realize it.

☐ 2. He has better absorption of calcium now than before the accident.

☐ 3. His kidneys are not clearing calcium as well as before surgery.

☐ 4. The lack of stress on the long bones causes demineralization and increases the amount of calcium to be cleared by the kidneys.

353. Mr. Reed asks how the injury is going to affect his sexual function. The nurse's response would include which of the following?

☐ 1. Normal sexual function is not possible.

☐ 2. His sexual functioning should not be impaired at all.

☐ 3. He will probably be able to have erections.

☐ 4. Ejaculation will be normal.

Eunice Raye, a 30-year-old homemaker, fell asleep while smoking a cigarette. She sustained severe burns of the face, neck, anterior chest, and both arms and hands.

354. Using the "rule of nines," which of the following is the best estimate of total body-surface area burned?

☐ 1. 18%.

☐ 2. 22%.

☐ 3. 31%.

☐ 4. 40%.

355. The nurse determines that Mrs. Raye has second- and third-degree burns. Which of the following would be characteristic of a fresh, second-degree burn?

☐ 1. Absence of pain and pressure sense.

☐ 2. White or dark, dry, leathery appearance.

☐ 3. Large, thick blisters.

☐ 4. Visible, thrombosed small vessels.

356. Because of the location of Mrs. Raye's burns, what is the nurse's primary concern?

☐ 1. Debride and dress the wounds.

☐ 2. Initiate and administer antibiotics.

☐ 3. Frequently observe for hoarseness, stridor, and dyspnea.

☐ 4. Obtain a thorough history of events leading to the accident.

357. A narcotic IV was ordered to control Mrs. Raye's pain. Why was the IV route selected?

☐ 1. Burns cause excruciating pain, requiring immediate relief.

☐ 2. Circulatory blood volume is reduced, delaying absorption from subcutaneous and muscle tissue.

☐ 3. Cardiac function is enhanced by immediate action of the drug.

☐ 4. Metabolism of the drug would be delayed because of decreased insulin production.

358. A major goal during the first 48 hours is to prevent hypovolemic shock. Which of the following would *not* be a useful guide to fluid restitution during this period?

☐ 1. Elevated hematocrit.

☐ 2. Urine output of 30 ml/hr.

☐ 3. Change in sensorium.

☐ 4. Estimate of fluid loss through the burn eschar.

359. Mafenide acetate (Sulfamylon) is applied to Mrs. Raye's wounds every 12 hours. The nurse's assessment would include observation for which of the following side effects of this drug?

☐ 1. Metabolic acidosis.

☐ 2. Discoloration of the skin.

☐ 3. Maceration of the skin.

☐ 4. Dehydration and electrolyte loss.

360. Eventually, autografts are done. Care of the donor site would *not* include

☐ 1. Changing the dressing every shift.

☐ 2. Reporting any odor to the physician.

☐ 3. Using a heat lamp to dry the wound.

☐ 4. Exposing the mesh-covered wound to the air.

361. Contractures are among the most serious of the long-term complications of a burn. Because of the location of these burns, which of the following nursing measures would most likely cause Mrs. Raye to have contractures?

☐ 1. Change the location of the bed or the TV set, or both, daily.

☐ 2. Encourage her to chew gum and blow up balloons.

☐ 3. Avoid using a pillow or place the head in a position of hyperextension.

☐ 4. Help her to assume a position of comfort.

362. What is the primary aim of all burn-wound care?

☐ 1. To debride the wound of dead tissue and eschar.

☐ 2. To limit fluid loss through the skin.

☐ 3. To prevent growth of microorganisms.

☐ 4. To decrease formation of disfiguring scars.

Arnold Hamilton, age 63, has recently received a diagnosis of Parkinson's disease.

363. The pathophysiology in parkinsonism is commonly believed found in which part of the brain?
- ☐ 1. Medulla oblongata.
- ☐ 2. Thalamus.
- ☐ 3. Basal ganglia.
- ☐ 4. Brainstem.

364. Parkinsonism is best characterized by
- ☐ 1. Ptosis of both eyelids.
- ☐ 2. Visual impairment and slurred speech.
- ☐ 3. Involuntary resting tremor.
- ☐ 4. Vertigo.

365. A client's motor function can be best assessed in which of the following ways?
- ☐ 1. Check Babinski's reflex.
- ☐ 2. Have the client count backward from 100 by sevens.
- ☐ 3. Have the client walk the length of the room.
- ☐ 4. Test the knee-jerk reflex.

366. There are several forms of parkinsonism. The most common etiological classification is
- ☐ 1. Idiopathic.
- ☐ 2. Postencephalitic.
- ☐ 3. Atherosclerotic.
- ☐ 4. Drug induced.

367. Mr. Hamilton has recently been placed on levodopa (Levopa), 250 mg BID. Which of the following would indicate that a therapeutic response had been achieved?
- ☐ 1. Decrease in bradykinesia and rigidity.
- ☐ 2. Decrease in tics.
- ☐ 3. Presence of hypotension.
- ☐ 4. Increased appetite.

Leonard Vernon is a 30-year-old, admitted with a diagnosis of multiple sclerosis and worsening of symptoms.

368. In taking a history, which of the following complaints would the nurse consider most *atypical?*
- ☐ 1. Tremors.
- ☐ 2. Pain.
- ☐ 3. Incontinence.
- ☐ 4. Numbness of hands.

369. Mr. Vernon is started on a prednisone regimen. He states he has never been treated with this drug before and asks for general information. Which of the following pieces of information would *not* be correct to give?
- ☐ 1. The drug should make him feel better.
- ☐ 2. He will be taking it the rest of his life.
- ☐ 3. It might be working by decreasing edema around involved areas of the nervous systems.
- ☐ 4. The way in which it improves symptoms in multiple sclerosis is unknown.

A nurse in a department store notices a group of people gathered around a person lying on the floor having a seizure.

370. The best immediate response would be to
- ☐ 1. Cradle the person's head in your lap.
- ☐ 2. Place something in the person's mouth.
- ☐ 3. Hold the person's arms down.
- ☐ 4. Move the person to a place of safety.

371. Which type of seizure is frequently preceded by an aura?
- ☐ 1. Jacksonian (focal motor).
- ☐ 2. Petit mal (absence).
- ☐ 3. Grand mal (tonic-clonic).
- ☐ 4. Myoclonic.

372. All but one of the following statements concerning epilepsy (recurrent seizures) are true. Identify the *false* statement.
- ☐ 1. Epilepsy is a disease that afflicts about one in every 200 Americans.
- ☐ 2. Epilepsy can be controlled by medications in all cases.
- ☐ 3. There is still a stigma connected with the term "epilepsy."
- ☐ 4. The causes of most cases of epilepsy remain unknown.

373. Which of the following tests furnishes the best diagnostic information about seizures?
- ☐ 1. Pneumoencephalogram.
- ☐ 2. Electroencephalogram.
- ☐ 3. Cerebral angiogram.
- ☐ 4. Cerebral tomography.

374. What is the most common reason why clients suffer from sudden seizure recurrence?
- ☐ 1. Extreme physical or emotional stress.
- ☐ 2. Alcoholic beverages in excess.
- ☐ 3. Premenstrual fluid retention.
- ☐ 4. Noncompliance with medication schedules.

375. When one seizure after another occurs without the client's regaining consciousness between seizures, it is called
- ☐ 1. Frequent seizures.
- ☐ 2. Febrile seizures.
- ☐ 3. Status epilepticus.
- ☐ 4. Petit mal seizures.

Foster Williams, a 55-year-old black man, is admitted to the hospital in acute respiratory distress. His condition has previously been diagnosed as myasthenia gravis.

376. The emergency room treatment of a client with severe weakness related to myasthenia gravis would focus on
- ☐ 1. Renal failure.
- ☐ 2. Reversing coma.

3. Restoring blood volume.

4. Ventilation.

377. Which of the following is *not* a reliable assessment parameter for cyanosis in dark-skinned persons?

  1. Conjunctiva and oral mucosa.

  2. Nail beds.

  3. Hard palate.

  4. Behavioral responses to hypoxia.

378. What is the primary nursing approach in the care of Mr. Williams?

  1. Prevent contractures and atrophy of muscles.

  2. Decrease environmental stimuli.

  3. Maintain open and optimal respirations.

  4. Foster communication with significant others.

379. An IV was started on Mr. Williams in the emergency room, but he started to complain of pain at the site upon admission to the unit. Which of the following is not likely to be an indication of an infiltrated IV in this client?

  1. Pain on touch.

  2. Redness at the IV site.

  3. Edema at the site.

  4. No blood return when lowering the IV bottle.

380. The following day, the physician orders hydrocortisone sodium succinate (Solu-Cortef). What is the purpose of this medication in this situation?

  1. Decrease hypercapnia.

  2. Relax smooth muscle and produce diuresis.

  3. Support the body through crisis by reducing the inflammatory response.

  4. Decrease client anxiety.

381. Cholinergic drugs act directly and indirectly to produce the same effects as which neurohormone?

  1. Norepinephrine.

  2. Acetylcholine.

  3. Epinephrine.

  4. Acetylcholinesterase.

382. Cholinergic agents act on effector organs to produce three of the following reactions. Which one is *not* an outcome of cholinergic drug administration?

  1. Increased motility and tone of smooth muscles in the gastrointestinal tract.

  2. Increased mucus secretion, sweating, and salivation.

  3. Increased heart rate and constriction of blood vessels.

  4. Miosis and a reduction in intraocular pressure.

The head nurse of an eye and ear clinic is orienting nursing students.

383. Normal visual acuity as measured with a Snellen eye chart is 20/20. What does a visual acuity of 20/30 indicate?

  1. At 20 feet, an individual can only read letters large enough to be read at 30 feet.

  2. At 30 feet, an individual can read letters small enough to be read at 20 feet.

  3. An individual can read 20 out of 30 total letters on the chart.

  4. An individual can read 30 out of 50 total letters on the chart at 20 feet.

384. Damage to the visual area of the occipital lobe of the cerebrum, on the *left* side, would produce what type of visual loss?

  1. Left eye only.

  2. Right eye only.

  3. Medial half of the right eye and lateral half of the left eye.

  4. Medial half of the left eye and lateral half of the right eye.

385. The anterior chamber of the eye refers to all the space in what area?

  1. Anterior to the retina.

  2. Between the iris and the cornea.

  3. Between the lens and the cornea.

  4. Between the lens and the iris.

386. What condition results when rays of light are focused in front of the retina?

  1. Myopia.

  2. Hyperopia.

  3. Presbyopia.

  4. Emmetropia.

387. As the person grows older, the lens loses its elasticity, causing which kind of farsightedness?

  1. Emmetropia.

  2. Presbyopia.

  3. Diplopia.

  4. Myopia.

388. If a person has a foreign object of unknown material that is not readily seen in one eye, what would the first action be?

  1. Irrigate the eye with a boric acid solution.

  2. Examine the lower eyelid and then the upper eyelid.

  3. Irrigate the eye with copious amounts of water.

  4. Shield the eye from pressure, and seek medical help.

389. A sudden loss of an area of vision, as if a curtain were being drawn, is a principal symptom of

  1. Retinal detachment.

  2. Glaucoma.

  3. Cataract.

  4. Keratitis.

390. Postoperative care for a client following a stapedectomy would *not* include which of the following?

  1. Out of bed as desired.

  2. No moisture in the affected ear.

☐ 3. Avoid sneezing.
☐ 4. No bending over or lifting of heavy objects.

391. Dimenhydrinate (Dramamine) is given after a stapedectomy
☐ 1. To accelerate the auditory process.
☐ 2. To dull the pain experienced when the semicircular canal is disturbed.
☐ 3. To minimize the sensations of equilibrium disturbances and imbalance.
☐ 4. To prevent an increased tendency toward nausea.

392. Why is there no hearing loss after a myringotomy?
☐ 1. The procedure involves just washing out the ear.
☐ 2. The procedure involves removing fluid from the outer ear.
☐ 3. The procedure involves cutting the tympanic membrane, but it heals very quickly.
☐ 4. The procedure requires removing the tympanic membrane and putting a new membrane in.

393. A client with Ménière's syndrome is extremely uncomfortable because of which of these?
☐ 1. Severe earache.
☐ 2. Many perceptual difficulties.
☐ 3. Vertigo and resultant nausea.
☐ 4. Facial paralysis.

Ona Clark is admitted for cataract extraction.

394. What is a cataract of the eye?
☐ 1. Opacity of the cornea.
☐ 2. Clouding of the aqueous humor.
☐ 3. Opacity of the lens.
☐ 4. Papilledema.

395. Treating a cataract primarily involves which of the following?
☐ 1. Instillation of miotics.
☐ 2. Instillation of mydriatics.
☐ 3. Removal of the lens.
☐ 4. Enucleation.

396. Preoperative instruction will *not* need to include
☐ 1. Type of surgery.
☐ 2. How to use the call bell.
☐ 3. How to prevent paralytic ileus.
☐ 4. How to prevent respiratory infections.

397. In preparing to teach Mrs. Cook about adjustment to cataract lenses, the nurse needs to know that the lenses will
☐ 1. Magnify objects by one-third with central vision.
☐ 2. Magnify objects by one-third with peripheral vision.
☐ 3. Reduce objects by one-third with central vision.
☐ 4. Reduce objects by one-third with peripheral vision.

398. In the immediate postoperative period, the one action that is contraindicated for Mrs. Clark compared with clients after most other operations is which of the following?
☐ 1. Coughing.
☐ 2. Turning on the unoperative side.
☐ 3. Measures to control nausea and vomiting.
☐ 4. Eating after nausea passes.

399. Immediate nursing care following cataract extraction is directed primarily toward preventing
☐ 1. Atelectasis.
☐ 2. Infection of the cornea.
☐ 3. Hemorrhage.
☐ 4. Prolapse of the iris.

400. Mrs. Clark is confused during her first night after eye surgery. What would the nurse do?
☐ 1. Tell her to stay in bed.
☐ 2. Apply restraints to keep her in bed.
☐ 3. Explain why she cannot get out of bed, keep side rails up, and check her frequently.
☐ 4. Sedate her.

401. Discharge teaching for Mrs. Clark would probably *not* need to include
☐ 1. Staying in a darkened room as much as possible.
☐ 2. Avoiding alcoholic drinks; limiting the use of tea and coffee.
☐ 3. Using no eye washes or drops unless they were prescribed by the physician.
☐ 4. Avoiding being excessively sedentary.

402. Mrs. Clark also needs to be instructed to limit
☐ 1. Sewing.
☐ 2. Watching TV.
☐ 3. Walking.
☐ 4. Weeding her garden.

Helen Kowalski visits her ophthalmologist and receives a mydriatric drug in order to facilitate the examination. After returning home, she experiences severe eye pain, nausea and vomiting, and blurred vision. During a visit to the emergency room, a diagnosis of acute glaucoma is made.

403. Mrs. Kowalski's glaucoma has been caused by
☐ 1. Blockage of the outflow of aqueous humor by the dilatation of the pupil.
☐ 2. Blockage of the outflow of aqueous humor by the constriction of the pupil.
☐ 3. Increased intraocular pressure resulting from the increased production of aqueous humor.
☐ 4. Decreased intraocular pressure resulting from decreased production of aqueous humor.

404. Intraocular pressure is measured clinically by a tonometer. What tonometer reading would be indicative of glaucoma?
☐ 1. Pressure of 10 mm Hg.
☐ 2. Pressure of 15 mm Hg.
☐ 3. Pressure of 20 mm Hg.
☐ 4. Pressure of 25 mm Hg.

405. Which cranial nerve transmits visual impulses?
   □ 1. I (olfactory).
   □ 2. II (optic).
   □ 3. III (oculomotor).
   □ 4. IV (abducens).

406. Untreated or uncontrolled glaucoma damages the optic nerve. Three of the following signs and symptoms result from optic nerve atrophy; which one does *not*?
   □ 1. Colored halos around lights.
   □ 2. Severe pain in the eye.
   □ 3. Dilated and fixed pupils.
   □ 4. Opacity of the lens.

407. Glaucoma is conservatively managed with miotic eye drops. Mydriatic eye drops are contraindicated for glaucoma. Which of the following drugs is a mydriatic?
   □ 1. Neostigmine.
   □ 2. Pilocarpine.
   □ 3. Physostigmine.
   □ 4. Atropine.

408. Glaucoma may require surgical treatment. Preoperatively, the client would be taught to expect which of the following postoperatively?
   □ 1. Cough and deep-breathe qh.
   □ 2. Turn only to the unaffected side.
   □ 3. Medication for severe eye pain.
   □ 4. Restriction of fluids for the first 24 hours.

Allen James, a 55-year-old man, is admitted to the hospital with wide-angle glaucoma.

409. What was the symptom that probably brought Mr. James to the ophthalmologist initially?
   □ 1. Decreasing vision.
   □ 2. Extreme pain in the eye.
   □ 3. Redness and tearing of the eye.
   □ 4. Seeing colored flashes of light.

410. The teaching plan for Mr. James would include which of the following?
   □ 1. Reduce fluid intake.
   □ 2. Add extra lighting in the home.
   □ 3. Wear dark glasses during the day.
   □ 4. Avoid exercise.

411. Miotics are used in the treatment of glaucoma. What is an example of a commonly used miotic?
   □ 1. Atropine.
   □ 2. Pilocarpine.
   □ 3. Acetazolamide (Diamox).
   □ 4. Scopolamine.

412. What is the rationale for using miotics in the treatment of glaucoma?
   □ 1. They decrease the rate of aqueous humor production.
   □ 2. Pupil constriction increases outflow of aqueous humor.

   □ 3. Increased pupil size relaxes the ciliary muscles.
   □ 4. The blood flow to the conjunctiva is increased.

413. When instilling eye drops for a client with glaucoma, what procedure would the nurse follow?
   □ 1. Place the medication in the middle of the lower lid, and put pressure on the lacrimal duct after instillation.
   □ 2. Instill the drug at the outer angle of the eye; have client tilt head back.
   □ 3. Instill the drug at the innermost angle; wipe with cotton away from inner aspect.
   □ 4. Instill medication in middle of eye; have client blink for better absorption.

414. Carbonic anhydrase inhibitors are sometimes used in the treatment of glaucoma because they
   □ 1. Depress secretion of aqueous humor.
   □ 2. Dilate the pupil.
   □ 3. Paralyze the power of accommodation.
   □ 4. Increase the power of accommodation.

415. Teaching a client with glaucoma will *not* include which of the following?
   □ 1. Vision can be restored only if the client remains under a physician's care.
   □ 2. Avoid stimulants (e.g., caffeine).
   □ 3. Take all medications conscientiously.
   □ 4. Prevent constipation, and avoid heavy lifting and emotional excitement.

416. Glaucoma is a progressive disease that can lead to blindness. It can be managed if diagnosed early. Preventive health teaching would best include which of the following points?
   □ 1. Early surgical action may be necessary.
   □ 2. All clients over 40 years of age should have an annual tonometry exam.
   □ 3. The use of contact lenses in older clients is not advisable.
   □ 4. Clients should seek early treatment for eye infections.

417. A client with progressive glaucoma may be experiencing sensory deprivation. Which of the following actions would best minimize this problem?
   □ 1. Speak in a louder voice.
   □ 2. Ensure that a sedative is ordered.
   □ 3. Orient the client to time, place, and person.
   □ 4. Use touch frequently when providing care.

Brenda Bates is a 20-year-old college student who is self-conscious about the appearance of her nose. She is admitted to the hospital for an elective rhinoplasty.

418. Nursing management following rhinoplasty will *not* include which of the following?
   □ 1. Elevate the head of the bed.
   □ 2. Check the gag reflex.
   □ 3. Observe for frequent swallowing.
   □ 4. Monitor the HemoVac suction.

419. While caring for Mrs. Bates, the nurse observes one small, tarry stool. What is the most appropriate nursing action?
    - ☐ 1. Call the physician immediately.
    - ☐ 2. Administer analgesics.
    - ☐ 3. Observe for signs of fresh bleeding.
    - ☐ 4. Check her gag reflex.
420. Before her discharge, the nurse would instruct Mrs. Bates to
    - ☐ 1. "Avoid blowing your nose for 3 to 4 days."
    - ☐ 2. "Resume your prior activities immediately."
    - ☐ 3. "Limit your fluid intake for 1 week."
    - ☐ 4. "Take aspirin if you observe increased pain and swelling."

Claude Rollins is seen in the emergency room with the diagnosis of epistaxis.

421. It is unlikely that Mr. Rollins' history will include
    - ☐ 1. Minor trauma to the nose.
    - ☐ 2. A deviated septum.
    - ☐ 3. Acute sinusitis.
    - ☐ 4. Hypotension.
422. Which of the following medications would be used with Mr. Rollins in order to promote vasoconstriction and control bleeding?
    - ☐ 1. Epinephrine.
    - ☐ 2. Lidocaine (Xylocaine).
    - ☐ 3. Pilocarpine.
    - ☐ 4. Cyclopentolate (Cyclogyl).
423. Which of the following positions would be most desirable for Mr. Rollins?
    - ☐ 1. Trendelenburg's, to control shock.
    - ☐ 2. A sitting position, unless he is hypotensive.
    - ☐ 3. Side-lying, to prevent aspiration.
    - ☐ 4. Prone, to prevent aspiration.
424. The physician decides to insert nasal packing. Of the following nursing actions, which would have the highest priority?
    - ☐ 1. Encourage Mr. Rollins to breathe through his mouth, because he may feel panicky after the insertion.
    - ☐ 2. Advise Mr. Rollins to expectorate the blood in the nasopharynx gently and not to swallow it.
    - ☐ 3. Periodically check the position of the nasal packing, because airway obstruction can occur if the packing accidentally slips out of place.
    - ☐ 4. Take rectal temperatures, because he must rely on mouth breathing and would be unable to keep his mouth closed on the thermometer.
425. After bleeding has been controlled, Mr. Rollins is taken to surgery to correct a deviated nasal septum. Which of the following is a likely complication of this surgery?
    - ☐ 1. Loss of the ability to smell.
    - ☐ 2. Inability to breathe through the nose.

- ☐ 3. Infection.
- ☐ 4. Hemorrhage.
426. Upon his discharge, the nurse instructs Mr. Rollins on the use of vasoconstrictive nose drops and cautions him to avoid too frequent and excessive use of these drugs. Which of the following provides the best rationale for this caution?
    - ☐ 1. A rebound effect occurs in which stuffiness worsens after each successive dose.
    - ☐ 2. Cocaine, a frequent ingredient in nose drops, may lead to psychological addiction.
    - ☐ 3. These medications may be absorbed systemically, causing severe hypotension.
    - ☐ 4. Persistent vasoconstriction of the nasal mucosa can lead to alterations in the olfactory nerve.

Mary Hayes has had radical head and neck surgery for cancer of the larynx.

427. Mrs. Hayes has a tracheostomy. When suctioning the tracheostomy, which of the following is *not* correct?
    - ☐ 1. Use sterile technique.
    - ☐ 2. Turn head to right to suction left bronchus.
    - ☐ 3. Suction for no longer than 10 to 15 seconds.
    - ☐ 4. Observe for tachycardia.
428. Mrs. Hayes requires both nasopharyngeal suctioning and suctioning through the laryngectomy tube. When doing these two procedures at the same time, the nurse would *not* do which of the following?
    - ☐ 1. Use a sterile suction setup.
    - ☐ 2. Suction the nose first, then the laryngectomy tube.
    - ☐ 3. Suction the laryngectomy tube first, then the nose.
    - ☐ 4. Lubricate the catheter with saline.
429. A nasogastric tube is used to provide Mrs. Hayes with fluids and nutrients for approximately 10 days, for which of the following reasons?
    - ☐ 1. To prevent pain while swallowing.
    - ☐ 2. To prevent contamination of the suture line.
    - ☐ 3. To decrease need for swallowing.
    - ☐ 4. To prevent need for holding head up to eat.
430. Acidosis would most likely follow which condition?
    - ☐ 1. Excessive loss of sodium and potassium ions in diarrhea.
    - ☐ 2. Loss of hydrogen and chloride ions in vomiting.
    - ☐ 3. Excessive conservation of bicarbonate in urine.
    - ☐ 4. Increased loss of carbon dioxide with hyperventilation.
431. Mrs. Hayes' children are concerned about their own risk of developing cancer. All but one of the following are facts that describe malignant neoplasia and must be considered by the nurse in her responses. Which one is *incorrect*?

1. Familial factors may influence an individual's susceptibility to neoplasia.
2. Long-term use of corticosteroids enhances the body's defense against the development of cancer.
3. Sexual differences influence an individual's susceptibility to specific neoplasms.
4. Living in industrialized areas increases an individual's susceptibility to a malignant neoplasm.

432. When would Mrs. Hayes best begin speech rehabilitation?
   1. When she leaves the hospital.
   2. When the esophageal suture line is healed.
   3. Three months after surgery.
   4. When she regains all her strength.

David Wilson, a 24-year-old client, sustains a compound fracture of the shaft of the right femur in a motorcycle accident. Paramedics reach the scene and administer emergency treatment, which includes the application of a splint.

433. How should the splint be applied?
   1. Apply it while the limb is in good alignment.
   2. Apply it to the limb in the position in which it is found.
   3. Extending from the fracture site downward.
   4. Extending from the fracture site upward.
434. Mr. Wilson is brought to the emergency room. What is the first thing the emergency room nurse should do?
   1. Cover the open wounds.
   2. Take his blood pressure.
   3. Clean the fracture site.
   4. Assess his respiratory status.
435. After an open reduction of his fracture, Mr. Wilson displayed the following symptoms postoperatively: an increase in blood pressure, signs of confusion, and increased restlessness. Which one of the following would the nurse most likely suspect?
   1. Concussion.
   2. Impending shock.
   3. Fat emboli.
   4. Anxiety.

Henry Kahn, age 45, is in an auto accident and suffers a fracture of the tibia and fibula. He is taken to surgery for an open reduction with internal fixation. He arrives in the orthopedic unit with a plaster-of-paris cast extending from above the knee to below the ankle.

436. Mr. Kahn is cautioned to be careful of the cast until it is dry. A dry cast has which of the following characteristics?
   1. Gray, dull, and a musty odor.
   2. Gray, shiny, and a musty odor.
   3. White, shiny, and odorless.
   4. White, dull, and tends to flake off when scratched.

437. Which of the following is the recommended method of drying Mr. Kahn's cast?
   1. Place a radiation heat lamp about 1 foot from the cast.
   2. Cover the extremity with an electric heat cradle.
   3. Place an electric fan at the foot of the bed.
   4. Leave the cast uncovered in a well-ventilated room.
438. Which of the following is an *inappropriate* nursing action during the first 24 to 48 hours?
   1. Handle the cast with the palms of the hand.
   2. Place the casted extremity in normal alignment.
   3. Place rubber-covered pillows under the cast.
   4. Elevate the entire extremity.
439. When Mr. Kahn returns from surgery, there are two small bloodstains on the cast. Four hours later, the stains double in size. What should the nurse do?
   1. Call the physician.
   2. Outline the spots with a pencil; note the time and date on the cast.
   3. Cut a window in the cast to observe the site.
   4. Record the amount of bleeding in the nurses' notes only.
440. On the first postoperative day, Mr. Kahn complains of a burning pain in one spot under the cast. The nurse should suspect which of the following as the source of the discomfort?
   1. Skin irritation from a pressure spot.
   2. A burn from the cast.
   3. An infection in the operative site.
   4. Hemorrhage from the incision.
441. The first indication of an infection in Mr. Kahn's leg would most likely be
   1. An elevated temperature.
   2. An unpleasant odor.
   3. Redness and heat above and below the cast.
   4. Purulent drainage on the cast.
442. Mr. Kahn is at risk for peroneal nerve palsy. Which of the following is *not* characteristic of this complication?
   1. Inability to dorsiflex foot and extend toes.
   2. Numbness in the webbed space between the first and second toe.
   3. Inability to touch the heel to the floor when standing.
   4. Cyanotic toes.
443. Before discharge, Mr. Kahn asks how to clean his cast. How should the nurse reply?
   1. "Cover the soiled area with shoe polish."
   2. "Spray the cast with shellac."
   3. "Wipe the soiled area with a cloth moistened with alcohol."

☐ 4. "Clean soiled areas with a small amount of Bon Ami and a damp cloth."

Megan Carey slips on some grease on her kitchen floor and fractures the proximal end of the ulna. There is extensive soft tissue damage in the fracture area. A cast is applied in the emergency department.

444. Because of the location and type of fracture, Mrs. Carey is most at risk for the complication of compartment syndrome. Which of the following would be the earliest indication of this phenomenon?
☐ 1. Absence of the pulse distal to the fracture.
☐ 2. Pallor of the extremity.
☐ 3. Paralysis of the hand.
☐ 4. Progressive pain unrelieved by analgesics.

445. If Mrs. Carey experiences the symptoms of compartment syndrome, which of the following is the recommended course of action?
☐ 1. Bivalve the cast, and wrap it loosely with an elastic bandage.
☐ 2. Apply hot packs to improve venous circulation.
☐ 3. Administer diuretics to reduce edema.
☐ 4. Encourage flexion and extension of the fingers on the affected arm.

446. If compartment syndrome is not recognized and treated early, what is the probable outcome?
☐ 1. Gangrene will develop.
☐ 2. A paralyzed and deformed arm with a clawlike hand results (Volkmann's contracture).
☐ 3. Healing of the fracture is delayed.
☐ 4. Cast syndrome will result.

Elaina Balinski is a 78-year-old woman admitted to the hospital because of dehydration. In the hospital, she reaches for a glass of water and falls out of bed, fracturing the neck of the femur.

447. Mrs. Balinski is at risk of suffering serious complications. What assessments are characteristic of a fat embolus after a fracture?
☐ 1. Severe, stabbing chest pain 10 days after the fracture.
☐ 2. Frothy sputum.
☐ 3. Petechiae across the chest and shoulders 24 hours after the fracture.
☐ 4. Hypertension and coma.

448. What is the most common reason why elderly women sustain hip fractures?
☐ 1. Decreased intake of calcium.
☐ 2. Lack of muscles.
☐ 3. Decreased production of bone marrow.
☐ 4. Osteoporosis.

449. Buck's extension is applied to Mrs. Balinski's fractured leg. Which of the following is an *inappropriate* reason for using Buck's traction?

☐ 1. Reduces muscle spasms and pain.
☐ 2. Prevents further soft-tissue damage.
☐ 3. Reduces the fracture.
☐ 4. Immobilizes the leg while the dehydration is being treated.

450. Buck's traction would be contraindicated if Mrs. Balinski experiences which of the following?
☐ 1. Arthritis.
☐ 2. Bilateral lower leg ulcers.
☐ 3. Pelvic pain.
☐ 4. Deformity of the affected leg.

451. A plan of care for Mrs. Balinski would include which of the following?
☐ 1. Remove the traction every shift to observe for pressure areas and provide skin care.
☐ 2. Turn her to the unaffected side for back care.
☐ 3. Elevate the head of the bed to apply countertraction.
☐ 4. Raise the knee gatch to prevent her sliding down in bed.

452. When a client is immobilized, what is the most appropriate plan to prevent constipation?
☐ 1. Encourage daily laxative use.
☐ 2. Limit fluid intake.
☐ 3. Encourage frequent periods of sitting on the bedpan.
☐ 4. Increase the fiber in the client's diet.

453. Which of the following is an *inappropriate* statement concerning avascular necrosis of the femoral head?
☐ 1. It is often a complication of total hip replacement.
☐ 2. It results from impaired circulation.
☐ 3. Pain in the groin may be the first symptom in adults.
☐ 4. Restriction of abduction and internal rotation can occur.

Jenna Sam has had a right hip nailing.

454. When planning postoperative care, the nurse includes which of the following actions?
☐ 1. Prevent internal rotation of the affected extremity.
☐ 2. Prevent external rotation of the affected extremity.
☐ 3. Prevent hip flexion of greater than 10°.
☐ 4. Prevent hip flexion of greater than 30°.

455. Where would the nurse place the trochanter rolls on the affected extremity to prevent external rotation?
☐ 1. From the hip to the ankle.
☐ 2. From the hip to the knee.
☐ 3. From the knee to the ankle.
☐ 4. From the knee to the midcalf.

456. Mrs. Sam complains of severe burning in her right leg on the second postoperative day. The nurse assesses the pulses, sensation, and movement of both legs as well as vital signs. What is the next best action?
- ☐ 1. Give the prn medication.
- ☐ 2. Notify the physician.
- ☐ 3. Continue to monitor the assessments q5min.
- ☐ 4. Reassure Mrs. Sam that this is a normal response after this type of surgery.

457. Mrs. Sam is now learning to walk with the use of a walker. Which of the following best describes the correct use of a walker?
- ☐ 1. Always walk into the walker when all four of its legs are on the floor.
- ☐ 2. Always walk into the walker when two of its legs are on the floor and the other two are off the floor.
- ☐ 3. Always have the walker legs at least 2 inches off the floor.
- ☐ 4. Always lift the walker up and down with each step.

Nathan Tool falls and breaks his hip. He is taken to surgery and receives a hip prosthesis.

458. Positioning Mr. Tool the first day postoperatively is best described by which of the following?
- ☐ 1. Prevent external rotation and abduction of the affected extremity.
- ☐ 2. Prevent external rotation and adduction of the affected extremity.
- ☐ 3. Prevent internal rotation and adduction of the affected extremity.
- ☐ 4. Prevent internal rotation and abduction of the affected extremity.

459. The second day after surgery, Mr. Tool complains of the sudden onset of severe pain in the operative site. Assessment reveals the affected extremity has a pulse, the color is pink, and the skin is warm. What is the next best action?
- ☐ 1. Notify the physician.
- ☐ 2. Give morphine as ordered.
- ☐ 3. Reposition the extremity.
- ☐ 4. Provide diversional activity.

460. Five days after surgery, Mr. Tool asks to use the bedpan. Which of the following approaches would be the best for the nurse to use?
- ☐ 1. Have Mr. Tool lift up by using the overhead trapeze.
- ☐ 2. Have Mr. Tool use the bedside commode.
- ☐ 3. Have Mr. Tool flex his legs and lift up his buttocks to slide the bedpan under him.
- ☐ 4. Get another nurse to help turn Mr. Tool to his unaffected side. Place the bedpan under him and roll him back onto the pan.

Arnold Jessup has a standard above-the-knee amputation (AKA) with an immediate prosthesis fitting.

461. The surgeon's final decision on the level of Mr. Jessup's amputation is based on
- ☐ 1. Saving all possible length and tissue of the extremity.
- ☐ 2. Results of diagnostic tests such as an arteriography.
- ☐ 3. Observation of vascularity of tissue during surgery.
- ☐ 4. The best level to facilitate fitting with a prosthesis.

462. During Mr. Jessup's fifth postoperative day, his rigid dressing falls off. What is the nurse's first course of action?
- ☐ 1. Call the physician.
- ☐ 2. Apply an elastic bandage firmly.
- ☐ 3. Apply a saline dressing.
- ☐ 4. Elevate the limb on a pillow.

463. The nurse includes the important measures for stump care in the teaching plan for Mr. Jessup. Which measures would be *inappropriate* for the teaching plan?
- ☐ 1. Wash, dry, and inspect the stump daily.
- ☐ 2. Treat superficial abrasions and blisters promptly.
- ☐ 3. Apply a "shrinker" bandage with tighter turns around the proximal end of the affected limb.
- ☐ 4. Toughen the stump by pushing it against a progressively harder substance (e.g., pillow on a footstool).

Ron Gillman's left arm is badly mutilated in a boating accident and is amputated just below the shoulder.

464. While the nurse is checking Mr. Gillman's dressing, he says he is anxious and asks to have both his hands held. Which of the following is the nurse's best response?
- ☐ 1. "Mr. Gillman, I'm holding your hand."
- ☐ 2. "Your left hand and arm were amputated the day of the boating accident."
- ☐ 3. "Your dressing is dry and clean where the doctors removed your arm."
- ☐ 4. "Many persons think their missing extremity is still present immediately after surgery."

465. How can the nurse best help Mr. Gillman adapt to his new body image?
- ☐ 1. Have him think of how he would like to look.
- ☐ 2. Talk to his wife about his change in body image.
- ☐ 3. Have him write about his feelings.
- ☐ 4. Have him touch and reorient himself to his body.

Alice Balio, 65 years old, comes to the clinic for a routine checkup. She is 5 feet 4 inches tall and weighs 180

pounds. Her major complaint is pain in her joints. She is retired and has had to give up her volunteer work because of her discomfort. She was told her diagnosis was osteoarthritis about 5 years ago.

466. Which of the following is *least* characteristic of osteoarthritis?
   □ 1. It most commonly affects the weight-bearing joints.
   □ 2. Stiffness lasts about 15 minutes after a period of inactivity.
   □ 3. Joint effusion and crepitus are often present.
   □ 4. Inflammation and systemic symptoms are apparent.

467. Which of the following would be *inappropriate* to include on the care plan for Mrs. Balio?
   □ 1. Decrease the calorie count of her daily diet.
   □ 2. Take warm baths when arising.
   □ 3. Slide items across the floor rather than lift them.
   □ 4. Place items so that it is necessary to bend or stretch to reach them.

468. The drug of choice for the treatment of arthritis is aspirin. Mrs. Balio's knowledge concerning aspirin is correct if she states which of the following?
   □ 1. Avoid enteric-coated aspirin if gastrointestinal discomfort occurs.
   □ 2. Take as many as 12 to 16 tablets every day on a regularly scheduled basis.
   □ 3. Increase the amount taken if there is ringing in the ears.
   □ 4. Absence of sensitivity to aspirin over time ensures continued safety with no risk of reactions.

Matt Flore is admitted from the emergency department with severe pain and edema in the right foot. His diagnosis is gouty arthritis.

469. Which of the following is most characteristic of gout?
   □ 1. It may be a familial metabolic disorder of purine metabolism.
   □ 2. Ninety-five percent of the clients with gout are men between ages 18 and 30.
   □ 3. Urate crystal deposits cause a foreign body reaction in the plasma.
   □ 4. It usually occurs in previously traumatized joints.

470. When developing a plan of care, which of the following would have the highest priority?
   □ 1. Apply hot compresses to the affected joints.
   □ 2. Stress the importance of maintaining good posture to prevent deformities.
   □ 3. Administer salicylates to minimize the inflammatory reaction.
   □ 4. Ensure an intake of at least 3000 ml fluid/day.

471. Which of the following dietary practices would be most appropriate for Mr. Flore?
   □ 1. Permanently eliminate foods high in purine.
   □ 2. Eliminate foods high in purine only during the acute phase.
   □ 3. Permanently eliminate ingestion of alcohol and all rich foods.
   □ 4. Ingest foods that will keep the urine acidic.

472. Allopurinol (Zyloprim) is prescribed for Mr. Flore. Which of the following information is appropriate to include in discharge planning?
   □ 1. He should drink at least 1000 ml fluids/day.
   □ 2. He should eliminate all foods with purine for the rest of his life.
   □ 3. He should take the medication before meals.
   □ 4. He should take the medication immediately after eating.

473. When teaching Mr. Flore the side effects of this medication, the nurse should be sure to include monitoring for the first sign of a severe hypersensitivity reaction, which is
   □ 1. Dizziness.
   □ 2. A skin rash.
   □ 3. Aplastic anemia.
   □ 4. Agranulocytosis.

Harvey Daniel had a laminectomy and spinal fusion yesterday.

474. Which of the following statements is *incorrect* to include in the plan of care?
   □ 1. Before log rolling, place a pillow under the client's head and a pillow between the client's legs.
   □ 2. Before log rolling, remove the pillow from under the client's head and use no pillows between the client's legs.
   □ 3. Keep the knees slightly flexed while the client is lying in semi-Fowler's position in bed.
   □ 4. Keep a pillow under the client's head as needed for comfort.

The nurse in a cancer prevention and screening clinic is responsible for health education.

475. Which of the following is *not* one of the seven warning signs of cancer cited by the American Cancer Society?
   □ 1. Indigestion or difficulty swallowing.
   □ 2. Unusually slow healing sore.
   □ 3. Unusual bleeding or discharge.
   □ 4. Unusual tenderness in breast tissue.

476. In the health education class, the American Cancer Society Guidelines for early detection of cancer are discussed. Which response from a group member indicates correct understanding of these guidelines?
   □ 1. "I should have a cancer-related checkup every 5 years after I reach age 50."

☐ 2. "Women should have a baseline mammogram taken between the ages of 45 and 50."

☐ 3. "Adults over the age of 50 should have a guaiac test done on a yearly basis."

☐ 4. "A Pap smear needs to be done only on sexually active women."

477. A 40-year-old woman in the class asks what part of her body the cell sample is taken from for her yearly Pap smear. The nurse replies that the cells are scraped from the

☐ 1. Cervix.

☐ 2. Uterus.

☐ 3. Cul-de-sac.

☐ 4. Fallopian tubes.

478. If a client receives a Pap smear report that is class 1, what should the nurse advise?

☐ 1. Call the physician to discuss treatment options.

☐ 2. Prepare to go to the hospital for surgery.

☐ 3. Refrain from sexual activity.

☐ 4. Return for another Pap smear in 1 to 3 years, as directed by physician.

479. One of the best screening procedures for colorectal cancer is a

☐ 1. Barium enema for change in bowel pattern.

☐ 2. Home Hemoccult test.

☐ 3. Yearly proctosigmoidoscopy.

☐ 4. Digital rectal self-examination.

John Lark, a 67-year-old man, is admitted to the hospital with a tentative diagnosis of bronchogenic carcinoma. His chief complaint is dyspnea and a chronic cough.

480. Mr. Lark's physician orderes a sputum sample for cytological testing. Important nursing implications involved with obtaining a sputum sample for cytology should include which of the following?

☐ 1. Obtain the specimen in the evening hours.

☐ 2. Collect the specimen before the client eats and drinks.

☐ 3. Have the client brush his teeth before collection of the specimen.

☐ 4. Keep the client NPO for 24 hours before collection of the specimen.

481. Three of the following statements are true regarding lung cancer. Which one is *incorrect?*

☐ 1. The 5-year survival rate depends on tumor histology and disease stage at the time treatment is initiated.

☐ 2. Small-cell lung cancer has an excellent prognosis.

☐ 3. The 5-year survival rate for lung cancer is less than 15%.

☐ 4. Lung cancer is usually widespread by the time it is detected on chest x-ray.

482. Mr. Lark is scheduled for external radiation treatment. The most common systemic side effects of external radiation include all the following *except*

☐ 1. Anorexia.

☐ 2. Fatigue.

☐ 3. Malaise.

☐ 4. Dry desquamation of the skin.

483. When teaching Mr. Lark about his upcoming external radiation treatments, the nurse should stress the importance of

☐ 1. Massaging the area daily.

☐ 2. Exposing the area to sunlight or a heat lamp.

☐ 3. Not bathing the treatment area.

☐ 4. Applying powder to the area as needed.

484. Which of the following medications would be used to decrease Mr. Lark's nausea and vomiting?

☐ 1. Dexamethasone (Decadron).

☐ 2. Methylcellulose (Citrucel).

☐ 3. Phentolamine mesylate (Regitine).

☐ 4. Metoclopramide (Reglan).

Robert Varella is 54 years old and is admitted to the hospital for suspected colon cancer.

485. During the preoperative period, what is the most important aspect of Mr. Varella's nursing care?

☐ 1. Assure Mr. Varella that he will be cured of cancer.

☐ 2. Assess understanding of the procedure and expectation of bodily appearance after surgery.

☐ 3. Maintain a cheerful and optimistic environment.

☐ 4. Keep visitors to a minimum, so that he can have time to think things through.

486. Mr. Varella is found to have adenocarcinoma of the rectum. An abdominoperineal resection with a colostomy will be done. What surgical principle is applied when surgery is performed to cure or control cancer?

☐ 1. A margin of normal, healthy tissue must surround the tumor at the time of resection.

☐ 2. More tissue than necessary is removed to ensure that the cancer does not spread.

☐ 3. Surgery is usually done only as a last resort, after failure of radiation and chemotherapy.

☐ 4. The more radical the surgery, the better the prognosis.

487. During surgery, it is found that Mr. Varella has positive peritoneal lymph nodes. The next most likely site of metastasis would be the

☐ 1. Brain.

☐ 2. Bone.

☐ 3. Liver.

☐ 4. Mediastinum.

488. A chemotherapeutic agent, 5-fluorouracil (5-FU) is ordered for Mr. Varella as an adjunct measure to surgery. Which of the following statements about chemotherapy is true?

☐ 1. It is a local treatment affecting only tumor cells.
☐ 2. It is a systemic treatment affecting both tumor and normal cells.
☐ 3. It has not yet been proven an effective treatment for cancer.
☐ 4. It causes few if any side effects.

489. Mr. Varella develops stomatitis during his course of 5-fluorouracil (5-FU). Nursing care for this problem should include

☐ 1. A soft, bland diet.
☐ 2. Restricting fluids to decrease salivation.
☐ 3. Avoiding topical anesthetics, because they alter taste sensations.
☐ 4. Encouraging the client to drink hot liquids.

490. Mr. Varella asks the nurse why these sores developed in his mouth. What is the most appropriate response?

☐ 1. "Don't worry; it always happens with chemotherapy."
☐ 2. "Your oral hygiene needs improvement."
☐ 3. "It is a sign that the medication is effective."
☐ 4. "The sores result because the cells in the mouth are sensitive to the chemotherapy."

Susan Allen is a 24-year-old woman who has a diagnosis of acute granulocytic leukemia. She has an acute upper respiratory infection and bleeding gums.

491. When Mrs. Allen's husband is told that she has leukemia, he insists that she not be told her diagnosis. Which approach is best?

☐ 1. Tell her husband that it is her right to be told.
☐ 2. Suggest that he talk with the hospital chaplain.
☐ 3. Allow him to express his feelings and explain how his wife can benefit from being told.
☐ 4. Be patient with him, hoping he will feel differently when his anger subsides.

492. Mrs. Allen begins a regimen of chemotherapy. Her platelet count falls to 98,000. Which action is *not* necessary at this time?

☐ 1. Test all excreta for occult blood.
☐ 2. Use a soft toothbrush or foam cleaner for oral hygiene.
☐ 3. Implement reverse isolation.
☐ 4. Avoid IM injections.

493. High uric acid levels may develop in clients who are receiving chemotherapy. This is caused by

☐ 1. The inability of the kidneys to excrete the drug metabolites.
☐ 2. Rapid cell catabolism.
☐ 3. Toxic effects of the prophylactic antibiotics that are given concurrently.
☐ 4. The altered blood pH from the acid medium of the drugs.

494. The drug of choice to decrease uric acid levels is

☐ 1. Prednisone (Colisone).
☐ 2. Allopurinol (Zyloprim).
☐ 3. Indomethacin (Indocin).
☐ 4. Hydrochlorothiazide (HydroDIURIL).

495. Nursing care for the client undergoing chemotherapy includes assessment for signs of bone marrow depression. Which of the following accounts for some of the symptoms related to bone marrow depression?

☐ 1. Erythrocytosis.
☐ 2. Leukocytosis.
☐ 3. Polycythemia.
☐ 4. Thrombocytopenia.

Upon admission to the hospital, Joanne Day describes symptoms of intermenstrual bleeding and a foul-smelling vaginal discharge. An outpatient punch biopsy confirms cervical cancer.

496. Which of the following is *not* a predisposing factor for cervical cancer?

☐ 1. Early sexual experience with multiple partners.
☐ 2. History of genital herpes, chronic cervicitis, or venereal disease.
☐ 3. Family history of cervical cancer.
☐ 4. Multiple pregnancies at an early age.

497. Medical treatment for Mrs. Day will include a hysterectomy followed by internal radiation. Although she is 32 years old and has three children, Mrs. Day tells the nurse that she is anxious regarding the impending treatment and loss of her femininity. Which of the following interactions is most appropriate?

☐ 1. Tell Mrs. Day that now she does not have to worry about pregnancy.
☐ 2. Provide Mrs. Day with adequate information about the effects of treatment on sexual functioning.
☐ 3. Refer her to the physician.
☐ 4. Avoid the question. Nurses are not specialists in providing sexual counseling.

498. Mrs. Day receives a cervical intracavity radium implant as part of her therapy. A common side effect of a cervical implant is

☐ 1. Creamy, pink-tinged vaginal drainage.
☐ 2. Confusion.
☐ 3. Constipation.
☐ 4. Xerostomia.

499. Mrs. Day's care plan during the time that she has the cervical implant in place would include which of the following interventions?

☐ 1. Frequent ambulation.
☐ 2. Unlimited visitors.
☐ 3. Low-residue diet.
☐ 4. Vaginal irrigations every shift.

500. Which of the following is a long-term side effect of a cervical radium implant?
- ☐ 1. Shortening and narrowing of the vagina.
- ☐ 2. Nausea.
- ☐ 3. Uterine cramping.
- ☐ 4. Constipation.

Phyllis Newsberg, a 34-year-old client, has recently had a mastectomy.

501. Before discharge from the hospital, the nurse encourages Mrs. Newsberg to look at the incision. She turns her head and cries, "It is horrible." How should the nurse respond?
- ☐ 1. "I know, I'd feel the same way, too."
- ☐ 2. "It's OK, you can look at it anytime."
- ☐ 3. "Your feelings are normal; it's all right to cry."
- ☐ 4. "I know this is depressing, but it's not that terrible."

502. An important part of Mrs. Newsberg's long-term rehabilitation is teaching her the techniques of breast self-examination (BSE). Why is this important?
- ☐ 1. Breast cancer can be bilateral.
- ☐ 2. It will help the client confront the deformity.
- ☐ 3. It helps the client to focus on the possibility of future metastasis.
- ☐ 4. Teaching BSE really is not important as long as the client visits her physician regularly.

Two days before 65-year-old Delores Wu and her husband were to leave on a trip to Florida, she found a lump in her breast. She is admitted for a biopsy of the right breast with possible mastectomy and node dissection. While the nurse is doing preoperative teaching, Mrs. Wu says, "I'm sure this surgery will make me look like half a woman."

503. What is the most appropriate nursing response?
- ☐ 1. "I'm sure no one will know you've had a mastectomy."
- ☐ 2. "Today's prosthetic devices are very realistic."
- ☐ 3. "You're concerned about how you'll look after surgery?"
- ☐ 4. "You're going to be the same person after surgery that you are now."

504. What does the nurse do after having premedicated Mrs. Wu for surgery?
- ☐ 1. Check her vital signs, and document them on the chart.
- ☐ 2. Have Mrs. Wu sign the operative permit.
- ☐ 3. Have Mrs. Wu void.
- ☐ 4. Put the side rails up.

505. Mrs. Wu's postoperative diagnosis is breast cancer, treated with a right, modified mastectomy. She returns from the recovery room in supine position, with an IV infusing, an elastic bandage wrapped around her chest, and a HemoVac in place. The nurse monitors Mrs. Wu's vital signs and her dressing. Which part of the dressing does the nurse particularly observe for drainage?
- ☐ 1. Back.
- ☐ 2. Front.
- ☐ 3. Left side.
- ☐ 4. Right side.

506. Which of the following discharge instructions is essential for the nurse to give Mrs. Wu?
- ☐ 1. "Don't shave your right axilla."
- ☐ 2. "Don't wear your bra until after the first visit to your doctor's office."
- ☐ 3. "Increase your sodium and fluid intake."
- ☐ 4. "Wash the incision every day with a soft cloth and an antiseptic solution."

Forty-year-old Rita Goldfarb recently visited her gynecologist for her annual examination. During the visit, the nurse practitioner palpated a lump in Mrs. Goldfarb's right breast. She has now been admitted to the hospital for a breast biopsy.

507. Which of the following is *not* necessary to include in the admission assessment data?
- ☐ 1. Prior sexual relationships.
- ☐ 2. Quality of present sexual relationship.
- ☐ 3. Body image.
- ☐ 4. Occupational role.

508. During her admission interview, Mrs. Goldfarb states, "This is really nothing to worry about. After all, I had a normal checkup last year. I expect to be back home tomorrow night." Mrs. Goldfarb is most likely experiencing which of the following?
- ☐ 1. Anger.
- ☐ 2. Denial.
- ☐ 3. Depression.
- ☐ 4. Loss.

509. Depression may follow the mastectomy. Which of the following observations would most alert the nurse to depression in this client?
- ☐ 1. Disorientation during afternoon hours.
- ☐ 2. Increased agitation or restlessness.
- ☐ 3. Verbalization of hopelessness or helplessness.
- ☐ 4. Increased desire to sleep.

510. Which of the following nursing diagnoses is this client most likely to have following her mastectomy?
- ☐ 1. Disturbance in self-concept.
- ☐ 2. Self-care deficit.
- ☐ 3. Impaired verbal communication.
- ☐ 4. Alteration in cardiac output.

511. Lymphedema is the most common postoperative complication following axillary lymph node dissection. Which of the following actions would minimize this problem?

☐ 1. Avoid blood pressure measurements and constrictive clothing on the affected arm.

☐ 2. Allow a liberal fluid and sodium intake.

☐ 3. Discourage feeding, washing, or hair combing with the affected arm.

☐ 4. Place the affected arm in a dependent position, below the level of the heart.

512. It has been decided that Mrs. Goldfarb will have antineoplastic chemotherapy after surgery. Which of the following purposes of this chemotherapy will also help best explain to the client the possible side effects of the therapy?

☐ 1. It offers the only hope of cure.

☐ 2. It attacks the fastest growing cells of the body.

☐ 3. It is always indicated after a mastectomy.

☐ 4. It is a new treatment with few side effects.

513. Since Mrs. Goldfarb's left breast is free of tumor, the nurse reviews the technique of breast self-examination with her before discharge. When would be the most appropriate time for this client to perform this examination?

☐ 1. Just before the time of menstruation.

☐ 2. The day menstruation begins.

☐ 3. One week after the start of each menstrual period.

☐ 4. Varying times throughout the month.

Jean Chambers has had a mammogram and biopsy for bleeding from the nipple of her left breast. The physician diagnosed intraductal breast cancer and explained a modified mastectomy is necessary. Mrs. Chambers has agreed to the surgery, which is scheduled for the following morning.

514. What would be the most important aspect of the nurse's preoperative teaching?

☐ 1. Discuss with the client how her sexual relations will be altered.

☐ 2. Discuss the skin graft that will be necessary.

☐ 3. Explore the client's feelings and expectations about the surgery and correct any misconceptions.

☐ 4. Explain that most breast masses are benign, and hers will most likely be nonmalignant.

515. A HemoVac suction apparatus is in place at the surgical site postoperatively. Which of the following nursing actions would be incorrect when caring for the HemoVac?

☐ 1. Report bright-red, bloody drainage to the physician immediately.

☐ 2. Maintain aseptic technique.

☐ 3. Curl the tubing, and tape firmly against the skin.

☐ 4. Check the HemoVac drum frequently, and empty it when half full.

516. In the early postoperative period, the surgeon encourages Mrs. Chambers to begin using her left arm. She tells the nurse it hurts too much to move.

What would be the best nursing action to reinforce the physician's instructions?

☐ 1. Put the left arm in a sling to provide support.

☐ 2. Initiate slow, passive range-of-motion exercises.

☐ 3. Teach the client full, active range of motion.

☐ 4. Have the client do stretching exercises.

517. Which of the following nursing actions is least appropriate in planning for Mrs. Chambers' discharge from the hospital?

☐ 1. Provide information on a local "Reach to Recovery" group.

☐ 2. Discuss plans for obtaining a permanent prosthesis.

☐ 3. Discuss the possibility of a breast reconstruction in the future.

☐ 4. Discuss activities the client will need to discontinue.

April Hart is 21 years old and is admitted to the hospital for suspected Hodgkin's disease.

518. Which one of the following statements is correct concerning Hodgkin's disease?

☐ 1. It is a malignancy of the lymphoid system.

☐ 2. It is a malignant neoplasm of the plasma cells.

☐ 3. It is a syndrome characterized by a defect in cell-mediated immunity.

☐ 4. It is a malignant disease that is associated with diffuse abnormal growth of leukocyte precursors in the bone marrow.

519. During the nursing history, Miss Hart's chief complaints are night sweats, not feeling hungry, not eating as well, frequent abdominal cramps, diarrhea, and enlarged lymph nodes in her neck. Which one of the following symptoms is not considered a sign or symptom of Hodgkin's disease?

☐ 1. Night sweats.

☐ 2. Anorexia.

☐ 3. Diarrhea.

☐ 4. Enlarged lymph nodes.

520. Miss Hart is scheduled for a lymphangiography. To prepare her for the procedure the nurse would tell her that

☐ 1. She will be NPO after midnight.

☐ 2. She will be allowed to move about freely during the examination.

☐ 3. She will need to keep her leg in a dependent position after the procedure.

☐ 4. Her stools and urine will be blue-tinged for several days.

Max Evans, a 24-year-old man, makes an appointment at the health clinic for his complaints of fatigue, diarrhea, and weight loss. He is concerned that he might have acquired immunodeficiency syndrome (AIDS).

521. Which one of the following statements is correct regarding AIDS?

- ☐ 1. It is caused by a retrovirus that destroys T4 lymphocytes.
- ☐ 2. It is a malignancy of the lymphoid tissue.
- ☐ 3. It is caused by a bacterial infection that produces fatal endotoxins.
- ☐ 4. It is a malignancy of the skin.

522. The initial screening test for AIDS is

- ☐ 1. Lymphangiography.
- ☐ 2. Enzyme-linked immunosorbent assay (ELISA).
- ☐ 3. Western blot assay.
- ☐ 4. Schilling test.

523. Which of the following is an opportunistic disease frequently seen in AIDS clients?

- ☐ 1. Pancreatitis.
- ☐ 2. Prostatic cancer.
- ☐ 3. Hodgkin's disease.
- ☐ 4. *Pneumocystis carinii* pneumonia (PCP).

524. Mr. Evans is diagnosed as being HIV positive. When preparing for discharge, an important nursing goal is that he be knowledgeable about methods to prevent HIV transmission to others. Which response from Mr. Evans indicates that he has a correct understanding of this?

- ☐ 1. "I can donate blood 1 year after my therapy with zidovudine (Retrovir) is started."
- ☐ 2. "I should avoid casual contact with all males."
- ☐ 3. "I need to wear gloves and a mask at all times."
- ☐ 4. "I should not donate my plasma, sperm, or organs."

References

Barrick, B. (1988). Caring for A.I.D.S. patients: A challenge you can meet. *Nursing88, 18*(11), 50–59.

Bullock, B.L., & Rosendahl, P.P. (1988). *Pathophysiology: Adaptations and alterations in function* (2nd ed.). Glenview, IL: Scott, Foresman.

Pagana, K.D., & Pagana, T.J. (1990). *Diagnostic testing and nursing implications: A case study approach* (3rd ed.). St. Louis: Mosby–Year Book.

Skidmore-Roth, L. (1988). *Mosby's nursing drug reference*. St. Louis: Mosby–Year Book.

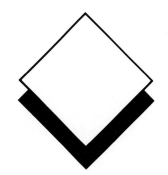

Correct Answers

1. no. 2.	**40.** no. 1.	**79.** no. 2.	**118.** no. 4.
2. no. 2.	**41.** no. 4.	**80.** no. 3.	**119.** no. 1.
3. no. 4.	**42.** no. 4.	**81.** no. 2.	**120.** no. 2.
4. no. 4.	**43.** no. 4.	**82.** no. 1.	**121.** no. 2.
5. no. 1.	**44.** no. 4.	**83.** no. 4.	**122.** no. 3.
6. no. 4.	**45.** no. 3.	**84.** no. 3.	**123.** no. 4.
7. no. 3.	**46.** no. 1.	**85.** no. 1.	**124.** no. 1.
8. no. 1.	**47.** no. 3.	**86.** no. 4.	**125.** no. 2.
9. no. 4.	**48.** no. 2.	**87.** no. 2.	**126.** no. 2.
10. no. 3.	**49.** no. 1.	**88.** no. 4.	**127.** no. 4.
11. no. 1.	**50.** no. 3.	**89.** no. 2.	**128.** no. 2.
12. no. 2.	**51.** no. 1.	**90.** no. 4.	**129.** no. 2.
13. no. 1.	**52.** no. 2.	**91.** no. 1.	**130.** no. 3.
14. no. 3.	**53.** no. 1.	**92.** no. 3.	**131.** no. 2.
15. no. 1.	**54.** no. 3.	**93.** no. 2.	**132.** no. 3.
16. no. 1.	**55.** no. 3.	**94.** no. 3.	**133.** no. 1.
17. no. 4.	**56.** no. 2.	**95.** no. 2.	**134.** no. 3.
18. no. 1.	**57.** no. 2.	**96.** no. 2.	**135.** no. 4.
19. no. 3.	**58.** no. 4.	**97.** no. 2.	**136.** no. 1.
20. no. 4.	**59.** no. 4.	**98.** no. 2.	**137.** no. 4.
21. no. 1.	**60.** no. 2.	**99.** no. 1.	**138.** no. 4.
22. no. 2.	**61.** no. 2.	**100.** no. 4.	**139.** no. 4.
23. no. 4.	**62.** no. 2.	**101.** no. 1.	**140.** no. 3.
24. no. 2.	**63.** no. 2.	**102.** no. 3.	**141.** no. 2.
25. no. 2.	**64.** no. 3.	**103.** no. 4.	**142.** no. 4.
26. no. 3.	**65.** no. 2.	**104.** no. 2.	**143.** no. 4.
27. no. 3.	**66.** no. 1.	**105.** no. 2.	**144.** no. 3.
28. no. 3.	**67.** no. 2.	**106.** no. 4.	**145.** no. 2.
29. no. 2.	**68.** no. 3.	**107.** no. 2.	**146.** no. 2.
30. no. 3.	**69.** no. 2.	**108.** no. 2.	**147.** no. 1.
31. no. 2.	**70.** no. 3.	**109.** no. 3.	**148.** no. 3.
32. no. 1.	**71.** no. 3.	**110.** no. 2.	**149.** no. 1.
33. no. 3.	**72.** no. 1.	**111.** no. 2.	**150.** no. 4.
34. no. 1.	**73.** no. 1.	**112.** no. 1.	**151.** no. 2.
35. no. 2.	**74.** no. 2.	**113.** no. 2.	**152.** no. 3.
36. no. 3.	**75.** no. 3.	**114.** no. 3.	**153.** no. 4.
37. no. 3.	**76.** no. 4.	**115.** no. 3.	**154.** no. 1.
38. no. 3.	**77.** no. 2.	**116.** no. 2.	**155.** no. 4.
39. no. 4.	**78.** no. 3.	**117.** no. 2.	**156.** no. 2.

157. no. 3.	213. no. 2.	269. no. 3.	325. no. 3.
158. no. 2.	214. no. 4.	270. no. 1.	326. no. 2.
159. no. 2.	215. no. 4.	271. no. 3.	327. no. 1.
160. no. 1.	216. no. 4.	272. no. 1.	328. no. 3.
161. no. 2.	217. no. 1.	273. no. 4.	329. no. 4.
162. no. 3.	218. no. 4.	274. no. 2.	330. no. 2.
163. no. 3.	219. no. 3.	275. no. 1.	331. no. 4.
164. no. 2.	220. no. 4.	276. no. 1.	332. no. 1.
165. no. 4.	221. no. 3.	277. no. 1.	333. no. 3.
166. no. 1.	222. no. 3.	278. no. 1.	334. no. 2.
167. no. 2.	223. no. 1.	279. no. 2.	335. no. 2.
168. no. 3.	224. no. 4.	280. no. 3.	336. no. 2.
169. no. 2.	225. no. 2.	281. no. 1.	337. no. 4.
170. no. 4.	226. no. 1.	282. no. 3.	338. no. 1.
171. no. 1.	227. no. 1.	283. no. 4.	339. no. 2.
172. no. 4.	228. no. 2.	284. no. 3.	340. no. 4.
173. no. 2.	229. no. 4.	285. no. 2.	341. no. 3.
174. no. 4.	230. no. 2.	286. no. 1.	342. no. 1.
175. no. 4.	231. no. 3.	287. no. 2.	343. no. 4.
176. no. 2.	232. no. 3.	288. no. 3.	344. no. 4.
177. no. 2.	233. no. 4.	289. no. 3.	345. no. 3.
178. no. 4.	234. no. 4.	290. no. 1.	346. no. 2.
179. no. 2.	235. no. 2.	291. no. 4.	347. no. 3.
180. no. 2.	236. no. 1.	292. no. 2.	348. no. 4.
181. no. 4.	237. no. 3.	293. no. 3.	349. no. 3.
182. no. 2.	238. no. 1.	294. no. 1.	350. no. 2.
183. no. 4.	239. no. 3.	295. no. 3.	351. no. 3.
184. no. 4.	240. no. 3.	296. no. 4.	352. no. 4.
185. no. 2.	241. no. 1.	297. no. 3.	353. no. 3.
186. no. 1.	242. no. 2.	298. no. 4.	354. no. 3.
187. no. 3.	243. no. 2.	299. no. 2.	355. no. 3.
188. no. 2.	244. no. 3.	300. no. 3.	356. no. 3.
189. no. 3.	245. no. 1.	301. no. 2.	357. no. 2.
190. no. 3.	246. no. 4.	302. no. 1.	358. no. 4.
191. no. 3.	247. no. 4.	303. no. 2.	359. no. 1.
192. no. 2.	248. no. 3.	304. no. 2.	360. no. 1.
193. no. 2.	249. no. 1.	305. no. 3.	361. no. 4.
194. no. 2.	250. no. 2.	306. no. 2.	362. no. 3.
195. no. 3.	251. no. 1.	307. no. 1.	363. no. 3.
196. no. 1.	252. no. 2.	308. no. 4.	364. no. 3.
197. no. 3.	253. no. 4.	309. no. 3.	365. no. 3.
198. no. 1.	254. no. 1.	310. no. 1.	366. no. 1.
199. no. 4.	255. no. 1.	311. no. 1.	367. no. 4.
200. no. 2.	256. no. 4.	312. no. 3.	368. no. 2.
201. no. 4.	257. no. 1.	313. no. 1.	369. no. 2.
202. no. 1.	258. no. 2.	314. no. 2.	370. no. 1.
203. no. 3.	259. no. 1.	315. no. 2.	371. no. 3.
204. no. 4.	260. no. 2.	316. no. 1.	372. no. 2.
205. no. 1.	261. no. 3.	317. no. 2.	373. no. 2.
206. no. 2.	262. no. 2.	318. no. 1.	374. no. 4.
207. no. 3.	263. no. 4.	319. no. 4.	375. no. 3.
208. no. 4.	264. no. 2.	320. no. 2.	376. no. 4.
209. no. 1.	265. no. 4.	321. no. 4.	377. no. 3.
210. no. 4.	266. no. 4.	322. no. 4.	378. no. 3.
211. no. 3.	267. no. 2.	323. no. 3.	379. no. 2.
212. no. 2.	268. no. 4.	324. no. 2.	380. no. 3.

381. no. 2.
382. no. 3.
383. no. 1.
384. no. 3.
385. no. 3.
386. no. 1.
387. no. 2.
388. no. 4.
389. no. 1.
390. no. 1.
391. no. 3.
392. no. 3.
393. no. 3.
394. no. 3.
395. no. 3.
396. no. 3.
397. no. 1.
398. no. 1.
399. no. 4.
400. no. 3.
401. no. 1.
402. no. 4.
403. no. 1.
404. no. 4.
405. no. 2.
406. no. 4.
407. no. 4.
408. no. 2.
409. no. 1.
410. no. 2.
411. no. 2.
412. no. 2.
413. no. 1.
414. no. 1.
415. no. 1.
416. no. 2.

417. no. 4.
418. no. 4.
419. no. 3.
420. no. 1.
421. no. 4.
422. no. 1.
423. no. 2.
424. no. 3.
425. no. 4.
426. no. 1.
427. no. 4.
428. no. 2.
429. no. 2.
430. no. 1.
431. no. 2.
432. no. 2.
433. no. 2.
434. no. 4.
435. no. 3.
436. no. 3.
437. no. 4.
438. no. 3.
439. no. 2.
440. no. 1.
441. no. 2.
442. no. 4.
443. no. 4.
444. no. 4.
445. no. 1.
446. no. 2.
447. no. 3.
448. no. 4.
449. no. 3.
450. no. 2.
451. no. 1.
452. no. 4.

453. no. 1.
454. no. 3.
455. no. 2.
456. no. 3.
457. no. 2.
458. no. 4.
459. no. 4.
460. no. 4.
461. no. 2.
462. no. 1.
463. no. 4.
464. no. 2.
465. no. 4.
466. no. 2.
467. no. 2.
468. no. 2.
469. no. 2.
470. no. 1.
471. no. 3.
472. no. 1.
473. no. 4.
474. no. 2.
475. no. 4.
476. no. 3.
477. no. 1.
478. no. 4.
479. no. 2.
480. no. 2.
481. no. 2.
482. no. 4.
483. no. 3.
484. no. 4.
485. no. 2.
486. no. 1.
487. no. 3.
488. no. 2.

489. no. 1.
490. no. 4.
491. no. 3.
492. no. 4.
493. no. 2.
494. no. 2.
495. no. 3.
496. no. 3.
497. no. 2.
498. no. 1.
499. no. 3.
500. no. 1.
501. no. 3.
502. no. 1.
503. no. 3.
504. no. 4.
505. no. 1.
506. no. 1.
507. no. 1.
508. no. 2.
509. no. 3.
510. no. 1.
511. no. 1.
512. no. 2.
513. no. 3.
514. no. 3.
515. no. 3.
516. no. 2.
517. no. 4.
518. no. 1.
519. no. 3.
520. no. 4.
521. no. 1.
522. no. 2.
523. no. 4.
524. no. 4.

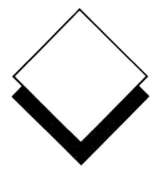

Correct Answers with Rationales

Editor's note: Three pieces of information are supplied at the end of each rationale. First, you will find a reference to a section in the *AJN/Mosby Nursing Boards Review* where a more complete discussion of the topic may be found, should you desire more information. A second reference indicates what part of the nursing process the question addresses. The third piece of information describes the appropriate client need category.

KEY TO ABBREVIATIONS
Section of the Review Book

A = Adult
  H = Healthy Adult
  S = Surgery
  O = Oxygenation
  NM = Nutrition and Metabolism
  E = Elimination
  SP = Sensation and Perception
  M = Mobility
  CA = Cellular Aberration

Nursing process category

AS = Assessment
AN = Analysis
PL = Plan
IM = Implementation
EV = Evaluation

Client need category

E = Safe, Effective Care Environment
PS = Physiological Integrity
PC = Psychosocial Integrity
H = Health Promotion and Maintenance

1. no. 2. Hyperextending the neck can cause a spinal injury if the vertebrae have been fractured. The other options are correct, based on CPR standards. A/O, IM, PS

2. no. 2. The mouth is kept closed during inspiration. No more force than normal is required. The victim's neck is extended, not hyperextended. In both approaches, the mouth is open during expiration. A/O, IM, PS

3. no. 4. Using one hand, only approximately 400 ml of air can be delivered. Almost 1000 ml can be delivered if both hands are used. A/O, AN, PS

4. no. 4. Fluid volume is the first priority after adequate ventilation. The blood pressure and pulse indicate that the client is in a volume-depleted state. Sodium bicarbonate may be given only following arterial blood gas results. Options no. 2 and no. 3 are not considerations of therapy in arrest situations. A/O, PL, PS

5. no. 1. The type of instrument involved (blunt vs. sharp) and where it hit is information of the most value, since it will help define the type of injury. A sharp injury tends to bleed more quickly; a blunt injury tends to leak or ooze. Options no. 2 and no. 3 are important, but not specific to blood loss. Option no. 4 is irrelevant. A/O, AS, PS

6. no. 4. With a negative thoracentesis and a rising central venous pressure, the only reasonable conclusion is that cardiac tamponade is the cause. Bleeding into the pericardial sac causes both decreased blood pressure and increased central venous pressure. Options no. 1, no. 2, or no. 3 tend to have no effect on central venous pressure. A/O, AN, PS

7. no. 3. When the systolic blood pressure falls below 80 mm Hg, circulation to the vital organs is markedly compromised. A/O, AS, PS

8. no. 1. Increased levels of angiotensin and renin result in vasoconstriction of the peripheral vessels; thus, blood is more available for the brain, heart, and kidneys. Options no. 3 and no. 4 are incorrect; these substances do not affect the respiratory center. A/O, AN, PS

9. no. 4. Although dopamine is a potent vasopressor, kidney perfusion can be maintained in the mild to moderate dosage range. In low doses (2-5 μg/kg/min), dopamine dilates renal, cerebral, and coronary blood vessels. In moderate doses (5-10 μg/kg/min), dopamine increases myocardial contractility. In high-dose ranges (over 10 μg/kg/min), dopamine constricts renal vessels. Untoward effects include dysrhythmias, angina, and pulmonary congestion. A/O, AN, PS

10. no. 3. A urine output of 30 ml/hr indicates there is adequate kidney perfusion. In selected cases, systolic pressure of 90 or 100 mm Hg would not ensure adequate renal perfusion. The minimum for adequate urine output is 30 ml/hr. A/O, AS, PS

11. no. 1. The most precise measurement of hemodynamic status would be used, particularly in an older client. These two factors reflect fluid volume adequate enough to perfuse the kidneys. CVP readings would best reflect response to treatment as well as hourly urine output. Recommended urine output is 30 ml/hr for at least 2 consecutive hours. A/O, EV, PS

12. no. 2. As sympathomimetics, adrenergic agents cause vasoconstriction. Options no. 1 and no. 3 are incorrect and not desirable for the client in shock. Option no. 4 has no relationship to adrenergic agents. A/O, AN, PS

13. no. 1. Adrenalin is a potent cardiac stimulant. It does not cause any of the effects listed in the other options. A/O, AN, PS

14. no. 3. As sympathomimetics, adrenergics can cause overstimulation of the heart and dysrhythmias. The other side effects listed are not considered serious. A/O, AS, PS

15. no. 1. These values indicate metabolic acidosis, as evidenced by low pH, normal P_{CO_2}, and low bicarbonate level. Low bicarbonate levels reflect a metabolic disturbance. P_{O_2} has no bearing on determining type of acidosis or alkalosis. A/O, AN, PS

16. no. 1. Any extreme in pH will inhibit enzyme activity with resulting loss of total body functioning. A/O, AN, PS

17. no. 4. The blood buffers (oxyhemoglobin, phosphates, carbonates) are the first line of defense. These tend to be quicker responses. Retention of bicarbonate by the kidneys is a slow process; this usually takes at least 24 hours to be effective. A/O, AN, PS

18. no. 1. A client receiving chronic steroid therapy is very prone to a relative insufficiency when stressed, because the adrenals cannot produce extra amounts of cortisol as required. Addison's disease is a primary adrenocortical insufficiency. Azotemia is the condition of abnormally high levels of nitrogenous wastes. A/NM, AN, PS

19. no. 3. These symptoms are typical of disseminated intravascular coagulation. A/O, AN, PS

20. no. 4. This client will have a relative deficiency of glucocorticoids and mineralocorticoids when under stress, requiring replacement drugs. A/NM, AN, PS

21. no. 1. Although hemorrhage is a symptom seen in disseminated intravascular coagulation, the problem is really one of microcoagulation. Heparin would be used cautiously because it blocks the subsequent formation of microemboli by inhibiting thrombin activity. PRBC will replace those lost. A/O, AN, PS

22. no. 2. The first phase of disseminated intravascular coagulation (DIC), hypercoagulation, results in the formation of microthrombi. Renal failure can result from thrombosis of the microcirculation of the kidneys. Options no. 1, no. 3, and no. 4 have no relationship to DIC. A/O, AN, PS

23. no. 4. Remove hypothermia equipment when the client is one degree above the recommended temperature, because an additional temperature drop may occur after discontinuance. A/O, IM, PS

24. no. 2. Decreasing his pain is the most important priority at this time. As long as the pain is present, there is the danger of extension of the infarcted area. Starting an IV is a second action, especially if the medication is ordered IV. A/O, IM, PS

25. no. 2. An infarction results in anoxia of the involved tissue. This anoxia results in ischemic tissue with irritation of the nerve endings in the infarcted area. Pain is the clinical presentation. A/O, AN, PS

26. no. 3. The left ventricle of the heart, which contributes most to contraction, is most frequently the site of the myocardial infarction. Because of this, the nurse monitors myocardial infarction clients for left-sided congestive heart failure. A/O, AN, PS

27. no. 3. Keeping family and significant others informed of client progress is of paramount importance and is therapeutic for the client. A/O, IM, H

28. no. 3. Denial is the most common reason for not seeking medical attention. The client may fear the consequences and thus uses denial as a defense mechanism. A/O, AN, PC

29. no. 2. Establishing an airway is the primary objective and action in any emergency, especially in a cardiopulmonary arrest. Initiating cardiac massage and calling a physician follow next in order of priority. A/O, IM, PS

30. no. 3. Presence of a carotid pulse represents adequate vascular perfusion and myocardial oxygenation because he had cardiac arrest. Options no. 1 and no. 2 indicate adequate perfusion to the pupils and periphery. Option no. 4 is an abnormal re-

sponse that may be a manifestation of a pyramidal tract lesion. A/O, EV, PS

31. no. 2. Chest pain in an acute myocardial infarction is intense and severe and is not relieved by nitroglycerin or rest. Nitroglycerin is the drug of choice for angina pectoris. A/O, AS, PS

32. no. 1. Morphine sulfate is the drug of choice in this situation, because it has a rapid action, is potent, has a diuretic effect, results in slight coronary vasodilatation, and is helpful in relieving anxiety. These are all particularly beneficial outcomes for the myocardial infarction client. Options no. 3 and no. 4 are not usually used for chest pain. Meperidine (Demerol) tends to lower the blood pressure. A/O, AN, PS

33. no. 3. With an infarction, anoxia of the myocardium occurs. Administration of oxygen will help relieve dyspnea and cyanosis associated with the pain, but the primary purpose is to increase oxygen concentration in the damaged tissue of the myocardium. A/O, AN, PS

34. no. 1. The first 24 to 48 hours is a very dangerous period, because of the extreme irritability of the heart. The irritability comes from the ischemic area surrounding the infarcted dead-tissue area. A/O, AN, PS

35. no. 2. The heart is very irritable at this time, and ventricular dysrhythmias are most common and very serious. The other options listed are serious, but not as commonly associated with myocardial infarction as dysrhythmias are. A/O, AN, PS

36. no. 3. The mortality rate is 80% for all clients who go into cardiogenic shock. Even sophisticated drugs and intraaortic balloon pumping may not be able to help the client who has lost the pumping action of the heart. A/O, AN, PS

37. no. 3. Whenever there is tissue death, certain enzymes are released. Creatine kinase-MB isoenzyme (CK-MB) and lactic dehydrogenase (LDH_1) isoenzymes are specific for cardiac muscle; typically, the higher the level of enzyme elevation, the greater the damage to the muscle. A 12-lead ECG is used to determine the location of a myocardial infarction. A/O, AN, PS

38. no. 3. Lidocaine decreases ventricular irritability and thereby reduces premature ventricular contractions. Procainamide and phenytoin are second-choice drugs if lidocaine is ineffective. Digoxin is used to slow the heart rate and increase contractility. A/O, AN, PS

39. no. 4. Sedation is a more common side effect of lidocaine. It actually may be a positive action, since it helps the client to relax; however, it must be assessed so that central nervous system depression does not progress. A/O, AS, PS

40. no. 1. Administration of laxatives can prevent straining on defecation. Straining results in Valsalva's maneuver. Options no. 2 and no. 4 may stimulate Valsalva's maneuver. Liquids at room temperature neither prevent nor stimulate Valsalva's maneuver. A/O, IM, PS

41. no. 4. There is a high probability that her husband may die, and she needs to prepare for that. Actions in options no. 1, no. 2, and no. 3 would tend to facilitate movement through the grief experience. Letting her know the nurses are competent may reassure her, but it will not help with anticipatory grieving. A/O, IM, H

42. no. 4. Allowing Mr. Mung to express his concerns is the initial priority. A one-on-one teaching approach is advisable for this delicate subject. When he feels comfortable, a teaching session with his wife may be planned. A/O, PL, H

43. no. 4. Liver is an organ meat high in cholesterol; tuna and shellfish have minimal cholesterol. Rice has the lowest amount. A/O, AN, H

44. no. 4. Taking aspirin daily prevents platelet aggregation and may decrease the risk of myocardial infarction. Family history of cardiovascular disease, diabetes, and smoking increases the risk. A/O, AS, PS

45. no. 3. This represents the most reasonable amount of activity. Walking up stairs significantly increases the work load of the heart. The physician will determine how and when the client can undertake this activity. A/O, IM, H

46. no. 1. Congestive heart failure results from circulatory congestion, and the characteristic symptom is dyspnea. Bronchi are not obstructed by mucoid secretions. Secretions are very watery and voluminous. It is unlikely that the heart will dilate to the point of lung-tissue compression severe enough to cause dyspnea. This client is in left-sided heart failure; ascites is a manifestation of right-sided heart failure. A/O, AN, PS

47. no. 3. Venous pressure increases and stasis occurs, promoting the extravasation of fluid from the vascular space into the tissue. Diffusion results when solid particles in solution move from an area of higher concentration to lower concentration; osmosis is fluid moving from an area of lower solute concentration to higher concentration. Neither of these describes the cause of edema. The capillary bed does dilate, but it is the increased venous pressure that causes the edema. A/O, AN, PS

48. no. 2. Because of gravity, dependent edema, especially in the feet, occurs in cardiac failure. The edema is pitting and nonpainful in nature. Periorbital edema usually occurs as a result of head trauma or renal failure. A/O, AS, PS

49. no. 1. *Left-sided* congestive heart failure produces pulmonary symptoms because the blood is in the pulmonary system before entering the left heart chambers. The other symptoms listed are systemic ones associated with *right-sided* congestive heart failure. A/O, AS, PS

50. no. 3. Potassium affects neuromuscular activity. Hyperkalemia (serum potassium greater than 5.5 mEq/L) often results in ventricular fibrillation, leading to death. A/O, AN, PS

51. no. 1. Respirations in congestive heart failure are rapid and shallow because a shift of fluid from extravascular to the vascular space results in increased venous return and greater work load on the heart and lungs. Wheezing does not occur from heart failure alone; however, if a client also has chronic obstructive pulmonary disease, then wheezing might be heard. Cheyne-Stokes respirations are seen in the later stages of congestive heart failure. A/O, AS, PS

52. no. 2. The client with congestive heart failure can breathe more easily in a Fowler's or semi-Fowler's position because gravity promotes drainage of secretions from the pulmonary bed and pooling of blood in the extremities. Also, maximal lung expansion is permitted, because there is less pressure from the abdominal organs. A/O, IM, PS

53. no. 1. Circulation is decreased in congestive heart failure; thus, drug absorption and distribution are slowed. A/O, AN, PS

54. no. 3. Furosemide (Lasix) causes loss of potassium. Hypokalemia increases the effect of digoxin and increases the risk of digitalis toxicity. A/O, PL, PS

55. no. 3. Rotating tourniquets are used to decrease venous return to the right side of the heart, thus relieving some of the congestion in the heart and lungs. A/O, AN, PS

56. no. 2. This ensures that no single extremity is compressed for more than 45 minutes. In the elderly client, this procedure may be modified by rotating tourniquets at 5-minute intervals rather than 15-minute intervals. A/O, IM, E

57. no. 2. Canned tuna is highly salted (628 mg sodium per 3¼ oz). Unsalted nuts are not contraindicated on a sodium-restricted diet. Whole milk and eggs are not allowed on a low-cholesterol, low-polysaturated-fat diet, but they are allowed on a 2000-mg sodium diet. Low-sodium milk is used only on a *severely* sodium-restricted diet (200 to 500 mg sodium). A/O, IM, H

58. no. 4. Breads and cereals contain almost no potassium. A/O, IM, H

59. no. 4. Thrombophlebitis is the occlusion of a vessel with inflammation and thrombus formation. It results in such signs and symptoms as a positive Homans' sign, history of leg pain, redness, and unilateral swelling. A/O, AS, PS

60. no. 2. In order to prevent dislodgment of a thrombus, maintain bed rest for 5 to 10 days, elevate the legs, apply warm, moist packs to the involved site, and provide range-of-motion exercises to the *unaffected* extremity at least two times per shift. A/O, PL, PS

61. no. 2. Heparin inactivates thromboplastin and thrombin that forms. Neither parenteral nor oral anticoagulants affect existing thrombi. A/O, AN, PS

62. no. 2. Monitor the partial thromboplastin time (PTT) when clients are receiving parenteral anticoagulants. Prothrombin times are monitored when a client is on warfarin (Coumadin) or dicumarol. A/O, IM, PS

63. no. 2. A positive Homans' sign is pain in the calf when the foot is dorsiflexed. It is a sign of phlebitis. A/O, AS, PS

64. no. 3. Protamine sulfate is the antidote for heparin sodium; vitamin K is the antidote for warfarin (Coumadin). A/O, AN, PS

65. no. 2. Mrs. Avery should avoid using any product that increases anticoagulation (e.g., aspirin) or causes bleeding (e.g., a hard toothbrush). She should notify her physician at once of any signs and symptoms of bleeding such as hematuria or melena. A/O, IM, E

66. no. 1. A pulmonary embolus causes hyperventilation. This lowers the P_{CO_2} and produces respiratory alkalosis. A/O, AN, PS

67. no. 2. Hyperventilation and lowered P_{CO_2} are common after a pulmonary embolus. A/O, AS, PS

68. no. 3. Central cyanosis would indicate a serious drop in the P_{O_2}. It is the most significant sign of hypoxia. A/O, AS, PS

69. no. 2. The ratio is 1 part of carbonic acid (P_{CO_2}) to 20 parts of base bicarbonate (HCO_3). A/O, AN, PS

70. no. 3. Cor pulmonale is a complication of obstructive pulmonary disease. Hypertrophy of the right side of the heart resulting from pulmonary hypertension causes the signs and symptoms of right-sided heart failure. A/O, AN, PS

71. no. 3. For clients with a long-standing history of chronic obstructive pulmonary disease, hypoxemia is the major stimulus to respiration. If oxygen is administered in high concentrations, it will eliminate this hypoxic drive, and the rate and depth of respirations will decrease. A/O, IM, PS

72. no. 1. Pursed-lip breathing prevents bronchiolar collapse, which results in air trapping. A/O, AN, PS

73. no. 1. Hemoptysis indicates bleeding, and percussion could exacerbate this condition. The condi-

tions indicated in no. 2, no. 3, and no. 4 would benefit from percussion because there is the possibility of retained secretions in all. A/O, AN, PS

74. no. 2. Hyperkalemia always occurs with acidemia. A/O, AS, PS

75. no. 3. Pneumonia is characterized by these symptoms. Anginal pain is not usually influenced by coughing or associated with a productive cough. Pulmonary edema is associated with frothy pink, blood-tinged sputum. A/O, AN, PS

76. no. 4. The pneumococcal bacteria account for the majority of pneumonia cases, and the resulting infection is characterized by rust-colored sputum. Sputum color varies with different types of organisms. A/O, AS, PS

77. no. 2. Respirations are usually rapid and shallow in pneumonia, because of pain on deep inspiration. Tachycardia often occurs with the fever; breath sounds would be diminished on the right side; and a pleural friction rub would be auscultated. A/O, AS, PS

78. no. 3. Dullness is of medium-intensity pitch and is elicited over areas of mixed solid and lung tissues, as with the consolidated lung tissue in pneumonia. Tympanic sounds are drumlike, as heard when a gas-filled bowel is percussed. Resonance is the normal sound heard when normal lung tissue is percussed. Hyperresonance is heard over an emphysematous lung. A/O, AS, PS

79. no. 2. Splinting occurs when the chest is held rigid to prevent pain on respiratory movement. A/O, AS, PS

80. no. 3. Increased fluids are needed to help liquefy secretions; no history of cardiac problems has been given that would contraindicate this action. Analgesics (though not necessarily narcotics) are given so the discomfort associated with coughing, deep breathing, percussion, and postural drainage every 2 to 4 hours can be tolerated. A/O, PL, E

81. no. 2. Venturi masks can control oxygen delivery at 24%, 28%, 31%, 35%, and 40% with a great deal of accuracy. A/O, AN, PS

82. no. 1. Gentamicin is an aminoglycoside. This group of antibiotics is nephrotoxic, and BUN and creatinine must be monitored to assess for any decrease in renal function as shown by an increase in BUN and creatinine. A/O, AS, PS

83. no. 4. Atelectasis is a complication of pneumonia; it is treated with tracheal suctioning, effective coughing, and deep breathing. A/O, AN, PS

84. no. 3. Measures to prevent hypoxemia during suctioning include preoxygenation and limiting each suctioning to 10 to 15 seconds. A/O, IM, E

85. no. 1. Tuberculosis is an infectious disease caused by the bacteria *Mycobacterium tuberculosis*. A/O, AN, E

86. no. 4. The PPD skin test is specific for tuberculosis and is considered positive when there is induration of 10 mm or larger. A/O, AS, PS

87. no. 2. The PPD skin test is used to determine presence of tuberculous antibodies; it indicates, when positive, that a person has been exposed to *Mycobacterium tuberculosis*. Further studies are needed to determine the presence of an active infection. A/O, AN, PS

88. no. 4. In the treatment of tuberculosis, drugs are often given in combination with other drugs to delay development of resistance and to increase tuberculostatic effects. A/O, AN, PS

89. no. 2. The most common and important untoward effect of isoniazid (INH) is peripheral neuritis. A/O, AS, PS

90. no. 4. The peripheral neuritis that occurs with isoniazid therapy can be controlled with the administration of vitamin B_6 (pyridoxine), because the neuritis is a result of pyridoxine deficiency. A/O, AN, PS

91. no. 1. A fairly common side effect of rifampin (Rimactane) therapy is reddish-orange urine, saliva, and sputum. A/O, IM, H

92. no. 3. Isoniazid (INH) is used as preventive therapy in household members of newly diagnosed clients. It is effective and inexpensive and is given orally. A/O, AN, PS

93. no. 2. Because isoniazid (INH) is known to cause hepatitis in some persons, liver function tests may be done before the client starts taking the drug. A/O, AS, PS

94. no. 3. Histoplasmosis has many of the same symptoms as tuberculosis, but is caused by a fungus. A/O, AN, PS

95. no. 2. The fungus is responsive to amphotericin B, not to the other drugs listed. A/O, AN, PS

96. no. 2. This position promotes maximal ventilation of the affected lung. Positioning on the operative side would inhibit thoracic excursion and, therefore, ventilation. Fowler's position increases the intrathoracic space, which allows maximal ventilation. A/O, PL, PS

97. no. 2. Continuous bubbling could indicate an air leak in the system. Bubbling should be intermittent, and it indicates the expulsion of air from the pleural space. There should be fluctuation in the water-seal tube with respiration. Suction is not used in a one-bottle setup. A/O, AS, PS

98. no. 2. Water-seal drainage means that the chest tube is under a water seal to prevent air from entering the chest cavity. Chest-tube drainage setups must be kept below chest level at all times. The chest tube must not be attached to any tube or drainage bottle that would be open to air. A/O, AN, PS

99. no. 1. The fluid in the tube oscillates with inspiration and expiration when the water-seal apparatus is functioning properly. On inspiration the fluid will rise; on expiration the fluid will fall. A/O, AN, PS

100. no. 4. The most common symptom of bronchogenic carcinoma is the development of a cough or change in the severity of a chronic cough. There are no early signs of lung cancer. A/O, AS, PS

101. no. 1. The client will be kept NPO until the gag reflex returns in 2 to 4 hours. A/O, PL, PS

102. no. 3. The less pain the client experiences, the more effectively he can cough and deep-breathe. The other options are very good, but cannot be effective unless the client's postoperative pain is controlled. A/O, IM, PS

103. no. 4. The long tube submerged 3 to 5 cm below the fluid level acts as a one-way valve, permitting air and fluid to drain out of the pleural space while preventing influx of air. A/O, AN, PS

104. no. 2. Continuous bubbling in the water-seal bottle during inspiration and expiration may indicate an air leak. Bubbling should be intermittent. A/O, AN, PS

105. no. 2. After the specimen is obtained, apply pressure to the area for 5 minutes to prevent bleeding and hematoma formation. A/O, IM, E

106. no. 4. Normal values are as follows: pH 7.35 to 7.45, Po_2 80 to 100 mm Hg, Pco_2 35 to 45 mm Hg, oxygen saturation 95% to 98%. A/O, AS, PS

107. no. 2. The client should be less confused because all the blood-gas values have improved. Confusion usually results when the Po_2 falls below 50. A/O, EV, PS

108. no. 2. Effects of gravity are lost when lying or bending, and gastric reflux occurs more easily. Increased stress may increase stomach acid; however, position changes along with this increased acid would result in a report of symptoms being worse. Position changes that counteract the effects of gravity are a priority. A/NM, AS, PS

109. no. 3. Esophagus-sphincter pressure is increased by gastrin in the stomach and decreased by fatty foods, secretin, and cholecystokinin from the small intestine. A/NM, AS, PS

110. no. 2. Smoking and alcohol aggravate and contribute to the condition. The head of the bed should be raised. Increased weight, especially in the abdominal area, may aggravate the symptoms by pushing upon the esophageal sphincter. A/NM, PL, H

111. no. 2. The late development of symptoms coupled with early lymphatic spread means that metastasis has probably occurred by the time the disease is diagnosed. Thus prognosis is poor at the time of diagnosis. A/NM, AN, PS

112. no. 1. Clients are advised to eat small meals to prevent excessive gastric distension and to avoid eating before going to bed or lying down. Swallowing air and belching tend to increase gastric regurgitation. A/NM, IM, H

113. no. 2. A local anesthetic is given to deaden the gag reflex. Do not give oral fluids until this reflex returns. Without a gag reflex, risk of aspiration is high. A/NM, IM, PS

114. no. 3. Guaiac testing is done to detect presence of occult (not visible) blood. Hydrochloric acid is tested by measuring the pH of the stomach aspirate. A pH of less than 5 is usually associated with a lower risk of ulcer development. A/NM, AN, PS

115. no. 3. Duodenal ulcer pain occurs when excess hydrochloric acid irritates an empty stomach. Typically, pain with a gastric ulcer usually follows the ingestion of food; options no. 1, no. 2, and no. 4 would apply. A/NM, AS, PS

116. no. 2. Nicotine stimulates the secretory cells and increases gastric acidity, thus enhancing symptoms. All of the other options are incorrect. A/NM, IM, H

117. no. 2. Coffee, even when decaffeinated, is thought to stimulate gastric acidity. Coffee may increase systolic pressure; however, option no. 4 is not specific to the question. A/NM, IM, H

118. no. 4. A subtotal gastrectomy (Billroth I or II) involves removal of one-half to two-thirds of the lower stomach. This area is the gastric-producing portion of the stomach. A Billroth I is a gastro-duodenostomy; Billroth II is a gastrojejunostomy. A/NM, AN, E

119. no. 1. The vagus nerve stimulates secretion of hydrochloric acid. The other options do not describe functions of the vagus nerve. A/NM, AN, PS

120. no. 2. The secretion of bile is blocked if the duodenum is removed. A/NM, AN, PS

121. no. 2. The high incision causes pain that, in turn, limits chest expansion. Options no. 1, no. 3, and no. 4 are incorrect. A/NM, AN, PS

122. no. 3. When bowel sounds return to normal, peristalsis has returned, and the nasogastric tube can be removed. Passage of numerous liquid stools may indicate a hyperactive bowel or other problems. Passage of flatus along with the return of bowel sounds after the procedure indicates a safe time to remove NG tubes. A/NM, AN, PS

123. no. 4. After a subtotal gastrectomy, food can move quickly into the jejunum in a highly concentrated form, causing what is known as the dumping syndrome. Client teaching should include the avoidance of concentrated sweets and liquids during mealtimes to avert symptoms. Eating slowly is also recommended. Since carbohydrates leave the stomach more quickly, diet guidelines include low car-

bohydrates and high protein and fat. A/NM, AN, PS

124. no. 1. Aluminum hydroxide gel (Amphogel) coats the gastrointestinal mucosa, but it is not absorbed systemically. Constipation may result from the aluminum. Phosphorus excretion is enhanced; it binds the phosphorus from the serum and is lost in the stool. Both constipation and phosphorus excretion may be dose related. The other options are incorrect. A/NM, AN, PS

125. no. 2. The diet for the treatment of dumping syndrome is high protein and fat and low carbohydrates. Refined or concentrated carbohydrates should be avoided because they leave the stomach more quickly, pull fluid into the intestine, and increase insulin release. Thus, the symptoms occur for dumping syndrome. A/NM, EV, PS

126. no. 2. Of all the options, no. 2 has all correct data. The other options all contain clinical signs and symptoms that may occur with dumping syndrome except loss of appetite, hypertension, and headache. Borborygmi are noises made from gas passing through the small intestine. A/NM, EV, PS

127. no. 4. Propantheline bromide (Pro-Banthine), an anticholinergic, promotes urinary retention as well as inhibiting gastrointestinal mobility and gastric secretions. A dry mouth is a side effect of Propantheline bromide (Pro-Banthine); however, it is not dose limiting. A/NM, AN, PS

128. no. 2. A fecalith obstructs the lumen of the appendix, leading to inflammation. A/NM, AN, PS

129. no. 2. The colon is filled with bacteria that invade the peritoneal cavity after the appendix ruptures. Digestive juices are not found in the appendix. A/NM, AN, PS

130. no. 3. Vitamin C is important in the formation of granulation and collagen tissue. Vitamin E has no known special role; vitamin B_1 may have a role in antibody formation and WBC function; vitamin D is necessary for absorption, transport, and metabolism of calcium. A/NM, AN, PS

131. no. 2. Until the client is responsive, she should be placed in a side-lying position to prevent aspiration of secretions or vomitus. All other options are correct. A/NM, IM, E

132. no. 3. Pain is a subjective experience. Clients' reactions to pain vary widely, depending upon such factors as training, culture, and previous experiences. How a client exhibits pain is not always a reliable indicator of how much pain is being experienced. A/NM, AS, PS

133. no. 1. Cholecystectomy clients have an increased susceptibility to respiratory complications. Because of the subcostal incision and the discomfort associated with the incision site, they tend to breathe shallowly. Postoperative pain should be treated and controlled in a timely manner. This will facilitate coughing and deep-breathing to prevent hypostatic pneumonia. A/NM, PL, E

134. no. 3. An output of 30 ml or less per hour is indicative of inadequate fluid-volume replacement after surgery. Options no. 1, no. 2, and no. 4 are expected outcomes after this surgery. A/NM, AS, PS

135. no. 4. Factors that contribute to delayed wound healing in obese clients are limited vascularity of adipose tissue, dead spaces in adipose tissue left during suturing, and increased tension on sutures. A/NM, AS, H

136. no. 1. Following discharge, the client who has had abdominal surgery is usually permitted activity as tolerated. The only restriction is to avoid heavy lifting, pushing, and pulling. A/NM, EV, PS

137. no. 4. Signs and symptoms consistent with a diagnosis of cholecystitis include fullness, eructation, and dyspepsia following fat ingestion; abdominal pain, usually in the right upper quadrant; and nausea and vomiting. A/NM, AS, PS

138. no. 4. You would verify the order with the physician who wrote it. Meperidine (Demerol) is usually ordered, because morphine tends to cause spasms of the bile ducts, which may result in increased pain. A/NM, IM, E

139. no. 4. A cholecystogram is an x-ray visualization of the gallbladder and biliary tract following oral ingestion of iodine dye. An allergy history is important. If she is allergic to any shellfish, she may be allergic to iodine. A/NM, AS, PS

140. no. 3. A T-tube is inserted whenever the common bile duct is explored. The other options describe a standard cholecystectomy, which does not require placement of a T-tube. A/NM, AN, PS

141. no. 2. You would irrigate a nasogastric tube only with normal saline and as ordered to keep it patent. Using distilled water can cause electrolyte depletion in the postoperative client. In these clients the nasogastric tube should not be repositioned without a physician's order because of the risk of damage to the internal operative site. A/NM, IM, PS

142. no. 4. This answer provides Mrs. Belzer with specific information. A/NM, IM, E

143. no. 4. The nurse would notify her physician because drainage should be 200 to 500 ml per day for the first several days. T-tubes are usually not irrigated. Continued drainage after 3 days may indicate blockage of the common bile duct. A/NM, IM, PS

144. no. 3. A T-tube is usually removed 10 to 12 days after surgery, following a T-tube cholangiogram, to determine the status of the common bile duct, which should be patent. The other options are incorrect. A/NM, AN, E

145. no. 2. Common causes associated with pancreatitis are trauma, infection, alcohol abuse, and biliary tract disease. Alcoholism and biliary tract disease are the most common factors. These disorders can cause fibrosis and edema of the pancreas, which results in inadequate digestion of fats and proteins. The pancreatic enzymes, unable to follow their normal course, build up in the ducts and eventually rupture the ducts and result in autodigestion of the pancreas. A/NM, AS, PS

146. no. 2. The exocrine function of the pancreas is to secrete three digestive enzymes—amylase, lipase, and trypsin. Secretion of insulin is an endocrine function. A/NM, AN, PS

147. no. 1. By keeping the client NPO, digestive activity is decreased, and there is less pancreatic stimulation. The other options are appropriate secondary goals. A/NM, PL, PS

148. no. 3. Propantheline bromide (Pro-Banthine) is an anticholinergic drug useful as an antispasmodic to relieve pancreatic pain. A/NM, AN, PS

149. no. 1. The serum amylase is the first of the pancreatic enzymes to rise in pancreatitis, and the level is used most frequently to diagnose and to evaluate response to treatment. AST is the former serum glutamic-oxalacetic transaminase (SGOT). A/NM, EV, PS

150. no. 4. The serum transaminases, AST and ALT (alanine aminotransferase, formerly serum glutamic-pyruvic transaminase [SGPT]) are the first to show an elevation. Abnormal serum ammonia, bilirubin, or prothrombin time are all indicative of more advanced, serious liver disease. A/NM, AS, PS

151. no. 2. Bed rest with bathroom privileges is recommended to promote liver regeneration. Options no. 1 and no. 3 would be appropriate but not priority. Option no. 4 is incorrect since rest is needed; however, diversional activity while on bed rest would be desirable. A/NM, PL, E

152. no. 3. Adequate calories either in the diet or through intravenous therapy are necessary for the liver to regenerate. Most clients tolerate a low-fat, high-carbohydrate diet best, with the largest meal in the morning when energy level is greatest. Liquids of 2500-3000 ml/day are recommended to prevent dehydration. A/NM, PL, PS

153. no. 4. In cirrhosis, the liver cells develop fatty infiltrates and degenerate by an inflammatory process. Therefore, there are fewer liver cells available to accommodate the volume of blood. The inflammatory process also increases the congestion in the liver, which inhibits blood flow. This results in venous back-up causing dilatation of the esophageal vessels. A/NM, AN, PS

154. no. 1. It is important for the nurse to elicit an alcohol-consumption history from the client in order to accurately observe withdrawal during hospitalization. The items in the other options may be interventions only after mutual planning with the client. A/NM, PL, E

155. no. 4. A quiet, calm environment with even lighting minimizes the chance of creating shadows and reactions such as alcoholic hallucinations. Unusual noise, restraints, or lighting may increase or stimulate agitation. Side rails that are up would be appropriate. Restraints, usually soft, might be used only if the client is in danger of harming himself. A/NM, IM, E

156. no. 2. Portal hypertension is common in cirrhosis and causes these problems. Spider angiomas and palmar erythema are believed to be caused by an increase in estrogen levels found in alcoholics. A/NM, AS, PS

157. no. 3. Prothrombin time increases in clients with cirrhosis; it takes blood longer to clot when there is liver failure. Leukopenia is to be expected with cirrhosis. A/NM, AS, PS

158. no. 2. Portal hypertension causes blood to accumulate in the weaker vessels of the esophagus, causing them to become distended. These vessels can rupture if the distension becomes too great. The other options do not contribute to the formation of esophageal varices. A/NM, AN, PS

159. no. 2. Portal hypertension will not cause pulmonary edema. Pulmonary edema is usually due to left-sided heart failure. A/NM, AN, PS

160. no. 1. Insertion of any tube through the esophagus traumatizes the distended vessels, making reinsertion for a faulty tube undesirable. Therefore, checking the balloons for leaks before insertion is a priority. Labeling the lumens of the tube prevents confusion after the tube has been inserted. Both balloons are always inflated with air, never fluid, and are inflated after placement. A/NM, IM, E

161. no. 2. Administering a neomycin enema may be done at a later time to decrease ammonia production in the bowel and to prevent hepatic coma. A/NM, IM, E

162. no. 3. The client should be placed in a semi-Fowler's position (not supine) to promote ventilation and prevent gastric reflux and aspiration. Side-lying with the head up is also acceptable. With this tube in place, the client is not able to swallow anything, including saliva. Thus, actions in option no. 1 are correct. A/NM, IM, E

163. no. 3. Upward dislodgment of the gastric balloon may result in respiratory obstruction. Upward dislodgment is more likely because tension is used with this tube to put pressure on the esophageal-gastric junction from the gastric balloon. Ulceration is not likely because the tube is used for a short term, and the esophageal balloon is usually deflated every 12 hours and the gastric balloon every 24-36

hours. If pressure on the balloons is checked periodically, esophageal rupture can be prevented. A/NM, AN, PS

164. no. 2. Vasopressin is a potent vasopressor; optimally, it results in constriction of the esophageal veins. It can be given IV or through the nasogastric tube port. A/NM, IM, PS

165. no. 4. Clients with Sengstaken-Blakemore tubes should be sedated cautiously because of the risk of aspiration and respiratory insufficiency. A/NM, PL, E

166. no. 1. This client needs a diet to correct the negative nitrogen balance and malnutrition, to promote liver regeneration, and to avoid fluid retention. He needs a low-sodium diet to decrease his ascites, which results from portal hypertension. A/NM, IM, H

167. no. 2. Hepatic encephalopathy occurs frequently in clients with severe liver disease, especially if therapy is neglected. A/NM, AN, PS

168. no. 3. In hepatic encephalopathy, the liver is unable to detoxify ammonia and convert it to urea. The ammonia levels build, and ammonia crosses the blood-brain barrier, causing decreased mentation. A/NM, AN, PS

169. no. 2. The central venous pressure will give the best and quickest indication of circulating volume. Normal is 4-12 cm of water pressure; less than 4 cm indicates hypovolemia, and greater than 12 cm indicates hypervolemia. A baseline reading immediately after inserting the line is a priority. This information is an indirect assessment of the adequacy of renal perfusion. A low CVP, reflecting hypovolemia, puts the client at risk for inadequate renal perfusion. A/NM, IM, PS

170. no. 4. Exophthalmos occurs primarily with hyperthyroidism; it is not a sign or symptom of hepatic encephalopathy. A/NM, AS, PS

171. no. 1. Neomycin decreases the ammonia-forming bacteria in the intestinal tract, thus decreasing the serum ammonia level. Lactulose decreases the pH of the colon, which allows ammonias to diffuse into the colon from the blood to form nonabsorbable ammonium ions. These are then eliminated in the stool. The medications in no. 3 and no. 4 are given for seizure activity. Protein–tube feeding is not given; proteins form ammonia in the process of breaking down, which is to be avoided in this case. A/NM, AN, PS

172. no. 4. Normal bacteria found in the gastrointestinal tract cause ammonia to form. The antibacterial effect of neomycin reduces the intestinal flora; thus, it decreases levels of ammonia. The client's level of consciousness will improve when serum ammonia levels are reduced. A/NM, PL, PS

173. no. 2. Proteins (amino acids) break down in the body to form ammonia; therefore, a low-protein

diet will help prevent the buildup of ammonia. A/NM, PL, E

174. no. 4. Water intake is restricted to control ascites. A/NM, IM, H

175. no. 4. Esophageal varices are observed only with an x-ray or by direct visualization through an endoscope. A/NM, AS, PS

176. no. 2. The nutritional inadequacies are easier to correct by teaching about nutrition and diet. Long-term substance-abuse problems are difficult to control. The alcoholic client has nutritional deprivation, especially a decrease in protein intake. This deprivation results in Laënnec's cirrhosis. A/NM, AN, PS

177. no. 2. He was admitted after having vomited large quantities of blood. Oral hygiene is most likely to make him comfortable. A/NM, IM, E

178. no. 4. Dimenhydrinate (Dramamine) is the best selection. The other medications rely on the liver for detoxification. Caution must be taken when administering antiemetics to clients with liver damage. A/NM, PL, PS

179. no. 2. Pruritus is a result of bile salt excretion through the skin. Soap, perfumed lotion, and rubbing alcohol should be avoided because they cause further drying of the skin. Moisturizing lotions may be beneficial. Assess for scratching, which can cause subcutaneous bleeding. The skin should be patted and not rubbed during the bath. A/NM, AS, PS

180. no. 2. Weight loss or gain directly reflects water loss or gain and is the best parameter for measuring fluid balance in the body. A/NM, AS, PS

181. no. 4. Gynecomastia is an endocrine problem (estrogen excess) commonly seen in clients with cirrhosis of the liver, but it is not preventable with nursing actions. A/NM, AN, E

182. no. 2. For small tumors, an incision is made here. For larger tumors a transfrontal craniotomy may be used. Other surgical postoperative assessments would include looking for signs and symptoms of meningitis, optic nerve damage, and hypopituitarism. A/NM, AS, PS

183. no. 4. Prolactin is secreted by the pituitary gland in pregnant and nursing women to produce lactation. A pituitary tumor can produce an excess of this hormone, causing galactorrhea (excessive or abnormal lactation). A/NM, AN, PS

184. no. 4. A serum calcium will give no information about the type of tumor or size of the lesion, whereas the other studies will. CT scans help to determine bone changes. Visual field testing is performed to determine if the tumor is pressing on the optic chiasm. Hormone levels would typically be elevated. A/NM, AS, PS

185. no. 2. Diabetes insipidus is a frequent temporary complication following a hypophysectomy. Large

volumes of urine may be excreted, causing critical problems if not treated. The other options listed would be contraindicated because they might increase intracranial pressure or cause cerebrospinal fluid leaks into the sinuses. A/NM, PL, E

186. no. 1. Hypopituitarism is a common problem with clients who have had hypophysectomies, since the anterior pituitary gland has been affected. Pituitary hormone replacements may have to be given. Cushing's disease results from excess steroid production. A/NM, AN, PS

187. no. 3. The gonadal-stimulating hormones from the pituitary gland that affect pregnancy may be deficient, but replacements can be administered. A/NM, IM, H

188. no. 2. Tingling of the toes, fingers, or around the mouth is the first sign of hypocalcemia, which can lead to tetany. Thyroid surgery clients are at high risk for this problem because of the possibility of removal of or damage to the parathyroid gland. A/NM, AS, PS

189. no. 3. Help Mrs. Schiller use the semi-Fowler's position with her neck supported for optimal ventilation and to avoid strain on the neck muscles. A/NM, IM, E

190. no. 3. Hypoparathyroidism leads to hypocalcemia, which causes increased neuromuscular irritability and laryngospasm. Chvostek's sign is a contraction of the facial muscles elicited in response to a light tap over the facial nerve in front of the ear. Trousseau's sign is a carpopedal spasm induced by inflating a blood pressure cuff above the client's systolic pressure. A/NM, AS, PS

191. no. 3. Respiratory distress from edema or hemorrhage is a potential complication of a subtotal thyroidectomy, so a tracheostomy set is kept at Mrs. Schiller's bedside. The thyroid is very vascular. A total thyroidectomy does not have as high a risk of bleeding because no thyroid tissue remains. A/NM, IM, E

192. no. 2. Hypocalcemia can result from the accidental removal of one or two parathyroid glands, so calcium gluconate must be kept on hand. Calcium gluconate is more readily used than calcium chloride if given IV. Calcitonin is given in hypothyroid conditions to inhibit bone resorption (loss of calcium from the bone). SSKI is an antithyroid drug used to treat hyperthyroidism. A/NM, AN, PS

193. no. 2. Flexing or hyperextending the neck puts excessive tension on the surgical site. Two or three pillows would strain the incision. The other options are all appropriate nursing actions. A/NM, IM, E

194. no. 2. Before instructing the client on self-care related to diabetes, the nurse must establish a baseline regarding the client's knowledge of diabetes.

Assessment of client knowledge is the priority before teaching. A/NM, AS, E

195. no. 3. Diabetes is a chronic disorder of carbohydrate metabolism and is one of the leading causes of death in the United States. It is not a curable illness. Diabetes responds to diet and exercise as well as insulin. A/NM, AN, PS

196. no. 1. In diabetes, insulin deficiency results in hyperglycemia. Glucose is excreted in the urine and, acting as an osmotic diuretic, carries water and electrolytes with it. All the other options are incorrect. A/NM, AN, PS

197. no. 3. In addition, more rapid absorption can occur in unaffected sites, leading to hypoglycemia. All the other options are incorrect. A/NM, AN, H

198. no. 1. Peak hours of action for regular insulin are 2 to 4 hours after administration. Breakfast is usually served between 8 and 9 AM. A hypoglycemic reaction would occur between 9:30 to 11:30 AM, especially if the client has not eaten much at breakfast. It is extremely important for the nurse to monitor food intake at meals when regular insulin is given before meals according to a sliding scale. A/NM, AN, PS

199. no. 4. The other options are symptoms of hyperglycemia. Other symptoms of hypoglycemia are mild sweating, hunger, tremor, anxiety, weakness, nausea, complaints of nightmares, and restless sleep. Major symptoms are perioral paresthesia, headache, visual changes, mental confusion, personality changes, depression, and loss of consciousness. A/NM, AS, PS

200. no. 2. Exercise is important for diabetic clients and is planned according to age and interests and in balance with the prescribed insulin and diet regimen. A/NM, AN, H

201. no. 4. Hunger is characteristic, but because the glucose cannot be used, weight loss occurs. A/NM, AS, PS

202. no. 1. Warm, flushed, dry skin indicates dehydration. This is the major initial problem caused by polyuria requiring treatment. A/NM, AS, PS

203. no. 3. The client has a fluid deficit of 8 to 12 L, and replacement is a priority to be carried out as rapidly as tolerated. Generally, 0.9% saline solution is used initially, then 0.45% saline and water. Regular insulin may be given via IV continuous low-dose infusions with bolus SC as needed hourly based on serum blood glucose values. A/NM, PL, PS

204. no. 4. This is the most therapeutic and most honest response. All other options do not support or address the client's comment and are incorrect. A/NM, IM, PC

205. no. 1. Intermittent claudication is pain in the extremity with exercise, usually walking. When the

energy demands exceed the oxygen supply, pain is experienced. Peripheral parasthesias reflect nerve problems and may be the result of poor circulation, but are not classic findings. Skin may be shiny and atrophic over the ankle area in arterial insufficiency. Pain on dorsiflexion of the foot indicates venous thrombophlebitis. A/NM, AS, PS

206. no. 2. Keeping the feet covered with socks will keep the feet warm and not compromise circulation any further. Using external heat, such as hot water bottles, increases oxygen consumption and impairs arterial flow even more. Massaging the feet or flexing the toes are inappropriate actions that would do nothing for arterial circulation. A/NM, IM, PS

207. no. 3. It is important for her to talk about her fears of body changes and loss, even if she will never need an amputation. This response acknowledges that the nurse heard the statement, and it encourages client verbalization. A/NM, IM, PC

208. no. 4. Even though Mrs. Carter is a type II diabetic, the stress of surgery may cause her blood glucose to rise for a short time; thus, it should be controlled with short-acting insulin administered according to the client's needs as determined by monitoring serum glucose levels. A/NM, IM, PS

209. no. 1. Irritability is often the first sign of hypoglycemia, particularly in the morning when the client has not had anything to eat for several hours. The nurse should also check prior glucose levels and when the last insulin was given in order to assess for insulin-induced hypoglycemia. A/NM, IM, PS

210. no. 4. Complex carbohydrates have much value in the diabetic diet since they are a good source of energy and keep the blood sugar more stable. The other options are incorrect. A/NM, IM, H

211. no. 3. Elevating the legs is indicated for venous, not arterial, problems of the extremities. Mrs. Carter had an arterial problem. A/NM, IM, H

212. no. 2. Weakness and weight loss are symptoms of adrenocortical insufficiency. Increased skin pigmentation results as adrenal insufficiency allows melanocyte-stimulating hormone levels to increase. A/NM, AS, PS

213. no. 2. Stress of any type increases the client's weakness. The client is vulnerable to stress, because she lacks the protection of the adrenal hormones—Addison's disease is hypofunction of the adrenal glands. Exertion is a type of physiological stress. A/NM, PL, E

214. no. 4. Addison's disease is characterized by inadequate amounts of cortisol, which results in hypotension. All the other options are correct. A/NM, PL, E

215. no. 4. Critical deficiency of glucocorticoids leads to vascular collapse, hypotension, and diminished urine output. A/NM, AS, PS

216. no. 4. The client with Addison's disease can live a normal life, provided the client takes the daily medications without exception. A/NM, IM, H

217. no. 1. Clients at high risk for septic shock include the very young, the very old, those with genitourinary infections who undergo cystoscopy, and those with severe gastrointestinal blood loss. A/E, AS, PS

218. no. 4. This answer gives Mr. Thomas an opportunity to express his concerns and fears. The other options do not acknowledge his concerns. A/E, IM, PC

219. no. 3. Septic shock is insidious in onset, and slight changes in vital signs may be the only warning. Therefore, check the vital signs again in 15 minutes for any changes. A/E, IM, PS

220. no. 4. Restlessness is an early sign of septic shock. Hypotension and cool, clammy skin are late signs. In early septic shock, urinary output is slightly decreased. A/E, AS, PS

221. no. 3. Dried apricots are high in potassium and low in sodium; the other choices are high in sodium. A/E, EV, H

222. no. 3. It is important that the client with high blood pressure stop smoking. The other options are not correct statements. A/E, EV, H

223. no. 1. Forcing fluids serves as an internal irrigant, flushes the urinary tract, and decreases burning. Options no. 2 and no. 4 are important but focused more on prevention. Option no. 1 is most important for *treating* the infection. A/E, IM, H

224. no. 4. This is a sign of possible anaphylaxis. The client should be informed about the other reactions, which are normal. A/E, AS, E

225. no. 2. Activity aids in passage of the calculus. Even though she may need pain relief and will have to strain her urine, these do not aid in passage of stones. A/E, IM, E

226. no. 1. Calculi readily develop in immobile clients, and especially in those with multiple myeloma, because the diseased bones release calcium, leading to the formation of calculi. Options no. 2, no. 3, and no. 4 will decrease the possibility of renal calculi. A/E, AN, PS

227. no. 1. The etiology of bladder cancer is related to cigarette smoking and exposure to dyes used in rubber and cable industries. A/E, AS, E

228. no. 2. Painless, gross hematuria is the most common clinical finding and the first sign in 75% of clients with carcinoma of the bladder. A/E, AS, PS

229. no. 4. Gentle acceptance of the client's anxiety and open-ended questioning allows the client the opportunity to express his feelings and concerns. The other options do not encourage the client to discuss his feelings. A/E, IM, PC

230. no. 2. Instruct the client to do range-of-motion exercises for his legs and teach him to keep his legs uncrossed. These activities decrease the risk of thrombophlebitis. A/E, IM, PS

231. no. 3. A nasogastric tube may become obstructed with mucus, sediment, or old blood. It can be checked for patency by irrigating with 30 ml of normal saline. One indicator of obstruction is nausea. Administering an antiemetic may be unnecessary if irrigating the nasogastric tube relieves the nausea. Repositioning will not help the client's nausea. A/E, IM, PS

232. no. 3. There is a risk of paralytic ileus when part of the bowel is removed. A nasogastric tube is used for 3 to 5 days or until bowel sounds return. A/E, AN, PS

233. no. 4. The urinary stoma should be dark-pink to red. A dark-red color is indicative of inadequate circulation. A/E, AS, PS

234. no. 4. Intramuscular or subcutaneous injections should not be administered because of the vasoconstriction in hypotension. Medications may not be absorbed and might accumulate; then, when perfusion improves, the client could experience an overdose. A/E, IM, PS

235. no. 2. Normal potassium is 3.5 to 5.0 mEq/L. Hyperkalemia can cause lethal cardiac dysrhythmias if not promptly treated. A/E, AS, PS

236. no. 1. Fluid restriction is indicated during the oliguric phase of renal failure, when fluid overload is a problem. The sodium value in this client reflects dilution. By decreasing the fluid overload, you will increase the sodium value. A/E, AN, PS

237. no. 3. Trousseau's sign is an indication of tetany, which results from the increased neuromuscular irritability caused by hypocalcemia. The method of eliciting this sign is to constrict the radial or brachial artery and observe the hand and fingers for spasm. The constriction can be done with a blood pressure cuff. A/E, AN, PS

238. no. 1. This is the only correct group of actions. In addition, bed rest should be maintained to reduce the buildup of lactic acid, which is released with muscle activity. Restrict fluids to reduce hypervolemia. A/E, IM, E

239. no. 3. The diuretic phase of acute renal failure causes loss of circulating volume, potassium, and sodium. This phase is exacerbated by the buildup of urea during the oliguric phase, which acts as a natural diuretic. A/E, AS, PS

240. no. 3. The blood urea nitrogen becomes elevated because functioning nephrons are damaged and the body is unable to get rid of waste products through the kidneys. A/E, AN, PS

241. no. 1. A diet high in calories and low in protein is prescribed. The protein should be of high biological value to prevent catabolism of body protein. A/E, IM, H

242. no. 2. Careful monitoring of the client's intake and output is important, as fluid replacement is often based on the output. A/E, PL, E

243. no. 2. These laboratory findings are consistent with renal failure. A decreased serum calcium results from both a decreased gastrointestinal absorption of calcium and an elevated serum phosphorus. The inability of the kidneys to excrete the potassium raises the potassium as well as the hydrogen-ion level, and results in acidosis. A/E, AS, PS

244. no. 3. A likely cause of Mr. Brown's decreased serum calcium is an elevated serum phosphorus. Remember that his kidneys are unable to excrete phosphorus, and there is an inverse relationship of calcium and phosphorus. Nutritional deficiencies would be an unlikely cause. A/E, AN, PS

245. no. 1. The kidneys are unable to excrete the hydrogen ion or reabsorb the bicarbonate ion. The result is acidosis, for which the lungs attempt to compensate by blowing off excess hydrogen ion (carbon dioxide). A/E, AN, PS

246. no. 4. Phosphorus and calcium are inversely related. Potassium levels are usually inversely related to sodium. A/E, AN, PS

247. no. 4. Aluminum hydroxide antacids bind with the phosphate ion and are then excreted in the stool. A/E, AN, PS

248. no. 3. A client treated with peritoneal dialysis may need to be dialyzed three to five times per week for 8 to 12 hours each time. Vascular access is required for hemodialysis only. Hepatitis is more problematic with hemodialysis. A/E, AN, PS

249. no. 1. Respiratory distress may indicate a fluid shift and pulmonary edema, requiring immediate attention. Hemorrhage is less likely once the catheter is in place; abdominal pain and peritonitis may also occur, but breathing is the first priority. A/E, AN, PS

250. no. 2. The life span of the shunt is 6 to 12 months. Major complications are clotting and infections, which are avoided by not using the arm for taking blood pressure or blood drawing. Daily heparinization is not common practice. Changing the Silastic tube is not possible since it would cause hemorrhage. A/E, IM, PS

251. no. 1. These are symptoms of the disequilibrium syndrome. It occurs when urea is removed more rapidly from the blood than the brain. The osmotic gradient caused by urea results in fluid passing to cerebral cells; thus, cerebral edema occurs. A/E, IM, PS

252. no. 2. The Foley catheter is inserted to maintain urinary flow. Monitor intake and output throughout Mr. Rasmussen's preoperative and postoperative periods. A/E, PL, PS

253. no. 4. A transurethral resection is the only type of prostatic surgery not requiring an incision through the skin. A/E, IM, E

254. no. 1. If increased blood is seen, first increase the speed of the irrigation. If this is not effective, notify the physician. Do not alter the traction on the Foley, since its purpose is to put pressure on the prostatic bed. Manual irrigation is done mainly for clots and requires a physician order. A/E, IM, PS

255. no. 1. The large balloon on the Foley can stimulate spasms; therefore, administer narcotics plus anticholinergic drugs as ordered. Providing a sitz bath and decreasing the speed of irrigation will not decrease the bladder spasms. Never decrease the traction on the Foley. A/E, IM, PS

256. no. 4. Nursing strategies that can help prevent thrombophlebitis include helping with leg exercises and taking deep breaths, and obtaining an order for antiembolism stockings for the client. Nursing actions cannot prevent epididymitis, osteitis pubis, or urinary incontinence. A/E, AN, PS

257. no. 1. Mr. Rasmussen should refrain from sexual intercourse for approximately 6 weeks after surgery. In addition, he should avoid heavy lifting, straining at stool, and driving a car for approximately 6 weeks. A/E, IM, H

258. no. 2. Instruct Mr. Rasmussen to monitor his urine at home; it should be continually clear. A/E, EV, H

259. no. 1. A man with an enlarged prostate has difficulty emptying his bladder and has to strain to urinate. The stream lacks force and becomes weak, and dribbling occurs. Initiating a stream may also be a problem. A/E, AS, PS

260. no. 2. Prostatic hypertrophy can be diagnosed by rectal digital exam. Gloves and lubricant are needed. A/E, AS, E

261. no. 3. The kidneys are located in the retroperitoneum, and the bowel must be cleared of any gas or fecal material that would obscure their visualization. Additional preparation for an intravenous pyelogram includes restricting food and fluids from midnight before the exam. A/E, IM, E

262. no. 2. Continuous bladder irrigation with saline or other solutions is done to remove clotted blood from the bladder. Blood and clots are normal in the first 24 to 48 hours after TURP. A/E, PL, PS

263. no. 4. A Foley catheter can irritate the bladder mucosa, causing bladder spasms. The catheter must also be checked to ensure patency, but these sensations may be present with a patent catheter. A/E, AN, PS

264. no. 2. Temporary urinary frequency or incontinence, or both, can occur after removal of the catheter. A/E, AN, PS

265. no. 3. Race is not a factor in the client's ability to undergo surgery. It does have implications in the nursing care following surgery, especially in the assessment phase of the nursing process. A/E, AS, E

266. no. 4. There is postoperative pain with this procedure, but it can be managed with analgesics. A/E, IM, E

267. no. 2. The rectal area is less than 1 inch from the incision and prostatic bed; taking a rectal temperature could cause trauma. An air ring can cause venous stasis and edema; a hard surface may increase pain. A/E, IM, PS

268. no. 4. Sexual impotence is expected in suprapubic and retropubic prostatectomies, but not following transurethral resections. However, in the immediate postoperative period, it is too early to assess this activity. A/E, IM, E

269. no. 3. This requires a physician's order. In the early postoperative period, active exercise is usually limited to leg dangling and brief ambulation. Passive exercise, however, is imperative for Mr. Lacona. A/E, PL, E

270. no. 1. Any invasive procedure on the urinary tract increases the risk of urinary tract infections. A/E, AN, PS

271. no. 3. After removal of the catheter, incontinence is common in the older client undergoing a prostatectomy because a Foley catheter decreases the contractility of the bladder muscle. A/E, PL, H

272. no. 1. The lower gastrointestinal tract must be clear for the exam. Cathartics are given at least 12 hours before the test, along with enemas until the bowel is clear on the morning of the exam. A/E, IM, E

273. no. 4. The knee-chest position provides maximum exposure for the proctosigmoidoscopy. A/E, IM, E

274. no. 2. No anesthetic is given and the client must relax, not bear down. The procedure is not painful, but it is uncomfortable. A/E, IM, E

275. no. 1. Stool samples for amoebae must be tested while they are warm and fresh, or the amoebae will die. A/E, IM, PS

276. no. 1. Ulcerative colitis is characterized by very frequent diarrhea with mucus and blood, caused by inflammation of the colonic mucosa. A/E, AS, PS

277. no. 1. Vitamin K, vital to the formation of prothrombin, is normally absorbed in the colon. A/E, AN, PS

278. no. 1. Sedation and decreased bladder tone may occur, but these drugs are given to decrease gastrointestinal motility. A/E, AN, PS

279. no. 2. An ileostomy involves removal of the whole colon and formation of an ileal stoma. A/E, AN, PS

280. no. 3. An ileostomy has liquid, almost continuous drainage. Weight gain may result from new-found food tolerance. The drainage containing enzymes is irritating to the skin. A/E, AS, PS

281. no. 1. Research indicates that virtually 100% of colon polyps are premalignant and can be expected to become cancerous if not excised. Colitis and amebiasis cause chronic irritation and therefore may predispose the client to colon cancer. A/E, AS, PS

282. no. 3. Palpation is done last, because it can stimulate bowel sounds. Percussion usually does not stimulate bowel sounds because the technique is superficial to the bowel. A/E, AS, PS

283. no. 4. Signs and symptoms of mechanical obstruction of the colon include decreased bowel sounds, abdominal distension, decreased flatus, and projectile vomiting. A/E, AS, PS

284. no. 3. Fluid and electrolyte deficiency is the major problem, if the intestinal blood supply is not compromised. A/E, AN, PS

285. no. 2. The Miller-Abbott tube is an intestinal tube with an inflated bag designed to advance into the intestine. Taping it could traumatize nasal tissue as well as prevent further advance of the tube. A/E, IM, E

286. no. 1. Review deep-breathing exercises. Mr. Hawkins's weight and a probable abdominal incision predispose him to postoperative pulmonary complications. Preoperatively, a distended abdomen may prevent him from doing a return demonstration of deep-breathing exercises. A/E, IM, E

287. no. 2. Feces become increasingly firm as they progress through the colon because of water being reabsorbed back into the body. Stool in the transverse colon is mushy to semiformed, depending on the specific location. A/E, AS, PS

288. no. 3. Colostomy irrigations should be done only once a day. A/E, IM, E

289. no. 3. The area around the stoma must be kept dry and oil free in order for the colostomy appliance to adhere. A/E, IM, PS

290. no. 1. Eating a balanced diet will provide proper stool consistency. A colostomy can be irrigated at any time that is convenient for the client. A/E, AN, H

291. no. 4. Gradual involvement of the client in his ostomy care is more likely to increase acceptance. A/E, PL, PC

292. no. 2. A nasogastric tube attached to suction keeps the stomach drained and decompressed. This prevents the risk of aspiration before, during, and after surgery. A/E, AN, PS

293. no. 3. Although the catheter can be used to check renal function, the proximity of the rectum and sigmoid colon to the bladder makes avoidance of injury a prime concern. A/E, AN, PS

294. no. 1. Colon tumors metastasize to other areas within the colon by direct extension. Enough colon needs to be removed so that the specimen margins are clear of any tumor cells. A/E, AN, PS

295. no. 3. Tube feedings circumvent swallowing, anorexia, and the gag reflex and can be administered regardless of appetite or level of consciousness; but the gastrointestinal tract distal to the feeding must be intact and functioning. A/E, AN, PS

296. no. 4. Talking to a person who has a colostomy and has it well under control can be very encouraging for the new ostomate. A/E, IM, E

297. no. 3. Warm tap water will cause the least irritation, while at the same time stimulating evacuation of the colon. A/E, IM, PS

298. no. 4. The client must be relaxed for successful irrigation. A/E, AN, PS

299. no. 2. Excessive flatus is not symptomatic of colon cancer. A change in bowel habits is more common with left-sided lesions, while pain and obstructive symptoms are more common with right-sided lesions. A/E, AS, PS

300. no. 3. While the carcinoembryonic antigen has been used in recent years to aid in diagnosing colon cancer, it is not as conclusive as a biopsy of the lesion. A/E, AN, PS

301. no. 2. Neomycin is given to achieve bowel sterilization. It destroys the normal flora of the bowel and will result in some loose stools. This enhances the bowel cleansing and is the desired outcome. A/E, IM, PS

302. no. 1. The colostomy will be permanent since the cancerous rectum will be removed. Denial or lack of understanding may be the problem. In either case, further teaching is needed. A/E, E, H

303. no. 2. Getting Mr. Simms to talk about his fears and concerns before he is discharged is the priority right now. A/E, IM, PC

304. no. 2. Bone marrow depression and stomatitis are the main side effects from this drug. A decreased white blood cell count can make him more prone to infection. A/E, AN, PS

305. no. 3. Diverticulitis is an inflammatory condition manifested by crampy lower left quadrant pain, diarrhea with blood and mucus, weakness, and anemia. Characteristic signs and symptoms of appendicitis are right lower quadrant or periumbilical pain and rebound tenderness; for cholecystitis they are nausea, vomiting, and pain and tenderness in the right subcostal region or in the epigastric region; and for pancreatitis they are vomiting and localized pain to epigastrium or left upper quadrant with radiation of pain to the back and flanks as the pain progresses. A/M, AN, PS

306. no. 2. Diverticula often perforate. These are signs and symptoms of perforation and peritonitis. Op-

tions no. 1 and no. 3 are found in obstructive gall-bladder disease. A/M, AS, PS

307. no. 1. Diverticula are usually located in the sigmoid colon. Because a diagnosis of diverticulitis has not been previously established, an x-ray examination of the entire lower gastrointestinal tract will be done, and the entire colon will be examined to rule out other abnormalities. Option no. 2 items are done for ulcer disease. Option no. 3 items are done for gallbladder disease. A Schilling test is used to assess B_{12} problems. A/NM, AN, PS

308. no. 4. Clients with diverticulitis may benefit from a high-residue diet and should avoid foods that are highly refined and processed, since they predispose the clients to this condition. Bulk-forming medications (e.g., Psyllium hydrophilic mucilloid [Metamucil]) are helpful. Stress-management techniques are most helpful for upper-GI disturbances or colitis. A/NM, IM, H

309. no. 3. Insulin shock must be ruled out as a cause when dealing with a comatose client with no signs of injury. A/SP, PL, PS

310. no. 1. Vital signs can reflect a client's increasing intracranial pressure. A lumbar puncture is contraindicated in a client with possible increased intracranial pressure. A quick reduction of pressure in the spinal column caused by the lumbar puncture may cause herniation of the brain. A Levin tube is not required at the time. In addition, a complication of Levin-tube insertion is that flexing the client's neck may increase intracranial pressure. Although Biot's respirations indicate increased intracranial pressure, they are not an indication for an emergency tracheostomy. A/SP, PL, PS

311. no. 1. Ketoacidosis will not cause unequal pupillary light reflexes. In an unconscious client, unequal pupils can result from oculomotor nerve compression, hypothalamic damage, and midbrain damage. A brain contusion, epidural hematoma, or brain tumor all could cause unequal and sluggish pupillary responses. A/SP, AN, PS

312. no. 3. Biot's respirations are characterized by several short breaths followed by long, irregular periods of apnea. They are common in clients with severe, persistent, increased intracranial pressure. Option no. 4 is seen with Kussmaul's respirations. Option no. 2 is bradypnea. Option no. 1 indicates Cheyne-Stokes respirations. A/SP, AS, PS

313. no. 1. In decerebrate posturing there is rigid extension of both the upper and lower extremities. In decorticate posturing there is flexion of the upper extremities and extension of the lower extremities. Options no. 3 and no. 4 are not signs of neurological posturing. A/SP, AS, PS

314. no. 2. The most likely cause of Mrs. Swan's condition is an aneurysm; hypertension is a predis-posing factor, and headaches may be a symptom. A cerebral concussion will not usually cause Biot's respirations and decerebrate posturing. Meningitis is usually characterized by fever, convulsions, and positive Kernig's and Brudzinski's signs. Diabetic ketoacidosis would not cause unequal pupillary reactions and Biot's respirations. A/SP, AN, PS

315. no. 2. A neurological baseline must be established so that significant postoperative changes will not be overlooked. Notifying relatives and obtaining a complete history and physical are important, but they are not the first priority. The medical team is responsible for the diagnostic workup that will establish the location of the lesion. A/SP, PL, PS

316. no. 1. The pupil and neurological checks are important; however, maintaining respiratory status is the highest priority. Vital signs and dressing checks will be performed more frequently in the initial postoperative period. A/SP, PL, PS

317. no. 2. Pooling of secretions occurs when the client is in a side-lying position. These need to be suctioned before the client is repositioned. A/O, IM, PS

318. no. 1. A tracheostomy is performed when an endotracheal tube is required for a long time in order to prevent tracheal necrosis. Postural drainage is done before or at least 2 hours after meals to prevent regurgitation. Options no. 2 and no. 3 are not correct. A/O, AN, PS

319. no. 4. The trachea is suctioned first using a sterile catheter. To suction the mouth first would contaminate the equipment. Remember the rule: *clean to dirty*. One to 3 ml sterile normal saline may be required to help remove thick, tenacious secretions. Instructing the client to cough can help raise secretions that are deep in the lower lobes of the lung. A/O, IM, PS

320. no. 2. If the pharynx is not suctioned first, the secretions will be aspirated into the trachea when the cuff is deflated. A hissing sound around the stoma, nose, or mouth indicates an air leak. Air is used to inflate a tracheostomy cuff. A/O, IM, PS

321. no. 4. Xerostomia (dry mouth) is not a complication of a tracheostomy tube. Tracheal stenosis and tracheoesophageal fistulas can occur when there is excessive pressure on the trachea from the cuff. Pulmonary infections are a risk because of altered ciliary function and trauma to the mucosa caused by suctioning, intubation, and colonization of the airway with infectious microorganisms. A/O, AN, PS

322. no. 4. Restraints will likely increase client resistance. A/SP, IM, PS

323. no. 3. Of the options listed, only antiinflammatory drugs do not have respiratory depression as a side effect. A/SP, AN, PS

324. no. 2. Diabetes insipidus occurs when there is suppression of antidiuretic hormone (ADH), leading to uncontrolled diuresis. Cerebral edema, contusion, and concussion will not directly affect urine output. A/SP, AN, PS

325. no. 3. ADH is stored and secreted by the posterior pituitary lobe. It is produced in the hypothalamus. A/SP, AN, PS

326. no. 2. The uncontrolled diuresis leads to loss of water and washout of most electrolytes. The diuresis will not increase intracranial pressure; it may even decrease it. Diuresis is not associated with cerebral infection and retrograde amnesia. A/SP, AN, PS

327. no. 1. Diabetes insipidus causes polyuria, leading to urine output of 5 to 20 L/day. The urine will have an abnormally low specific gravity (1.001 to 1.005) because the urine is so dilute, almost like water. A/SP, AS, PS

328. no. 3. Tachycardia is a symptom of cardiac dysfunction. The options are related to the neurological system. A/SP, AS, PS

329. no. 4. Of the options listed, only a cerebral arteriogram is an invasive procedure. A/SP, AN, PS

330. no. 2. Personality, higher-level functioning, concentration, and storage of information occur in the cortex of the frontal lobe. The temporal lobes are the primary auditory receptive areas. The occipital area is the primary receptive area for vision. The parietal lobes are the primary sensory cortex. A/SP, AN, PS

331. no. 4. Any changes in mental functioning in a head-injury client are significant and require constant monitoring. Confusion and personality changes will also put the client at high risk for injury, so the paramount consideration is frequent monitoring and safety interventions. The other three options may be appropriate at a later time. A/SP, PL, E

332. no. 1. All options are important to monitor; however, adequacy of respirations always has the priority. A/SP, AS, PS

333. no. 3. The blood pressure is markedly abnormal, particularly the diastolic reading. The three other options are considered predisposing or risk factors, not direct causes. A/SP, AN, PS

334. no. 2. It is important to first assess functions necessary for maintenance of life. A/SP, AS, E

335. no. 2. A suction machine will allow the nurse to maintain a patent airway. Maintaining adequate oxygenation is a basic goal for all acutely ill clients. The second priority with a client whose mobility is impaired is correct positioning. A/SP, PL, E

336. no. 2. Mouth breathing commonly occurs during a coma. Even clients who are NPO can be properly hydrated, and there is no evidence to suggest option no. 3. Option no. 4 is not correct. A/SP, AN, PS

337. no. 4. Although all options are appropriate, turning the client is the best way to prevent decubitus ulcers. A/SP, IM, PS

338. no. 1. Stroke clients who are not correctly positioned and exercised tend to develop flexion contractures because flexor muscles are generally stronger than extensors. The fingers should never be tightly flexed. The footboard will not be effective in preventing a plantar flexion contracture if it is flush with the mattress. A/SP, AN, E

339. no. 2. Although an increasing temperature may indicate an infectious or healing process, the changes in pulse and respirations indicate a more fundamental problem is occurring. These signs suggest increasing intracranial pressure or damage to the vital areas of the brainstem. A/SP, AN, PS

340. no. 4. Allowing her uppermost shoulder to fall out of alignment during the procedure could cause injury. Options no. 1 and no. 2 are advisable, but are not critical to the procedure. A/SP, IM, E

341. no. 3. Normal cerebrospinal fluid should contain no red blood cells. The presence of less than five lymphocytes per mm^3 is normal. The normal color of CSF is clear or colorless, and the normal glucose level is 50 to 75 mg/dl. A/SP, AS, PS

342. no. 1. Emotional lability often follows this type of cerebral insult. This is the only correct option. A/SP, H

343. no. 4. Movement of the head, neck, and back may cause further trauma, so it is essential that the entire spinal cord be immobilized. Although it is always important to explain procedures, the client who is paralyzed cannot assist in the transfer. The back will not be supported with pillows. Option no. 1 is appropriate, but it is not the most important consideration. A/SP, PL, E

344. no. 4. Spinal shock refers to the effects that result from spinal cord transection. It involves the suppression of all reflex activity below the level of the injury. Tendon reflexes diminish and temperature control and vasomotor tone are lost. Paralysis of the bladder results in urinary retention. Flaccid paralysis, not spastic paralysis, will occur. Blood pressure will be low and unstable. There is a loss of ability to perspire below the level of the injury so the skin will feel warm, not damp, with diaphoresis. A/SP, AS, PS

345. no. 3. This is the top priority. With a C3-4 injury, paralysis of the diaphragm is likely. Options no. 1, no. 2, and no. 4 are appropriate, but maintaining the airway and adequate ventilation is the most important nursing action. A/SP, PL, PS

346. no. 2. In early stages of injury, no reflexes will be present, and the client will have an atonic bladder. The bladder will become increasingly distended if the client is not catheterized. This alteration occurs with spinal shock. The bladder is not spastic. A/SP, AN, PS

347. no. 3. The sympathetic system controls the "flight or fight" response. The parasympathetic system is more concerned with normal body function. A/SP, AN, PS

348. no. 4. A reflex is a quick stimulus-response act such as a "hand-on-hot-stove" response. A/SP, AN, PS

349. no. 3. Spinal shock usually occurs 30 to 60 minutes after the cord injury and usually resolves in several months, depending on the severity of the injury. Recovery is a gradual process where the spinal neurons regain their excitability. Partial or complete return of reflexes is possible. On average, the duration of spinal shock is 1 to 6 weeks. A/SP, AN, PS

350. no. 2. The person with spinal cord injury above T6 has sympathetic fibers that can be stimulated by ascending information entering the cord below the level of lesion (i.e., sacral cord). The sympathetics are stimulated to fire, and since the cord is cut off from higher centers, firing is uncontrolled. This mechanism is triggered by a noxious stimulus (e.g., distended bladder). The symptoms given are classic for autonomic hyperreflexia. A/SP, AN, PS

351. no. 3. The clamping of the Foley catheter could have precipitated bladder distension. Fear does not stimulate autonomic hyperreflexia. There are no data to suggest that bowel distension may be present. A/SP, AN, PS

352. no. 4. Demineralization is a major problem with lack of stress on the long bones. Absorption is not changed. Option no. 1 is not based on an objective assessment and therefore may be inaccurate. A/SP, AN, H

353. no. 3. Erection can be stimulated by stroking the genitalia or other parts of the body, because it is a reflex action. Ejaculation may not be present with a complete injury, but may be possible with an incomplete injury. Orgasms may occur but will be different. A/SP, IM, H

354. no. 3. Face and neck (approximately) 4%; anterior chest (approximately) 9%; arms and hands 18% (9% each): total = 31%. C/SP, AS, PS

355. no. 3. Options no. 1, no. 2, and no. 4 are characteristic of third-degree burns. C/SP, AS, PS

356. no. 3. Persons with orofacial burns are at risk of developing upper airway edema. Options no. 1, no. 2, and no. 4 are important; however, airway management always takes first priority. C/SP, PL, PS

357. no. 2. Blood volume is reduced from the burn's fluid loss, resulting in poor peripheral absorption. Burn clients need effective pain relief. C/SP, AN, PS

358. no. 4. More accurate measures are necessitated by the severity of the problem. C/SP, EV, PS

359. no. 1. Sulfamylon is a carbonic anhydrase inhibitor and can lead to impairment of the renal buffering system. Options no. 2, no. 3, and no. 4 are side effects of silver nitrate. C/SP, AS, PS

360. no. 1. Dressings on the donor site are never disturbed without a specific order. C/SP, PL, PS

361. no. 4. A position of comfort often leads to a contracture, because clients tend to flex joints near the burn. Extension is a better position. C/SP, PL, E

362. no. 3. Since the major cause of death in burn clients is infection, this is the primary goal; however, all the options listed are important goals. C/SP, PL, PS

363. no. 3. Parkinson's disease is a chronic, degenerative disorder of the basal ganglia. The other three options are incorrect. A/SP, AN, PS

364. no. 3. Clients with Parkinson's disease have a classic resting tremor of the upper extremities (pill rolling). These tremors are only present when the hand is at rest; they disappear with sleep and with active movement of the hands. Ptosis, visual impairment, and vertigo are not signs of Parkinson's disease. A/SP, AS, PS

365. no. 3. Motor function is tested by observing muscular movement, such as when the client walks. Options no. 1 and no. 4 test reflex function; no. 3 tests cognitive function. A/SP, AS, PS

366. no. 1. There is no known cause for most cases of Parkinson's disease. Drugs and arteriosclerosis are implicated only in some cases. A/SP, AN, PS

367. no. 4. Tremors are the first symptom to appear and the last to be controlled. A/SP, EV, PS

368. no. 2. Pain is the only option listed that is not commonly experienced by persons with multiple sclerosis. A/SP, AS, PS

369. no. 2. There is no known benefit to long-term corticosteroid therapy in treating multiple sclerosis. The other options given are all true. A/SP, IM, H

370. no. 1. This will prevent head injury. Once the seizure has begun, trying to place something in the mouth is dangerous. A person having a seizure should not be moved unless there is an immediate danger. After the seizure, the person can be turned on one side to facilitate the drainage of secretions. The nurse should guide a client's movements to avoid injury, but a client should not be restrained. A/SP, IM, PS

371. no. 3. Grand mal seizures (also known as tonic-clonic seizures) are commonly preceded by a brief aura consisting of a specific movement or unnatural sensation. The three other seizure types are not characterized by auras. A/SP, AN, PS

372. no. 2. Most, but not all, cases of epilepsy can be controlled by medication. A/SP, AN, H

373. no. 2. This test measures the electrical activity of the brain. Since epilepsy is caused by an abnormal discharge of the neurons, this test is the most specific. A/SP, AS, PS

374. no. 4. Since seizures are controlled when clients take medication, they often begin to believe they are "cured" and stop taking the drugs, at which time the seizures recur. Although the other options may precipitate a seizure in an epileptic client, the effects are not consistent or common. A/SP, AS, PS

375. no. 3. The definition of status epilepticus is continuous seizures. Consciousness is not regained until the seizures have been controlled. A/SP, AN, PS

376. no. 4. Myasthenia gravis is a chronic progressive muscle disease that affects muscles of the eye, face, neck, diaphragm, and intercostal region. When the muscles of respiration are affected, the subsequent respiratory weakness can lead to death. Restoring or maintaining ventilation has priority in the emergency room. The other three options are not associated with myasthenia gravis. A/SP, PL, PS

377. no. 3. Assessment of the hard palate in dark-skinned persons is done to observe early signs of jaundice. There is not enough vascular tissue in this area for cyanosis to be evident. A/SP, AS, PS

378. no. 3. In myasthenia gravis, loss of voluntary breathing is a high risk. The other goals are important, but not priorities. A/SP, PL, E

379. no. 2. Pain, edema, and lack of a blood return are all signs of an infiltrated IV. Redness, which usually indicates inflammation or infection, is difficult to detect in dark-skinned individuals. A/SP, PL, PS

380. no. 3. This is the only correct action for hydrocortisone sodium succinate (Solu-Cortef) listed and describes the reason for administration. A/SP, AN, PS

381. no. 2. Cholinergic drugs act in the same way as acetylcholine. A/SP, AN, PS

382. no. 3. Cholinergic drugs cause vasodilatation, not vasoconstriction. A/SP, EV, PS

383. no. 1. The standard distance from an eye chart has been set at 20 feet. At this distance, letters of a certain size can be identified by a normal eye. Thus a person who reads the 20-feet line at a distance of 20 feet is said to have 20/20 vision. If a person can read only a line with larger letters (e.g., the 30-feet line), the visual acuity is 20/30, and so forth. A/SP, AN, PS

384. no. 3. The left occipital visual area contains fibers from the lateral half of the right retina. Thus damage to the left occipital visual area produces the pattern of blindness described in option no. 3. The reverse pattern of blindness results from damage to the right occipital visual area. A/SP, AS, PS

385. no. 3. This is the area defined as the anterior chamber. A/SP, AN, PS

386. no. 1. In myopia (nearsightedness) light rays converge anterior to the retina, causing distant objects to be blurred. In hyperopia (farsightedness) the light rays focus posterior to the retina. Presbyopia, an age-related change, is a loss of the ability to focus on objects close to the eye. In emmetropia, light rays focus exactly on the retina. A/SP, AN, PS

387. no. 2. Presbyopia is an age-related change in which the ability to focus on objects close to the eye is lost. It usually occurs after age 40. Emmetropia is normal vision; diplopia is double vision; myopia is nearsightedness. A/SP, AN, PS

388. no. 4. Foreign bodies embedded in the eye must be removed by a physician or ophthalmologist. Rubbing the eye may abrade the corneal tissue and cause the particle to become further embedded. The eye needs to be protected from pressure or rubbing. After examination by the ophthalmologist, the eye may be irrigated with normal saline, not with water or boric acid. A/SP, IM, PS

389. no. 1. A sudden loss of an area of vision is associated with retinal detachment. Glaucoma is associated with a peripheral vision loss. Cataract is associated with a clouding of vision. Keratitis is associated with blurred vision and photophobia. A/SP, AN, PS

390. no. 1. Bed rest is required so that healing can occur. A/SP, PL, E

391. no. 3. This is an antiemetic, but it is specific for motion sickness and acts on the inner ear. The use of dimenhydrinate (Dramamine) is not associated with the other three options. A/SP, PL, PS

392. no. 3. The small incision to decrease pressure in the middle ear and prevent rupture of the eardrum heals quickly. A/SP, AN, PS

393. no. 3. Vertigo and nausea are classic signs of this syndrome. The remaining options are not characteristic of Ménière's syndrome. A/SP, AS, PS

394. no. 3. The lens is the area of the eye affected by cataracts. A/SP, AS, PS

395. no. 3. The opacity cannot be treated except by surgical removal of the lens. A/SP, AN, PS

396. no. 3. Paralytic ileus is not a complication that generally occurs following cataract extraction. How to use the call bell will be important because of postoperative positioning and eye patches. Respiratory infections must be avoided since coughing and sneezing can increase intraocular pressure. A/SP, PL, E

397. no. 1. This option correctly describes the effects of cataract lenses. The client will need time to

adjust to the distortion resulting with cataract lenses; new safety measures must be learned since peripheral vision will be very distorted. A/SP, AN, H

398. no. 1. Coughing increases intraocular pressure and is contraindicated for clients after eye surgery. Turning and positioning will only be allowed with the head of the bed elevated 30° and with the client lying either supine or on the unoperated side to maintain intraocular pressure and to minimize swelling. Nausea and vomiting need to be prevented because vomiting can increase intraocular pressure. A/SP, PL, PS

399. no. 4. Prolapse of the iris can precipitate acute glaucoma. This is the most common postoperative complication following lens extraction. A/SP, AN, E

400. no. 3. Postoperative confusion is a frequent complication of eye surgery, especially with elderly clients. The nurse should reorient the client frequently, explain all procedures, and keep the side rails up and call light within easy reach. Restraints are contraindicated because they increase client anxiety and can increase intraocular pressure if the client strains against them. Telling the client to stay in bed is often inadequate when the client is confused. Giving a client a sedative can further increase confusion in the elderly. A/SP, IM, E

401. no. 1. There is no reason to stay in a darkened room. In fact, this combined with impaired vision can lead to injury. A/SP, PL, H

402. no. 4. Weeding requires bending, which increases intraocular pressure. The other options are all acceptable activities. A/SP, PL, H

403. no. 1. Mydriatic drugs cause dilatation of the pupil. A dilated pupil can block the outflow of aqueous humor and increase intraocular pressure. A/SP, AN, PS

404. no. 4. Normal intraocular pressure, measured by a tonometer, is 12 to 20 mm Hg. Glaucoma is a disease in which the intraocular pressure increases to pathologic levels, sometimes as high as 85 to 90 mm Hg. A/SP, AS, PS

405. no. 2. The optic nerve is the sensory cranial nerve that controls visual acuity and visual fields. The olfactory nerve (I) is responsible for the sense of smell. Cranial nerve III controls pupillary reactions and external muscles of the eye. Cranial nerve IV controls external muscles of the eye. A/SP, AN, PS

406. no. 4. Lens opacity is characteristic of cataracts. In addition to options no. 1 through no. 3, optic nerve atrophy produces diminishing vision (first peripheral, then finally central vision). A/SP, AS, PS

407. no. 4. Atropine sulfate is an anticholinergic drug that dilates the pupil secondary to inhibition of the parasympathetic nervous system. Neostigmine, pilocarpine, and physostigmine are all miotics and are used in the treatment of glaucoma. A/SP, AN, PS

408. no. 2. Routine care following eye surgery includes no coughing, no turning or turning only to the *unaffected* side, and adequate fluid intake. The client should not experience severe eye pain. A/SP, PL, E

409. no. 1. Usually the first symptom to be noted is decreasing peripheral vision. There may be some mild aching but generally no pain. Severe pain is characteristic of *acute* glaucoma. In the late stage, the client may see halos around lights. A/SP, AS, PS

410. no. 2. Mr. James's vision in dark places may be decreased when using miotics to control the glaucoma; for safety reasons, more light is needed. Moderate exercise is indicated to promote better circulation, but excessive exercise would be contraindicated. A/SP, PL, H

411. no. 2. Pilocarpine is the miotic that is commonly used in the medical management of glaucoma. Atropine is an anticholinergic drug that dilates the pupil secondary to inhibition of the parasympathetic nervous sytem. Acetazolamide (Diamox) is a carbonic anhydrase inhibitor that reduces intraocular pressure. Scopolamine is a mydriatic that is used to treat uveitis and iritis. A/SP, AN, PS

412. no. 2. Miotics constrict the pupil and contract the ciliary muscles increasing the outflow of aqueous humor, thus decreasing intraocular pressure. Mydriatics (drugs that dilate the pupil) such as atropine can precipitate an acute episode of glaucoma. A/SP, AN, PS

413. no. 1. Putting pressure on the lacrimal duct at the inner canthus of the eyes is important to prevent systemic effects of miotics. A/SP, IM, E

414. no. 1. Reduction of aqueous humor is desirable. Acetazolamide (Diamox) is the drug commonly used to do this. Carbonic anhydrase inhibitors do not dilate the pupil or affect accommodation. A/SP, AN, PS

415. no. 1. Once vision has been lost, it cannot be restored. Treatment for glaucoma is aimed at preventing the loss of vision. A/SP, PL, H

416. no. 2. A tonometry exam measures the intraocular pressure and can reveal early glaucoma. Treatment can then be initiated. Surgical procedures are avoided if possible, since most of the filtering procedures can cause cataract formation. A/SP, PL, H

417. no. 4. Touching will provide stimulation and enhance the senses, one means to help prevent further

regressive behaviors. Speaking in a louder voice is not necessary. Visual loss does not affect hearing. A sedative would cause further sensory deprivation. Orienting the client would be appropriate; however, frequent touch will be more effective in minimizing sensory deprivation. A/SP, IM, E

418. no. 4. Nasal packing and splinting are used to prevent postoperative edema and bleeding after a rhinoplasty. A HemoVac suction is never used. Frequent swallowing is a sign of bleeding that should be monitored frequently. The head of the bed should be elevated to prevent aspiration. The gag reflex should be checked to ensure the client will not aspirate bloody drainage. A/SP, PL, PS

419. no. 3. Initial stools may be tarry as a result of swallowed blood. Since it may also indicate hemorrhage, further assessment is in order. The physician will not be called until after the nursing assessment is completed. Options no. 2 and no. 4 are not indicated. A/SP, IM, PS

420. no. 1. Blowing the nose is contraindicated because it can cause bleeding. Increased pain and swelling are signs of infection and should be reported to the physician immediately. Rest, activity limitation, and adequate food and fluid intake help to prevent infection. Aspirin should be avoided if pain relief is necessary because of its effects on coagulation. A/SP, IM, H

421. no. 4. A history of hypertension is common with the occurrence of epistaxis. Trauma, acute sinusitis, nasal surgery, and deviated septum are all risk factors for epistaxis. A/SP, AS, PS

422. no. 1. Epinephrine is applied locally to create vasoconstriction and hemostasis. Lidocaine is an antidysrhythmic and a topical anesthetic. Pilocarpine is a miotic used to treat glaucoma. Cyclopentolate is a mydriatic that results in pupil dilatation. A/SP, AN, PS

423. no. 2. The sitting position will prevent the client from swallowing blood and secretions. A/SP, PL, E

424. no. 3. All the options are correct, but keeping the airway open is the main priority. A/SP, PL, PS

425. no. 4. The nose is a vascular area; thus, hemorrhage is the most common complication. Infection is possible but not a likely complication. Altered smell and inability to breathe through the nose are not complications. A/SP, AN, PS

426. no. 1. Vasoconstrictive nose drops stimulate the sympathetic nervous system. This is followed by relaxation of these vessels, accompanied by nasal stuffiness. Therefore, after the nose is temporarily relieved by the nose drops, it becomes more stuffy than it was before. Phenylephrine (Neo-Synephrine) is a commonly used vasoconstrictive nasal spray. This drug may be absorbed systemi-

cally but does not cause hypotension. It does not contain cocaine and will not affect the olfactory nerve. A/SP, AN, PS

427. no. 4. Vagal stimulation may produce dysrhythmias and bradycardia, not tachycardia. All other options are appropriate for tracheal suctioning. A/SP, IM, PS

428. no. 2. The laryngectomy tube enters directly into the trachea and is considered sterile; it should be suctioned first. The nose can be suctioned last using the same suction catheter. A sterile setup should always be used for suctioning, and the catheter should always be lubricated with saline before suctioning. A/SP, IM, E

429. no. 2. The nasogastric tube prevents food and fluid from contaminating the pharyngeal and esophageal suture line. A/SP, PL, E

430. no. 1. In addition to potassium and sodium loss, bicarbonate is also lost in diarrhea. The result is acidosis. Options no. 2, no. 3, and no. 4 will cause alkalosis. A/SP, AN, PS

431. no. 2. Predisposing factors of cancer are known to be influenced by familial factors, sex differences, and environment, Long-term use of corticosteroids is associated with a higher incidence of cancer. A/CA, AS, H

432. no. 2. Speech rehabilitation can be started as soon as the esophageal suture line has healed. A/SP, PL, H

433. no. 2. Immediate first aid at the scene of the accident requires fractures to be immobilized in the position in which the fracture is found, in order to prevent further injury. Options no. 3 and no. 4 do not describe adequate splinting. A/M, IM, PS

434. no. 4. Initial assessments of any injured client with a fracture would first rule out any life-threatening injuries before dealing with the fracture. Covering open wounds, taking blood pressure, and cleaning the fracture site are all appropriate interventions, but airway and breathing always take first priority. A/M, IM, PS

435. no. 3. Increased blood pressure, confusion, and restlessness in a young adult are some of the first signs of fat emboli. Shock manifests with a decrease in blood pressure. A concussion presents signs of lethargy and possibly other signs of increased intracranial pressure. A/M, AN, PS

436. no. 3. Any malodor indicates a potential infection. A plaster cast color other than white indicates presence of drainage. The cast should not flake when dry. A plaster cast usually dries in 8 to 10 hours. It takes longer for larger casts such as long-leg or body casts. Weight bearing with short-leg plaster casts is usually possible 24 to 48 hours after application. Fiberglass casts may be different colors;

they dry within minutes and can usually bear weight within 30 minutes. A/M, AS, E

437. no. 4. The other options tend to dry the cast from the outside, leaving the inside damp and crumbly with the potential of skin irritation. Options no. 1 and no. 2 risk burning the client's exposed skin. An electric fan may cause drying from the outside to the inside, resulting in too-early weight bearing when the outside is hard but the inside is soft. This creates the potential for indentations and the development of pressure sores. A/M, IM, E

438. no. 3. Rubber makes the pillow hard, which can cause dents in the cast. The other options are correct. A/M, IM, E

439. no. 2. This is a good way of assessing the amount of bleeding. As described, the bleeding is not excessive, so the physician need not be notified. With internal fixation, some slight bleeding is normal. The amount or size of bleeding should also be charted in the nurses' notes. A/M, IM, PS

440. no. 1. An infection would not be apparent on the first postoperative day. Hemorrhage would not be painful. After the first postoperative day, the cast would be almost dry; thus this pain could be from pressure. Casts are warm during the drying process but do not get hot enough to burn. A/M, AN, PS

441. no. 2. An unpleasant odor indicates infection. It need not include drainage. Temperature may not be elevated in local sites of infection. Option no. 3 is incorrect. A/M, AS, PS

442. no. 4. Cyanosis is the result of poor circulation, not nerve damage. All the other options reflect peroneal nerve palsy. A/M, AS, PS

443. no. 4. Shoe polish and alcohol might soften the cast. Shellac prevents evaporation of body moisture. Option no. 4 is correct. A/M, IM, H

444. no. 4. Pain unrelieved by analgesics is an early sign of compartment syndrome. Clients with this problem tend to complain of severe pain upon passive movements of the digits. Then they may be unable to move the digits of the affected extremity. Absence of the pulse and pallor may be present but are not reliable signs, because deep circulation may still be intact. Paralysis indicates nerve damage. A/M, AS, PS

445. no. 1. Bivalving the cast (i.e., cutting it lengthwise into two equal parts) will reduce the external constriction, which is the critical problem; the other options are inappropriate. A/M, IM, PS

446. no. 2. Unrelieved pressure on nerves and vessels entering and leaving the compartments of the arm can cause paralysis and deformity of the arm and hand. Irreversible muscle damage can occur within 6 hours if untreated. Within 24 to 48 hours, permanent deformity with scarring, contractures, pa-

ralysis, and loss of sensation can occur. Impaired circulation would be detected before development of gangrene. A/M, AN, PS

447. no. 3. Fat emboli cause petechiae, usually across the chest and shoulders. When they occur, it is within 12 to 36 hours after fracturing a long bone. Frothy sputum indicates pulmonary embolus. Hypertension and coma indicate cerebral embolism. A/M, AS, PS

448. no. 4. After menopause, osteoporosis becomes a problem for many women as a result of estrogen deficiency. Additionally, calcium absorption in both men and women over 65 declines as part of the aging process. Older women with this problem are at particular risk for fractures. A/M, AN, PS

449. no. 3. Buck's traction does not reduce the fracture; the pull is minimal, usually with less than 10 pounds. The use of Buck's traction is usually intermittent. Skeletal traction is used to reduce fractures. C/M, AN, PS

450. no. 2. The traction is applied directly to the skin, so it would irritate any existing ulcers. Other contraindications are a rash in the area to be covered, an allergy to the materials used for wrapping, and a neurovascular problem in the affected extremity (e.g., paralysis, phlebitis). The other options are not contraindications. C/M, AN, PS

451. no. 1. The traction device can cause irritation and skin breakdown if skin care is neglected. The bed acts as a splint when the client is turned on her affected side. Options no. 3 and no. 4 will cause the loss of countertraction and the effectiveness of the traction. C/M, PL, E

452. no. 4. High dietary fiber is a natural way to prevent constipation. Fluid intake should be encouraged. Medication should be used if fluids and increased fiber fail to obtain results. A/M, PL, E

453. no. 1. Total hip replacement is the treatment for avascular necrosis, which requires replacement of the femoral head. The other options are true of avascular necrosis. A/M, AN, PS

454. no. 2. The lower extremities usually rotate externally when a person is lying in bed. In addition, this client has had surgery on the thigh area, and this weakens the muscles in the extremity and further promotes external rotation. The other options are incorrect. A/M, PL, E

455. no. 2. This is the only option that will prevent external rotation. A/M, IM, E

456. no. 2. After assessment of the client, the physician should be notified of the findings. Severe pain is not normal after a hip nailing. The other options are incorrect. A/M, AS, PS

457. no. 1. The walker should always be walked into when all four legs are on the floor. The other options are incorrect. A/M, EV, E

458. no. 3. These should be prevented because both can promote dislodgment of the hip prosthesis. The affected extremity is to be abducted by the use of an abductor pillow. The other options are incorrect. A/M, IM, E

459. no. 1. The sudden onset of severe pain in the hip prosthesis site indicates dislodgment. The physician should be notified once the nurse has completed an assessment of the extremity. The other options are incorrect interventions at this time. A/M, IM, PS

460. no. 4. This is the best choice. He probably still has the abduction pillow in place. He must avoid flexing the hip greater than 90° in order to prevent prosthesis displacement. A/M, IM, E

461. no. 3. Adequate blood supply is required for tissue to heal and survive; thus the decision regarding the level of an amputation depends on the quality of vascularity of the tissue. This is best evaluated at the time of the surgery. A/M, AN, PS

462. no. 2. Firm application of an elastic bandage is necessary to prevent fluid accumulation and to continue to mold the limb if the rigid dressing comes off, at which time the physician is notified. Elevating the limb on the fifth day is contraindicated. Elevation of a lower extremity after amputation is only done for the first 24 hours postoperatively. After that, elevation promotes flexion contractures, the most common complication after amputation of lower extremities. A saline dressing is used in the event of evisceration. A/M, IM, PS

463. no. 3. A "shrinker" bandage is properly applied with tighter turns around the distal end of the affected limb to promote venous return and stump molding. The other options are appropriate. A/M, IM, H

464. no. 2. The nurse should be direct and honest with the client concerning the accident and outcome of the surgery. The first step in the grieving process is acknowledgment of the loss. This option facilitates acknowledgment. Option no. 1 is not truthful and avoids the issue. Option no. 3 also avoids the issue of the loss of the arm. Option no. 4 is incorrect since phantom limb sensation is a feeling process; the sensation is related to the severing of the nerves at the amputation site. It is not a thinking process. Also, the sensation that the limb is present occurs after surgery and may last for as long as 6 months. A/M, IM, PC

465. no. 4. The client needs to identify his new body boundaries by touching and reorienting himself to his body. This will facilitate the rehabilitation process, especially acceptance of a changing body image. A/M, IM, PC

466. no. 4. Inflammation and systemic symptoms are characteristic of rheumatoid arthritis. Osteoarthritis is characterized by local symptoms and usually no systemic symptoms such as fever and elevated sedimentation rate. A/M, AS, PS

467. no. 4. Clients with osteoarthritis should conserve energy when possible. Mrs. Balto is overweight and needs to achieve her ideal body weight in order to decrease the stress on her joints. Warm baths will decrease the discomfort and facilitate increased movement. Sliding items across the floor requires less energy than lifting and carrying them. A/M, IM, E

468. no. 2. The usual dose range of aspirin to treat inflammation is 3 to 5 grams/day. Regularly scheduled intake provides a constant plasma level and increases effects. Ringing in the ears is a first sign of overdose of aspirin. Enteric-coated tablets (e.g., Ecotrin) are helpful in preventing gastrointestinal distress. A hypersensitivity reaction can occur at any time. A/M, EV, H

469. no. 1. This is the only correct option. Gout occurs in the small joints and results when urate crystals are deposited in the joints. The most common age group is 30- to 40-year-old men. Option no. 4 is characteristic of osteoarthritis. A/M, AN, PS

470. no. 4. Fluid intake is increased to prevent the precipitation of urate in the kidneys. Clients often cannot tolerate the pressure of compresses on the affected areas. Salicylates antagonize the action of some uricosuric drugs. Aspirin and other salicylates at low doses (300 to 600 mg) inhibit uric acid secretion. Acetaminophen could be substituted for simple pain relief. Deformities are rare in gout. A/M, PL, E

471. no. 2. Dietary restrictions of purine are usually initiated after the acute attack. The disease can be well-controlled with dietary management and medications. Dietary management includes limiting high-purine foods and alcohol ingestion and maintaining an ideal body weight. Foods high in purine are organ meats, yeast, anchovies, sardines in oil, and meat extracts. The urine should be kept alkaline to prevent stone formation. This may be achieved by an alkaline-ash diet that includes milk, vegetables, and fruits (except for cranberries, prunes, and plums). A/M, PL, H

472. no. 4. Allopurinol (Zyloprim) is irritating to the intestinal tract. It is best to take the medication during or after the meal, since medication taken on an empty stomach is more likely to cause gastrointestinal irritation. The other options are incorrect information. Fluids are usually encouraged with a minimum of 2000 ml/day. Foods with purine are usually limited or restricted, but are not totally eliminated. A/M, PL, E

473. no. 2. A skin rash is the first sign of a severe hypersensitivity reaction. The other options are side effects of allopurinol (Zyloprim). A/M, IM, E

474. no. 2. This is the incorrect option. Option no. 1 is the appropriate action to plan. Keeping the knees slightly flexed while the client is in semi-Fowler's position will decrease muscle strain in the lower back. Keeping a pillow under the head for comfort will cause no harm and will promote comfort. A/M, PL, E

475. no. 4. A thickening or lump noted in the breast is one of the signs of cancer cited by the American Cancer Society. A tumor itself does not cause pain; pain results from pressure exerted on surrounding tissue when the tumor enlarges and would be a later sign of cancer. Options no. 1, no. 2, and no. 3 are three of the seven warning signs for cancer cited by the American Cancer Society. A/CA, AN, H

476. no. 3. According to the most recent guidelines established by the American Cancer Society, a guaiac test and a cancer-related check-up should be done yearly after the age of 50. A baseline mammogram should be done between the ages of 35 and 39. A Pap smear is done every 3 years after three initial negative tests that are done 1 year apart, or as directed by the physician. A/CA, EV, H

477. no. 1. A Pap smear is obtained to detect neoplastic cells in the cervical and vaginal secretions that have been shed by cervical and endometrial neoplastic cells. Material is collected by scraping the cervical canal and the squamocolumnar junction with a spatula or a cotton swab moistened with saline. The Pap smear does not directly evaluate the uterus, the fallopian tubes, or the cul-de-sac (the peritoneal space between the rectum and the uterus). The fallopian tubes are usually examined with a laparoscopy or culdoscopy. A/CA, AN, H

478. no. 4. A class-1 Pap smear indicates absence of atypical or abnormal cells. After three initial negative tests taken 1 year apart, Pap smears are done every 3 years or as directed by a physician. Classes 2 to 4 require more extensive evaluation to determine if a malignancy exists. Class 5 cytological findings indicate malignancy and require treatment. Following a class-1 finding, surgery, treatment, or refraining from sexual activity is not indicated. A/CA, IM, H

479. no. 2. The Hemoccult test is an excellent screening device for the general public; it can be done in the privacy of the home and has a low rate of false-negative results (i.e., if there is blood in the stool, this test will detect it most of the time). A barium enema is not a recommended screening test. A proctosigmoidoscopy should be done every 3 to 5 years, and the digital rectal exam should be conducted by a skilled practitioner, not by a lay person. A/CA, AS, H

480. no. 2. Sputum samples should be collected early in the morning before the client eats or drinks. The client is not required to be NPO for 24 hours before the procedure. Using toothpaste or mouthwash should be avoided because they can affect the sample. The sample should be coughed up from deep within the lungs. Saliva should not be collected. A/CA, IM, H

481. no. 2. Small-cell lung cancer has a very poor prognosis because it is rarely diagnosed in a limited and localized state. Even with treatment the client has only a 20% chance for 2-year survival. At advanced stages most clients die within 6 months. The 5-year survival rate depends on the type of lung cancer (non–small-cell cancer has a somewhat better 5-year survival rate) and stage (cancer is easier to treat in an earlier stage when the cancer is localized). Usually by the time a lung tumor is detected on x-ray, about 75% of the disease course has elapsed. Eighty-seven percent of lung cancer clients die within 5 years. A/CA, AS, PS

482. no. 4. Options no. 1, no. 2, and no. 3 are all common systemic side effects of external radiation therapy. Dry desquamation of the skin is a common localized side effect. A/CA, AS, PS

483. no. 3. Skin markings over the treatment area should not be washed off for the duration of the therapy unless special permission is given because they are important reference marks for the radiation beams. The area should be left open to air, but sunlight should be avoided. The skin should not be massaged, and lotions, cosmetics, and powder should not be applied. These interventions will reduce the problems associated with dry desquamation of the skin. A/CA, IM, E

484. no. 4. Metoclopramide (Reglan) is a cholinergic medication used to prevent the nausea and vomiting associated with chemotherapy and delayed gastric emptying. Phentolamine mesylate (Regitine) is an alpha-adrenergic blocker used for treating hypertension. Methylcellulase (Citrucel) is a bulk laxative. Dexamethasone (Decadron) is a corticosteroid used to treat cerebral edema. A/CA, AN, PS

485. no. 2. False reassurance that everything will be all right is inappropriate. The client should understand the extent of surgery as well as the type and care of the ostomy. Although a cheerful, optimistic environment is important, it is essential that Mr. Varella understand the proposed surgical treatment.

Visitors should not be restricted. Family and friends can provide valuable emotional support to the client. A/CA, PL, E

486. no. 1. A margin of uninvolved tissue must be excised, but only as much tissue as necessary is removed. Wider or more radical excisions generally do not improve prognosis. Surgery is the treatment of choice for colon cancer. Radiation and chemotherapy may also be used in conjunction with surgery. Surgery is usually not considered a last resort. A/CA, AN, PS

487. no. 3. Colon tumors tend to spread through the lymphatics and portal vein to the liver. While metastasis to the other sites listed is possible, the liver is most likely the first to be affected. A/CA, AN, PS

488. no. 2. 5-fluorouracil (5-FU) is an antineoplastic, antimetabolic drug that inhibits DNA synthesis and interferes with cell replication. It is given intravenously and acts systemically. It affects all rapidly growing cells, both malignant and normal. It is used as adjuvant therapy for treating cancer of the colon, rectum, stomach, breast, and pancreas. This drug has many side effects, including thrombocytopenia, leukopenia, myelosuppression, anemia, anorexia, stomatitis, and renal failure. A/CA, AN, PS

489. no. 1. Bland foods of moderate temperature facilitate swallowing and decrease pain. Fluids should be encouraged to keep oral membranes moist and to decrease side effects of chemotherapy. Topical anesthetics such as viscous lidocaine (Xylocaine) should be encouraged to decrease oral discomfort. However, commercial mouthwashes should be avoided because of their alcohol content. A/CA, PL, E

490. no. 4. Epithelial cells are extremely sensitive to chemotherapy because of their normally high rate of cell turnover. Options no. 1, no. 2, and no. 3 are not as appropriate because they do not address the client's concern. The client is requesting factual information. In addition, no. 1 negates the client's concerns. A/CA, IM, E

491. no. 3. It is important for the significant other to express anger, but allowing the client to know the diagnosis and treatment options cannot be delayed. Although clients have the right to know their diagnosis, no. 1 is not correct because it does not address the issue of why the husband wants the diagnosis kept from his wife. The situation will be difficult to resolve unless the husband's rationale is known. A/CA, IM, PC

492. no. 4. Option no. 1 will detect internal occult bleeding. Options no. 2 and no. 4 will decrease the risk of bleeding. Option no. 3 is not necessary because it will not affect the risk of hemorrhage. Reverse

isolation would be implemented for a granulocyte count below 2000 mm³. A/CA, PL, PS

493. no. 2. When chemotherapy is initiated, there is a breakdown of many cancer cells. Uric acid is a cell metabolite. A/CA, AN, PS

494. no. 2. Allopurinol is an antigout drug that decreases uric acid formation. Prednisone is a corticosteroid used for immunosuppression and severe inflammation. Indomethacin inhibits prostaglandin synthesis; it is effective as an analgesic, antiinflammatory, and antipyretic agent. Hydrochlorothiazide is a thiazide diuretic that is effective in hypertension and edema. A/CA, AN, PS

495. no. 3. Thrombocytopenia is an abnormal decrease in the number of platelets, which results in bleeding tendencies. Erythrocytosis is an abnormal increase in the number of circulating red blood cells. Leukocytosis is an increase in the number of white blood cells in the blood. Polycythemia is also an excess of red blood cells and is a synonym for erythrocytosis. With chemotherapy there is a decrease in red and white blood cells, not an increase. A/CA, AS, PS

496. no. 3. A positive family history has not been identified as a risk factor for cervical cancer. The other three options are all considered to be risk factors for cervical cancer. A/CA, AS, PS

497. no. 2. Many women with cervical cancer fear a loss of femininity. It is important to discuss the effects of treatment to enable the client to prepare for changes in sexual functioning. Although telling Mrs. Day that she does not have to worry about pregnancy is accurate, it is not a therapeutic response. Nurses are capable of answering questions regarding sexuality. The client will need to be referred to other resources if the client's concerns cannot be addressed by the nurse. The physician should be notified of the client's concerns, but not necessarily as a referral. A/CA, IM, PC

498. no. 1. Vaginal drainage will usually persist for 1 to 2 months after removal of a cervical implant. Diarrhea, not constipation, is usually a side effect of cervical implants. Confusion and xerostomia are not side effects of cervical implants. A/CA, IM, PS

499. no. 3. Clients with cervical implants require a low-residue diet (and often antidiarrheal medications) to reduce the frequency of defecation. Defecation may cause accidental dislodgment of the implant from straining and sitting on a bedpan. Frequent ambulation is contraindicated because it will dislodge the implant. Bed rest in a supine or low-Fowler's position should be maintained. Visitors should be limited to one 15-minute visit a day, and no pregnant women or children should be allowed because of the radiation exposure. Vaginal irrigations are contraindicated during this period of time. A/CA, IM, E

500. no. 1. Shortening and narrowing of the vagina is a distressing long-term complication of cervical implants. Women need to use a vaginal dilator twice a week to stretch the tissue. Uterine cramping is a temporary side effect that occurs only if the implant extends into the uterus. Nausea and constipation may occur during the initial treatment but are not long-term side effects. A/CA, AS, PS

501. no. 3. It is important to allow the client to express grief over the loss of her breast. False assurance will impede further communication. A/CA, IM, PC

502. no. 1. A significant breast cancer risk factor is a history of previous breast cancer. Breast cancer can develop bilaterally, so it is imperative that the client be instructed to perform breast self-exams on the remaining breast. A/CA, AN, H

503. no. 3. Although no. 1 and no. 2 are technically correct, they do not address the client's feelings about her body image. Mrs. Wu needs to express her feelings and concerns before effective teaching can be accomplished. A/CA, IM, PC

504. no. 4. Raising the side rails after premedication is an essential safety measure that needs to be done immediately after administration. Options no. 1, no. 2, and no. 3 should not be done before premedicating the client. Mrs. Wu should be maintained on bed rest and should not get up to void because her gait may be unstable. Operative permits are not valid if obtained following administration of narcotics or consciousness-altering medications. A/CA, IM, E

505. no. 1. Check under Mrs. Wu's back for drainage, since gravity will draw it toward the back. A/CA, IM, PS

506. no. 1. The right axilla should not be shaved because of the risk of cutting the skin and subsequent infection development. Lymphedema following a mastectomy will increase this risk of infection. Sodium intake should not be increased because it will further increase lymphedema. A client can wear her own bra with padding upon discharge or use a "Reach to Recovery" prosthesis. The incision should be gently cleansed with mild soap and warm water, not an antiseptic solution. A/CA, IM, H

507. no. 1. The other three options have been identified as influencing a couple's sexual adaptation to mastectomy, something that must be assessed in this case. A/CA, AS, PS

508. no. 2. Denial is often the first response to a crisis or grief reaction. It is a defense against more anxiety than the client can cope with at the time. Mrs. Goldfarb may experience the other phenomena later, but her comments do not at present suggest them. A/CA, AN, PC

509. no. 3. Expressions of hopelessness or despair, or both, are defining characteristics of reactive (situational) depression. P/E, AS, PC

510. no. 1. This diagnosis reflects an actual change in the structure and function of a body. Impaired verbal communication and alteration in cardiac output will not occur with an uncomplicated mastectomy. The client may have a temporary self-care deficit if the pectoralis muscle is removed or damaged. However, this aggressive surgery is not done as frequently today. A/CA, AN, PS

511. no. 1. These safety measures must be instituted to promote adequate drainage and prevent infection in the affected arm. The other choices listed would actually contribute to tissue edema. A/CA, PL, E

512. no. 2. Cancer cells are generally the most rapidly dividing in the body. Healthy tissues such as bone marrow, gastrointestinal epithelium, and hair follicles are also rapidly proliferating and thus bear the brunt of the effects of many of the cytotoxic drugs. A/CA, AN, E

513. no. 3. Some women have engorgement of the breasts premenstrually, which usually disappears a few days after the onset of menstruation. Because of this possible change, it is important that the breasts be examined at the same point in the menstrual cycle each month, ideally when the hormonal influences on the breast are the smallest. CBF/W, IM, H

514. no. 3. A woman who is having a breast removed has many fears related to sexual and social acceptance, disfigurement, and death. Many women have been unable to discuss these feelings with significant others. The nurse can help the client verbalize her feelings and understand what the surgery means to her as a person. The client has a need to be understood and accepted by the nurse. The nurse can clarify any misconceptions and reduce the client's anxiety preoperatively. Sexual relations need not be altered as a result of the surgery, and a skin graft is not needed with a modified radical mastectomy. A/CA, PL, E

515. no. 3. Curling the tubing impedes free flow of the drainage and puts pressure on the skin. The skin will become irritated and could slough. In general, the wound exudate is a straw-colored fluid that is initially blood tinged. Obvious bleeding is bright-red and should be immediately reported to the surgeon. To maintain suction, empty the HemoVac reservoir when it is half full and reestablish the negative pressure. A/CA, IM, PS

516. no. 2. Because movement of the arm is painful, the nurse should support the arm the first few times the arm is exercised. Abduct and adduct it slowly;

flex and extend the elbow, wrist, and fingers. Gentle exercises help reduce muscle dysfunction. The nurse's assistance helps to assure the client that movement of the arm will not cause any harm. Slings are to be avoided, and full range of motion cannot be achieved this early in the postoperative period. A/CA, IM, H

517. no. 4. Clients should be encouraged to resume normal activities after returning home. The nursing care goals are to strengthen self-esteem and contribute to restoring normal function with no activity restrictions after the wound is healed. A/CA, IM, H

518. no. 1. Hodgkin's disease is a malignancy of the lymphoid system that is characterized by a generalized painless lymphadenopathy. It has a 5-year survival rate of 90%. Option no. 2 refers to a multiple myeloma, no. 3 refers to AIDS, and no. 4 refers to leukemia. A/CA, AN, PS

519. no. 3. Diarrhea and abdominal cramps are not indicative of Hodgkin's disease. The other three options frequently occur with the disease. A/CA, AS, PS

520. no. 4. Lymphangiography provides an x-ray examination of the lymphatic system. A bluish contrast medium is injected into a lymphatic vessel in each foot or hand. The blue dye will give skin a bluish tinge and will discolor the stools and urine for several days. The client must lie very still during the procedure. After the procedure, the affected extremity will need to be elevated to prevent edema. A/CA, IM, PS

521. no. 1. AIDS is a syndrome characterized by a defect in cell-mediated immunity. It is caused by the human immunodeficiency virus (HIV), which is a retrovirus that destroys T4 lymphocytes. It does not affect the lymphoid tissues. Kaposi's sarcoma is an opportunistic disease that causes multiple areas of cell proliferation in the skin and eventually in other body sites, but the disease itself is not a malignancy of the skin. AIDS is not a bacterial infection; however, a number of bacterial infections occur as opportunistic diseases. A/CA, AN, PS

522. no. 2. The ELISA measures antibodies to HIV in serum or plasma and is the most widely used screening test for AIDS. The Western blot assay is a *supplemental* test conducted to validate the findings of the ELISA. Lymphangiography is a diagnostic procedure that detects disease of the lymphoid tissue. A Schilling test is used to detect vitamin B_{12} absorption. A/CA, AS, H

523. no. 4. *Pneumocystis carinii* pneumonia is a protozoal disease frequently seen in AIDS clients. The other three options are not considered opportunistic diseases of AIDS. Although non-Hodgkin's lymphoma is a cancer seen in HIV infection, Hodgkin's disease is not. A/CA, AN, PS

524. no. 4. Clients who are HIV positive should not donate blood, plasma, sperm, or body organs. They do not have to avoid casual contact with anyone and do not need to wear gloves or a mask. A/CA, EV, H

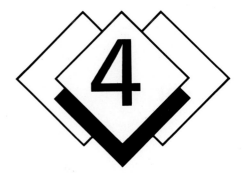

Nursing Care of the Childbearing Family

Coordinator

Francene M. Weatherby, PhD, RNC

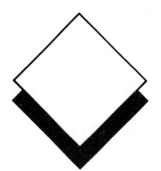

Questions

Juanita Romero has been married 1½ years. She stopped taking oral contraceptives several months ago and now suspects she is pregnant. She is being seen by her physician for the first time.

1. Mrs. Romero has numerous common signs and symptoms associated with pregnancy. Which of the following signs suggests she is probably pregnant?
- ☐ 1. Amenorrhea.
- ☐ 2. Frequent micturition.
- ☐ 3. Enlarged and tender breasts.
- ☐ 4. Goodell's sign.

2. Mrs. Romero's last menstrual period was from November 10-15. She had intercourse on November 17. Her expected date of delivery is
- ☐ 1. July 21.
- ☐ 2. Aug. 17.
- ☐ 3. Aug. 22.
- ☐ 4. Aug. 24.

3. Which of the following is true of pregnancy tests done on urine samples?
- ☐ 1. A positive test is based on increased estrogen excretion in the urine.
- ☐ 2. They are 100% accurate if done 10 to 14 days after fertilization.
- ☐ 3. A positive test is based on the excretion of chorionic gonadotropin in the urine.
- ☐ 4. Home pregnancy tests are not accurate, and clients should be cautioned not to use them.

4. Mrs. Romero is concerned about eating the proper foods during her pregnancy. Which of the following nursing actions is the most appropriate initially?
- ☐ 1. Give her a list of foods to refer to in planning her meals.
- ☐ 2. Emphasize the importance of limiting highly seasoned and salty foods.
- ☐ 3. Ask Mrs. Romero to list her food intake for the last 3 days.
- ☐ 4. Instruct her to continue her usual diet, since she appears to be nutritionally fit.

5. Mrs. Romero has a low hemoglobin. When counseling her to increase her iron intake, which of the following meals would the nurse recommend to her?
- ☐ 1. Ham sandwich, corn pudding, and tossed salad.
- ☐ 2. Hamburger, green beans, and fruit cup.
- ☐ 3. Chicken livers, sliced tomatoes, and dried apricots.
- ☐ 4. Omelet with mushrooms and spinach salad.

6. The nurse would instruct Mrs. Romero to notify the physician immediately if which of the following symptoms occur?
- ☐ 1. Swelling of the face.
- ☐ 2. Frequent urination.
- ☐ 3. Increased vaginal discharge.
- ☐ 4. The presence of chloasma.

7. Which of the following changes is a pregnant woman most likely to notice in her breasts?
- ☐ 1. Darkening of the areolas, tingling sensations, and engorgement.
- ☐ 2. Lightening of the areolas, colostrum, and increased size.
- ☐ 3. Colostrum, tingling sensations, and darkening of the areolas.
- ☐ 4. Increased size, tenderness, and flattening of the nipples.

8. Mrs. Romero is treated for syphilis during the first trimester with intramuscular injections of penicillin. The baby's diagnosis at birth would most likely be
- ☐ 1. Congenital syphilis.
- ☐ 2. Stillborn.
- ☐ 3. Normal newborn.
- ☐ 4. Premature newborn.

9. Constipation during pregnancy is best treated by
- ☐ 1. Regular use of a mild laxative.
- ☐ 2. Increased bulk and fluid in the diet.
- ☐ 3. Limiting excessive weight gain.
- ☐ 4. Regular use of bisacodyl (Dulcolax) suppositories.

10. Which of the following symptoms would be

considered normal if found while assessing Mrs. Romero?

☐ 1. Vaginal bleeding and 1 + albuminuria.
☐ 2. Oliguria and glycosuria.
☐ 3. In the urine, 1 + sugar and urinary frequency.
☐ 4. Swelling of the face and increased vaginal discharge.

Sharon Webb, age 24, is delighted with confirmation of her first pregnancy, since she and her husband of 2 years hope to have a large family. Initial assessments indicate she is in good health and eager to learn about her needs during pregnancy. Richard Webb participates in the discussion, emphasizing their desire to adapt their life-styles to promote the health of the baby.

11. Mrs. Webb has a history of 28-day, regular menstrual cycles. At which point in Mrs. Webb's cycle was the mature ovum released from the ovarian follicle?
☐ 1. On the first or second day.
☐ 2. On the tenth or eleventh day.
☐ 3. On the fourteenth or fifteenth day.
☐ 4. Release of the ovum is unpredictable.

12. The young expectant father asks about leisure activities he can enjoy with his wife during pregnancy. Which response by the nurse best indicates an understanding of the needs of the couple during pregnancy?
☐ 1. "Although she may tire easily, you can continue most activities you have enjoyed in the past."
☐ 2. "You should explore more sedentary recreation now, since active exercise needs to be limited."
☐ 3. "You may wish to continue with your hobbies, and allow your wife to enjoy leisure with her friends."
☐ 4. "This is a time to prepare yourselves for the role of new parents, rather than thinking of yourselves."

13. The nurse determines that Mrs. Webb is in her tenth week of gestation. Which of the following signs of pregnancy would the nurse expect to observe?
☐ 1. Breast tenderness.
☐ 2. Quickening.
☐ 3. Dyspnea.
☐ 4. Dependent edema.

14. The nurse instructs Mrs. Webb what to do if vaginal bleeding occurs. Which of the following actions indicates that she understands prenatal instructions?
☐ 1. She considers it normal, especially if bleeding occurs at the time of her usual period.
☐ 2. She records the date and amount of bleeding and reports it on her next visit.
☐ 3. She phones the physician to give duration and amount of bleeding.

☐ 4. She remains on complete bed rest until the bleeding ceases.

15. After two clinic visits, Mrs. Webb seems discouraged. She tells you, "I guess I am pleased to be pregnant, but these visits are so routine. It's hard for me to take time from work to sit in the waiting room for just a urine check and weigh-in." What teaching would be most emphasized with this client?
☐ 1. "Although pregnancy is normal, one must be prepared for any problems."
☐ 2. "These routine visits are essential to the fetus and to your health."
☐ 3. "Perhaps you might weigh yourself at home each week and call us."
☐ 4. "Have you considered resigning from your job at this time?"

16. In Mrs. Webb's fourth lunar month of pregnancy, the physician advises her to adjust her daily routine as a typist. The nurse discusses her activities in the office and the nature of her work. Which one of the following tasks needs to be modified for her to promote a healthy pregnancy?
☐ 1. Sitting in one position for 6 hours without a break.
☐ 2. Delivering messages to several adjacent departments each day.
☐ 3. Answering phones as relief for the receptionist 1 hour each day.
☐ 4. Filing vouchers for sales personnel for 2 hours daily.

17. Mrs. Webb calls the clinic to report that her younger sister has toxoplasmosis. In assessing the risk to Mrs. Webb, which factor is most critical?
☐ 1. There has been no direct contact with her sister in 5 days.
☐ 2. The client has a cat that recently gave birth to kittens.
☐ 3. Both wife and husband are strict vegetarians.
☐ 4. The client, at present, feels very well.

18. After a thorough assessment and lab work, it is determined that the client has no signs of toxoplasmosis. The physician is concerned about mild anemia, however, and asks the nurse to discuss dietary modifications with Mrs. Webb. Considering that she usually avoids meat and poultry, which foods would be included when planning a healthy daily diet?
☐ 1. Egg yolks and dried fruit.
☐ 2. Cereal and yellow vegetables.
☐ 3. Leafy green vegetables and oranges.
☐ 4. Fish and dairy products.

19. As the client approaches full term, the nurse discusses with Mr. and Mrs. Webb the antepartal classes they have attended. They tell the nurse of their participation in Lamaze classes with 10 other

couples. Which statement by this couple best indicates understanding of key concepts?

- ☐ 1. "Being well prepared will ensure delivery without anesthesia."
- ☐ 2. "Self-hypnosis is the key to pain-free birth."
- ☐ 3. "We will avoid all pain medication in labor."
- ☐ 4. "We plan to continue using a wall hanging for a focal point."

20. Mrs. Webb calls the prenatal clinic and states that she thinks she is in labor. Which of the following signs would indicate that she is in true labor?

- ☐ 1. Walking eases her contractions.
- ☐ 2. She has urinary frequency and urgency.
- ☐ 3. She thinks that the baby has dropped because she can breathe better.
- ☐ 4. Her contractions are increasing in frequency and duration.

One of the components of antepartal care is provision of childbirth education. The antepartal-care nurse is planning to conduct eight weekly classes for women in their third trimester.

21. What is the main objective of this program according to modern concepts of childbirth education in the United States?

- ☐ 1. A painless childbirth experience.
- ☐ 2. The participation of both parents in the birth process.
- ☐ 3. The elimination of medication in labor and delivery.
- ☐ 4. An emotionally satisfying birth experience.

22. During the first childbirth class, one of the participants states, "I cannot relax! Just thinking of going through labor makes me tense all over." Which response is most appropriate?

- ☐ 1. "Labor pains don't hurt as much as you have been led to believe. Childbirth can be a really enjoyable experience."
- ☐ 2. "Once you understand the importance of natural childbirth, you will begin to relax, and your fears will disappear."
- ☐ 3. "It is quite common for women to be anxious about labor and delivery. Women can learn to relax through education and physical training."
- ☐ 4. "Fear causes tension, which results in pain. When you learn about childbirth, your fear will be eliminated, and pain will not occur."

Claire Ostrow, a primigravida, has encouraged her husband to attend prenatal classes with her. Although he has two children from a previous marriage, he did not participate in classes. Now he is eager to learn and is enthusiastic when practicing breathing techniques. At the last class a film on childbirth is shown. After class the couple expresses concerns about the pain of labor and delivery.

23. It is recognized that the perception of pain during childbirth is influenced by many factors, including culture, education, and anxiety. How can the nurse best assess the level of pain experienced by the laboring client?

- ☐ 1. Analyze objective and subjective data.
- ☐ 2. Correlate dilatation and effacement with assessment.
- ☐ 3. Consider gravity and parity as a variable.
- ☐ 4. Use past experience as a guide to assessment of pain.

24. Two weeks later, Mrs. Ostrow begins labor, and the couple goes to the birthing center. Upon admission they seem very frightened. How would the nurse most effectively support the couple during early labor?

- ☐ 1. Give a condensed course in childbirth education.
- ☐ 2. Ask the couple what would help them at this time.
- ☐ 3. Demonstrate comfort measures the father may use.
- ☐ 4. Assure them that most first-time parents are nervous at this time.

25. As the nurse teaches this couple about the birth process, which of the following is most appropriate?

- ☐ 1. Assess present knowledge of couple.
- ☐ 2. Teach at learners' level of understanding.
- ☐ 3. Use a standard teaching plan.
- ☐ 4. Reinforce key concepts as necessary.

26. When she reaches transition, Mrs. Ostrow tells her husband to leave her alone. What is the best nursing action at this time?

- ☐ 1. Ask the father to leave the nurse and the client alone.
- ☐ 2. Urge the client to remain quiet at this time.
- ☐ 3. Explore their feelings for one another.
- ☐ 4. Accept this behavior as normal in this situation.

27. Sibling visitation is arranged for Mrs. Ostrow's stepchildren. Upon visiting the infant, the 2-year-old sister seems uninterested and asks to go home. The nursing student asks the nurse if this is related to the family situation. What explanation to the student would be most appropriate?

- ☐ 1. "The parents may not have prepared the child well."
- ☐ 2. "The 2-year-old probably resents the stepmother."
- ☐ 3. "The social worker should assess the family situation."
- ☐ 4. "This behavior is common for this child's developmental level."

28. Later that evening, the client is informed that her stepdaughter has a fever and a tentative diagnosis of rubella. What statement made by the mother best

indicates an understanding of the implications of this viral infection?

- ☐ 1. "I'll remind my mother to give her aspirin for the fever."
- ☐ 2. "My sister is 2 months pregnant; I'll ask her to stay away from our home."
- ☐ 3. "If our infant catches the infection, she won't need a vaccination."
- ☐ 4. "It's good that my husband and I both had German measles as children."

29. When counseling Mrs. Ostrow about the signs of ovulation, which of the following points is most appropriate to include in the discussion?

- ☐ 1. Ovulation comes predictably 14 days after onset of menses.
- ☐ 2. Lower abdominal pain may be experienced at the time of rupture of the follicle.
- ☐ 3. The cervical mucus becomes thick and sticky at ovulation.
- ☐ 4. A slight rise in temperature occurs before ovulation.

30. Mrs. Ostrow indicates that she understands the ovulation method correctly now and wonders if she should douche after intercourse for added precaution against pregnancy. How would the nurse respond to Mrs. Ostrow?

- ☐ 1. "I wouldn't recommend that. It would greatly increase your chances for a vaginal infection."
- ☐ 2. "That would be very helpful, since douching will wash the sperm from your vaginal canal."
- ☐ 3. "Douching is not an effective method of contraception and may even facilitate fertilization if a mature egg is available."
- ☐ 4. "That's a good idea, since failure rates with natural planning alone are quite high."

31. Mrs. Ostrow confides that her husband wants her to have a tubal ligation in the future. Which statement most indicates a *lack* of understanding of this type of contraception?

- ☐ 1. "I know it can be reversed later if I change my mind."
- ☐ 2. "He tells me it involves just a few days of hospitalization."
- ☐ 3. "My doctor says it is almost as safe as a vasectomy."
- ☐ 4. "It will remove all worry about pregnancy from our marriage."

A telephone call is received in the antepartal clinic from 18-year-old Susan Winter, who has recently been diagnosed as being approximately 10 weeks pregnant. The nurse is told by a sobbing Mrs. Winter, "I am losing my baby! I am bleeding uncontrollably."

32. Which one of the following would be the most appropriate initial nursing response?

- ☐ 1. "You must be quite upset right now. Why don't you come to the clinic immediately?"
- ☐ 2. "Go to bed immediately with your feet elevated. I will call for an ambulance."
- ☐ 3. "It is very common for women to have some bleeding during early pregnancy."
- ☐ 4. "Can you describe the bleeding to me and tell me when it first became apparent?"

33. When Mrs. Winter is seen by the physician in the emergency room, her cervix is found to be 2 cm dilated, and she is having moderate, bright-red vaginal bleeding. Which term best describes her condition?

- ☐ 1. Incomplete abortion.
- ☐ 2. Inevitable abortion.
- ☐ 3. Threatened abortion.
- ☐ 4. Missed abortion.

34. Mrs. Winter is admitted to the hospital. Her initial nursing management would include which of the following?

- ☐ 1. Examine all perineal pads for tissues and clots.
- ☐ 2. Place the bed in Trendelenburg's position.
- ☐ 3. Prepare her for a Shirodkar procedure.
- ☐ 4. Restrict all physical activity and fluid intake.

35. Mrs. Winter overhears the physician telling her roommate that she has had "a missed abortion." Mrs. Winter asks the nurse to explain what this means. Which response is most appropriate?

- ☐ 1. "It's another name for a miscarriage."
- ☐ 2. "The baby is deformed, resulting in an abortion".
- ☐ 3. "The baby is no longer alive and growing, but the body hasn't expelled it yet."
- ☐ 4. "There was no pregnancy; her body just responded as if there were."

James and Anne Collins have been trying to have a baby for 4 years. Mrs. Collins has been pregnant three times, but all three times she aborted between the third and fourth months. A medical diagnosis of incompetent cervical os was made.

36. Mrs. Collins is told that she will have McDonald's procedure when she gets pregnant again. She asks the nurse about the procedure. Which of the following statements best explains the procedure?

- ☐ 1. "It is a suture that is put around the cervix around 24 weeks' gestation."
- ☐ 2. "The suture around the cervix means that a cesarean section will be performed at term."
- ☐ 3. "The suture is temporary and will be removed at term. You may be able to have a vaginal delivery if all goes well."
- ☐ 4. "You will have to spend most of the pregnancy in bed, but the suture will enable you to carry the baby to term."

37. After McDonald's procedure is done, it will be especially important for Mrs. Collins to receive discharge instructions regarding which one of the following?
- ☐ 1. Abstinence from intercourse until after the suture is removed.
- ☐ 2. Recognition of the signs and symptoms of labor.
- ☐ 3. Avoidance of infection.
- ☐ 4. Monitoring of fetal activity.

Sara Burns, in her first trimester of pregnancy, is seen in the antepartal clinic. An ectopic pregnancy is suspected.

38. Which of the following symptoms would the nurse most likely expect to be present in an ectopic pregnancy?
- ☐ 1. Spotting and lower abdominal pain radiating to the shoulders.
- ☐ 2. Excruciating pelvic pain and an enlarged uterus.
- ☐ 3. Leukorrhea and an enlarged uterus.
- ☐ 4. Headache, profuse bleeding, and lower abdominal pain.

39. Which of the following factors is *not* considered a high-risk factor for ectopic pregnancy?
- ☐ 1. History of infertility.
- ☐ 2. History of pelvic inflammatory disease.
- ☐ 3. History of gonorrhea.
- ☐ 4. History of three consecutive spontaneous abortions.

40. The client with an ectopic pregnancy is a high-risk client. Which of the following reasons best accounts for this?
- ☐ 1. Surgery is required to treat this complication.
- ☐ 2. Hemorrhage is a major problem.
- ☐ 3. Removal of the fallopian tube may result in sterility.
- ☐ 4. The ovum may abort into the abdominal cavity.

Wi-Li Chin, who has completed 37 weeks of gestation, calls the clinic where she has been receiving antepartal care. She tells the nurse that there is a small amount of bright-red blood coming from her vagina, but that she has no pain.

41. Based on the information given, what would the nurse best conclude?
- ☐ 1. Lacerated vaginal mucosa.
- ☐ 2. Premature labor.
- ☐ 3. Abruptio placentae.
- ☐ 4. Placenta previa.

42. Mrs. Chin is hospitalized. Which of the following nursing actions is most important at this time?
- ☐ 1. Assess the degree of cervical dilatation.
- ☐ 2. Estimate amount of blood loss.
- ☐ 3. Take vital signs every 15 minutes.
- ☐ 4. Determine fetal scalp blood pH.

43. In caring for Mrs. Chin, the nurse would
- ☐ 1. Prepare for a vaginal examination.
- ☐ 2. Expect an emergency cesarean birth.
- ☐ 3. Keep her on bed rest.
- ☐ 4. Administer an enema.

44. Which of the following is most important for the nurse to teach Mrs. Chin?
- ☐ 1. Increase ambulation.
- ☐ 2. Decrease protein consumption.
- ☐ 3. Limit physical activity.
- ☐ 4. Avoid emotional upset.

45. Mrs. Chin tells the nurse that she was dancing the night before the bleeding began, and she feels responsible for her current condition. What would be the most appropriate response for the nurse?
- ☐ 1. "Don't feel guilty. It wasn't your fault."
- ☐ 2. "It's too late to change anything now."
- ☐ 3. "This was caused by an abnormal implantation of the placenta."
- ☐ 4. "No one knows why this happens."

Jayne Simmons, gravida 3, para 2, is admitted to the labor room in early labor. She has a history of precipitate deliveries and has had an elevated blood pressure since 28 weeks' gestation. She is leaking amniotic fluid and currently has a blood pressure of 150/100 mm Hg.

46. Mrs. Simmons begins to have a vaginal discharge of bright-red blood. The nurse recognizes that this could be related to placenta previa or to abruptio placentae. Which of the following predisposing factors to abruptio placentae does Mrs. Simmons have?
- ☐ 1. Chronic hypertension.
- ☐ 2. Pregnancy-induced hypertension.
- ☐ 3. Multiple pregnancy.
- ☐ 4. Rapid decrease in uterine volume.

47. To further assess Mrs. Simmons, which of the following would be done?
- ☐ 1. Monitor urine output by inserting a Foley catheter.
- ☐ 2. Do a vaginal examination to evaluate progression of labor.
- ☐ 3. Check her vital signs every 30 minutes.
- ☐ 4. Conduct an abdominal examination for signs of tenderness or rigidity.

48. In providing care for Mrs. Simmons, which of the following measures would be most appropriate for the situation and be of most benefit to the fetus?
- ☐ 1. Turn Mrs. Simmons.
- ☐ 2. Administer oxygen.
- ☐ 3. Estimate amount of blood loss.
- ☐ 4. Observe for changes in the pattern of uterine contractions.

49. The systemic effects of blood loss on both mother and fetus and the possibility of abruptio placentae are primary concerns when caring for Mrs. Simmons. What complication of abruptio placentae is of most concern?

☐ 1. Disseminated intravascular coagulation syndrome.

☐ 2. Pulmonary embolus.

☐ 3. Hypocalcemia.

☐ 4. Urinary tract infection.

50. Which of the following findings would indicate that Mrs. Simmons might be developing complications from an abruptio placentae?

☐ 1. Mrs. Simmons' temperature is 100° F (38.3° C).

☐ 2. Fluid-filled vesicles appear in the vaginal discharge.

☐ 3. A venipuncture site continues to bleed for 15 minutes.

☐ 4. Urinary output is approximately 50 ml/hr.

51. Mrs. Simmons' vaginal discharge begins showing meconium staining. What would be the most appropriate initial nursing action?

☐ 1. Begin preparing Mrs. Simmons for an emergency cesarean birth.

☐ 2. Contact the physician immediately to report fetal distress.

☐ 3. Record a careful description of the vaginal discharge and of Mrs. Simmons' vital signs.

☐ 4. Check fetal heart tones and apply an external fetal monitor, if it has not already been applied.

Harriet Morton, age 40, is hospitalized for severe pregnancy-induced hypertension (PIH). She is in her eighth month of pregnancy and has gained 66 pounds.

52. Which nursing action would occur first after Mrs. Morton has been admitted?

☐ 1. Start an IV for oxytocin administration.

☐ 2. Record baseline vital signs.

☐ 3. Administer antihypertensive drugs.

☐ 4. Call the lab to draw blood.

53. Which of the following nursing actions would reduce the possibility of a convulsion?

☐ 1. Keep the side rails padded and up.

☐ 2. Place the client in the room closest to the nurse's station.

☐ 3. Keep the room dimly lit.

☐ 4. Stay with the client at all times.

54. The main purpose of bed rest as a treatment for PIH is to

☐ 1. Reduce blood pressure by lowering body metabolism.

☐ 2. Conserve energy in view of the impending labor.

☐ 3. Lower the incidence of headaches.

☐ 4. Limit contact with other clients.

55. The nurse administers magnesium sulfate to Mrs. Morton. What medication would the nurse have available to counteract toxicity?

☐ 1. Sodium chloride.

☐ 2. Calcium gluconate.

☐ 3. Epinephrine (Adrenalin).

☐ 4. Sodium bicarbonate.

56. Mrs. Morton asks the nurse if the magnesium sulfate will affect her baby. What would be the best response?

☐ 1. "No, the placenta acts as a barrier to the medication."

☐ 2. "The doctor wouldn't order it if it would hurt the baby."

☐ 3. "It has a minor effect; however, the effects of a convulsion are much more severe."

☐ 4. "We don't know if this drug crosses the placental barrier."

Sally Dunsmore is a gravida 2, para 0, Class C diabetic. She is at 34 weeks' gestation. At her weekly prenatal visit, her physician decides to hospitalize her because her fasting blood glucose is 325. Mrs. Dunsmore's previous fasting blood glucose test results have all been within normal limits.

57. Which of the following is true regarding insulin needs during pregnancy?

☐ 1. Insulin needs during pregnancy will be essentially the same as before pregnancy, as long as the client maintains a well-balanced diet.

☐ 2. Insulin needs will vary throughout the pregnancy and will need to be watched closely. It is not possible to predict when insulin needs will be greatest.

☐ 3. With a proper balance of nutrition and exercise, the client may not need insulin during pregnancy, since the baby will be producing insulin, which will be available for the mother's body to use.

☐ 4. Insulin needs will vary throughout the pregnancy. Need is likely to decrease during the first trimester and then continue to increase throughout the remainder of the pregnancy.

58. Mrs. Dunsmore inquires about how her baby will be delivered. Which of the following is the best response?

☐ 1. "You will probably have either a cesarean section or have labor induced at about 37 weeks' gestation."

☐ 2. "You will probably have a cesarean section to decrease the stress of delivery on the baby."

☐ 3. "Your insulin needs will be carefully monitored; and, if they follow a normal pattern, your pregnancy will probably be allowed to progress to term with labor occurring naturally."

☐ 4. "Your pregnancy will be carefully monitored

with the best time for delivery chosen on the basis of your status and tests of placental function and fetal maturity."

59. Baby Boy Dunsmore weighs 9 pounds 6 ounces at birth. Which of the following characteristics would the nurse expect to find in this infant?
   ☐ 1. Postmature.
   ☐ 2. Active and alert.
   ☐ 3. Tremors.
   ☐ 4. Hypobilirubinemia.

60. When caring for Baby Dunsmore in the delivery room, what is the nurse's first priority?
   ☐ 1. Ensure proper identification.
   ☐ 2. Establish a warm environment.
   ☐ 3. Maintain a patent airway.
   ☐ 4. Facilitate parental bonding.

61. Which of the following is of high priority when caring for Baby Dunsmore in the nursery?
   ☐ 1. Maintain hydration.
   ☐ 2. Assess gestational age.
   ☐ 3. Initiate early feeding.
   ☐ 4. Monitor bilirubin levels.

62. Mrs. Dunsmore wants to breastfeed her baby. The nurse plans a response based on which of the following facts?
   ☐ 1. Insulin does not pass into breast milk.
   ☐ 2. Breastfeeding predisposes the mother to infection.
   ☐ 3. The breastfeeding mother has a markedly decreased caloric demand.
   ☐ 4. The infant of the diabetic mother is often hypoactive.

63. In preparing Mrs. Dunsmore for discharge, the nurse includes infant-care teaching. Which of the following is most important for this mother to know?
   ☐ 1. Although the baby has a problem, he is normal and should be treated like any infant.
   ☐ 2. Give the child 24 calories per ounce of formula to counteract hypoglycemia.
   ☐ 3. See a pediatrician regularly throughout infancy and childhood.
   ☐ 4. Feed the child skim milk to maintain weight in infancy.

Shelly and Mark Novak have been married for 5 years and have avoided pregnancy during that time on the advice of her physician. Mrs. Novak had corrective heart surgery as an infant, and there was fear that pregnancy might be unwise. After consultation with a cardiologist, the couple were advised that conception would be safe, and with regular care during the pregnancy, problems could be avoided. Mrs. Novak has visited the physician every 2 weeks and complies with dietary advice, and her blood pressure remains stable.

64. Which of the following would most likely indicate potential problems for a pregnant client with a history of heart disease?
   ☐ 1. Reduced tolerance of activity.
   ☐ 2. Polyhydramnios.
   ☐ 3. Frequent urinary tract infections.
   ☐ 4. Frequent heartburn.

65. Mrs. Novak delivers a healthy 7-pound son in a forceps-assisted delivery. Mother and infant remain in the recovery room for several hours for observation. The nurse notes that the mother's pulse rate is stable at 66. She received no medication other than oxytocin. What is the appropriate nursing action?
   ☐ 1. Notify the physician immediately.
   ☐ 2. Continue to assess vital signs routinely.
   ☐ 3. Observe for toxicity to oxytoxic drugs.
   ☐ 4. Monitor the level of consciousness.

66. In the first 48 hours postpartum, which physiological adaptation would increase stress on this mother's heart?
   ☐ 1. Moderate diaphoresis.
   ☐ 2. Release of prolactin.
   ☐ 3. Uterine contractions.
   ☐ 4. Increased blood volume.

Juanita Lopez, a 15-year-old gravida 1 para 0, registers for antepartal care at 10 weeks' gestation.

67. Which of the following is a priority for high-risk clients in a prenatal clinic?
   ☐ 1. Encourage regular prenatal care.
   ☐ 2. Encourage acceptance of the pregnancy.
   ☐ 3. Arrange for financial support.
   ☐ 4. Recommend genetic screening.

68. Juanita is facing the psychological task of accepting her pregnancy and "incorporating the fetus into her body image," as identified by Rubin. Which of the following behaviors best characterizes this?
   ☐ 1. Acknowledging the surprise she experiences at being in the pregnant state.
   ☐ 2. Planning for a Lamaze childbirth experience.
   ☐ 3. Arranging a baby nursery in the home.
   ☐ 4. Talking about the responsibilities of motherhood.

69. During the initial antepartal appointment, which of the following nursing actions would most encourage Juanita in developing a positive response to her new, changing physical status?
   ☐ 1. Discuss clients' rights and explain informed consent.
   ☐ 2. Provide a description of the scope of available services.
   ☐ 3. Stay with Juanita and listen to her concerns.
   ☐ 4. Reassure Juanita that many teenagers experience a temporary uneasiness at this time.

70. Basic nutritional counseling is an important component of Juanita's nursing care. Guidance in diet planning for pregnant teenagers differs from that of pregnant adults because of which basic consideration?
   1. The nutritional needs of pregnant women decline with advancing age.
   2. Metabolic alterations increase nutrient catabolism in pregnant adolescents.
   3. Postpubescent women have an increase in protein deposition.
   4. There is a pubertal acceleration in growth of pregnant adolescents.
71. Based upon the clinical findings of Juanita's examination at 32 weeks' gestation, it is determined that she has iron-deficiency anemia. Which one of these findings supports the diagnosis?
   1. Hemoglobin less than 10 g.
   2. Hematocrit less than 40%.
   3. Hemoglobin less than 14 g.
   4. Hematocrit less than 36%.
72. The increased demand for iron during pregnancy is most likely caused by
   1. A decrease in hematopoiesis occurring in the third trimester.
   2. The rise in hemoconcentration occurring between 24 and 32 weeks' gestation.
   3. An expansion in total blood cell volume and hemoglobin mass by approximately 25% to 50% during pregnancy.
   4. A decreased efficiency of iron absorption during pregnancy and fetal inability to absorb the mineral.
73. The nurse asks Juanita to select foods that best meet her dietary needs for increased iron. Juanita's knowledge of foods highest in iron would be accurate if she selected which of these meals for lunch?
   1. A peanut-butter–and–jelly sandwich, ½ cup cooked carrots, and 1 cup whole milk.
   2. An 8-ounce strawberry yogurt, one banana, and 1 cup apple juice.
   3. Enriched macaroni, broccoli, and 1 cup orange juice.
   4. One-half chicken breast, split peas, and 1 cup prune juice.

Donna Walsh, a 16-year-old primigravida, is completing 28 weeks' gestation. She has received no prenatal education and began receiving prenatal care only 2 weeks ago.

74. Which of the following best describes obstetrical hazards experienced by the pregnant adolescent?
   1. They have an increased mortality rate and an increased incidence of anemia, vaginitis, urinary tract infections, and pregnancy-induced hypertension.
   2. They have decreased cognitive development, have little emotional support available, and display childlike behaviors, which may cause conflict.
   3. They usually experience economic and social handicaps leading to an unsafe physical environment.
   4. They usually have low self-esteem; therefore, they have a decreased ability to establish meaningful relationships.
75. Donna reaches 40 weeks' gestation. She arrives at the hospital with complaints of uterine contractions crying, "It's time to have the baby." Which of the following nursing actions would be first?
   1. Assess her contractions.
   2. Take a nursing history.
   3. Call the physician.
   4. Start an IV.
76. Donna has received no childbirth preparation. When will she be most receptive to learning breathing techniques?
   1. Any time between contractions.
   2. During the contractions for simultaneous theory and practice.
   3. When her anxiety has been reduced.
   4. Early, when she is most alert and comfortable.
77. During a strong contraction, Donna's membranes rupture. What nursing assessment is most important at this time?
   1. Color of amniotic fluid.
   2. Extent of cervical dilatation.
   3. Change in baseline maternal vital signs.
   4. Donna's psychological response to this event.
78. Donna delivers a 5-pound daughter after a difficult labor. She was alone during labor. She has spoken to the social worker about adoption, but has not made a final decision. She asks few questions of the staff and sleeps most of the time. The labor room nurse visits to follow up on the care of the previous day. Donna seems eager to talk about what she should do with her baby. Which of the following statements made by the nurse is most appropriate?
   1. "Adoption is really the best solution to your situation."
   2. "It must be difficult to be in this position."
   3. "Was this pregnancy planned or unplanned?"
   4. "What would your parents like you to do?"
79. The nursing student expresses concern that the client continues to care for and feed the infant while remaining ambivalent about an adoption decision. On what knowledge would the nurse base a response to the student?
   1. Such behavior is typical of adolescence.

☐ 2. This care giving indicates guilt feelings.
☐ 3. Such actions contribute to a healthy grieving response.
☐ 4. Caring for the infant delays decision making.

80. Donna agrees to sign the papers for adoption. After Donna has been discharged, the adoptive parents and social worker visit the 5-day-old newborn in the nursery. Based upon an understanding of the process of attachment, what would the nurse teach the adoptive parents?
☐ 1. "Hold the infant and talk to her often."
☐ 2. "Sleep with the baby to enhance bonding."
☐ 3. "Learn basic infant care skills quickly."
☐ 4. "It is too late to attach, but you'll learn to care."

81. While dressing the infant, which observation by the adoptive father is the most positive sign of early parenting?
☐ 1. "Look at her watch me as I talk to her!"
☐ 2. "See how great this pink sweater looks on her!"
☐ 3. "Her eyes don't look much like anyone in the family."
☐ 4. "I read that hiccoughs are normal for a newborn."

Jan Rondinelli, a 26-year-old primigravida at 40 weeks' gestation, is admitted to the labor area. She has had no antepartal care. She is accompanied by her husband. Her membranes ruptured in the car on the way to the hospital.

82. Which of the following initial nursing assessments would be *least* important during her admission?
☐ 1. Type of anesthesia requested for delivery.
☐ 2. Location, rate, and rhythm of fetal heart tones.
☐ 3. Maternal vital signs.
☐ 4. Onset, duration, and frequency of contractions.

83. The admitting vaginal exam reveals that Mrs. Rondinelli's cervix is 6 cm dilated and 100% effaced. The fetus is at 1 + station and left occiput anterior. She is having difficulty coping with her contractions, which are occurring every 3 minutes. Which of these nursing actions is appropriate during her next contraction?
☐ 1. Encourage her to bear down with the contraction.
☐ 2. Check the perineum for crowning.
☐ 3. Provide direct coaching using chest-abdominal breathing techniques.
☐ 4. Show her husband how to apply firm pressure to her sacral area.

84. The nurse knows that Mrs. Rondinelli is in the transition phase of labor when she
☐ 1. Begins accelerated breathing.
☐ 2. Requests pain medication.
☐ 3. Becomes irritable and frightened.
☐ 4. Complains of rectal pressure.

85. Mrs. Rondinelli is in the transitional phase of labor.

Her contractions are lasting 75 seconds and occurring every 2 minutes. She begins to grunt and says she has to push. Upon vaginal exam, the nurse finds her cervix is dilated 9 cm. What is the most appropriate immediate nursing action?
☐ 1. Roll her on her side and tell her to breathe slowly.
☐ 2. Tell her to blow out until the urge passes.
☐ 3. Explain in careful detail that pushing will cause the cervix to swell and delay dilatation.
☐ 4. Tell her to push with each contraction.

86. Mrs. Rondinelli begins to show symptoms of hyperventilation with her rapid panting during contractions. The nurse instructs her to slow down her breathing and breathe into her cupped hands. Which of the following would best indicate effectiveness of this action?
☐ 1. Dizziness and finger tingling subside.
☐ 2. Nausea increases.
☐ 3. Amnesia between contractions lessens.
☐ 4. The urge to push subsides.

87. Mrs. Rondinelli has now progressed to full cervical dilatation and effacement without perineal bulging. The nurse would
☐ 1. Prep and drape her for delivery.
☐ 2. Coach her how to push effectively with contractions.
☐ 3. Provide privacy for her and her husband.
☐ 4. Administer a narcotic analgesic.

88. Mrs. Rondinelli has an uneventful vaginal delivery with a midline episiotomy done under local anesthesia. During the fourth stage of labor, the nurse would include which of the following in the nursing care plan?
☐ 1. Massage the fundus constantly.
☐ 2. Monitor temperature every 30 minutes.
☐ 3. Palpate the uterus to check muscle tone every 15 minutes.
☐ 4. Monitor blood pressure every 5 minutes.

89. Baby Girl Rondinelli weighed 6 pounds at birth and received routine care. Her eyes were treated prophylactically with 1% silver nitrate. This treatment is done to prevent
☐ 1. Chemical conjunctivitis.
☐ 2. Neonatal syphilis.
☐ 3. Herpes infection.
☐ 4. Ophthalmia neonatorum.

The professional nurse assigned to the labor and delivery unit of a hospital is required to manage care for a group of clients. The application of the nursing process in such a setting involves setting priorities as a part of decision making. The use of electronic fetal monitoring has enhanced the assessment of fetal response to labor, yet the nurse must constantly apply knowledge to interpret the tracings.

90. The nurse is going to care for Mrs. Sanchez, a multigravida, in the labor room. During an assessment the nurse notes a change in fetal-heart-rate variability on the monitor. Previous variability was 10 to 15 beats; it is now 2 to 3 beats over several minutes. Contractions are mild. What is the best analysis of these data?
   □ 1. The change is within normal limits.
   □ 2. There is indication of potential hypoxia.
   □ 3. Such variability is common in the fetus of a multigravida.
   □ 4. True variability can only be assessed with the external monitor.

91. The nurse sees that there are many variable decelerations on Mrs. Sanchez's fetal monitor strip. Variable decelerations most likely are due to
   □ 1. Head compression.
   □ 2. Cord compression.
   □ 3. Uteroplacental insufficiency.
   □ 4. Posterior presentation.

92. Which of the following readings would be considered a normal finding?
   □ 1. Late decelerations and good variability.
   □ 2. Early decelerations and no variability.
   □ 3. Early decelerations and good variability.
   □ 4. Variable decelerations and no variability.

93. After asking the physician to examine Mrs. Sanchez, the nurse is called to a second labor room. The expectant father has noticed that the fetal heart rate drops slightly just before his wife's contraction, then recovers at the end of the contraction. What is the most appropriate *initial* nursing action?
   □ 1. Assess maternal vital signs.
   □ 2. Administer oxygen.
   □ 3. Notify the physician.
   □ 4. Reassure him that this is normal.

94. The physician orders an internal electrode for Mrs. Sakolov. The nurse is asked to assist in placement of the scalp electrode. This technique
   □ 1. Is an invasive procedure.
   □ 2. Routinely follows amniotomy.
   □ 3. Is an extraordinary assessment.
   □ 4. Is risk free.

95. Mrs. Sakolov is in the second stage of labor. Which of the following patterns would necessitate immediate action?
   □ 1. Baseline fetal heart rate between 120 and 130.
   □ 2. Fetal heart rate that drops to 100 during contractions and returns to baseline when the contraction ends.
   □ 3. An increase in baseline fetal heart rate to 150 just before the contraction.
   □ 4. Fetal heart rate that drops to 120 during the contraction and returns to baseline 1 minute after the contraction ends.

96. The nursing student asks the nurse to check her client. "The baseline fetal heart rate has gradually decreased from 140 to 120. But I know that is within normal range," says the student. What is the appropriate nursing action?
   □ 1. Confirm that this is within a normal heart rate range.
   □ 2. Notify the physician immediately.
   □ 3. Elevate the foot of the bed in Trendelenburg's position.
   □ 4. Take the client's blood pressure and temperature.

97. Late decelerations are observed on the fetal heart rate monitor; what would the first nursing action be?
   □ 1. Turn off the oxytocin.
   □ 2. Change the client's position.
   □ 3. Administer oxygen.
   □ 4. Inform the physician.

Marianne Stoner, age 41, is admitted to the labor and delivery unit at 4 PM. While taking the history, the nurse notes the following: gravida 8, para 7; 41 weeks of completed gestation; membranes ruptured at 10 AM. that day; contractions occur every 3 minutes; strong intensity with a duration of 60 seconds.

98. What nursing action would take highest priority at this time?
   □ 1. Get blood and urine samples.
   □ 2. Do perineal prep and give enema.
   □ 3. Attach monitors to client.
   □ 4. Determine extent of cervical dilatation.

99. Mrs. Stoner has just been given an epidural anesthetic. What is the most important assessment at this time?
   □ 1. Maternal blood pressure.
   □ 2. Fetal heart rate.
   □ 3. Maternal level of consciousness.
   □ 4. Fetal position.

100. Mrs. Stoner has a normal spontaneous delivery. Why would she be considered at risk for development of postpartal hemorrhage?
   □ 1. Grand multiparity.
   □ 2. Premature rupture of membranes.
   □ 3. Postterm delivery.
   □ 4. Anesthesia.

101. Mrs. Stoner asks to be discharged after 24 hours, and her physician agrees. What is most important for the nurse to include in the discharge instructions?
   □ 1. Family planning information.
   □ 2. Newborn care information.
   □ 3. Need to have infant tested for phenylketonuria.
   □ 4. Referral to social service.

A nurse is summoned to the home of a neighbor, a multigravida, during a severe snowstorm. She appears to be in active labor. Both she and her husband are very apprehensive.

102. The initial nursing action would be to
- ☐ 1. Call the hospital for an ambulance.
- ☐ 2. Calm both parents.
- ☐ 3. Prepare a clean delivery field.
- ☐ 4. Assess the mother's status.

103. The assessment reveals the infant in a vertex presentation, crowning. As the nurse assists in the delivery of the head, which would be the most appropriate instruction to the mother?
- ☐ 1. Push during the contraction to aid in delivery.
- ☐ 2. Pant during contractions to avoid forceful expulsion.
- ☐ 3. Bear down continuously to assist the abdominal muscles.
- ☐ 4. Breathe slowly and deeply to ensure proper oxygenation of the fetus.

104. Before help arrives, it appears that the newly delivered mother is bleeding excessively. What nursing action is most appropriate at this time?
- ☐ 1. Put the infant to the breast.
- ☐ 2. Place sandbags on the fundus.
- ☐ 3. Pack the vagina with a towel.
- ☐ 4. Apply vigorous pressure to the uterus.

Tracy Stepanich is a primipara admitted for an elective cesarean delivery. Mrs. Stepanich crushed her pelvis in an automobile accident as a teenager. This pelvic damage led to an extremely narrow pelvic outlet, resulting in dystocia. The pregnancy has been normal.

105. Which of the following would *not* be included in preparation for the elective cesarean delivery?
- ☐ 1. Insert a Foley catheter.
- ☐ 2. Do an abdominal prep.
- ☐ 3. Ensure that blood has been typed and cross-matched.
- ☐ 4. Insert an internal fetal monitor.

106. Mrs. Stepanich asks what is the most common reason for a cesarean delivery. Which of the following is the best explanation?
- ☐ 1. Hemorrhage.
- ☐ 2. Toxemia.
- ☐ 3. Dysfunctional labor.
- ☐ 4. Cephalopelvic disproportion.

107. After the cesarean delivery, Mrs. Stepanich will need the usual postoperative care as well as the usual postpartum care. Which of the following is true in this regard?
- ☐ 1. Fundal height should not be checked because of the location of the abdominal incision.
- ☐ 2. Lochia flow will be checked less frequently since the uterus is cleansed more thoroughly during a cesarean delivery.
- ☐ 3. Perineal checks are less important since there should not have been any perineal trauma.
- ☐ 4. The surgical incision will not need to be checked

frequently since increased vascularity in the area will speed healing.

108. Mrs. Stepanich indicates she wants to breastfeed her newborn, but is uncertain if she can. The nurse's response would include which of the following?
- ☐ 1. Following a cesarean delivery, the mother's limited oral intake during the first 2 days will inhibit the production of milk.
- ☐ 2. She is likely to stay in the hospital for more than a week, but the baby does not need to stay this long.
- ☐ 3. Breastfeeding is not contraindicated by a surgical delivery.
- ☐ 4. The abdominal incision will make it very uncomfortable for her to breastfeed.

Judy Harris, age 31, gravida 2, para 1, delivered her first child by cesarean birth because the newborn was a footling breech. She is admitted for a planned, repeat cesarean delivery under regional anesthesia. During the initial assessment, she comments on the thrill she anticipates in watching the birth. Reviewing the prenatal record, the nurse notes that she kept her prenatal appointments.

109. Each of the following is noted on the chart. Which would be reported to the anesthesiologist before delivery?
- ☐ 1. Corrective surgery for scoliosis at age 14.
- ☐ 2. Trace of glucose in urine throughout pregnancy.
- ☐ 3. Hemoglobin 12 g; hematocrit 39%.
- ☐ 4. Acute episode of herpes type II before pregnancy.

110. The physician orders an IV of 5% dextrose in normal saline to be infused over 6 hours before surgery. The IV inadvertently infuses more rapidly than desired. What assessments are most essential when fluids are administered too rapidly?
- ☐ 1. Pulse and temperature.
- ☐ 2. Blood pressure and fetal heart rate.
- ☐ 3. Respirations and pulse rate.
- ☐ 4. Level of consciousness and hematocrit.

111. The cesarean delivery proceeds normally under general anesthesia, and a healthy 6-pound son is delivered. As Mrs. Harris recovers from surgery in the postanesthesia recovery unit, which of the following assessments is most significant?
- ☐ 1. Blood pressure is stable at 100/72 mm Hg.
- ☐ 2. Respirations are 32 and shallow.
- ☐ 3. Temperature is constant at 99.8° F (37.6° C) orally.
- ☐ 4. Pulse is 68 and regular.

112. On the second postoperative day, Mrs. Harris asks to have the infant room-in with her. In planning for her comfort and for the safety of the newborn, which nursing action is most appropriate?

☐ 1. Suggest she delay breastfeeding for several days.

☐ 2. Ask the father to room-in with mother and infant.

☐ 3. Inform her that the nurse is available to assist her.

☐ 4. Place the signal light near her chair.

113. One evening during visiting hours, Mrs. Harris tells the nurse that she is afraid her 3-year-old son will be jealous of the new baby. The nurse would suggest that the parents take which of the following actions?

☐ 1. "Ignore him; he will outgrow his jealousy."

☐ 2. "Tell your son that he will learn to love their new baby."

☐ 3. "Leave your son with his grandparents until the new baby is settled at home."

☐ 4. "Bring your son a baby doll or other toy at the time the baby is taken home."

114. The parents notice a dark pigmented area on their son's lower back and buttocks. Which notation on the chart will best explain this observation?

☐ 1. Positive rubella titer.

☐ 2. AB blood type.

☐ 3. Ethnic background: black.

☐ 4. Genetic screening positive for sickle-cell disease.

115. Both Mr. and Mrs. Harris are sickle-cell carriers. The mother asks the nurse about the probability of inheritance of sickle-cell disease. What response would be most appropriate to give?

☐ 1. "It is not possible to predict."

☐ 2. "There is a 25% probability."

☐ 3. "There is no risk with two carriers."

☐ 4. "Fifty percent of your offspring will have the disease."

116. On the third day, the nurse observes Mrs. Harris and the infant during feeding. The nurse notices that the infant nurses at the breast for a few minutes, then falls asleep. What other assessments are indicated?

☐ 1. Observe the sleep periods.

☐ 2. Note the mother's apprehension.

☐ 3. Record the intake and output.

☐ 4. Assess infant satisfaction.

Anna Wolinski had a low-segment cesarean delivery last evening for failure to progress in labor. It has been 12 hours since the operation. Mrs. Wolinski has an intravenous infusion with 1000 ml of 5% dextrose in water running at 150 ml/hr.

117. What primary advantage does the low-segment cesarean delivery have, compared with the classic cesarean delivery?

☐ 1. Easier delivery of a fetus in a transverse lie.

☐ 2. Greater safety for delivery with an anterior placenta previa.

☐ 3. Simpler procedure to perform operatively.

☐ 4. Lower incidence of postoperative infection and a smaller amount of blood loss.

118. Mrs. Wolinski had an intrathecal injection for anesthesia. To prevent the occurrence of a headache, what would the nurse do during the first 8 hours postoperatively?

☐ 1. Maintain an indwelling catheter.

☐ 2. Ambulate her progressively.

☐ 3. Administer analgesics and antiemetics.

☐ 4. Maintain bed rest in a recumbent position.

Inga Swenson, age 32, is admitted for induction of labor. It is estimated by ultrasound that the fetus is at 42 weeks' gestation. She is very impatient for the birth of this planned child. The physician elects to rupture the membranes artificially. Subsequently, fetal heartbeat is stable at 144. Amniotic fluid is clear.

119. As the nurse continues to care for Mrs. Swenson, she experiences sudden onset of dyspnea, cyanosis, and severe apprehension. This is followed by severe chest pain. Which of the following conditions is suggested by these data?

☐ 1. Acute myocardial infarction.

☐ 2. Pulmonary embolus.

☐ 3. Hysterical reaction.

☐ 4. Massive infection.

120. As Mr. Swenson watches, his wife is transferred to the intensive care unit (ICU). He remains in the waiting room, stunned. He refuses to talk to the resident and insists he will wait there for the safe delivery of his child. How could the nurse best meet his needs at this time?

☐ 1. Insist that he go to ICU.

☐ 2. Remain with him for the next few minutes.

☐ 3. Allow him privacy and leave him alone.

☐ 4. Ask the attending physician to see him later.

121. After 30 minutes, the husband joins his wife in the ICU. She is unresponsive. There is evidence of massive internal hemorrhage associated with disseminated intravascular coagulation. The physician orders immediate transfusions, but the husband refuses on religious grounds. Which action by the nurse is *least* appropriate at this time?

☐ 1. Call the clergyman to speak with the father.

☐ 2. Emphasize that religious values are not as important as saving lives.

☐ 3. Clarify the physician's explanation of the situation.

☐ 4. Ask the father if he wishes to consult with his family.

122. While awaiting a decision on the use of blood transfusions, the client's status is best evaluated by which of the following?

□   1. Level of consciousness.
□   2. Blood pressure and pulse.
□   3. Observation of bleeding.
□   4. Repeated hematocrit levels.

123. After discussion with clergy and physicians, Mr. Swenson agrees to life-saving measures and transfusions. However, the client does not respond to therapy, and both mother and fetus die. Which statement made to the distraught father by the nurse is most appropriate?
□   1. "I am so sorry."
□   2. "Try not to feel guilty."
□   3. "It must be very difficult for you."
□   4. "At least you have other children at home."

Suzanne Phillips is a 14-year-old, newly delivered primipara. She has just been admitted to her postpartum room after having been in the recovery room for 8 hours because of fluctuating blood pressure. She had a saddle block for delivery.

124. Suzanne has an IV infusing to which 10 ml of oxytocin (Pitocin) has been added. The rationale for administering oxytocin after delivery of the placenta is to
□   1. Shorten the third stage of labor.
□   2. Control postpartal bleeding.
□   3. Stabilize the mother's blood pressure.
□   4. Inhibit lactation in the bottle-feeding mother.

125. Suzanne states that her bladder feels full and that she needs to void but cannot. The nurse would
□   1. Walk her to the bathroom and encourage her to try to void.
□   2. Insert a Foley catheter to prevent postpartum cystitis.
□   3. Administer ergonovine maleate (Ergotrate) as ordered.
□   4. Place her on a bedpan, dabble her fingers in water, and run water in the bathroom loud enough for her to hear.

126. Suzanne begins to tremble and shake. She states she is cold and cannot control her shaking. Nursing actions would include which of the following?
□   1. Cover her with a warm blanket.
□   2. Notify the physician immediately.
□   3. Administer a tranquilizer.
□   4. Discontinue the IV (oxytocin).

127. Two days postpartum, Suzanne complains of perineal pain. Observing her midline episiotomy, the nurse sees that it is edematous but healing. Which of the following might help her?
□   1. Apply ice packs to the perineal area.
□   2. Encourage sitz baths as desired.
□   3. Administer chlorotrianisene (TACE) as ordered.
□   4. Encourage postpartal Kegel exercises.

Sally Noyamba is a primipara who is trying to breast-feed her infant for the first time.

128. Milk production after delivery is a direct result of
□   1. A decrease in estrogen and progesterone.
□   2. An increase in estrogen and progesterone.
□   3. A decrease in oxytocin.
□   4. An increase in prolactin.

129. Which of the following would be *least* helpful to Mrs. Noyamba?
□   1. Stimulate the infant to suck by rubbing her cheek on the side closest to the nipple.
□   2. Use nipple rolling to get the nipple erect.
□   3. Use a breast pump to bring the milk forward to the areola.
□   4. Place most of the areola in the infant's mouth.

130. After 3 days, Mrs. Noyamba asks which type of contraceptive is acceptable to use before her first postpartal check. The nurse would advise which of the following?
□   1. Birth control pills.
□   2. IUD.
□   3. Condoms.
□   4. Diaphragm and jelly.

131. Which of the following statements by Mrs. Noyamba would indicate that she may need more teaching before her discharge?
□   1. "I know how and when to bathe the infant."
□   2. "I know that if my lochia becomes bright-red I will need to rest and call my doctor."
□   3. "I need to increase my calorie intake by 500 calories."
□   4. "I plan on doing push-ups and sit-ups when I return home."

Sylvia Martino has just delivered a 10-pound girl.

132. In assessing Mrs. Martino immediately after delivery, which of the following would the nurse most likely find?
□   1. Fundus located halfway between the symphysis pubis and the umbilicus; lochia rubra.
□   2. Fundus displaced to the right and 3 cm above the umbilicus; lochia serosa.
□   3. Fundus located at the umbilicus; lochia rubra.
□   4. Fundus located halfway between the symphysis pubis and the umbilicus; lochia serosa.

133. Mrs. Martino is having vaginal bleeding of bright-red blood that is continuously trickling from the vagina. Her fundus is firm and in the midline. What is the most likely cause of this bleeding?
□   1. Lacerations.
□   2. Subinvolution.
□   3. Uterine atony.
□   4. Retained placental fragments.

134. Which of the following conditions predisposes a client to postpartal hemorrhage?

1. Twin pregnancy.
2. Breech presentation.
3. Premature rupture of membranes.
4. Cesarean birth.

135. Twenty-four hours later, Mrs. Martino has a temperature of 100° F (37.8° C) and has voided 2000 ml since delivery, and her skin is diaphoretic. Nursing actions would include which of the following?
   1. Notify the physician of the findings.
   2. Notify the nursery to feed the baby in the nursery, since the mother has a fever.
   3. Explain to Mrs. Martino that these symptoms are all very normal for a woman who has just delivered.
   4. Suspect a postpartal infection, and isolate mother and newborn.

136. Mrs. Martino's sister warns her to expect afterpains. The nurse's teaching is based on the knowledge that the most likely candidate for afterpains is the
   1. Primipara who is bottle feeding.
   2. Grand multipara who is breastfeeding twin boys.
   3. Primipara who delivers prematurely and who is pumping her breasts.
   4. Adolescent primipara who is breastfeeding.

137. Mrs. Martino is bottle feeding her baby and asks when she should expect her first menses. The appropriate response would be
   1. "It usually takes at least 3 months before menstruation resumes after delivery."
   2. "Because you aren't breastfeeding, it should occur in 4 to 6 weeks."
   3. "Two weeks is the average time for menses to return."
   4. "Ask your doctor. I'm sure that after doing a pelvic exam, she can tell you."

138. What modifications are made in formula to make it more comparable with breast milk?
   1. Water and simple carbohydrates are added.
   2. Simple carbohydrates are added.
   3. Water is added.
   4. Casein is added.

139. While attempting to diaper her baby, Mrs. Martino observes her infant crying. Her response is, "He can cry!" And with this, her eyes fill with tears. The tears shed by this mother are probably caused by
   1. Relief that the child could function normally.
   2. Fear that the child was sick.
   3. Concern that she was not handling the child correctly.
   4. Belief that the child did not like her.

Valerie Jackson, gravida 5 para 5, is in the fourth stage of labor after delivering a 9-pound 14-ounce baby. The nurse has been checking her blood pressure, pulse, fundus, lochia, and perineum every 15 minutes for the past 45 minutes. The blood pressure has remained stable at 114/60 mm Hg, pulse 76, respirations 12. Her uterus tends to become boggy between checks, but firms readily with manual massage. Lochia is moderate and rubra. As the nurse approaches for the fourth check, she notices some large new bloodstains on the top sheet. The nurse immediately removes the top sheet and blanket to discover Mrs. Jackson lying in a pool of blood that covers the Chux pad.

140. What would the nurse's first action be?
   1. Take her blood pressure.
   2. Start an IV.
   3. Give her oxygen through a mask at 7 L.
   4. Find and massage the uterus.

141. The most frequent cause of early postpartum hemorrhage and probably the cause of Mrs. Jackson's bleeding is uterine
   1. Atony.
   2. Inertia.
   3. Lacerations.
   4. Dystocia.

142. Mrs. Jackson has experienced a postpartal hemorrhage based upon her total blood loss in the first 24 hours. How much blood must be lost to be considered hemorrhage?
   1. 1000 ml.
   2. 800 ml.
   3. 500 ml.
   4. 300 ml.

143. Mrs. Jackson's hemoglobin is 8.5 g/dl, and her hematocrit is 25%. She has a further diagnosis of anemia secondary to postpartum hemorrhage. Which of the following would *not* be included in discharge planning and teaching?
   1. Eat a diet high in protein and iron-rich foods.
   2. Take ferrous sulfate tablets as ordered by the physician.
   3. Stop breastfeeding the infant until the anemia is gone.
   4. Expect to feel tired for possibly 2 to 4 months.

Rosita Javier, a 1-day postpartum primipara, is Rh negative and has delivered an Rh-positive, 7-pound daughter.

144. Mrs. Javier is to receive Rh_0 (D) immune globulin (RhoGAM). Which action is essential before administration?
   1. Determine if Mrs. Javier's Coombs' test results are negative.
   2. Reverify the baby's blood type.
   3. Assess the paternal Rh factor.
   4. Assess maternal temperature.

145. Which of the following best describes how RhoGAM acts in the maternal system?

☐ 1. RhoGAM attaches to maternal anti-Rh antibodies and directly destroys them.

☐ 2. RhoGAM suppresses the immunological production of maternal antibodies.

☐ 3. RhoGAM destroys fetal Rh-positive red blood cells in the maternal circulation before sensitization occurs.

☐ 4. RhoGAM prevents fetal-maternal bleeding episodes from occurring at the former placenta site.

146. Mrs. Javier asks if there is a danger of this problem occurring in future pregnancies. Which of these understandings about Rh factor is most important for the nurse to communicate to Mrs. Javier?

☐ 1. This administration of RhoGAM will provide lifelong immunity against fetal Rh disease.

☐ 2. If Mrs. Javier delivers another Rh-positive infant, she will require a subsequent dose of RhoGAM.

☐ 3. The protective antibodies formed during this pregnancy increase the risk of hemolytic disease in future infants.

☐ 4. It is safe to assume that future infants have a 50% chance of being Rh negative.

Mindy Lowell, age 21, is admitted in active labor. Prenatal history indicates she has taken heroin regularly during the past 3 years. Two months ago she attempted to change to methadone maintenance, but was not compliant in keeping appointments. Initial observations include jaundiced sclera and skin. Lab data confirm a diagnosis of hepatitis B secondary to substance abuse.

147. A priority of nursing care for this client focuses on

☐ 1. Maintaining strict enteric isolation.

☐ 2. Using mask, gown, and gloves during care.

☐ 3. Disposing of syringes and needles appropriately.

☐ 4. Taking no extraordinary precautions.

148. Following delivery of a 6-pound infant, the client is transferred to a medical unit and placed in isolation. Which of the following menus would meet Mrs. Lowell's needs as she recovers from hepatitis and adapts to the postpartal period?

☐ 1. Orange juice, eggs, wheat toast, and tea with sugar.

☐ 2. Grapefruit juice, prunes, eggs, and tea with honey.

☐ 3. Pineapple slices, sweet roll, bacon, and tea with cream.

☐ 4. Applesauce, pancakes, sausage, and tea with milk.

149. Which of the following signs observed in a newborn nursery would be indicative of withdrawal if the newborn is drug addicted?

☐ 1. Dyspnea, bradycardia, restlessness.

☐ 2. Hyperactivity, irritability, tremors.

☐ 3. Pallor, subnormal temperature, weak cry.

☐ 4. Petechiae, limpness, high-pitched cry.

150. Baby Boy Lowell is placed in the isolation nursery for observation for several days. The pediatrician administers hyperimmune gamma globulin to the infant and plans to discharge him to his grandmother. What assessment of the family system is most important at this time?

☐ 1. Does the grandmother express an interest in the client and infant?

☐ 2. Has the cause of substance abuse been identified for this client?

☐ 3. Is the infant's father involved in plans for care?

☐ 4. Does the home situation appear to be adequate and safe for the infant?

151. While in the newborn nursery, the most significant postnatal problem Baby Boy Lowell might experience is narcotic withdrawal. With heroin addiction, signs of withdrawal are most likely to

☐ 1. Appear within the first 4 hours after birth.

☐ 2. Occur 1 to 2 days after delivery.

☐ 3. Be delayed up to 5 days postnatally.

☐ 4. Be eliminated or greatly reduced if the newborn receives a narcotic antagonist such as naloxone immediately after delivery.

Amy Williams is a gravida 1 para 1, 3 weeks postpartum. She calls the postpartum unit with questions about breastfeeding while she has the flu. During the conversation, she tells the nurse her temperature is 103° F and that she has a persistent headache and feels exhausted.

152. Which of the following topics concerning possible mastitis would the nurse want to elicit more information about first?

☐ 1. Breast tenderness.

☐ 2. Quality of sleep pattern at night.

☐ 3. Character and amount of lochia.

☐ 4. Status of the baby.

153. Which of the following statements would *not* be included when counseling Mrs. Williams about her problem?

☐ 1. Take antibiotics and analgesics as ordered by the physician.

☐ 2. Wash the hands well before and after handling the breasts.

☐ 3. Breastfeeding will need to be discontinued indefinitely.

☐ 4. Apply heat locally, and wear a supportive bra to decrease discomfort.

154. Which of the following nursing actions would most likely prevent the problem?

☐ 1. Administer prophylactic antibiotics.

☐ 2. Decrease the frequency of nursing.

☐ 3. Encourage abrupt weaning.
☐ 4. Give prompt attention to cracked nipples.

Baby Speier is 3 hours old. As the nurse gives the initial bath, she conducts a physical assessment of the newborn.

155. In assessing Baby Speier's skin, which of the following observations would most likely require special attention?
☐ 1. Cyanosis of the hands and feet.
☐ 2. Vernix caseosa.
☐ 3. Harlequin sign.
☐ 4. Jaundice.

156. In comparing Baby Speier's head and chest measurements, which of the following observations would the nurse expect to find?
☐ 1. The chest circumference is approximately 1 inch smaller than the head circumference.
☐ 2. The chest circumference is approximately 1 inch larger than the head circumference.
☐ 3. The head and chest circumference are equal.
☐ 4. The chest circumference is approximately 3 inches smaller than the head circumference.

157. If one of the following were found on Baby Speier, which one would require special attention?
☐ 1. Erythema toxicum neonatorum.
☐ 2. "Stork-bite" marks.
☐ 3. Impetigo.
☐ 4. Mongolian spots.

158. The nurse assesses Baby Speier's eyes. Which condition, if found, would most likely require special attention?
☐ 1. Transient strabismus.
☐ 2. Subconjunctival hemorrhage.
☐ 3. Swelling and a watery discharge following administration of silver nitrate.
☐ 4. Opacity of a pupil.

159. The nurse assessing Baby Speier's trunk at birth makes the following observations. Which one would alert the nurse to carry out further assessment?
☐ 1. Breast engorgement.
☐ 2. Audible bowel sounds.
☐ 3. Palpable liver and kidneys.
☐ 4. Umbilical cord with one artery and one vein.

160. Which of the following assessments would the nurse report to the physician concerning Baby Speier's ears?
☐ 1. The upper part of the ears is on a plane with the angle of the eyes.
☐ 2. The ears are set low on the head.
☐ 3. Incurving of the pinna and instant recoil.
☐ 4. Responds to sound with a startle or blink.

Juan and Conchita Hernandez are proud parents of 3-day-old Feliz. They have planned to have this first child for the past several years. The nurse on the postpartum unit notices that they are very careful with Feliz and tend to handle him with much anxiety, but they are interested in getting acquainted with their son and initiating play activities.

161. Mrs. Hernandez asks the nurse when she can "play" with Feliz. Which reply represents an understanding of developmental needs in infancy?
☐ 1. "When do you think it would be appropriate?"
☐ 2. "After he receives his first immunizations from the physician."
☐ 3. "As soon as you feel comfortable with him, he is ready."
☐ 4. "Babies should not be played with during the first month because they require a great deal of uninterrupted sleep."

162. What is the newborn's visual capacity at birth?
☐ 1. Long-distance vision.
☐ 2. Short-distance fixation.
☐ 3. Convergence of the eyes.
☐ 4. Coordinated peripheral vision.

163. What are the most appropriate stimuli for the nurse to recommend for the first parent-child play activity?
☐ 1. Rattles and small stuffed toys.
☐ 2. Books and pictures.
☐ 3. Swings and cradles.
☐ 4. Human faces and black-and-white objects.

164. It would be most appropriate for the nurse to suggest the parents play with Feliz by which method?
☐ 1. Turning him from his abdomen to his back.
☐ 2. Moving his arms and legs through the range of motion.
☐ 3. Stroking him gently from head to toe.
☐ 4. Rocking him 3 to 4 hours during the day.

165. To check the palmar grasp reflex in the newborn, the nurse would implement which of the following actions?
☐ 1. Stroke either corner of the mouth.
☐ 2. Apply pressure to the ball of the foot at the base of the toes.
☐ 3. Rotate the head to one side and then the other.
☐ 4. Exert pressure on the palm at the base of the digits.

166. To elicit Moro's reflex, the nurse would implement which of the following actions?
☐ 1. Shake the infant rapidly from head to toe.
☐ 2. Hold the infant in both hands and lower both hands rapidly about an inch.
☐ 3. Place the infant in the prone position and observe posture.
☐ 4. Stroke the lateral plantar surface of the infant's foot.

Baby Girl Young is a 10-pound 2-ounce, 38-week-gestation infant of a diabetic mother. The Apgar scores

were 7 at 1 minute and 9 at 5 minutes. After spending some time with her mother in the recovery room, she is transferred to the nursery.

167. Which of the following problems would the nurse be most alert for in this infant?
   □ 1. Hypoglycemia.
   □ 2. Hyperglycemia.
   □ 3. Meconium aspiration.
   □ 4. Generalized sepsis.

168. Which of the following orders would be included when planning care for an infant of a diabetic mother?
   □ 1. Provide extra stimulation.
   □ 2. Use oil on the body after bathing.
   □ 3. Give early feeding of glucose water.
   □ 4. Start early infusion of insulin.

169. How would the nurse record information about this infant's gestational age?
   □ 1. Premature, large for gestational age.
   □ 2. Term, appropriate for gestational age.
   □ 3. Premature, appropriate for gestational age.
   □ 4. Term, large for gestational age.

170. Mrs. Young asks the nurse if her baby has diabetes. What would be the nurse's best response?
   □ 1. "No, we are giving your baby medication to prevent that from occurring."
   □ 2. "No; however, she will probably become diabetic sometime in childhood."
   □ 3. "No, there is no connection between your diabetes and your baby."
   □ 4. "No; however, you need to make regular visits to your pediatrician."

171. On the third day of life, Baby Girl Young acquires hyperbilirubinemia and is placed under phototherapy. Which of the following would *not* be included in the nurse's plan of care?
   □ 1. Cover her eyes with soft material.
   □ 2. Keep the infant covered and warm.
   □ 3. Give additional fluids.
   □ 4. Record the type and amount of stools.

Following morning report, the head nurse and the nursing instructor take a group of students on rounds to orient them to the newborn nursery.

172. Which of the following infants would be at *lowest* risk for hypoglycemia?
   □ 1. A 2-hour-old full-term neonate whose mother's blood-glucose level was 350 mg/dl during labor.
   □ 2. A large-for-gestational-age neonate 10 hours after birth whose Dextrostix test shows a reading of 60 mg/dl.
   □ 3. A 32-week-gestation neonate 5 hours after birth.
   □ 4. A small-for-gestational-age neonate 12 hours

after birth who is NPO because of respiratory distress.

173. Which of the following best indicates that a neonate with an infection is *not* fully recovered?
   □ 1. Respiratory rate of 65 at rest.
   □ 2. Weight increase of 3 ounces on 2 successive days.
   □ 3. Axillary temperature of 98.6° F (37° C).
   □ 4. Hemoglobin of 20 g/dl of blood.

174. The mother of a boy born 2 days ago is refusing to care for her infant. Which of the following is the most appropriate action for the nurse to take?
   □ 1. Care for the infant in the mother's room without making any demands on the mother.
   □ 2. Encourage the mother to at least change the baby's diaper.
   □ 3. Speak to the baby's father and encourage him to get the mother to care for the infant.
   □ 4. Explain to the mother that corrective surgery will improve the infant's appearance.

175. A 34-week-gestation neonate in an incubator experiences sudden apnea. The nurse would first
   □ 1. Administer oxygen with positive pressure.
   □ 2. Call the pediatrician.
   □ 3. Increase the humidity in the incubator.
   □ 4. Gently shake the infant.

176. When examining the inside of a newborn's mouth, the nurse notices a small, raised white bump on the palate; it does not come off nor does it bleed when touched. Which of the following is the most likely diagnosis?
   □ 1. Milia.
   □ 2. Thrush.
   □ 3. Epstein's pearls.
   □ 4. Milk curd.

177. Which of the following fetal circulatory structures are *not* needed for extrauterine life?
   □ 1. Ductus arteriosus, foramen ovale, pulmonary artery, and hypogastric arteries.
   □ 2. Ductus venosus, foramen ovale, portal vein, and ductus arteriosus.
   □ 3. Foramen ovale, pulmonary artery, ductus venosus, and umbilical vein.
   □ 4. Umbilical vein, foramen ovale, ductus venosus, and ductus arteriosus.

178. Neonates often "spit up" small quantities following feedings. Which of the following conditions offers the best explanation for this behavior?
   □ 1. Immature cardiac sphincter.
   □ 2. Overfeeding by parents.
   □ 3. Activity of the infant during feeding.
   □ 4. Inadequate concentration of enzymes.

179. Which of the following skull bones form the posterior fontanel?
   □ 1. Frontal and parietal.
   □ 2. Parietal and occipital.

☐ 3. Temporal and frontal.

☐ 4. Frontal and occipital.

180. How might the nurse best promote bonding while an infant is in an Isolette?

☐ 1. Remind the mother that the staff is skillful.

☐ 2. Allow the mother to touch the infant.

☐ 3. Suggest the mother visit the intensive care unit occasionally.

☐ 4. Inform the mother that the infant will be at home soon.

References

Bobak, I., Jensen, M., & Zalar, M. (1989). *Maternity and gynecologic care*. St. Louis: Mosby–Year Book.

Olds, S., London, M., & Ladewig, P. (1986). *Maternal-newborn nursing*. Menlo Park, CA: Addison-Wesley.

Reeder, S., & Martin, L. (1987). *Maternity nursing* (16th ed). Philadelphia: Lippincott.

Whaley, L., & Wong, D. (1991). *Nursing care of infants and children* (4th ed.). St. Louis: Mosby–Year Book.

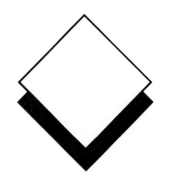

Correct Answers

1. no. 4.	**41.** no. 4.	**81.** no. 1.	**121.** no. 2.
2. no. 2.	**42.** no. 2.	**82.** no. 1.	**122.** no. 4.
3. no. 3.	**43.** no. 3.	**83.** no. 3.	**123.** no. 1.
4. no. 3.	**44.** no. 3.	**84.** no. 4.	**124.** no. 2.
5. no. 3.	**45.** no. 3.	**85.** no. 2.	**125.** no. 4.
6. no. 1.	**46.** no. 2.	**86.** no. 1.	**126.** no. 1.
7. no. 3.	**47.** no. 4.	**87.** no. 2.	**127.** no. 2.
8. no. 3.	**48.** no. 2.	**88.** no. 3.	**128.** no. 4.
9. no. 2.	**49.** no. 1.	**89.** no. 4.	**129.** no. 3.
10. no. 3.	**50.** no. 3.	**90.** no. 2.	**130.** no. 3.
11. no. 3.	**51.** no. 4.	**91.** no. 2.	**131.** no. 4.
12. no. 1.	**52.** no. 2.	**92.** no. 3.	**132.** no. 1.
13. no. 1.	**53.** no. 3.	**93.** no. 4.	**133.** no. 1.
14. no. 3.	**54.** no. 1.	**94.** no. 1.	**134.** no. 1.
15. no. 2.	**55.** no. 2.	**95.** no. 4.	**135.** no. 3.
16. no. 1.	**56.** no. 3.	**96.** no. 2.	**136.** no. 2.
17. no. 2.	**57.** no. 4.	**97.** no. 1.	**137.** no. 2.
18. no. 1.	**58.** no. 4.	**98.** no. 4.	**138.** no. 1.
19. no. 4.	**59.** no. 3.	**99.** no. 1.	**139.** no. 1.
20. no. 4.	**60.** no. 3.	**100.** no. 1.	**140.** no. 4.
21. no. 4.	**61.** no. 4.	**101.** no. 3.	**141.** no. 1.
22. no. 3.	**62.** no. 1.	**102.** no. 4.	**142.** no. 3.
23. no. 1.	**63.** no. 3.	**103.** no. 2.	**143.** no. 3.
24. no. 3.	**64.** no. 1.	**104.** no. 1.	**144.** no. 1.
25. no. 1.	**65.** no. 2.	**105.** no. 4.	**145.** no. 3.
26. no. 4.	**66.** no. 4.	**106.** no. 4.	**146.** no. 2.
27. no. 4.	**67.** no. 1.	**107.** no. 3.	**147.** no. 3.
28. no. 2.	**68.** no. 1.	**108.** no. 3.	**148.** no. 2.
29. no. 2.	**69.** no. 3.	**109.** no. 1.	**149.** no. 2.
30. no. 3.	**70.** no. 4.	**110.** no. 3.	**150.** no. 4.
31. no. 1.	**71.** no. 1.	**111.** no. 2.	**151.** no. 2.
32. no. 4.	**72.** no. 3.	**112.** no. 3.	**152.** no. 1.
33. no. 2.	**73.** no. 4.	**113.** no. 4.	**153.** no. 3.
34. no. 1.	**74.** no. 1.	**114.** no. 3.	**154.** no. 4.
35. no. 3.	**75.** no. 1.	**115.** no. 2.	**155.** no. 4.
36. no. 3.	**76.** no. 4.	**116.** no. 4.	**156.** no. 1.
37. no. 2.	**77.** no. 1.	**117.** no. 4.	**157.** no. 3.
38. no. 1.	**78.** no. 2.	**118.** no. 4.	**158.** no. 4.
39. no. 4.	**79.** no. 3.	**119.** no. 2.	**159.** no. 4.
40. no. 2.	**80.** no. 1.	**120.** no. 2.	**160.** no. 2.

161. no. 3.

162. no. 2.

163. no. 4.

164. no. 3.

165. no. 4.

166. no. 2.

167. no. 1.

168. no. 3.

169. no. 4.

170. no. 4.

171. no. 2.

172. no. 2.

173. no. 1.

174. no. 1.

175. no. 4.

176. no. 3.

177. no. 4.

178. no. 1.

179. no. 2.

180. no. 2.

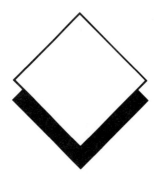

Correct Answers with Rationales

KEY TO ABBREVIATIONS
Section of the Review Book

CBF = Childbearing Family
  W = Women's Health Care
  A = Antepartal Care
  I = Intrapartal Care
  P = Postpartal Care
  N = Newborn Care

Nursing process category

AS = Assessment
AN = Analysis
PL = Plan
IM = Implementation
EV = Evaluation

Client need category

E = Safe, Effective Care Environment
PS = Physiological Integrity
PC = Psychosocial Integrity
H = Health Promotion and Maintenance

1. no. 4. Goodell's sign is the only probable sign; the other choices are presumptive signs. CBF/A, AS, PS
2. no. 2. Add 7 days, subtract 3 months, and add 1 year to the first day of the last menstrual period. This is Nägele's rule, which relates only to the first day of the menstrual cycle. There is no need for the client to consider the day of intercourse. CBF/A, AN, PS
3. no. 3. This is the only correct statement. HCG in the urine confirms the pregnancy. The urine test is 95% to 97% accurate. False positives and negatives are possible. Home tests are considered less accurate, most likely because of error in use. CBF/A, AN, PS
4. no. 3. The nurse must find out the eating habits of the pregnant client before she can teach or advise her. A basic principle of the teaching-learning process is to access the learner by obtaining a diet history. If the learner is knowledgeable, she simply may require reinforcement. Providing a list of foods does not ensure that she will comply with the suggested diet. Sodium is not restricted in pregnancy. CBF/A, IM, H
5. no. 3. Organ meats and dried fruits are high in iron. Spinach is also a good source, but option no. 3 lists two good sources. CBF/A, IM, H
6. no. 1. Swelling of the face is an indication of pre-eclampsia. The other symptoms are normal in pregnancy. Frequent urination is common in the first trimester because of pressure on the bladder from the uterus. Increased vaginal discharge is the result of an increase in glandular activity. Chloasma (also called the mask of pregnancy) results from an increased activity in the adrenal glands. CBF/A, IM, PS
7. no. 3. Slight temporary enlargement of the breasts may cause sensations of weight and tingling. As pregnancy advances, the areolas become darker in color. Colostrum, which is a precursor of breast milk, may appear spontaneously in the second half of pregnancy. Engorgement occurs after delivery when the mother's breasts begin to fill with milk. CBF/A, AS, PS
8. no. 3. There is a placental barrier to syphilis until the 18th week of pregnancy. If the mother is treated before the 18th week, the baby will not be affected.

However, titers will be positive at birth. CBF/A, AN, PS

9. no. 2. Bulk and fluid help increase peristalsis. Laxatives and suppositories should not be used in pregnancy. Prevention is more desirable than treatment. CBF/A, IM, PS

10. no. 3. Urinary frequency and the spilling of sugar in the urine are normal conditions, because of the pressure of the growing uterus on the bladder (frequency) and the increase in glomerular filtration rate (sugar in urine). Vaginal bleeding may indicate the possibility of an abortion. Albuminuria and facial swelling are associated with toxemia. Oliguria would indicate renal failure. CBF/A, AS, PS

11. no. 3. Ovulation occurs 14 days before the start of the next menstrual cycle. CBF/A, AN, PS

12. no. 1. The couple needs to continue to enjoy recreation together, and most activities can be continued during pregnancy. New sports should not be introduced at this time. CBF/A, IM, H

13. no. 1. Breast changes are expected to appear during the first trimester. Quickening, the feeling of movement experienced by the mother, occurs at 18 to 20 weeks' gestation. Dyspnea, caused by pressure on the enlarging uterus on the diaphragm, and dependent edema, caused by the enlarging uterus impeding venous return, are expected in the third trimester. CBF/A, AS, PS

14. no. 3. This may be a sign of threatened abortion. Remaining on bed rest is appropriate after the client's condition is assessed. CBF/A, EV, H

15. no. 2. Emphasis during antepartal care is on health promotion and early detection of problems. This option suggests a more positive approach than option no. 1. CBF/A, IM, PC

16. no. 1. To promote comfort and enhance venous circulation, she must change position more frequently than once every 6 hours. The other activities described are not a problem. CBF/A, AS, E

17. no. 2. Toxoplasmosis is a protozoan infection transmitted through cat feces and undercooked meat. However, the risk to this client is lower because she is in her second trimester. CBF/A, EAS

18. no. 1. Both of these foods are good sources of iron for the vegetarian. CBF/A, IM, H

19. no. 4. The chief concepts of Lamaze teaching include conditioned responses to stimuli through use of a focal point. An emotionally satisfying experience is promoted rather than discouraging use of analgesia and anesthesia. CBF/A, EV, H

20. no. 4. This is the only characteristic of true labor. Option no. 1 indicates false labor; options no. 2 and no. 3 are premonitory signs of labor. Walking has a tendency to increase true labor contractions. Urinary frequency is experienced after lightening or dropping of the fetus and is caused by uterine pressure on the bladder. Lightening occurs at approximately 38 weeks' gestation in the primipara. CBF/I, AS, PS

21. no. 4. Education for childbirth classes is designed to increase the clients' understanding of pregnancy and birth, and to promote the optimum health of mother and baby. Through use of relaxation and other techniques, pregnant women are helped to cope better with labor and achieve an emotionally satisfying experience. CBF/A, PL, H

22. no. 3. Fear is a major pain-producing agent in labor. Through childbirth education, pregnant women learn techniques to assist in relaxing and preventing the fear-anxiety-pain syndrome. Pain is subjective. Understanding alone will not produce relaxation, nor will education alone eliminate pain. CBF/A, IM, PC

23. no. 1. Although all responses are valid, option no. 1 is the best because it includes all possible assessments (i.e., what the client describes and physical and psychological changes). CBF/I, AS, PS

24. no. 3. Involve the father as much as possible by demonstrating comfort measures he can provide. If the couple is very frightened, attention span is reduced, and an explanation would not be effective. The couple that is not coping because of fear would be unable to verbalize their needs. CBF/I, IM, E

25. no. 1. Assessment of the learners is the priority. Teaching can then be directed at the learners' level of understanding and key concepts reinforced. A standard teaching plan is not appropriate. CBF/I, IM, E

26. no. 4. As transitional labor approaches, such behavior is very common. It is not appropriate to ask the husband to leave or withdraw his support at this most crucial time. A woman in transition is not able to explore feelings. CBF/I, IM, PC

27. no. 4. Sibling rivalry is normal. Grasping the reality of a new sibling is difficult for a child at this age. CBF/P, AN, PC

28. no. 2. Any woman in the first trimester of pregnancy is at risk if exposed to rubella. Fetal defects often result from such an infection. CBF/A, EV, PS

29. no. 2. "Mittelschmertz" may be experienced at the time of ovulation. Ovulation occurs approximately 14 days before the onset of menstruation. The cervical mucus becomes thicker following ovulation. A temperature rise follows ovulation. CBF/A, IM, H

30. no. 3. Douching is an ineffective method of contraception and may even facilitate conception by forcing sperm higher up into the female genital tract. CBF/A, IM, H

31. no. 1. Although it is possible to reverse a tubal ligation in some cases (a 12% success rate), it is

generally considered to be permanent sterilization. The other options are true. CBF/A, EV, E

32. no. 4. Bleeding during pregnancy is considered abnormal, but clients often overestimate the quantity of blood loss because of fear and lack of knowledge. As an initial response, the nurse should expand her data base by obtaining more specific information about the bleeding episode. Following complete assessment, a plan of care can be developed. CBF/A, IM, PS

33. no. 2. In an incomplete abortion the fetus is expelled, but parts are retained. The term inevitable abortion is used to describe pregnancies complicated by bleeding, cramping, and cervical dilatation (abortion is imminent). The term threatened abortion implies the pregnancy is jeopardized by bleeding and cramping, but the cervix is closed. In a missed abortion the fetus dies but is retained. CBF/A, AN, PS

34. no. 1. Because abortion is inevitable, all perineal pads must be inspected for the products of conception. Fluid replacement is necessary because of blood loss. There is no evidence of impending shock necessitating Trendelenburg's position. A Shirodkar procedure is done for an incompetent cervix, which is not the problem. CBF/A, IM, PS

35. no. 3. This is the definition of a missed abortion. Findings in a missed abortion include spotting and a uterus that is smaller than expected for the length of pregnancy. If spontaneous evacuation of the uterus does not occur within 1 month, a suction evacuation or D&C will be done to remove the products of conception. CBF/A, IM, H

36. no. 3. McDonald's procedure is application of a temporary suture at 14 to 18 weeks' gestation. The suture is removed at term. Vaginal delivery may be possible if all else stays well. Shirodkar's procedure is the application of a permanent suture necessitating cesarean delivery. CBF/A, IM, E

37. no. 2. A woman with a suture in place for incompetent cervix must especially be aware of the signs and symptoms of labor. When labor begins, the physician will remove the suture to avoid possible complications. CBF/A, IM, PS

38. no. 1. These findings are consistent with an ectopic pregnancy. The referred pain is the result of bleeding into the peritoneal cavity and overstimulation of the vagus nerve. Vaginal bleeding is not evident, nor is the uterus enlarged because the pregnancy is not implanted in the uterus. CBF/A, AS, PS

39. no. 4. A history of repeated spontaneous abortions is consistent with a diagnosis of an incompetent cervix. A history of infection, producing tubal scarring, is a consistent finding in an ectopic pregnancy. CBF/A, AS, PS

40. no. 2. Surgical intervention will be required; however, hemorrhage is the major life-threatening concern. If the tube ruptures in ectopic pregnancy, vascular collapse and hypovolemic shock may follow. The possibility of the ovum aborting into the abdominal cavity with a resulting abdominal pregnancy is rare. CBF/A, AN, PS

41. no. 4. Painless uterine bleeding occurring in the third trimester is a cardinal sign of placenta previa. CBF/A, AN, PS

42. no. 2. Persistent vaginal bleeding may seriously threaten the mother. Monitoring vital signs and fetal heart tones is important; however, significant changes may not occur until profound bleeding is present. Vaginal examination to assess cervical dilatation is never done when the woman presents with vaginal bleeding until the position of the placenta has been determined. CBF/A, IM, PS

43. no. 3. Because symptoms suggest a possible placenta previa, bed rest might help prevent further separation. Options no. 1 and no. 2 will cause further bleeding. Since she is in her eighth month and only bleeding a small amount, this client will most probably be kept under observation. CBF/A, IM, E

44. no. 3. Physical activity may increase bleeding. Decreasing anxiety is advisable, but bed rest is essential to limit the chances of her condition worsening. CBF/A, IM, E

45. no. 3. Location of the placenta and dilatation of the cervix are the causes of bleeding, and the condition cannot be prevented. Giving specifics is more useful than general reassurance. Options no. 2 and no. 4 imply that the client may have played a role. CBF/A, IM, PC

46. no. 2. Although all the factors listed are predisposing factors associated with abruptio placentae, Mrs. Simmons' history supports only pregnancy-induced hypertension, which occurs after 24 weeks. Vasoconstriction in the placenta causes placental separation. CBF/A, AS, PS

47. no. 4. Abdominal tenderness or rigidity or both are cardinal signs of abruptio placentae. A vaginal exam is definitely contraindicated. Options no. 1 and no. 3 are not specific for abruptio placentae. CBF/A, AS, PS

48. no. 2. The primary purpose of administering oxygen in this situation would be to increase the circulating oxygen in the mother to provide better oxygenation of the fetus. CBF/I, IM, E

49. no. 1. The hemorrhaging associated with abruptio placentae may deplete the woman's reserve of blood fibrinogen in the body's efforts to achieve clotting. Disseminated intravascular coagulation syndrome occurs when fibrinogen levels have been depleted. CBF/A, AN, PS

50. no. 3. Women with abruptio placentae are at risk for developing disseminated intravascular coagulation (DIC). DIC is an abnormal overstimulation of the coagulation process that ultimately leaves the woman with poorly clotting blood. Delayed clot formation at a venipuncture site is one manifestation of this condition. Fluid-filled vesicles passed vaginally are diagnostic of hydatidiform mole. The temperature and urine output given is in the normal range. CBF/I, AN, PS

51. no. 4. Meconium-stained fluid requires further assessment but is not necessarily an indication for emergency action. CBF/I, IM, PS

52. no. 2. Blood pressure should be monitored frequently in order to detect problems. Assessment of the client is a priority before designing a plan of care. CBF/A, IM, PS

53. no. 3. A loud noise or bright light may be enough to precipitate a convulsion because of the hyperactive nervous system. Keeping the side rails padded and up will protect the client, and careful monitoring of the client is in order; however, neither of these measures will reduce the possibility of convulsions. CBF/A, IM, E

54. no. 1. The client on bed rest has decreased physical activity and a reduced metabolic rate. There is also an increase in renal filtration rate. All of these physiological adaptations may improve circulation to the uteroplacental unit. CBF/A, PL, E

55. no. 2. Keep an ampule of calcium gluconate available when magnesium sulfate is being administered. CBF/A, AN, PS

56. no. 3. Magnesium sulfate is an excellent anticonvulsant and vasodilator that lowers blood pressure. Therapeutic doses of this drug are generally well tolerated by the fetus, although some respiratory depression may result. Option no. 2 does not answer the client's question. CBF/A, IM, PS

57. no. 4. Insulin needs do vary throughout pregnancy. The greatest incidence of insulin coma during pregnancy occurs during the second and third months; the greatest incidence of diabetic coma during pregnancy occurs around the sixth month. CBF/A, AN, PS

58. no. 4. Although a cesarean delivery at 37 weeks' gestation used to be common for diabetic mothers, current practice is to try achieving delivery at the optimum time for mother and infant. Stress for the infant is greater during a cesarean birth than during a vaginal delivery. Tests of placental function and of fetal maturity help determine the prognosis of the fetus at any given time. CBF/A, IM, E

59. no. 3. Newborn infants of diabetic mothers tend to be immature, lethargic, and hyperbilirubinemic and tend to have latent tetany, tremors, or neuromus-

cular irritability. These problems can be attributed to early delivery, hypoglycemia, and hypocalcemia. CBF/N, AS, PS

60. no. 3. Although all are correct, the priority is establishing and maintaining a patent airway. CBF/N, PL, E

61. no. 4. Excessive insulin may lead to hypoglycemia. Brain damage will result if not corrected. CBF/N, PL, E

62. no. 1. Because insulin does not pass into the breast milk, breastfeeding is not contraindicated for the mother with diabetes. Breastfeeding is encouraged because it decreases the insulin requirements for insulin-dependent clients. CBF/N, AN, PS

63. no. 3. This infant has the usual risk related to heredity for diabetes and should be seen regularly during childhood. CBF/N, IM, H

64. no. 1. Reduced activity tolerance is differentiated from the normal fatigue of pregnancy; it may be an early sign of congestive heart failure, a condition to which the cardiac client is highly predisposed. CBF/A, AS, PS

65. no. 2. This is a normal pulse rate for a newly delivered mother; continued routine assessments are all that is indicated. CBF/P, IM, PS

66. no. 4. A reduction in the pressure on the venous system allows fluid to move from the extravascular spaces into the bloodstream. This increased blood volume requires increased cardiac output. This is a normal adaptation for all new mothers, but could pose a risk after delivery for the woman with a cardiac problem. CBF/P, AN, PS

67. no. 1. Outcomes for the high-risk client and infant can be improved with regular prenatal care. CBF/A, PL, E

68. no. 1. During the first half of pregnancy, women question the reality of their condition and are often disbelieving. This may be expressed by "Now?", "Who, me?", or other statements of surprise. CBF/A, AS, PC

69. no. 3. It is most important for the nurse initially to establish rapport with the client by demonstrating a concerned and accepting attitude. CBF/A, IM, PC

70. no. 4. Adolescence is a time of great physical growth and development; to meet these needs as well as pregnancy needs, substantial nutritional intake is required. CBF/A, AN, PS

71. no. 1. The diagnosis of iron-deficiency anemia is made on the basis of a hemoglobin concentration value of 10 g/dl blood or less and a hematocrit value of 30% or less. CBF/A, AS, PS

72. no. 3. To meet increased circulatory needs, especially to the mother, fetus, and placenta, the blood volume increases starting at about 3 months' gestation. Beginning at about 6 months' gestation, the

total red blood cell volume and hemoglobin mass increase. CBF/A, AN, PS

73. no. 4. The iron content of prune juice is 10.5 mg/cup, and the iron content of split peas is 4.2 mg/cup; ½ breast of chicken contains 1.3 mg of iron. CBF/A, EV, PS

74. no. 1. The adolescent is prone to many complications during pregnancy. This can be attributed to lack of early prenatal care as well as to poor nutrition. The other options generally do not apply to the adolescent population. CBF/A, AS, H

75. no. 1. Assessment of the general situation is the first priority. What is important to know is how close the delivery is and how much time is available for preparation. Taking a nursing history, calling the physician, and starting an IV may follow assessment of contractions. CBF/I, IM, PS

76. no. 4. In early labor, motivation is high and readiness to learn is enhanced. As labor progresses, concentration becomes more difficult to maintain. CBF/I, AN, E

77. no. 1. Meconium-stained amniotic fluid frequently indicates fetal distress. CBF/I, AS, PC

78. no. 2. This therapeutic communication fosters open expression of feelings. The nurse can only offer alternatives. The ultimate decision lies with the client. CBF/P, IM, PC

79. no. 3. Considering crisis theory and the knowledge of the grieving process, allowing the relinquishing mother to provide care is considered healthy adaptation. CBF/P, AN, PC

80. no. 1. Adoptive parents, or any parent separated from the newborn in the period immediately following delivery, can still form a strong attachment to the infant. Encouragement and reinforcement of positive behaviors enhance such bonding. CBF/N, IM, H

81. no. 1. This option indicates the father is alert to cues and responds to them. This is the only option that demonstrates interaction between infant and parent. CBF/N, EV, PC

82. no. 1. The other assessments have priority upon admission in determining her current clinical condition. CBF/I, AS, PS

83. no. 3. Breathing techniques can help the laboring woman maintain control during contractions. The client should not bear down until she is completely dilated. Crowning will not occur until complete dilatation. Sacral pressure is a comfort measure used if the fetus is in a posterior position. CBF/I, IM, PS

84. no. 4. During transition, as dilatation nears completion, there is increased rectal pressure from the fetal presenting part. Accelerated breathing, irritability, fear, and the need for medication may occur at any time in active labor. CBF/I, AS, PS

85. no. 2. If the client blows, she will not be able to push, which is contraindicated at this point. Option no. 3 is correct information, but it is not appropriate to explain things to a client in transition. She needs direction because of her pain and emotional status during that phase of labor. CBF/I, IM, PS

86. no. 1. This action should reverse the initial symptoms of hyperventilation or carbon dioxide insufficiency (dizziness, tingling in the hands, or circumoral numbness) by enabling the client to rebreathe carbon dioxide and replace the bicarbonate ion. CBF/I, EV, PS

87. no. 2. It is now safe to assist the client with effective pushing techniques to bring the baby down to the perineum. Before complete dilatation, pushing results in cervical edema and increases the danger of cervical lacerations and fetal head trauma. Narcotics should not be given after full dilatation. The client now requires constant monitoring by the nurse. CBF/I, IM, E

88. no. 3. The uterus must be assessed every 15 minutes to ensure that it is well contracted, thus preventing hemorrhage. The fundus should not be massaged unless it is relaxed. Constant massaging would tire the uterine muscle, contributing to hemorrhage. Blood pressure is monitored every 15 minutes and temperature every hour unless there are significant changes. CBF/P, IM, E

89. no. 4. This treatment is to prevent gonorrheal ophthalmia neonatorum, which can lead to blindness. Chemical conjunctivitis may result from a reaction to the silver nitrate. Neonatal syphilis must be treated with penicillin. There is no cure for herpes. CBF/N, AN, E

90. no. 2. Absent variability is an ominous sign. Decreased or absent fluctuations indicate central nervous system depression. True variability can only be determined with internal monitoring. CBF/I, AN, PS

91. no. 2. Variable decelerations are the result of cord compression. Early decelerations result from head compression. Late decelerations result from uteroplacental insufficiency. Posterior positions should not affect fetal heart rate. CBF/I, AN, PS

92. no. 3. Early deceleration occurs in response to compression of the fetal head and does not indicate fetal distress. Lack of variability is considered a sign of possible fetal jeopardy. Fluctuations are caused by interplay of the parasympathetic and sympathetic components of the autonomic nervous system. When decreased variability is noted, the nurse must suspect compromise of these mechanisms. Variable decelerations result from cord compression and late decelerations result from uteroplacental insufficiency, both of which are abnormal. CBF/I, AS, PS

93. no. 4. Early deceleration is often caused by head compression; no action is needed. CBF/I, IM, PS

94. no. 1. This is an invasive technique requiring a written consent. Because internal monitoring is invasive, there is approximately a 17% chance of infection. CBF/I, AN, PS

95. no. 4. This signifies late decelerations, an ominous sign that indicates uteroplacental insufficiency. CBF/I, AS, PS

96. no. 2. Even though the fetal heart rate is still within a normal range, the change is significant and must be investigated. CBF/I, IM, PS

97. no. 1. Excessive oxytocin results in tetanic contractions that interfere with the fetal blood supply. It is necessary to stop the infusion to relax the uterine muscle. After turning off the oxytocin, changing the client's position and administering oxygen will help improve uteroplacental insufficiency. CBF/I, IM, PS

98. no. 4. Contractions that are strong, last 50 to 70 seconds, and occur every 2 to 3 minutes usually signal the second stage of labor. In light of this client's pregnancy history, assessment is in order. CBF/I, IM, PS

99. no. 1. Epidural anesthesia can cause maternal hypotension because of vasodilatation. CBF/I, IM, PS

100. no. 1. Uterine atony frequently occurs with older grand multiparas following spontaneous deliveries of full-term infants. Lack of muscle tone in the grand multipara predisposes to uterine relaxation. CBF/P, AN, PS

101. no. 3. Phenylketonuria (PKU) tests are not performed within the first 24 hours. The infant must have ingested formula or breast milk before the test results can be considered accurate. PKU is an inborn error of metabolism caused by autosomal recessive genes. These infants have a deficiency in the liver enzyme phenylalanine hydroxylase, which is required to convert the amino acid phenylalanine to tyrosine. When the converting ability is lacking, phenylalanine accumulates, leading to progressive mental retardation. CBF/I, IM, H

102. no. 4. Before taking any other action, assessment is a priority. The reaction of the mother is not necessarily reflective of the stage of labor she is in. CBF/I, IM, E

103. no. 2. The priority at this time is to prevent a precipitous delivery that may result in damage to the fetus as well as a perineal tear. The mother will experience the urge to push during the contraction, but panting will prevent her from doing so. It is important to deliver the baby in between contractions. CBF/I, IM, E

104. no. 1. The sucking of the infant triggers the release of oxytocin, which contracts the uterus. Fundal massage, not vigorous pressure, is also an important nursing action to stimulate contraction of the uterus. CBF/P, IM, PS

105. no. 4. There is no indication that Mrs. Stepanich's membranes are ruptured or that her cervix is dilated, both of which are necessary conditions for internal monitoring. If fetal monitoring is desired, an external monitor will be employed. CBF/I, IM, E

106. no. 4. Cephalopelvic disproportion is the most common indication for a cesarean delivery. The other conditions are less commonly encountered indications. CBF/I, AS, E

107. no. 3. This is the only true statement. Checking fundal height, uterine massage as indicated, monitoring lochia, and assessing the incisional site are all important nursing actions following a cesarean delivery. CBF/P, AN, E

108. no. 3. A cesarean delivery is not a contraindication to breastfeeding. Certain adjustments in position may be necessary, but these should not limit breastfeeding. Intravenous fluids will be given until oral intake is established. The mother and baby are generally discharged together. CBF/P, IM, PS

109. no. 1. Regional anesthesia may be contraindicated based on this surgical history. Blood and urine findings are normal. Active herpes at the time of delivery necessitates a cesarean delivery. CBF/I, AS, PS

110. no. 3. Rapid infusion of intravenous fluids may result in pulmonary edema if the heart is unable to adapt to the circulatory overload. CBF/I, AS, PS

111. no. 2. The respiratory assessment indicates a potential problem following general anesthesia and should be reported immediately. Other findings are within normal limits. CBF/P, AS, PS

112. no. 3. Although this may be quite early for rooming-in after a cesarean birth, with nursing assistance the client may be able to care safely for the infant. Asking the father to remain around-the-clock is ordinarily not feasible. The signal light should be placed close to the client. CBF/P, IM, E

113. no. 4. To help a 3-year-old adjust to a new sibling, a symbolic toy such as a baby doll may be provided. He may express his jealous feelings through symbolic play with this toy. CBF/P, IM, PC

114. no. 3. Parents of specific ethnic backgrounds (e.g., black, Asian, Mediterranean) often note Mongolian spots on their newborn. These are clusters of pigment cells, of no consequence, that disappear at school age. CBF/N, AN, PS

115. no. 2. Parents who are both carriers have a one-in-four chance of delivering a child with sickle-cell disease; they should be made aware of the genetic implications. A carrier of sickle-cell disease is heterozygous (Pp). A person with the disease is ho-

mozygous recessive (pp). Referral to a genetic counselor is appropriate. CBF/N, IM, H

116. no. 4. The infant weighed 6 pounds at birth. This behavior is often normal for a smaller infant on the first days of life. If the infant seems satisfied after feeding, sufficient milk is probably being obtained with nursing. Weight of the infant is also a factor, but that is not included among the listed options. CBF/N, IM, PS

117. no. 4. The incision is made in the lower segment of the uterus, the thinnest portion; thus there is minimal blood loss, and repair is simplified. The procedure is associated with a lower incidence of postoperative infection. CBF/I, AN, PS

118. no. 4. Headache after spinal anesthesia is often attributed to the leakage of spinal fluid through the puncture site of the dura. Therefore, maintaining the client in a recumbent position while the puncture hole is healing may prevent this complication. Option no. 1 has no effect on spinal headache occurrence; no. 3 is appropriate treatment, not prevention. CBF/P, IM, E

119. no. 2. After rupture of membranes, an amniotic fluid embolus may occur. In this case, the embolus apparently traveled to the lung. CBF/I, AN, PS

120. no. 2. The husband needs support during this time of crisis. He does not need to be left alone. A visit to the intensive care unit is probably not appropriate at this time. CBF/I, IM, PC

121. no. 2. It is never appropriate to argue with the value system of an individual or family. The other options listed encourage more thoughtful consideration of the choice the husband is making. CBF/I, IM, PC

122. no. 4. Hematocrit changes reflect blood loss most accurately and rapidly. Options no. 1 and no. 2 are important ongoing assessments, but option no. 4 is most specific. CBF/I, AS, PS

123. no. 1. A therapeutic response at this time is one that reflects empathy. Option no. 3 might be appropriate at some later stage of the grieving process. P/T, IM, PC

124. no. 2. Oxytocin is used to contract the uterus and minimize postpartal bleeding. CBF/P, AN, PS

125. no. 4. The bedpan and running water should be tried first. Eventually, the nurse may need to insert a catheter, but not as an initial action. Because of her fluctuating blood pressure and spinal anesthetic, it is not appropriate to get the client out of bed. CBF/P, IM, E

126. no. 1. Postpartum chills are a common occurrence following delivery. Possible causes are reaction to the anesthesia, exhaustion, and a decrease in intraabdominal pressure. Warming the client is the appropriate nursing action. CBF/P, IM, E

127. no. 2. Ice is used during the first 24 hours; then switch to heat (sitz baths), which promotes vasodilatation and healing. TACE is a lactation suppressant. Kegel exercises will increase vaginal tone but will not relieve pain and swelling. CBF/P, IM, PS

128. no. 4. Prolactin is the direct cause of milk production. The decrease in estrogen and progesterone following delivery of the placenta stimulates prolactin production. CBF/P, AN, PS

129. no. 3. Use of a breast pump is unnecessary when initiating feeding. The infant's sucking should stimulate the milk sufficiently. CBF/P, IM, PS

130. no. 3. The condom is the only safe, nonprescription contraceptive to use while a woman is lactating and before there is normal uterine involution. The intrauterine device is not inserted until healing takes place because of the increased risk of infection. Birth control pills are passed into breast milk. To be effective, a diaphragm must fit over the cervix, which has not undergone involution at this time. CBF/P, IM, H

131. no. 4. These activities are considered too strenuous the first week after delivery. CBF/P, EV, H

132. no. 1. Immediately after delivery, the fundus will be about halfway between the symphysis pubis and the umbilicus. Expect lochia rubra for about 3 days after delivery. CBF/P, AS, PS

133. no. 1. Suspect lacerations if the client is bleeding and the fundus is firm. Subinvolution as well as uterine atony indicate that the uterus is not contracting properly; thus, the fundus would not be firm. When placental fragments are retained, the uterus will not contract. CBF/P, AN, PS

134. no. 1. Overdistension of the uterus causes poor uterine-muscle tone, which in turn causes poor uterine contractions postpartum, leading to an increased risk of postpartum hemorrhage. CBF/P, AS, PS

135. no. 3. All these symptoms are expected for the first day postpartum. Maternal temperature during the first 24 hours following delivery may rise to 100.4° F (38° C) as a result of dehydration. The nurse can reassure the new mother that these symptoms are normal. CBF/P, IM, PS

136. no. 2. Afterpains are more common in the multipara and the nursing mother. Multiparas have poorer muscle tone, and the uterus has the tendency to contract and relax. Oxytocin is released during breastfeeding, causing the uterus to contract. CBF/P, AS, PS

137. no. 2. Menses return in 4 to 6 weeks in the nonnursing mother. CBF/P, IM, H

138. no. 1. Ready-prepared infant formulas have additional water and carbohydrates as compared with breast milk. Commercial formulas are also fortified with essential nutrients. The higher casein content

of formula makes it more difficult to digest than breast milk. CBF/P, AN, PS

139. no. 1. As an essential part of the attachment process, the mother begins to "discover" her infant. This includes identification of physical characteristics and bodily processes. Identifying and relating to her infant as a separate and healthy human being may be accompanied by a sense of emotional relief in the mother. CBF/P, AN, PC

140. no. 4. Of the options given, the only one that directly and immediately affects the bleeding is uterine massage. It would be important to start an IV with oxytocin at a rapid rate of flow and to give oxygen through a mask at 6 to 7 L/min. However, the first action is to initiate uterine massage and compression. CBF/P, IM, PS

141. no. 1. The three causes of early postpartum hemorrhage in order of frequency are uterine atony, birth-canal lacerations, and retained placental fragments. The client is a multipara who has given birth to a large baby, which results in decreased uterine tone. CBF/P, AN, PS

142. no. 3. Postpartal hemorrhage is defined as blood loss equal to or in excess of 500 ml in the first 24 hours following delivery. CBF/P, AS, PS

143. no. 3. There is no documentation in the literature that breastfeeding is contraindicated following a postpartum hemorrhage and its resultant anemia. It is very important, though, to replace the lost iron stores. This is accomplished by diet and ferrous sulfate or ferrous gluconate tablets. Fatigue is a problem common in the postpartum period and is aggravated by the anemia in this case. Until the blood tests are within normal range, Mrs. Jackson would be expected to be fatigued on exertion, light-headed when arising too quickly, and pale in appearance. CBF/P, IM, H

144. no. 1. The Rh-negative mother who has no titer (negative Coombs' test results, nonsensitized) and who has delivered an Rh-positive fetus is given an intramuscular injection of anti-Rh_0 (D) (RhoGAM). CBF/P, IM, E

145. no. 3. RhoGAM blocks antibody production by attaching to fetal Rh-negative blood cells in the maternal circulation before an immunological response is initiated. CBF/P, AN, PS

146. no. 2. RhoGAM must be administered to unsensitized postpartum women after the birth of each Rh-positive infant to prevent production of antibodies. If the father of future fetuses is Rh positive heterozygous, there is a 50% chance of an Rh-negative infant; if he is Rh positive homozygous, all infants will be Rh positive. CBF/P, IM, H

147. no. 3. Serum hepatitis is transmitted through blood; thus, needles and syringes must be disposed of properly. A/NM, PL, E

148. no. 2. This menu meets the required amounts of vitamin C, iron, carbohydrates, and protein. Since breastfeeding is contraindicated when the mother has hepatitis, milk does not need to be included in the meal. She can meet recommended daily allowances for milk without having a glass at every meal. CBF/P, IM, H

149. no. 2. These are signs of withdrawal in an addicted newborn. The onset of withdrawal usually occurs within 24 hours of birth. The newborn may be jittery and hyperactive. The cry is often shrill and persistent with yawning and sneezing. Tendon reflexes are increased, and Moro's reflex is decreased. CBF/N, AS, PS

150. no. 4. A home visit is essential when preparing to discharge an infant into the care of others. Other factors will be considered, but safety is the priority. CBF/N, AS, H

151. no. 2. For heroin-addicted newborns, a majority of withdrawal symptoms are seen within the first 24 to 48 hours. For barbiturate- and cocaine-addicted infants, withdrawal occurs several days after delivery. The use of narcotic antagonists to reverse respiratory depression in the drug-addicted neonate is contraindicated because these drugs may precipitate acute withdrawal in the neonate. CBF/N, AN, PS

152. no. 1. Mastitis most frequently occurs at 2 to 4 weeks postpartum with the initial symptoms of fever, chills, headache, breast tenderness, or a localized reddened area on the breast. The client may describe symptoms that are generally consistent with malaise. CBF/P, AS, H

153. no. 3. There is controversy about whether a woman should temporarily stop breastfeeding or continue to breastfeed when mastitis is present. There is no scientific reason that, once the infection has passed the acute phase and the woman is no longer febrile, breastfeeding cannot be resumed. During the acute phase, it is important that counseling be given on how to manually massage or use a breast pump to empty the breasts to prevent stasis and further engorgement. CBF/P, IM, H

154. no. 4. Cracked nipples provide a portal of entry for bacteria. Antibiotics are used to treat mastitis and would not be given routinely simply to prevent mastitis from occurring. Waiting too long between feedings and abrupt weaning may lead to clogged ducts, predisposing to mastitis. CBF/P, IM, PS

155. no. 4. Jaundice in the first 24 hours after birth is a cause for concern that requires further assessment. Possible causes of early jaundice are blood incompatibility, oxytocin induction, and severe hemolytic process. Acrocyanosis of the hands and feet is normal, resulting from sluggish peripheral circulation. Vernix caseosa is a white, creamy sub-

stance covering the fetus in utero and is a normal finding after delivery. Harlequin sign is a rare color change between the longitudinal halves of the infant (when the infant is on its side, the dependent half is noticeably pinker). CBF/N, AS, PS

156. no. 1. The head circumference is approximately 13 to 14 inches. The chest circumference is 1 inch smaller (12 to 13 inches). CBF/N, AS, PS

157. no. 3. Impetigo is a bacterial infection caused by staphylococci or streptococci, which can lead to a generalized infection, always serious in the newborn. Erythema toxicum is a normal newborn rash that disappears without treatment. Stork bites, or telangiectasia, are clusters of small, red, localized areas of capillary dilatation commonly found at the nape of the neck, upper eyelids, and bridge of the nose. They can be blanched with pressure of a finger and will disappear without treatment. Mongolian spots are bluish gray areas of pigmentation found over the lower back in black or Oriental infants. The spots fade within the first year or two of life. CBF/N, AS, PS

158. no. 4. An opaque pupil indicates a congenital cataract. Transient strabismus or nystagmus is present until the third or fourth month of life. Subconjunctival hemorrhage is due to the pressure sustained during birth and will resolve without treatment. The eyes may be irritated from the instillation of medication, causing some discharge. CBF/N, AS, PS

159. no. 4. The single artery is associated with an increased incidence of various congenital anomalies and with higher perinatal mortality. Breast engorgement may be present as the result of maternal hormones. Bowel sounds are present within 1 to 2 hours after birth. The liver is large in proportion to the rest of the body and is easily felt. Kidneys are more difficult to feel. CBF/N, AS, PS

160. no. 2. Ears that are set lower than usual on the head may be associated with a congenital renal disorder or autosomal chromosomal abnormality. Incurving of the pinna and instant recoil are signs of maturity. The infant hears immediately following birth, and hearing becomes acute as mucus from the middle ear is absorbed. CBF/N, AS, H

161. no. 3. During periods of alert activity, play can be initiated with young infants. In the taking-hold period, the mother is particularly receptive to instruction and assistance in learning play and other parenting skills. CBF/N, IM, PS

162. no. 2. Fixation is present at birth. The newborn can clearly see items that are within a visual field of 20 cm to 22 cm (about 9 inches). CBF/N, AN, PS

163. no. 4. Young infants respond well to human faces and black-and-white objects, because of the visual contrast they provide. Newborns may fixate on visual stimuli for periods of 4 to 10 seconds. CBF/N, IM, H

164. no. 3. Skin-to-skin touch provides a mild tactile stimulus appropriate for the infant. It can be accomplished by stroking the infant gently from head to toe. This procedure is very comforting and relaxing to the infant. CBF/N, IM, H

165. no. 4. This reflex is also known as the grasping reflex and is elicited if the palm of the hand is stimulated by touch. The fingers close. CBF/N, AS, PS

166. no. 2. The infant experiences a sensation of falling when held in both hands and lowered rapidly about 1 inch. This will cause abduction and extension of arms and spreading of fingers bilaterally. CBF/N, AS, PS

167. no. 1. Maternal glucose crosses the placental barrier and stimulates the fetal pancreas to produce large amounts of insulin. At birth, the excess insulin causes the blood glucose level to fall rapidly. CBF/N, AN, PS

168. no. 3. Hypoglycemia may be prevented by the oral administration of glucose water. Oral feeding should be started as soon as the infant's condition permits. CBF/N, IM, E

169. no. 4. A term infant is one born between 38 and 42 weeks' gestation; a weight of 10 pounds is above the 90th percentile. CBF/N, AN, PS

170. no. 4. There is an increased risk of development of diabetes later in life. CBF/N, IM, H

171. no. 2. Skin should be exposed to light to allow oxidation of bilirubin from the skin. The light may injure the delicate eye structures, particularly the retina, so the eyes are patched. The infant requires additional fluids to compensate for the increased water loss through the skin and loose stools. Stools and urine are evaluated for green color and amount. CBF/N, IM, E

172. no. 2. Although large-for-gestational-age infants are often prone to hypoglycemia, the Dextrostix reading in this situation indicates an adequate blood-glucose level. All the other situations are at risk for hypoglycemia. The infant who is exposed to high blood-glucose levels in utero may experience rapid and profound hypoglycemia after birth because of the cessation of a high in-utero glucose load. The small-for-gestational-age infant has used up glycogen stores as a result of intrauterine malnutrition and has blunted hepatic enzymatic response with which to carry out gluconeogenesis. The preterm infants have not been in utero for a sufficient period to store glycogen and fat. CBF/N, AS, PS

173. no. 1. Increased respirations indicate a high metabolic rate. This happens with an infection. The

other options are all within normal ranges. CBF/N, AS, PS

174. no. 1. The mother's behavior indicates she is grieving over the infant's appearance. The nurse demonstrates acceptance of her feelings if she makes no demands on her, but allows infant contact. CBF/N, IM, PC

175. no. 4. Periodic apnea is common in preterm infants. Usually, gentle stimulation is sufficient to get the infant to breathe. CBF/N, IM, PS

176. no. 3. Epstein's pearls are small, white cysts on the hard palate or gums of the newborn. They are not abnormal and will disappear shortly after birth. Milia are blocked sebaceous glands located on the chin and nose of the infant. Thrush is a fungal infection characterized by white patches that appear to be milk curd on the oral mucosa. They have a tendency to bleed when removal is attempted. Thrush is caused by a monilial infection in the mother. CBF/N, AN, PS

177. no. 4. The oxygenated blood flows up the cord through the umbilical vein; a fetal structure known as the ductus venosus shunts blood from the um-bilical vein to the inferior vena cava. From the inferior vena cava, the blood flows into the right atrium and goes directly into the left atrium through the foramen ovale. It then flows into the left ventricle and out through the aorta. A fetal structure known as the ductus arteriosus provides a direct communication between the pulmonary artery and aorta. CBF/N, AN, PS

178. no. 1. At birth, the newborn's cardiac sphincter is still immature, and the nervous control of the stomach is incomplete. As a result, some regurgitation may be observed, which may be minimized by small feedings and frequent bubbling. CBF/N, AN, PS

179. no. 2. The posterior fontanel is located at the intersection of the sagittal and lambdoid sutures of the skull. The sagittal suture is the space between the parietal bones; the lambdoid suture separates the two parietal bones and the occipital bone. CBF/N, AN, PS

180. no. 2. Parental contact promotes bonding and the parents' feeling that this is their infant. CBF/N, IM, PC

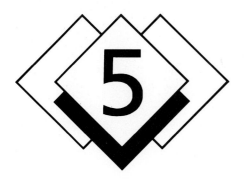

Nursing Care of the Child

Coordinator

Judith K. Leavitt, MEd, RN

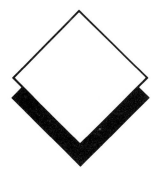

Questions

Toilet training is a problem for Mrs. Gates' daughter, 18-month-old Susie. She states that "Grandma says Susie should be potty trained by now, but she's still wearing diapers because she's stubborn and won't use the potty."

1. What is the nurse's best response to Susie's mother?
   - ☐ 1. "Most children are not ready to start toilet training until 18 months of age."
   - ☐ 2. "Susie should be potty trained by now, and she needs to be evaluated for developmental delay."
   - ☐ 3. "Keep her in diapers, and forget about toilet training; she'll train herself."
   - ☐ 4. "Susie is probably being stubborn."

2. The nurse plans to talk with Mrs. Gates about toilet training Susie, knowing that the most important factor in toilet training is which of the following?
   - ☐ 1. Mother's willingness to work at it.
   - ☐ 2. Starting early and being consistent.
   - ☐ 3. Approach and attitude of mother.
   - ☐ 4. Developmental readiness of child.

Kelly Patrick is sitting with her 18-month-old daughter, Kathy, at the well-baby clinic. She tells the nurse that Kathy has been "driving her crazy" by saying "no" to everything, and she needs help in handling her.

3. The nurse explains to Mrs. Patrick that Kathy's negativism is normal for a toddler and that this helps her daughter meet which of the following needs?
   - ☐ 1. Discipline.
   - ☐ 2. Independence.
   - ☐ 3. Trust.
   - ☐ 4. Consistency.

4. Mrs. Patrick states, "This morning I gave Kathy her orange juice and she said 'No.' I'm worried and frustrated. She needs her fluids. What should I do?" What is the nurse's best response?
   - ☐ 1. Offer her a choice of two juices to drink.
   - ☐ 2. Be firm, and hand her the glass.
   - ☐ 3. Distract her with solid food.
   - ☐ 4. Withhold fluids until she drinks the orange juice.

5. Before Mrs. Patrick leaves the clinic, the nurse tells her she can best help Kathy learn to control her own behavior at this age by
   - ☐ 1. Punishing her when she deserves it.
   - ☐ 2. Setting limits and being consistent.
   - ☐ 3. Allowing her to learn by her mistakes.
   - ☐ 4. Recognizing she is too young to be controlled.

A nurse-consultant for a preschool nursery is asked to speak to the parents' group. They ask a number of questions. In each situation, what is the nurse's best response?

6. "My 4-year-old is a picky eater and only wants peanut butter sandwiches. What can I do to get him to eat a more balanced diet?"
   - ☐ 1. "Serve him a balanced diet, and teach him to clean his plate."
   - ☐ 2. "Withhold between-meal foods and serve him only at family mealtime."
   - ☐ 3. "Offer him balanced meals and eliminate dessert if some of each food is not eaten."
   - ☐ 4. "Offer one small helping of each food at mealtime and two protein or fruit snacks."

7. "My 4-year-old refuses to go to sleep without a light on. How can I get him to give up the night-light?"
   - ☐ 1. "Tell him that he is too old for night-lights."
   - ☐ 2. "Let him go to bed with the night-light, then turn it off when he's asleep."
   - ☐ 3. "Give him a flashlight and tell him to use it to explore the dark room."
   - ☐ 4. "Let him turn the light on and off as he wishes. He will give it up when he does not need it any more."

8. "My 4-year-old is still wetting his bed almost every night. What can I do to train him?"

1. "Restrict all fluids after 5 PM, and remind him that he is too old to wet the bed."
2. "Get him up to urinate at midnight, and he will be able to stay dry until morning."
3. "Put him in diapers, and tell him to get up if he has to urinate."
4. "Limit fluids after dinner, and make sure he urinates before going to bed."

9. "My 4-year-old tells lies all the time. What can I do about this?"
   1. "Confront the child with this behavior, and let him know that lying is not acceptable."
   2. "The 4-year-old is old enough to tell the truth; ask him why he is not truthful."
   3. "The 4-year-old has a vivid imagination; ignore his lying and focus on reality."
   4. "Acknowledge his stories or fantasies by saying, 'What a nice story,' or, 'That's a pretend story.'"

10. "How should I respond to my 3½-year-old when he touches his genitals or masturbates?"
    1. "Permit the child to explore his body, but explain that masturbation is a private activity."
    2. "Distract him with other interests such as puzzles or books."
    3. "Set firm limits, and do not permit the child to indulge in this activity."
    4. "Masturbation may be a sign of an emotional disorder."

11. The parents of a 2-year-old express concern about their daughter's temper tantrums. The nurse would include which piece of information about the child's behavior?
    1. It indicates regression.
    2. It should be controlled by parental discipline.
    3. It is a normal expression of tension.
    4. It suggests an interference with development.

Kimberly, age 5, visits the pediatrician for her annual health visit. As an infant, she had the full recommended series of immunizations. Her last immunization was at 18 months.

12. Which of the following immunizations would Kimberly receive at this visit?
    1. DTP and OPV boosters.
    2. Tuberculin test.
    3. Measles, mumps, and rubella vaccine (MMR).
    4. No immunizations are indicated.

13. One day Kimberly's mother discovers Kimberly and her cousin, Will, age 7, undressed and curiously looking at and touching each other's bodies. What is Kimberly's mother's best initial response?
    1. "Will, it's time for you to go home."
    2. "Kimberly, we're going to have a talk when your daddy gets home."
    3. "Kimberly and Will, please put your clothes on. I'm going to wait in the kitchen for you."
    4. "What are you children doing?"

14. Kimberly asks about her grandmother's death. Which statement is most characteristic of the child between 5 and 8 years of age?
    1. Death is personified as a boogeyman.
    2. Death is considered to be reversible.
    3. Death is perceived as inevitable.
    4. The child recognizes that she will die.

Steve, age 8, and his brother Charlie, age 10, race to the breakfast table to see who gets a certain seat. This is usually followed by an argument.

15. Which of the following approaches is most effective in handling the above situation?
    1. Withhold breakfast until the boys come to agreement.
    2. Serve the boys away from the table.
    3. Assign the boys to places at the table.
    4. Solicit the boys' ideas as to how to resolve the problem.

16. Which of the following guidelines is *least* appropriate for parents of school-age children?
    1. Have the child eat most of the meal before offering second helpings or between-meal snacks.
    2. Avoid forcing the child to eat or using desserts as rewards for eating disliked foods.
    3. Deprive the child of a favorite food as punishment.
    4. Maintain good nutrition by having only fruit, vegetables, cheese, and protein snacks available.

17. Which of the following is the *least* effective approach to teaching nutrition to school-age children?
    1. Discuss nutrition without reference to "right" and "wrong."
    2. Present consequences of eating a balanced versus an unbalanced diet.
    3. Stress the importance of good table manners.
    4. Encourage children to keep a journal for 3 days to monitor types of food consumed.

18. What is the major psychosocial task for both Steve and Charlie, according to Erikson's theory of development?
    1. Trust vs. mistrust.
    2. Autonomy vs. shame and doubt.
    3. Industry vs. inferiority.
    4. Identity vs. role diffusion.

19. Both boys are in the stage of cognitive development defined by Piaget as
    1. Concrete operations.
    2. Symbolism.
    3. Preoperational thinking.
    4. Formal operations.

Marian Taylor is a 6-year-old with recurrent infection of the tonsils.

20. Mrs. Taylor was told by the surgeon that Marian would be scheduled for surgical removal of her tonsils and adenoids the following week. What can the nurse suggest to Marian's mother to facilitate Marian's adjustment to the hospital experience?
    ☐ 1. Explain about the surgery a week before her admission.
    ☐ 2. Admit her early on the day of admission to meet the staff.
    ☐ 3. Suggest that a friend schedule surgery at the same time.
    ☐ 4. Show pictures of the surgical procedure.

21. The nurse can anticipate that Marian's greatest fear will be
    ☐ 1. Separation from her parents.
    ☐ 2. A loss of control.
    ☐ 3. Body-image changes.
    ☐ 4. A strange environment.

22. Upon Marian's admission to the hospital, the laboratory technician visits Marian to obtain a sample of blood. Marian asks the nurse if the technician is going to hurt her. What is the best response?
    ☐ 1. "Of course not. You won't feel a thing."
    ☐ 2. "I don't know, but try to hold still."
    ☐ 3. "It will hurt a little bit, but we want to take good care of you."
    ☐ 4. "Yes, it will hurt, but we have to know your blood type if you should need a blood transfusion."

23. Which blood test is especially important preoperatively for Marian?
    ☐ 1. Bleeding and clotting time.
    ☐ 2. Eosinophil count.
    ☐ 3. Erythrocyte sedimentation rate (ESR).
    ☐ 4. Serum chloride levels.

24. Marian is noted to have a temperature of 100.8° F an hour before surgery. What action would the nurse take first?
    ☐ 1. Notify the physician immediately.
    ☐ 2. Call the operating room to cancel the surgery.
    ☐ 3. Administer acetaminophen prn as ordered.
    ☐ 4. Call Marian's parents.

25. Which position would Marian be placed in immediately postoperatively?
    ☐ 1. High-Fowler's position.
    ☐ 2. Semi-Fowler's position.
    ☐ 3. On her abdomen.
    ☐ 4. Trendelenburg's position.

26. What behavior of Marian's would the nurse be most concerned about 5 hours after surgery?
    ☐ 1. A very sore throat and a desire for cold drinks.
    ☐ 2. Frequent swallowing and restlessness.
    ☐ 3. Several attempts to void.
    ☐ 4. Difficulty speaking.

27. The evening of the day of surgery, Marian becomes restless and wants to get out of bed. What would the nurse do?
    ☐ 1. Allow Marian's mother to hold her.
    ☐ 2. Tell Marian to sit quietly in bed.
    ☐ 3. Permit Marian to walk in the halls.
    ☐ 4. Move Marian's bed near the nurse's station.

28. When the nurse prepares Marian and her parents for discharge, which instruction would be emphasized?
    ☐ 1. Notify the physician if bleeding occurs during the first 3 days.
    ☐ 2. Use saline gargles for comfort.
    ☐ 3. Remain out of school for 1 week.
    ☐ 4. Limit all activities for 1 month.

William Smith, 12 months old, has had an elevated temperature for 48 hours. There is evidence of nuchal rigidity, increasing lethargy, and nausea and vomiting. He is also dehydrated. Meningitis is suspected.

29. What classic sign in William would alert the nurse to confirm the diagnosis of meningitis?
    ☐ 1. Weight loss of 5%.
    ☐ 2. Urine specific gravity of 1.007.
    ☐ 3. Dry mucous membranes.
    ☐ 4. Bulging fontanel.

30. What equipment would the nurse have available at the bedside?
    ☐ 1. Thoracentesis set.
    ☐ 2. Lumbar puncture tray.
    ☐ 3. Nasogastric tube.
    ☐ 4. Foley catheter.

31. William's physician has ordered 5% dextrose in 0.33% normal saline with 20 mEq of potassium chloride (KCl) to infuse at 32 ml/hr. Which of the following would be brought to the physician's attention immediately?
    ☐ 1. William has not voided in 4 hours.
    ☐ 2. William has had three liquid green stools.
    ☐ 3. William has vomited 50 ml of mucus.
    ☐ 4. William is fussy and irritable when moved.

32. During the acute stages of William's illness, which nursing action would have the *least* priority?
    ☐ 1. Monitoring changes in his level of consciousness.
    ☐ 2. Maintaining the patency of the IV line.
    ☐ 3. Isolating him from other children.
    ☐ 4. Providing hourly tepid baths.

33. The priority nursing goal for William would be to
    ☐ 1. Administer antibiotics as soon as they are ordered.
    ☐ 2. Seek emotional support for William's parents.
    ☐ 3. Place him in isolation for 3 days.
    ☐ 4. Restrain all extremities to protect the IV.

Eight-year-old Carlos comes to the physician's office with a sore throat, enlarged cervical lymph nodes, elevated temperature, and malaise. He has a history of frequent streptococcal throat infections.

34. Carlos has bacterial pharyngitis and is put on a regimen of oral penicillin. Which of the following instructions to Carlos' parents is most important at this time?
    □ 1. Have him gargle with a saline solution.
    □ 2. Administer the full course of medication.
    □ 3. Provide a diet high in protein.
    □ 4. Encourage citric juices.

35. Carlos' mother asks the nurse what kind of books would be best for him to read. The best advice is
    □ 1. Small books, such as paperbacks.
    □ 2. Large-size print books.
    □ 3. Regular-size print books.
    □ 4. Picture books.

Four-year-old Judy is in a private room with "hand and linen precautions." She was admitted today for weight loss, anorexia, vaginitis, and insomnia. Lab tests include blood, urine, and stool tests. Results of lab tests are not on the chart yet. The nurse observes Judy scratching in the anal area at night.

36. Assessing the situation, the nurse suspects that Judy may have which one of the following conditions?
    □ 1. Ulcerative colitis.
    □ 2. Pinworms.
    □ 3. Salmonella.
    □ 4. Scabies.

37. Which test will confirm the diagnosis?
    □ 1. Sigmoidoscopic biopsy.
    □ 2. Cellophane tape over anus.
    □ 3. Microscopic exam of scrapings.
    □ 4. VDRL.

38. During nap time, Judy wets her bed. What action would the nurse take?
    □ 1. Change Judy's clothes and bed without comment.
    □ 2. Call her mother for suggestions.
    □ 3. Put her in diapers and note this in the Kardex.
    □ 4. Keep the bedpan in bed at nap time.

Carol Rauch yells for her nurse-neighbor to come look at 2-year-old Kirsten Rauch. The nurse finds the child sitting in the middle of the bathroom floor with several open medicine bottles strewn around the room. She is chewing on something and has white powder around her mouth.

39. Mrs. Rauch says, "Do something!" What would be the nurse's first action?
    □ 1. Call the poison control center.
    □ 2. Determine what Kirsten ate or drank.
    □ 3. Take Kirsten to the emergency room.

□ 4. Observe Kirsten closely to see if any symptoms develop.

40. The nurse determines that Kirsten ate only a few acetaminophen (Tylenol) tablets and a couple of her mother's arthritis capsules. The child is alert. The most appropriate nursing action would be to
    □ 1. Give her milk to coat her stomach and delay absorption.
    □ 2. Keep her NPO and observe her for symptoms.
    □ 3. Give 15 ml of syrup of ipecac with 15 ml of water.
    □ 4. Administer 15 g of activated charcoal.

41. When Kirsten is out of immediate danger, the nurse explores with Mrs. Rauch how to prevent another episode. Which of the following actions would be *least* appropriate?
    □ 1. Label all containers.
    □ 2. Lock up harmful substances.
    □ 3. Teach Kirsten to avoid poisonous substances.
    □ 4. Never refer to medicine as candy.

42. The best indicator that this teaching was successful is
    □ 1. Kirsten survives with no ill effects.
    □ 2. Mrs. Rauch knows the correct first aid for poisoning.
    □ 3. Kirsten returns to her normal activities.
    □ 4. the Rauch home is modified to prevent a recurrence of this situation.

43. Which observation by the nurse best indicates that Kirsten is at her normal developmental level?
    □ 1. Undresses herself, but needs help getting dressed.
    □ 2. Points to her body parts.
    □ 3. Puts smaller objects into larger holes.
    □ 4. Builds a tower out of two blocks.

Three-year-old Sandy has cerebral palsy, spastic type, with a severe motor impairment. Her mother has brought her to the clinic because she is having difficulty feeding Sandy.

44. What behaviors would the nurse observe in Sandy?
    □ 1. Hypotonic muscles.
    □ 2. Mental retardation.
    □ 3. Scissoring of legs.
    □ 4. Absent deep-tendon reflexes.

45. To improve Sandy's eating abilities, the nurse would counsel her mother to
    □ 1. Place Sandy in semi-Fowler's position with her head to one side, and allow her to suck liquids and pureed foods through a sturdy straw.
    □ 2. Encourage Sandy to feed herself to increase her independence.
    □ 3. Stand behind Sandy, support her jaw with one hand, and use the other hand to handle the cup or spoon to feed Sandy.
    □ 4. Place Sandy in a sitting position, tilt her head

slightly back, and use a Brecht feeder to give liquids and pureed foods.

46. Sandy's mother is pregnant and asks whether her second baby is likely to have cerebral palsy also. What is the nurse's best initial response?
   □ 1. "There is a strong possibility that your next baby may have cerebral palsy."
   □ 2. "Perhaps you were exposed to some illness or took some harmful medication when you were pregnant with your first baby."
   □ 3. "You're concerned that your next baby may have cerebral palsy."
   □ 4. "Attending prepared childbirth classes can lessen the possibility of birth trauma and decrease the risk of cerebral palsy."

Jessie, age 9 months, is admitted for severe burns of the face, neck, anterior chest, and hands, sustained when she grabbed a bowl of hot soup from the table.

47. The nurse determines the burns are primarily second degree because they appear to have
   □ 1. An absence of pain and pressure sensation.
   □ 2. White, dry, and leathery appearance.
   □ 3. Large, thick blisters.
   □ 4. Visible, thrombosed small vessels.

48. What would the priority nursing goal be on admission?
   □ 1. Debride and dress the wounds.
   □ 2. Administer antibiotics.
   □ 3. Observe for hoarseness, stridor, and dyspnea.
   □ 4. Obtain a complete history of the event.

49. A narcotic was ordered IV to control Jessie's pain. Why was the IV route selected?
   □ 1. For the fastest pain relief.
   □ 2. Circulatory blood volume is reduced, delaying absorption from the subcutaneous and muscle tissue.
   □ 3. Cardiac function is enhanced by the immediate action of the drug.
   □ 4. Decreased metabolism increases insulin production.

50. What would be considered an *unreliable* measure of fluid loss?
   □ 1. Hematocrit of 42.
   □ 2. Urinary output of 30 ml.
   □ 3. Change in LOC.
   □ 4. Leakage through the eschar.

51. Mafenide acetate (Sulfamylon) is applied to Jessie's wounds every 4 hours. What side effect would the nurse be most concerned about?
   □ 1. Metabolic acidosis.
   □ 2. Discoloration of the skin.
   □ 3. Vomiting and diarrhea.
   □ 4. Dehydration and electrolyte loss.

52. During this phase of wound management, what is the priority goal?

   □ 1. To debride the wound of dead tissue and eschar.
   □ 2. To limit fluid loss.
   □ 3. To prevent the growth of microorganisms.
   □ 4. To decrease formation of disfiguring scars.

53. As Jessie begins to improve she becomes interested in eating. What foods would be most appropriate for her?
   □ 1. Hot dog, french fries, and cooked spinach.
   □ 2. Hamburger, raisins, and cooked beans.
   □ 3. Omelet, mashed carrots, and crackers.
   □ 4. Pureed chicken, cooked peas, and bananas.

Suzi Jones is a newborn with Down syndrome. Her parents have been told the diagnosis and are in the process of trying to adjust.

54. Which of the following is most appropriate to include when counseling Mr. and Mrs. Jones?
   □ 1. Suzi's developmental potential is greatest during infancy.
   □ 2. Suzi will be severely retarded.
   □ 3. Suzi will have hyperreflexia.
   □ 4. Suzi will be as susceptible to colds as her older brother.

55. Which of the following is an *incorrect* statement regarding Down syndrome?
   □ 1. It is associated with a higher incidence of congenital heart disease.
   □ 2. It is associated with a higher incidence of gastrointestinal defects.
   □ 3. It is associated with a higher incidence of leukemia.
   □ 4. It is inherited as an autosomal recessive trait.

56. Which of the following measures is of primary importance for parents with a young, mentally retarded child at home?
   □ 1. Limit the amount of environmental stimulation to which the child is exposed.
   □ 2. Have the same parent teach the child new skills.
   □ 3. Teach the child socially acceptable behaviors.
   □ 4. Maintain a consistent routine for daily activities.

Baby Girl Carlton was born yesterday with a myelomeningocele, which is covered with a thin, fragile membrane. She is now in the special care nursery.

57. When her father visits for the first time, he is most likely to exhibit which grief reaction?
   □ 1. Anger.
   □ 2. Depression.
   □ 3. Disbelief.
   □ 4. Bargaining.

58. Mr. Carlton is standing hesitantly beside the Isolette. What is the nurse's best initial action?
   □ 1. Show Mr. Carlton how to stroke and talk to his daughter.
   □ 2. Give him a detailed explanation of his daughter's defect.

☐ 3. Ask if he wants to hold his daughter.

☐ 4. Ask him how his wife is doing.

59. Preoperatively, what is the priority nursing goal for Baby Girl Carlton?

☐ 1. Prevent contractures of her lower extremities.

☐ 2. Protect the sac from injury.

☐ 3. Promote parent-infant bonding.

☐ 4. Maintain adequate hydration.

60. Which of the following measures would be most comforting for Baby Girl Carlton?

☐ 1. Decorate her crib with brightly colored mobiles.

☐ 2. Hold her closely and rock her.

☐ 3. Place a music box in her crib.

☐ 4. Sit at her cribside and talk to her.

61. Which nursing measure for Baby Girl Carlton would be most dangerous preoperatively?

☐ 1. Place her in a prone position.

☐ 2. Massage her skin periodically with lotion.

☐ 3. Apply dry, sterile dressings on the sac.

☐ 4. Empty her bladder by applying downward pressure over the suprapubic area.

62. Baby Girl Carlton's defect is surgically closed. Postoperatively, it is imperative that the nurse assess her for

☐ 1. Increased head circumference.

☐ 2. Tachycardia.

☐ 3. Lower extremity movement.

☐ 4. Bladder function.

63. Postoperatively, Baby Girl Carlton's IV is prescribed to infuse at 8 ml/hr. How many drops per minute would the nurse regulate the microdrip to infuse?

☐ 1. 2.

☐ 2. 4.

☐ 3. 8.

☐ 4. 12.

64. Knowing the associated incidence of congenital hip dysplasia in infants with a myelomeningocele, Baby Girl Carlton's hips would be maintained in which position?

☐ 1. Adduction.

☐ 2. Abduction.

☐ 3. Internal rotation.

☐ 4. External rotation.

65. Baby Girl Carlton's parents have named her Natalie. Three days after surgery, while in her crib, Natalie begins to have a grand mal seizure with tonic and clonic movements. Which nursing measure would be implemented first?

☐ 1. Hold Natalie's arms close to her body.

☐ 2. Place a small padded tongue blade between her gums.

☐ 3. Administer oxygen by mask.

☐ 4. Put a blanket between Natalie and the crib rails.

66. Natalie is given phenytoin sodium (Dilantin) elixir. Children are generally given higher doses of phe-

nytoin per kilogram of body weight than adults. What is the reason for this?

☐ 1. Children excrete anticonvulsants more readily from the body.

☐ 2. Children's seizures are usually more severe.

☐ 3. Children are less likely to develop toxic reactions to anticonvulsants.

☐ 4. Higher doses are necessary to prevent paradoxical effects from occurring.

67. Natalie will be discharged on a regimen of phenytoin. It is important to teach her parents to observe for all of the side effects. Which of the following is *not* a side effect of this drug?

☐ 1. Gingival hypertrophy.

☐ 2. Skin rash.

☐ 3. Nausea and vomiting.

☐ 4. Excessive sleepiness.

68. After 1 month, Natalie is returned for an evaluation of her neurological status. The physician decides to admit her because a CT scan shows developing hydrocephalus. When assessing Natalie for signs of increased intracranial pressure, the nurse observes which of the following signs that indicate her pressure is increasing?

☐ 1. High-pitched cry.

☐ 2. Absence of neonatal reflexes.

☐ 3. Sunken fontanel.

☐ 4. Pinpoint pupils.

69. A ventriculoperitoneal (VP) shunt is done, and a Holter valve is surgically inserted. Postoperative nursing assessment and discharge teaching would be guided by the knowledge that which of the following are the most common complications of VP shunts?

☐ 1. Hemorrhage and subdural hematoma.

☐ 2. Ascites and peritonitis.

☐ 3. Obstruction and infection.

☐ 4. Catheter leakage.

70. The physician has written an order to pump Natalie's shunt four times each shift. Natalie's parents ask why this needs to be done. The nurse explains that the primary purpose of pumping the shunt valve is to

☐ 1. Maintain patency of the shunt.

☐ 2. Prevent Natalie from having seizures.

☐ 3. Minimize the possibility of the development of mental retardation.

☐ 4. Prevent infection of the shunt.

71. What is the postoperative nursing priority for Natalie?

☐ 1. Help Natalie's parents cope with having a disabled child.

☐ 2. Prevent skin breakdown of the scalp.

☐ 3. Prevent overhydration.

☐ 4. Promote adequate nutrition.

72. Which of the following is the best indicator of a successful outcome of Natalie's care?
☐ 1. The degree of attachment between Natalie and her parents.
☐ 2. Natalie's physical growth.
☐ 3. Natalie's cognitive and motor skills.
☐ 4. Natalie's temperament and social skills.

Foster McKay is a 9-year-old who is admitted to the hospital for evaluation of a seizure disorder.

73. During the history, Foster tells the nurse he sees weird lights before his eyes and then doesn't remember what happens afterward. The nurse would suspect he is
☐ 1. Hallucinating.
☐ 2. Experiencing an aura.
☐ 3. Trying to get his parents' attention.
☐ 4. Describing an absence seizure.

74. Which test would the nurse prepare Foster for?
☐ 1. Stress test.
☐ 2. Electroencephalogram.
☐ 3. Angiogram.
☐ 4. Echocardiogram.

75. Foster is placed on phenytoin (Dilantin). What statement indicates the parents have *not* understood the nurse's teaching?
☐ 1. "We shall only use the prescribed brand of the drug."
☐ 2. "The dosage may be changed during growth spurts."
☐ 3. "The medication can be discontinued if the seizures stop."
☐ 4. "Gum changes may occur after prolonged usage."

One morning, Doris and Carl Howard find their previously healthy 3-month-old daughter Hilary face down in her crib. She is not breathing and is limp. They rush her to the emergency room where Hilary is pronounced dead. The cause is attributed to sudden infant death syndrome (SIDS).

76. Which nursing action would be *inappropriate* at this time?
☐ 1. Provide the Howards with a fully detailed explanation of SIDS.
☐ 2. Allow the Howards to be alone with their daughter's body for a short time.
☐ 3. Call a relative or close friend to come to the hospital to be with them.
☐ 4. Place an arm around their shoulders and say, "I'm so sorry."

77. A short time later, Mr. Howard says, "She was so healthy. I just can't understand what would have caused this. What did we do wrong?" What is the most appropriate response?

☐ 1. "It sounds like you feel responsible for what happened to Hilary."
☐ 2. "Try not to blame yourself for Hilary's death."
☐ 3. "No one knows the cause of SIDS."
☐ 4. "Did Hilary seem sick before bedtime?"

78. While assessing the Howards during a follow-up home visit, what is the best indicator of their successful coping with the loss of their daughter?
☐ 1. Moving to a new residence.
☐ 2. Involving themselves in a SIDS support group.
☐ 3. Attending their church regularly.
☐ 4. Returning to work.

Six-month-old Jésus Sanchez is admitted to the pediatric unit with a diagnosis of bronchiolitis. He has a 2½-year-old sibling.

79. What behaviors would the nurse expect to observe in Jésus?
☐ 1. Diminished breath sounds.
☐ 2. Dry, hacky cough.
☐ 3. Serous nasal discharge.
☐ 4. Shortened expiratory phase.

80. Jésus is kept NPO because
☐ 1. Hypoxemia reduces gastrointestinal motility.
☐ 2. Oral fluids increase mucus production.
☐ 3. Tachypnea predisposes an infant to aspiration.
☐ 4. Hydration is not a concern with bronchiolitis.

81. Which measure is *inappropriate* for Jésus?
☐ 1. Use deep suction.
☐ 2. Place in a mist tent with oxygen.
☐ 3. Maintain adequate hydration.
☐ 4. Monitor for cor pulmonale.

82. How would Jésus be positioned during the acute stages of his illness?
☐ 1. Modified Sims' position.
☐ 2. Semi-Fowler's position.
☐ 3. Supine position.
☐ 4. Prone position.

83. Chest physical therapy with postural drainage has been ordered for Jésus TID. When would these treatments be administered?
☐ 1. Before meals.
☐ 2. After meals.
☐ 3. Every 8 hours.
☐ 4. When parents are present.

84. If Jésus' weight is 3.5 kg at birth, how much would he be expected to weigh at 6 months of age?
☐ 1. 5.15 kg.
☐ 2. 7 kg.
☐ 3. 8.6 kg.
☐ 4. 10.5 kg.

85. Once Jésus is able to tolerate feedings, which of the following foods would be most appropriate for meeting his developmental needs?

☐ 1. Chopped egg white.
☐ 2. Strained fruit.
☐ 3. Crackers.
☐ 4. Orange juice.

86. If there is a history of food allergies in the Sanchez family, which cereal would be most appropriate for Jésus?
☐ 1. Oatmeal.
☐ 2. Rice.
☐ 3. Mixed.
☐ 4. Barley.

87. Mrs. Sanchez tells you that Jésus' immunizations are up-to-date. Which of the following would Jésus receive next?
☐ 1. Diphtheria and tetanus.
☐ 2. Oral polio.
☐ 3. Measles, mumps, and rubella.
☐ 4. Tuberculin test.

Ten-year-old Pedro is admitted with airway obstruction.

88. A tracheostomy is performed; Pedro requires frequent suctioning. The physician orders the instillation of 2 to 3 ml of sterile saline into the tracheostomy tube before suctioning. Which client outcome indicates the saline was effective?
☐ 1. Loosened secretions and coughing.
☐ 2. A long period of uninterrupted sleep at night.
☐ 3. Increased fluid intake.
☐ 4. Moist tracheal mucosa.

89. Before suctioning Pedro's tracheostomy, which of the following actions would the nurse perform?
☐ 1. Loosen the tracheostomy tube to facilitate suctioning.
☐ 2. Ask him to hold his breath to promote lung expansion.
☐ 3. Listen to his chest with a stethoscope.
☐ 4. Position him in a chair supported with pillows.

90. The nurse caring for Pedro would know that oxygenation before suctioning is essential to
☐ 1. Loosen respiratory secretions.
☐ 2. Relax Pedro.
☐ 3. Restore oxygen lost during suctioning.
☐ 4. Remove sodium ions from respiratory tissue.

91. Which of the following nursing actions would be most appropriate while providing tracheostomy care to Pedro?
☐ 1. Use a sterile glove and catheter when suctioning.
☐ 2. Inject 5 ml of air into the cuff to prevent aspiration.
☐ 3. Cleanse the inner cannula with peroxide and sterile saline daily.
☐ 4. Remove the outer cannula at least every 8 hours for cleaning.

92. If suctioning was effective, the nurse listening to Pedro's chest would hear
☐ 1. Increased breath sounds.
☐ 2. Decreased breath sounds.
☐ 3. Fine, moist rales.
☐ 4. Coarse rhonchi.

Pedro's recovery is uneventful. His tracheostomy has been plugged and he is able to perform daily activities with minimal assistance. He has been taking ampicillin, 500 mg PO bid, cromolyn sodium (Intal) prn, and a regular diet.

93. The nurse would instruct Pedro's mother to include which of the following foods in his diet while he is taking ampicillin?
☐ 1. Honey.
☐ 2. Yogurt.
☐ 3. Bran.
☐ 4. Oranges.

94. Which statement about cromolyn sodium (Intal) is correct?
☐ 1. It enhances the release of histamine.
☐ 2. It is used during an acute asthmatic attack.
☐ 3. It is administered with milk PO qid.
☐ 4. It may cause irritation to the throat and trachea.

95. What statement best describes Pedro's developmental level?
☐ 1. He enjoys numbers and is able to do simple fractions.
☐ 2. He is clumsy handling a pencil and pen.
☐ 3. He is interested in girls.
☐ 4. He has a huge appetite.

Six-and-a-half-year-old Molly, a first-grader who has a history of asthma, is hospitalized with an acute episode.

96. Which of the following nursing actions is *contraindicated* during the acute phase of Molly's illness?
☐ 1. Keep Molly's room quiet.
☐ 2. Teach Molly to use her diaphragm for breathing.
☐ 3. Give Molly a cough suppressant.
☐ 4. Place Molly in a high-Fowler's position.

97. Molly's IV has infiltrated. When the nurse tries to apply a warm, moist washcloth to her swollen left forearm, she begins to whine and pull away. What would the nurse say to gain Molly's cooperation?
☐ 1. "I'll come back in a few minutes after you calm down."
☐ 2. "The doctor says this washcloth will make your arm feel better."
☐ 3. "Try not to cry while I put this on."
☐ 4. "This will feel warm. I'll show you on your other arm first."

98. Which drug would the nurse be prepared to give Molly after her IV is started?

☐ 1. Epinephrine.

☐ 2. Aminophylline.

☐ 3. Cromolyn sodium.

☐ 4. Penicillin.

99. While Molly is hospitalized, it is most important for the nurse to plan ways to

☐ 1. Promote her sense of control.

☐ 2. Maintain her gross motor skills.

☐ 3. Maintain her school work.

☐ 4. Promote attachment to her parents.

100. Molly is to be discharged tomorrow. What would be included in the discharge teaching plan for her parents?

☐ 1. Avoid frequent dusting of Molly's room.

☐ 2. Ensure that Molly's immunizations and flu shots are current.

☐ 3. Have Molly sleep with her window open during cold weather.

☐ 4. Allow Molly to participate in quiet activities only.

Twelve-year-old LaTania is admitted to the adolescent unit with sickle-cell disease. She is in vasoocclusive crisis. Her right elbow is edematous, and she states that it is very painful.

101. In addition to pain, which of the following symptoms would LaTania most likely manifest?

☐ 1. Dactylitis.

☐ 2. Chronic hemolytic anemia.

☐ 3. Brushfield's spots.

☐ 4. Jaundice followed by pallor after a sickling crisis.

102. LaTania asks her nurse what she thinks caused this crisis episode. The nurse's correct reply is

☐ 1. Physical exercise.

☐ 2. Developmental growth spurts.

☐ 3. Hot, humid weather.

☐ 4. A viral infection.

103. The most appropriate intervention for LaTania is

☐ 1. Wrap a heating pad around her elbow.

☐ 2. Set up necessary equipment for a blood transfusion.

☐ 3. Limit her daily fluid intake to 900 ml.

☐ 4. Apply ice to her arms.

104. LaTania's mother asks what test she should get for LaTania's 1-year-old brother to see if he might have sickle-cell disease. The nurse would recommend a(n)

☐ 1. Sickledex.

☐ 2. Amniocentesis.

☐ 3. Hemoglobin electrophoresis.

☐ 4. Complete blood count.

Fourteen-year-old Darryl has hemophilia. He is being seen in the clinic today for a periodic checkup.

105. When obtaining a history from Darryl and his father, which one of the following reported manifestations would be the greatest cause for concern?

☐ 1. Epistaxis.

☐ 2. Pallor.

☐ 3. Easy bruising.

☐ 4. Hemarthrosis.

106. Darryl's father tells the nurse privately that Darryl is "crazy about sports, especially football. He wants to try out for his junior high football team. My wife and I are having a hard time convincing him this is impossible." What would the nurse recommend?

☐ 1. Allow him to try out for the team as long as he wears a helmet and body pads at all times.

☐ 2. Start a collection of football memorabilia.

☐ 3. Develop an interest in swimming or table tennis.

☐ 4. Become team manager.

107. Darryl is admitted to the hospital with an acute bleeding episode in his right elbow that could not be controlled at home. Which of the following will *not* be used to control his bleeding?

☐ 1. Plasma.

☐ 2. Plasma concentrate.

☐ 3. Packed cells.

☐ 4. Cryoprecipitate.

108. During his bleeding episode, which one of the following nursing measures is indicated?

☐ 1. Apply a heating pad to the right elbow.

☐ 2. Keep the right elbow flexed and immobile.

☐ 3. Encourage Darryl to lie on his right side.

☐ 4. Administer aspirin, 10 grains orally q4h.

109. Darryl is recovering and will be discharged tomorrow. His father expresses concern about Darryl's future as a "family man." The nurse ascertains that Darryl's father is anxious to know if Darryl can have children who do not have hemophilia. Assuming that Darryl's future spouse is not a carrier of the disease, which explanation is most accurate?

☐ 1. All Darryl's children will be carriers.

☐ 2. Darryl's sons will have the disease and his daughters will be carriers.

☐ 3. There is a 50% chance that each of Darryl's children will have hemophilia.

☐ 4. Darryl's sons will be normal and his daughters will be carriers.

110. Which one of the following is the best indicator of a successful outcome of Darryl's long-term treatment?

☐ 1. Bleeding episodes are prevented or treated early.

☐ 2. Darryl is able to keep up with his peers academically.

☐ 3. Darryl's weight is maintained within age-appropriate ranges.

☐ 4. Darryl chooses a realistic career goal.

Angela Rodriguez brings her 1-year-old son, Miguel, in for a well-child examination.

111. Which of the following activities would Miguel be expected to do at this age?
    ☐ 1. Move around solid objects.
    ☐ 2. Walk well, forward and backward.
    ☐ 3. Have a vocabulary of three words.
    ☐ 4. Feed himself with a spoon.

112. Miguel receives a tuberculin skin test using purified protein derivative (PPD). The nurse instructs Mrs. Rodriguez to check the site in 48 hours and 72 hours. Which of the following most accurately describes a positive reaction?
    ☐ 1. A pruritic rash on the arm.
    ☐ 2. Fever and coughing.
    ☐ 3. Induration of 10 mm at the site.
    ☐ 4. 3-mm area of erythema and swelling.

113. Miguel is diagnosed with tuberculosis. The nurse can expect the physician's orders to include which medication?
    ☐ 1. Corticosteroid.
    ☐ 2. Isoniazid.
    ☐ 3. Ampicillin.
    ☐ 4. Vitamin K.

114. Which comment by Mrs. Rodriguez indicates that she understands the discharge instructions?
    ☐ 1. "Miguel will remain home from school until his x-rays are normal."
    ☐ 2. "Miguel must have weekly sputum tests."
    ☐ 3. "Miguel should have a low-protein, high-calorie diet."
    ☐ 4. "Miguel must take his medication for at least a year."

Four-year-old Barbara Watson was admitted to the hospital for diagnostic studies and heart surgery for repair of aortic stenosis.

115. A cardiac catheterization is ordered for Barbara. Barbara's mother asks the nurse about the procedure. Which one of the following statements is the *best* nursing response?
    ☐ 1. "A pushing sensation may be felt when the tube catheter goes into her arm."
    ☐ 2. "Barbara may feel pain around her heart."
    ☐ 3. "There will be bright lights and loud noises."
    ☐ 4. "Barbara will feel a tingling sensation in her hands and feet."

116. While doing morning care for Barbara, the nurse notes that the blanket that she brought from home is torn and tattered. What would the nurse do?
    ☐ 1. Keep it close to Barbara.
    ☐ 2. Ask her parents to take it home.
    ☐ 3. Give her a new blanket.
    ☐ 4. Send the blanket to the laundry for a good washing.

117. After dinner, Mrs. Watson tells the nurse she has to leave. Barbara hears her and begins to cry loudly. Which action by the nurse would be best at this time?
    ☐ 1. Walk Mrs. Watson to the elevator.
    ☐ 2. Ask Mrs. Watson to stay until Barbara goes to sleep.
    ☐ 3. Stay with Barbara and try to comfort her.
    ☐ 4. Encourage Mrs. Watson not to visit for a while.

118. Mrs. Watson brings Barbara in for her checkup after discharge and her older brother, Eric, for his 5-year checkup. When taking Eric's vital signs, the nurse notices he has a sinus dysrhythmia. Which of the following nursing actions would be carried out?
    ☐ 1. Notify the physician immediately.
    ☐ 2. Obtain a 12-lead ECG.
    ☐ 3. Ask Mrs. Watson if Eric has been taking digoxin.
    ☐ 4. Have Eric hold his breath while listening to his apical pulse.

Ronald Fulton, 2 years old, was brought by his parents to the emergency room because of respiratory distress, an elevated temperature, and nasal congestion. A loud systolic murmur was noted over the left sternal border. His diagnosis was a large ventricular septal defect.

119. Which abnormal condition results from this defect?
    ☐ 1. Peripheral hypoxia.
    ☐ 2. Elevated hemoglobin and hematocrit.
    ☐ 3. Volume overload in the lungs.
    ☐ 4. Decreased blood pressure.

120. Children with congenital heart disease are extremely susceptible to which of the following problems?
    ☐ 1. Gastrointestinal disorders.
    ☐ 2. Upper respiratory tract infections.
    ☐ 3. Urinary tract infections.
    ☐ 4. Allergic conditions.

121. Children with congenital heart disease are often less able to adapt positively to frustrating situations. Which of the following provides the best explanation for their behavior?
    ☐ 1. They have usually been spoiled by their parents.
    ☐ 2. They have had fewer opportunities to learn to deal with frustrations.
    ☐ 3. They can manipulate others by their reactions.
    ☐ 4. They are developmentally delayed in their socialization.

122. A cardiac catheterization confirms the diagnosis. Plans are made for Ronald to be followed up in an outpatient clinic and to return for corrective surgery when he is 3 years old. In discussing discharge plans with Ronald's parents, which of the following instructions would be most realistic?

1. No restrictions or limits are needed.
2. Diet should emphasize iron-rich meats and vitamins.
3. Ronald's contacts should be limited to healthy adults.
4. Ronald can set his own limits on exercise and activities.

When Ronald is 3 years old, he is readmitted to the hospital for repair of the ventricular septal defect. He is receiving a daily dose of digoxin and is admitted 3 days before the surgery.

123. Ronald is placed in an oxygen tent for short periods of time before cardiac surgery for which primary reason?
    1. To accustom him to the experience.
    2. To avoid contact with people who have upper respiratory infections.
    3. To keep the body temperature low.
    4. To reduce preoperative secretions from the respiratory tract.
124. The nurse notes Ronald's apical pulse is 70. Which action by the nurse is *most* appropriate?
    1. Call an emergency alert because the child is in heart block.
    2. Give the digoxin because the pulse is within normal range.
    3. Take the radial pulse and compare it with the apical pulse.
    4. Withhold the digoxin, and notify the physician.
125. The nurse must administer 0.06 mg of digoxin, which comes in a solution of 1 ml = 0.05 mg. How many minims would the nurse give?
    1. 16.
    2. 18.
    3. 20.
    4. 22.
126. Which response would be *unexpected* from digoxin?
    1. Slower heart rate.
    2. Greater force in cardiac contraction.
    3. Accelerated AV node conduction.
    4. Increased urinary output.
127. Hypothermia is used in open-heart surgery to
    1. Lessen the dangers of postoperative febrile episodes.
    2. Stop cardiac activity.
    3. Minimize respiratory action.
    4. Reduce overall body metabolism.
128. Postoperatively, Ronald has a water-seal chest drainage system. This action helps drain air and fluid from
    1. The abdominal cavity.
    2. The alveoli.
    3. The myocardial sac.
    4. The pleural cavity.

129. For which of the following conditions would the nurse clamp off Ronald's thoracotomy tube?
    1. Obstruction of the drainage flow because of clots.
    2. The appearance of large amounts of blood in the tubing.
    3. Disconnection of the tubing.
    4. Movement of the child from side to side.
130. Which of the following nursing actions would best facilitate Ronald to cough?
    1. Sit him straight up in bed.
    2. Encircle the chest with both hands.
    3. Stimulate the cough reflex with a catheter.
    4. Clamp off the thoracotomy tube.
131. The nurse notices Ronald sucking his thumb. Which action would be most appropriate?
    1. Discuss with the parents how to break this habit.
    2. Gently remove the thumb from his mouth while diverting his attention.
    3. Recognize his behavior is expected regression and allow him to continue.
    4. Request permission to give him ice chips or sips of water by mouth.
132. Ronald's cardiac surgery has been successful. During the convalescent period, the Fulton family will probably need special counseling in
    1. Becoming less protective.
    2. Planning Ronald's educational goals.
    3. Learning to avoid physical complications related to Ronald's childhood diseases.
    4. Maintaining Ronald's restricted life-style.
133. Ronald's parents share their frustration with the nurse about his temper tantrums at home. Which parental response to the tantrums would best indicate that they are handling him appropriately?
    1. Ignoring the tantrum.
    2. Reasoning with Ronald during the tantrum.
    3. Restraining Ronald during the tantrum.
    4. Placing Ronald alone after the tantrum.
134. The nurse suggests that Ronald use which of the following activities to help him express his angry feelings?
    1. Reading a book.
    2. Stacking blocks.
    3. Throwing a ball.
    4. Watching educational television.

Twelve-month-old Marcus has been referred to the pediatric clinic by the public health nurse because of suspected nonorganic failure-to-thrive syndrome. His mother is a 19-year-old single parent who lives alone with her son.

135. A first-year nursing student in the clinic asks what causes nonorganic failure-to-thrive syndrome. The best reply would be that the most common cause is

☐ 1. Intestinal malabsorption.

☐ 2. Sensory overload.

☐ 3. Parent's limited knowledge of feeding technique.

☐ 4. Disruption in parent-infant attachment.

136. Nursing assessment of Marcus is most likely to reveal

☐ 1. Intense eye-to-eye contact.

☐ 2. Stranger anxiety.

☐ 3. Hyperresponsiveness to sensory stimuli.

☐ 4. Stiff posture when held.

137. During the assessment of Marcus, the nurse observes that he has good head control and can roll over, but he cannot sit up without support or transfer an object from one hand to another. Based on this observation, the nurse concludes that Marcus is at what developmental age?

☐ 1. 3 to 4 months.

☐ 2. 5 to 6 months.

☐ 3. 7 to 8 months.

☐ 4. 9 to 10 months.

138. A plan of care to best meet the needs of this child would *not* include

☐ 1. A schedule of stimulation geared to the infant's present level of development.

☐ 2. A plan to teach the mother ways to provide stimulation.

☐ 3. A plan to have staff members pick him up and play with him whenever they can.

☐ 4. Consistency in care and caregiver.

139. Which nursing action would receive the highest priority in Marcus' nursing care plan?

☐ 1. Help his mother find a job.

☐ 2. Provide his mother with growth and development information.

☐ 3. Praise his mother's nurturing behaviors.

☐ 4. Limit his mother's time with Marcus.

140. Which toys are *least* appropriate for Marcus?

☐ 1. Stacking blocks.

☐ 2. Large rattles.

☐ 3. Colored mobiles.

☐ 4. Squeeze toys.

141. What is the best indication of Marcus' improvement?

☐ 1. Daily weight gain of 2 ounces.

☐ 2. Normal consistency of stool.

☐ 3. Crying when he is hungry.

☐ 4. Exploring the toys in his crib.

142. What is the best indicator that Marcus's failure to thrive is being resolved?

☐ 1. Marcus's mother keeps scheduled clinic appointments.

☐ 2. Marcus's physical growth shows a consistent pattern of improvement.

☐ 3. Marcus's sleeping, eating, and elimination patterns are predictable.

☐ 4. Marcus's mother verbally expresses her fears and frustrations about being a parent.

Three-year-old Cassie is admitted to the pediatric unit with diarrhea and mild dehydration. Her weight is 14 kg.

143. When performing an assessment of Cassie, which of the following would the nurse *not* expect to find?

☐ 1. Dry oral mucous membranes.

☐ 2. Low blood pressure.

☐ 3. Urine specific gravity of 1.032.

☐ 4. Tachycardia.

144. The physician orders an IV of 5% dextrose in .2% normal saline with 60 mEq of KCl/L to infuse at a rate of 60 ml/hr. Based on her developmental stage, Cassie is most likely to view the starting of her IV as

☐ 1. A sign of her powerlessness.

☐ 2. Necessary treatment to regain health.

☐ 3. Punishment for a previous misdeed.

☐ 4. An indicator that she is very sick.

145. Before adding potassium to Cassie's IV fluid, which of the following nursing assessments would be most important?

☐ 1. Urine output.

☐ 2. Respiratory rate.

☐ 3. Blood pressure.

☐ 4. Heart rate.

146. A nursing priority with Cassie has been maintaining strict intake and output. At 12 AM, the nurse notes that Cassie's urine output for the last 4 hours is 36 ml. The nurse would

☐ 1. Continue to monitor.

☐ 2. Notify the physician.

☐ 3. Check the urine's specific gravity.

☐ 4. Obtain Cassie's blood pressure.

147. Cassie continues to have frequent bouts of watery diarrhea. If this continues, what will occur?

☐ 1. Metabolic acidosis with slow, shallow respirations.

☐ 2. Metabolic alkalosis with deep, rapid respirations.

☐ 3. Metabolic alkalosis with slow, shallow respirations.

☐ 4. Metabolic acidosis with deep, rapid respirations.

148. Cassie is now recovering from her illness and has just begun eating again. Which of the following foods would *not* be acceptable to include in her diet?

☐ 1. Applesauce.

☐ 2. Ice cream.

☐ 3. Toast.

☐ 4. Bananas.

Brooke White, age 4, is admitted to the pediatrics unit with pneumonia and dehydration.

149. Brooke is put into a croup tent to relieve her respiratory distress. Which toy would be most suitable for her at this time?
☐ 1. Her favorite storybook.
☐ 2. Her favorite doll.
☐ 3. Her favorite puzzle.
☐ 4. Her favorite stuffed animal.

150. Brooke cries uncontrollably when placed in the tent. What is the best way to help Brooke adjust?
☐ 1. Have the nurse put her head in the tent with Brooke.
☐ 2. Place another child with a croup tent in the same room.
☐ 3. Call Brooke's mother for suggestions.
☐ 4. Place additional toys in the tent.

151. Brooke is to receive 250 ml of IV fluid over 8 hours. Using a microdrip, what is the desired rate of drops per minute?
☐ 1. 5.
☐ 2. 31.
☐ 3. 60.
☐ 4. 83.

152. Before administering the next dose of ampicillin, Brooke's mother informs the nurse that Brooke has begun to have diarrhea. What is the best response?
☐ 1. Change to a different antibiotic.
☐ 2. Discontinue the ampicillin.
☐ 3. Administer the dose and consult the physician.
☐ 4. Institute isolation precautions.

153. Brooke has been running a fever and is still having frequent stools. The physician orders Brooke's temperature to be monitored q2h. The nurse would take
☐ 1. Oral temperatures.
☐ 2. Rectal temperatures.
☐ 3. Axillary temperatures.
☐ 4. Either oral or rectal temperatures.

154. Gentamicin sulfate (Garamycin), 65 mg, was ordered for IM injection. The multidose vial is labeled 40 mg/ml. How many ml of the medication would Brooke receive?
☐ 1. 0.61 ml.
☐ 2. 1.22 ml.
☐ 3. 1.60 ml.
☐ 4. 3.20 ml.

155. Discharge teaching for Brooke's parents would include which of the following factors to ensure optimal absorption of the liquid form of ampicillin?
☐ 1. Administer on an empty stomach.
☐ 2. Administer with milk.
☐ 3. Avoid shaking the container.
☐ 4. Store at room temperature.

Two-year-old Peter was admitted to the hospital for the second surgical repair of his cleft palate. His mother cannot stay overnight with her son or visit because of unexpected illness.

156. What information on admission is most important in developing a care plan for Peter?
☐ 1. Peter's sleeping habits.
☐ 2. Peter's feeding habits and ability to drink from a cup.
☐ 3. Peter's toilet training status.
☐ 4. Peter's favorite activities.

157. On the morning after admission, Peter is standing in his crib crying. He refuses to be comforted and calls for his mother. The nurse approaches Peter to bathe him and he screams louder. She recognizes this behavior as which of the following stages of "settling in"?
☐ 1. Protest.
☐ 2. Depression.
☐ 3. Denial.
☐ 4. Bargaining.

158. What would be the most helpful nursing action at this time?
☐ 1. Pick him up and walk him around the room.
☐ 2. Be firm and begin with his bath.
☐ 3. Sit at the bedside and spend time with Peter until his anxiety has decreased.
☐ 4. Chart the behaviors and let the next shift bathe him.

159. Following surgical repair of his cleft palate, in which position would Peter be placed?
☐ 1. On his abdomen.
☐ 2. On his back.
☐ 3. Fowler's position.
☐ 4. Any position that is comfortable for him.

160. To prevent Peter from damaging the surgical repair, the nurse would apply
☐ 1. A Logan bow to his mouth.
☐ 2. Elbow restraints.
☐ 3. Wrist restraints.
☐ 4. Gauze wrapping on Peter's hands.

161. It is one day after Peter's surgery. Which activity is most appropriate for him?
☐ 1. Listen to a volunteer read a story.
☐ 2. Watch *Sesame Street* on television.
☐ 3. Play a toy piano.
☐ 4. Put together a puzzle with large pieces.

162. On the third postoperative day, Peter begins to regress and lies quietly in his crib with his blanket. The nurse recognizes that he is now in which stage of separation anxiety?
☐ 1. Denial.
☐ 2. Despair.
☐ 3. Mistrust.
☐ 4. Shock and disbelief.

163. By the end of the first week of hospitalization, Peter smiles easily, no longer cries when his father leaves after visiting hours, and goes to the nurses happily. He has not seen his mother since he was admitted to hospital. What would the nurse understand about Peter's present behavior?
□ 1. He feels better physically and so is behaving better.
□ 2. He has established a routine and likes the nurses.
□ 3. He is repressing feelings about his mother and has given up fighting separation.
□ 4. He is becoming more mature.

A mother brings her 6-week-old infant, Marty, to the emergency room because she says the infant seems very hungry but has been vomiting over the past 3 days. She says that Marty expels the vomitus 2 to 3 feet. The diagnosis of pyloric stenosis is made.

164. During the assessment of Marty, what would the nurse expect to find?
□ 1. Signs of metabolic acidosis, a palpable olive-shaped mass in the epigastric area, and scanty urination.
□ 2. Visible peristaltic waves passing from left to right over the epigastric area, dehydration, and weight loss.
□ 3. Liquid green stools, dehydration, and signs of metabolic acidosis.
□ 4. A palpable sausage-shaped mass in the left upper quadrant, weight loss, and signs of metabolic alkalosis.

165. Marty has corrective surgery (a pylorotomy). He is alert 6 hours following his operation and is ready for his first feeding with glucose water. What position will be best for Marty following his feeding?
□ 1. Prone.
□ 2. Semi-Fowler's on his right side.
□ 3. Flat on his right side.
□ 4. Semi-Fowler's on his left side.

Twelve-year-old Alisa is admitted to the pediatric intensive care unit in a diabetic coma.

166. Which of the following would *not* be an expected finding?
□ 1. Ketonuria.
□ 2. Metabolic acidosis.
□ 3. Low blood glucose.
□ 4. Glycosuria.

167. Alisa's mother is feeling very guilty because she did not realize that her daughter could have had diabetes. She asks about the early signs of insulin-dependent diabetes in children. Which would Alisa *not* have experienced?
□ 1. Increased thirst.
□ 2. Weight loss.

□ 3. Decreased appetite.
□ 4. Increased urinary frequency.

168. After 3 days in intensive care, Alisa is transferred to the pediatric unit for diabetic teaching. When discussing the use of glucagon, the family would be instructed that the purpose of this drug is the treatment of
□ 1. Hyperglycemia.
□ 2. Acidosis.
□ 3. Hypoglycemia.
□ 4. Glycosuria.

169. Alisa is a very active child. Her parents ask if any changes need to be made in Alisa's diet or insulin dosage when she exercises. The nurse tells them that
□ 1. Insulin dosage should be increased before exercise.
□ 2. There is no need to adjust insulin or food intake before exercise.
□ 3. Insulin dosage should be decreased before exercise.
□ 4. Extra caloric intake should be provided before exercise.

170. The nurse is teaching Alisa about the major signs and symptoms of hypoglycemia. Which of the following would *not* be included?
□ 1. Thirst.
□ 2. Tremors.
□ 3. Diaphoresis.
□ 4. Hunger.

171. Because of Alisa's developmental stage, her greatest fear in relation to her diabetes will most likely be
□ 1. Death.
□ 2. Daily insulin injections.
□ 3. Rejection by her peers.
□ 4. Inability to control her diet.

Fifteen-year-old Angela has recently been diagnosed with diabetes.

172. Which of the following situations would indicate that Angela is at greatest risk for a hypoglycemic reaction?
□ 1. She has not taken her insulin for 3 days.
□ 2. Her urine test is positive for acetone.
□ 3. Her urine test is negative for glucose.
□ 4. She had an injection of NPH insulin 30 minutes ago.

173. Angela is invited to a pajama party. Which option indicates the most appropriate action to meet her developmental needs?
□ 1. Keep Angela at home until she knows her diet restrictions.
□ 2. Have Angela explain to her friends that she is diabetic and will bring her own sugar-free drinks.

☐ 3. Adjust her diet and insulin before going to the party so she does not need to eat.

☐ 4. Have Angela's mother call her friend's mother to explain her condition.

Eight-year-old Matt received a diagnosis of cystic fibrosis at 9 months of age. He has done well since then, but he is currently hospitalized for evaluation of his treatment.

174. Which behavioral assessment is most age appropriate for Matt?

☐ 1. He has an imaginary friend named Germaine.

☐ 2. He enjoys riding his bicycle.

☐ 3. He overidentifies with his peers (clothes etc.).

☐ 4. He is afraid of monsters.

175. Which problem of cystic fibrosis is most likely to be present in Matt?

☐ 1. Frequent urinary tract infections.

☐ 2. Large, bulky stools.

☐ 3. Gastric indigestion.

☐ 4. Poor appetite.

176. The physician prescribes pancreatic enzymes (Pancrease) for Matt. Which of the following instructions is most essential regarding this medication?

☐ 1. Mix it with hot food or milk.

☐ 2. Give it q6h around-the-clock.

☐ 3. If Matt skips a meal, do not give the enzyme.

☐ 4. Give more enzymes in very hot weather.

177. Which information is most important for Matt and his family to know before discharge?

☐ 1. Restrict his fluids to reduce excessive sweating.

☐ 2. Encourage quiet activities.

☐ 3. High-salt foods such as pretzels should be a regular part of his diet.

☐ 4. His diet should be high in fat content.

178. Matt's long-term nursing care plan is aimed primarily at which of the following?

☐ 1. Thoroughly educating his parents about cystic fibrosis.

☐ 2. Preventing respiratory infections.

☐ 3. Following his medical regimen.

☐ 4. Teaching him how to live with cystic fibrosis.

Bob Lee, age 7, was admitted yesterday with acute glomerulonephritis and hematuria. He has orders for bed rest, intake and output, blood pressure q2h, a sodium-restricted diet, and daily weights. Bob is an only child, and his parents are almost always present, feeding him and caring for him. Bob seems embarrassed but complies.

179. What additional clinical sign would the nurse expect Bob to exhibit?

☐ 1. Severe, generalized edema.

☐ 2. Markedly decreased serum protein.

☐ 3. Weight loss.

☐ 4. Elevated blood pressure.

180. What nursing diagnosis has the highest priority?

☐ 1. Fluid volume excess related to decreased plasma filtration.

☐ 2. Potential impaired skin integrity related to lowered body defenses.

☐ 3. Fluid volume deficit (intravascular) related to protein loss.

☐ 4. Activity intolerance related to fatigue.

181. The nurse can expect which test result to be elevated?

☐ 1. Liver enzymes.

☐ 2. Serum albumin.

☐ 3. Serum ADH.

☐ 4. Antistreptolysin in O titer (ASO).

182. Choose the primary nursing action to use when working with Bob's mother.

☐ 1. Inform her that her son needs more independence, and encourage her to let him take care of himself.

☐ 2. Spend time at Bob's bedside to explain hospital rules or procedures, or answer any questions that the family may have.

☐ 3. Encourage Mrs. Lee to attend the classes in family health education.

☐ 4. Teach her the basic functions of the kidneys.

Cindy, age 12, reluctantly comes into the emergency room, brought by her mother. Cindy states, "I'm OK now, my stomach doesn't hurt as much." Her mother says that Cindy has been complaining of abdominal pain, has been vomiting for 8 hours, is anorexic, and has been walking with a slight limp. As they got into the car to drive to the hospital, Cindy said that the pain was better.

183. Which admitting order would the nurse question?

☐ 1. Admit for observation.

☐ 2. Give a clear-liquid diet.

☐ 3. Get a complete blood count.

☐ 4. Get an abdominal x-ray.

184. One day after surgical repair of a ruptured appendix, Cindy has a Penrose drain in her incision site and is NPO. Which nursing order is *incorrect*?

☐ 1. Maintain her in a semi-Fowler's position.

☐ 2. Position her on her right side.

☐ 3. Administer broad-spectrum antibiotics as ordered.

☐ 4. Change the dressing q24h.

185. Three days after surgery, Cindy is observed lying on her back with her knees drawn up. Her respirations are irregular, temperature is normal, and her skin is warm and dry. Her abdomen is distended. When Cindy sees the nurse, she cries, "I'm so miserable, the pain is terrible." What initial nursing action is most appropriate?

☐ 1. Call the physician immediately.

☐ 2. Calm Cindy down, and reevaluate her pain in 1 hour.

☐ 3. Insert a rectal tube per physician's order.
☐ 4. Administer an analgesic per physician's order.

186. In evaluating the effectiveness of the nursing action with Cindy, which of the following indicates relief?
☐ 1. Respirations regular.
☐ 2. Pulse full and regular.
☐ 3. Abdomen soft and flat.
☐ 4. Normal perspiration.

Hirschsprung's disease is a mechanical obstruction of the colon caused by a lack of colonic motility resulting from an absence of innervation by the autonomic parasympathetic ganglion cells of the mesenteric and submucosal plexuses.

187. Which of the following is *not* characteristic of a newborn who has Hirschsprung's disease?
☐ 1. Failure to pass meconium within 24 to 48 hours after birth.
☐ 2. Refusal to take liquids.
☐ 3. Abdominal distension.
☐ 4. Frequent, greenish stools.

188. Which of the following is *not* characteristic of Hirschsprung's disease in the older infant?
☐ 1. Failure to thrive.
☐ 2. Constipation.
☐ 3. Diarrhea and vomiting.
☐ 4. Steatorrhea.

189. Preoperative care for the older child with Hirschsprung's disease would include which of the following diets?
☐ 1. Low residue, high calorie, and high protein.
☐ 2. High residue and high calorie.
☐ 3. Clear liquids.
☐ 4. High sodium and low potassium.

190. When Hirschsprung's disease is not diagnosed in infancy, the nurse's role in later diagnostic workup would emphasize
☐ 1. Bowel habits.
☐ 2. Disposition.
☐ 3. Feeding habits.
☐ 4. Skin color.

191. Surgical treatment of Hirschsprung's disease is removal of the affected part of the colon with an accompanying colostomy. When explaining to the parents about the colostomy, the nurse would include which of the following?
☐ 1. The colostomy is usually temporary.
☐ 2. The colostomy is usually permanent.
☐ 3. The colostomy may not be necessary.
☐ 4. The child will have a colostomy until he or she is full-grown.

192. A double-barrel colostomy is frequently performed on children following resection of the affected part of the colon. The nurse accurately evaluates the functioning of this type of colostomy in which of the following ways?

☐ 1. Both the proximal end and the distal end excrete feces.
☐ 2. Only the proximal end excretes feces.
☐ 3. The proximal end allows for excretion of feces; the distal end excretes mucus.
☐ 4. The proximal end allows for excretion of mucus; the distal end excretes feces.

193. Initial postoperative care following colon resection does *not* include
☐ 1. A clear liquid diet.
☐ 2. Nasogastric suction.
☐ 3. Frequent abdominal dressing changes.
☐ 4. IV feedings to replace electrolytes.

194. A diet low in residue is encouraged postoperatively when full bowel function returns. A low-residue diet would *not* include which of the following foods?
☐ 1. Jams and preserves.
☐ 2. White bread.
☐ 3. Vanilla ice cream.
☐ 4. Spaghetti with cream sauce.

A school nurse is planning to screen a school population for scoliosis, beginning with the high-risk group.

195. Which group of students would the nurse begin screening?
☐ 1. Girls and boys 8 to 11 years of age.
☐ 2. Girls 10 to 15 years of age.
☐ 3. Girls 15 to 19 years of age.
☐ 4. Boys 12 to 16 years of age.

196. Scoliosis can be most easily detected if the students are asked to assume which position?
☐ 1. Bend at the waist, to the right, and then to the left.
☐ 2. Stand straight, and then face the nurse with arms raised overhead.
☐ 3. Bend forward at the waist with head and arms hanging freely.
☐ 4. Stand straight with back to the nurse, and arms held out in front of the body.

197. Tina Ford, age 12, was found to have scoliosis during the initial school screening of high-risk groups. Tina states emphatically that it is a waste of time to get her back checked because she will never consider wearing a brace or having surgery. Tina's comment most likely indicates which of the following major fears associated with her age group?
☐ 1. Intrusive procedures.
☐ 2. Body mutilation.
☐ 3. Change in body image.
☐ 4. Separation from her friends.

198. Tina has wide mood swings; she acts like an adult one minute and behaves like a child the next. Which of the following best explains Tina's present behavior fluctuations?

☐ 1. She has regressed because of her impending scoliosis treatment.

☐ 2. She is acting like a normal adolescent.

☐ 3. She fears disruption in identity formation.

☐ 4. She is reassessing her values.

199. Tina is fitted for a Milwaukee brace. When teaching Tina what to expect with the brace, the nurse would explain that

☐ 1. Treatment of scoliosis is short term; the brace will be required for only a few months.

☐ 2. Frequent adjustments of the brace will be needed, because of rapid growth rates during adolescence.

☐ 3. The brace is worn only at night.

☐ 4. A tight fit is necessary, regardless of the discomfort.

200. How does Tina's physical development probably compare to that of boys her age?

☐ 1. She is probably 2 years behind them.

☐ 2. She is developing at about the same rate.

☐ 3. She is probably 2 years ahead of most boys her age.

☐ 4. Since she has scoliosis, her physical development cannot be accurately assessed.

Mary Anderson, 13 years old, is seen in the outpatient clinic. Her mother states that Mary has been complaining of knee and ankle pain. She also seems to bruise easily and upon examination, numerous petechiae and hematomas are noted. Mary has been anorexic, listless, and lethargic. A diagnosis of acute lymphocytic leukemia is made, and Mary is hospitalized.

201. Which of the following roommates would be most appropriate for Mary?

☐ 1. A 12-year-old with an elevated temperature.

☐ 2. A 12-year-old with cystic fibrosis.

☐ 3. A 12-year-old with sickle-cell crisis.

☐ 4. A 12-year-old with a fractured femur.

202. Assuming Mary is a normal 13-year-old, which of the following areas will present the most problems for her?

☐ 1. Family roles.

☐ 2. Limit setting.

☐ 3. School work.

☐ 4. Body image.

203. Mary will require many diagnostic tests, including lumbar puncture and bone marrow aspiration. Which statement reflects an appropriate outcome regarding Mary's acceptance of these tests?

☐ 1. The parents should be present at all tests.

☐ 2. Eventually the tests will become routine and tolerable.

☐ 3. The tests do not involve any risk.

☐ 4. Mary and her parents need to express their feelings about the experience.

204. Which of the following solutions would be most appropriate to use when flushing the IV tubing following Mary's blood transfusion?

☐ 1. Dextrose and water.

☐ 2. Normal saline.

☐ 3. Salt-poor albumin.

☐ 4. Fresh frozen plasma.

205. Mary has a reaction to the transfusion. Which behavior is *not* indicative of a transfusion reaction?

☐ 1. Shivering.

☐ 2. Urticaria.

☐ 3. Hypertension.

☐ 4. Dyspnea.

206. What is the priority nursing action for Mary?

☐ 1. Cover her with a blanket.

☐ 2. Place her in Trendelenburg's position.

☐ 3. Stop the transfusion.

☐ 4. Monitor her pulse, respirations, and blood pressure.

207. Epistaxis could be a serious problem for Mary. If this should develop, what would be the best initial action?

☐ 1. Place her in semi-Fowler's or high-Fowler's position.

☐ 2. Place her in a supine position with a small pillow under her neck.

☐ 3. Administer oxygen through nasal cannula at 4 L/min.

☐ 4. Instruct her to gently blow her nose to dislodge the clot.

208. Mary spikes to a temperature of 104° F (40° C) orally. Which of the following nursing actions would be *contraindicated* for Mary?

☐ 1. Encourage clear fluids as tolerated.

☐ 2. Monitor vital signs qh to q2h.

☐ 3. Administer 2 adult-sized aspirin tablets.

☐ 4. Sponge-bathe her with tepid water.

209. While Mary is acutely ill, the nurse considers how she is likely to view death. Which statement is *inaccurate* about adolescents' concept of death?

☐ 1. They believe that death will not happen to them.

☐ 2. They feel decreased anxiety about death.

☐ 3. They may attempt to exert their own power over mortality by tempting fate.

☐ 4. They may exhibit marked interest in religious beliefs concerning death.

210. In discussing chemotherapy with Mary and her parents, what side effects would *not* be included?

☐ 1. Anorexia.

☐ 2. Alopecia.

☐ 3. Stomatitis.

☐ 4. Peeling skin.

211. Mary is receiving methotrexate. Which of the following is contraindicated with methotrexate administration?

☐ 1. Antibiotics.

☐ 2. Anticholinergic medications.

☐ 3. Vitamins with folic acid.

☐ 4. Antihistamines.

212. Mary is also receiving allopurinol. This drug is given to prevent

☐ 1. Hypokalemia.

☐ 2. Hyperkalemia.

☐ 3. Hypouricemia.

☐ 4. Hyperuricemia.

213. Which of the following nursing actions will be most appropriate for Mary while she is receiving allopurinol?

☐ 1. Encourage oral fluids.

☐ 2. Provide foods high in protein.

☐ 3. Monitor diet for sucrose intake.

☐ 4. Omit carbonated beverages.

214. Which of the following will be *contraindicated* for Mary until her disease is in remission?

☐ 1. Antibiotics.

☐ 2. Immunizations.

☐ 3. Corticosteroids.

☐ 4. Bronchodilators.

215. While Mary's bed is being changed, she cries out loudly and says, "Don't touch me." Which of the following represents an accurate interpretation of this behavior?

☐ 1. Children with leukemia have been overprotected by their parents.

☐ 2. Children with leukemia are easily upset by disruptions in their routine.

☐ 3. Children with leukemia are sensitive to touch and movement.

☐ 4. Children with leukemia tend to employ manipulative techniques.

216. Mary responds well to treatment and is sent home. She is being seen in the outpatient clinic once a week for IV vincristine. Several weeks after discharge, Mrs. Anderson calls the clinic to say that Mary is complaining of weakness in her hands and feet, numbness, tingling, and jaw pain. What is the nurse's best approach?

☐ 1. Tell her this is part of the disease process, and it will disappear in 4 to 6 months.

☐ 2. Recognize that Mary's mother will be very sensitive to any change in her condition.

☐ 3. Suggest that Mrs. Anderson mention this at Mary's next checkup.

☐ 4. Tell her to notify the physician because these are manifestations of vincristine toxicity.

Wilms' tumor is the most frequent intraabdominal tumor of childhood and the most common type of cancer of the kidney.

217. The highest occurrence of Wilms' tumor is at which age?

☐ 1. Birth to 2 years.

☐ 2. 3 to 4 years.

☐ 3. 6 to 8 years.

☐ 4. 7 to 10 years.

218. What is the most frequent sign of Wilms' tumor?

☐ 1. Increasing abdominal girth.

☐ 2. Decreased urinary output.

☐ 3. Hypertension.

☐ 4. Weight loss.

219. What is the best method of teaching the toddler about preoperative and postoperative care?

☐ 1. Mimicry using dolls.

☐ 2. Audiovisual devices.

☐ 3. Verbal explanations.

☐ 4. Peer play.

220. Preoperative nursing care for the child with Wilms' tumor does *not* include

☐ 1. Preparing the child and family for preoperative tests.

☐ 2. Carefully monitoring blood pressure.

☐ 3. Palpating the abdomen to identify the tumor size.

☐ 4. Planning for postoperative care.

221. What is the overall goal in planning for discharge?

☐ 1. Decreasing effects of chemotherapy.

☐ 2. Preventing nausea and vomiting.

☐ 3. Planning for psychological support.

☐ 4. Returning the child to a normal preoperative life-style.

222. Which of the following is most important in helping parents learn about postoperative home care needs for the child?

☐ 1. Include the parents in implementing the care plans while the child is still in the hospital.

☐ 2. Give the parents informative home care literature to read.

☐ 3. Save teaching until discharge is imminent.

☐ 4. Allow the parents free time before teaching is begun.

REFERENCES

Foster, R., Hunsberger, M., & Anderson, J. (1989). *Family-centered nursing care of children*. Philadelphia: Saunders.

Govoni, L., & Hayes, J. (1988). *Drugs and nursing implications*. Norwalk, CT: Appleton & Lange.

Pilitteri, A. (1987). *Child health nursing: Care of the growing family* (3rd ed.). Boston: Little, Brown.

Whaley, L., & Wong, D. (1991). *Nursing care of infants and children* (4th ed.). St. Louis: Mosby–Year Book.

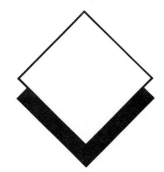

Correct Answers

1. no. 1.	**41.** no. 3.	**81.** no. 1.	**121.** no. 2.
2. no. 4.	**42.** no. 4.	**82.** no. 2.	**122.** no. 4.
3. no. 2.	**43.** no. 1.	**83.** no. 1.	**123.** no. 1.
4. no. 1.	**44.** no. 3.	**84.** no. 2.	**124.** no. 4.
5. no. 2.	**45.** no. 3.	**85.** no. 3.	**125.** no. 2.
6. no. 4.	**46.** no. 3.	**86.** no. 2.	**126.** no. 3.
7. no. 4.	**47.** no. 3.	**87.** no. 4.	**127.** no. 4.
8. no. 4.	**48.** no. 3.	**88.** no. 1.	**128.** no. 4.
9. no. 4.	**49.** no. 2.	**89.** no. 3.	**129.** no. 3.
10. no. 1.	**50.** no. 4.	**90.** no. 3.	**130.** no. 2.
11. no. 3.	**51.** no. 1.	**91.** no. 1.	**131.** no. 3.
12. no. 1.	**52.** no. 3.	**92.** no. 1.	**132.** no. 1.
13. no. 3.	**53.** no. 4.	**93.** no. 2.	**133.** no. 1.
14. no. 1.	**54.** no. 1.	**94.** no. 4.	**134.** no. 3.
15. no. 4.	**55.** no. 4.	**95.** no. 1.	**135.** no. 4.
16. no. 3.	**56.** no. 4.	**96.** no. 3.	**136.** no. 4.
17. no. 3.	**57.** no. 3.	**97.** no. 4.	**137.** no. 3.
18. no. 3.	**58.** no. 1.	**98.** no. 2.	**138.** no. 3.
19. no. 1.	**59.** no. 2.	**99.** no. 1.	**139.** no. 3.
20. no. 1.	**60.** no. 2.	**100.** no. 2.	**140.** no. 1.
21. no. 2.	**61.** no. 3.	**101.** no. 2.	**141.** no. 1.
22. no. 3.	**62.** no. 1.	**102.** no. 4.	**142.** no. 2.
23. no. 1.	**63.** no. 3.	**103.** no. 1.	**143.** no. 2.
24. no. 1.	**64.** no. 2.	**104.** no. 3.	**144.** no. 3.
25. no. 2.	**65.** no. 4.	**105.** no. 4.	**145.** no. 1.
26. no. 2.	**66.** no. 1.	**106.** no. 4.	**146.** no. 2.
27. no. 1.	**67.** no. 4.	**107.** no. 3.	**147.** no. 4.
28. no. 3.	**68.** no. 1.	**108.** no. 2.	**148.** no. 2.
29. no. 4.	**69.** no. 3.	**109.** no. 4.	**149.** no. 2.
30. no. 2.	**70.** no. 1.	**110.** no. 1.	**150.** no. 1.
31. no. 1.	**71.** no. 3.	**111.** no. 1.	**151.** no. 2.
32. no. 4.	**72.** no. 3.	**112.** no. 3.	**152.** no. 3.
33. no. 1.	**73.** no. 2.	**113.** no. 2.	**153.** no. 3.
34. no. 2.	**74.** no. 2.	**114.** no. 4.	**154.** no. 3.
35. no. 3.	**75.** no. 3.	**115.** no. 1.	**155.** no. 1.
36. no. 2.	**76.** no. 1.	**116.** no. 1.	**156.** no. 2.
37. no. 2.	**77.** no. 1.	**117.** no. 3.	**157.** no. 1.
38. no. 1.	**78.** no. 2.	**118.** no. 4.	**158.** no. 3.
39. no. 2.	**79.** no. 1.	**119.** no. 3.	**159.** no. 1.
40. no. 3.	**80.** no. 3.	**120.** no. 2.	**160.** no. 2.

161. no. 1.
162. no. 2.
163. no. 3.
164. no. 2.
165. no. 2.
166. no. 3.
167. no. 3.
168. no. 3.
169. no. 4.
170. no. 1.
171. no. 3.
172. no. 3.
173. no. 2.
174. no. 2.
175. no. 2.
176. no. 3.

177. no. 3.
178. no. 4.
179. no. 4.
180. no. 1.
181. no. 4.
182. no. 2.
183. no. 2.
184. no. 4.
185. no. 3.
186. no. 3.
187. no. 4.
188. no. 4.
189. no. 1.
190. no. 1.
191. no. 1.
192. no. 3.

193. no. 1.
194. no. 1.
195. no. 2.
196. no. 3.
197. no. 3.
198. no. 2.
199. no. 2.
200. no. 3.
201. no. 4.
202. no. 4.
203. no. 4.
204. no. 2.
205. no. 3.
206. no. 3.
207. no. 1.

208. no. 3.
209. no. 2.
210. no. 4.
211. no. 3.
212. no. 4.
213. no. 1.
214. no. 2.
215. no. 3.
216. no. 4.
217. no. 2.
218. no. 1.
219. no. 1.
220. no. 3.
221. no. 4.
222. no. 1.

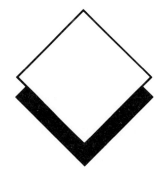

Correct Answers with Rationales

Editor's note: Three pieces of information are supplied at the end of each rationale. First, you will find a reference to a section in the *AJN/Mosby Nursing Boards Review* where a more complete discussion of the topic may be found, should you desire more information. A second reference indicates what part of the nursing process the question addresses. The third piece of information describes the appropriate client need category.

KEY TO ABBREVIATIONS
Section of the Review Book

C = Child
  H = Healthy Child
  I = Ill and Hospitalized Child
  SPP = Sensation, Perception, and Protection
  O = Oxygenation
  NM = Nutrition and Metabolism
  E = Elimination
  M = Mobility
  CA = Cellular Aberration

Nursing process category

AS = Assessment
AN = Analysis
PL = Plan
IM = Implementation
EV = Evaluation

Client need category

E = Safe, Effective Care Environment
PS = Physiological Integrity
PC = Psychosocial Integrity
H = Health Promotion/Maintenance

1. no. 1. Bowel control comes at about 18 months, depending on the developmental readiness of the child; readiness for daytime bladder training does not happen until the child is 2 to 3 years of age. C/H, IM, H
2. no. 4. Unless the child is developmentally ready, toilet training only serves to train the parent and may produce frustration. C/H, AN, H
3. no. 2. Autonomy and independence are the tasks of this age. Option no. 3 is a task of infancy; options no. 1 and no. 4 are strategies for task achievement. C/H, AN, H
4. no. 1. This answer gives the child a limited choice and avoids a "no" answer, at least most of the time. Option no. 4 is unacceptable because it is unnecessarily punitive. Although it is important to set consistent limits, option no. 2 will only increase her resistance. Option no. 3 does not address the need for fluids, and toddlers are usually picky eaters. C/H, IM, H
5. no. 2. Setting consistent limits teaches the child self-control and provides a sense of security. "Punishment" by removing the child from an undesirable situation is only effective if limits are known by the child beforehand. C/H, PL,
6. no. 4. Four-year-olds have a decreased appetite because their growth slows; they often pick a favorite food and need to choose the amount to eat. Small helpings at mealtime, plus nutritious snacks at midmorning and midafternoon, should be offered to them without bribes or threats. C/H, IM, H
7. no. 4. Lights help to decrease fears of the dark. Allowing the child to control the lights will enable him to control his fear. Exploring the room with a flashlight would increase fears at this age. Options no. 1 and no. 2 do not allow the child to get used to the dark and deal with his overactive imagination. C/H, IM, H
8. no. 4. Nighttime control is achieved between 4 and 5 years of age. This option is supportive and gently encouraging. Option no. 3 places all the responsibility on the child, at the same time indicating by the diapers that the child probably will not be successful. Option no. 2 sets unrealistic expectations. Option no. 1 is rigid and only emphasizes his "failure." C/H, IM, PS

9. no. 4. It is important to acknowledge the child's imagination; this will be the source of creativity in later life. Options no. 1 and no. 2 are not true; the child is not lying. Option no. 3 is all right, but it does not have the positive aspect that no. 4 has. C/H, IM, H

10. no. 1. Preschoolers need to explore their bodies, but they can begin to learn family and social limits at this age. Option no. 4 is untrue. Options no. 2 and no. 3 communicate to the child that masturbation is wrong. C/H, IM, PC

11. no. 3. Temper tantrums are the toddler's way of releasing tension and aggression and are used to gain control. It is a normal, age-appropriate behavior. C/H, IM, H

12. no. 1. According to the American Academy of Pediatrics recommended schedule, Kimberly should receive DTP and OPV boosters (these should be given once between 4 and 6 years of age). C/H, PL, PS

13. no. 3. This behavior is very normal at this age and should be handled matter-of-factly. However, Kimberly's mother should take the opportunity to explain to both children that there are other, more acceptable ways they can satisfy their curiosity, such as asking their parents questions or reading age-appropriate education materials. C/H, IM, PC

14. no. 1. Most children between 5 and 8 years of age are not aware that they themselves will die; this realization comes around age 9 to 10 years, along with the awareness that death is inevitable for everyone. Option no. 2 is typical of the preschool child who perceives death as sleeping. C/H, AN, H

15. no. 4. School-age children are old enough to learn to problem solve, cooperate, bargain, and compromise; the family is the most important place to learn these skills. To motivate school-age children, listen to their ideas and facilitate a problem-solving attitude. C/H, IM, H

16. no. 3. Depriving a child of food as punishment sets up a control struggle and is unnecessary; withholding other kinds of treats or using methods relevant to the causes of behavior is more effective in teaching healthy habits. C/H, PL, H

17. no. 3. Stressing the importance of good table manners is not effective. It is more effective to give information or teach the child to increase his own awareness by keeping a journal. C/H, PL, H

18. no. 3. According to Erikson, this is the task for the 6-to-12 age group. C/H, AN, PC

19. no. 1. Concrete operations covers the ages from 7 to 11. Preoperational thinking occurs in the preschool age, and formal operations is the final stage. C/H, AN, PC

20. no. 1. A 6-year-old has sufficient understanding of time to prepare cognitively for future events. The general guideline for children between ages 2 and 7 years is to tell them the number of days ahead for each year of age. The day of admission is too late to meet staff. Preadmission tours are advisable. Option no. 3 is unrealistic, and no. 4 would be too graphic and likely to increase fear. C/I, PL, PC

21. no. 2. For school-age children, loss of control and separation from peers are the major fears. Option no. 1 relates to toddlers, no. 3 to adolescents, and no. 4 relates to preschoolers because of their exaggerated fears and active imaginations. C/I, AN, PC

22. no. 3. This option gives the child realistic information; lying or telling the child not to complain will not help the child adjust. Suggesting the child might get very sick and need a blood transfusion is unnecessary and frightening. Unloaded, simple explanations are best. C/I, IM, E

23. no. 1. Tonsillectomy does not usually involve use of sutures, so the denuded area has the potential to bleed. The area is also highly vascular. Any bleeding dyscrasias must be checked preoperatively. Option no. 2 is elevated in allergic conditions, no. 3 is increased in chronic infections and arthritis, and no. 4 is altered in metabolic acidosis, none of which would be significant for a tonsillectomy. C/I, PL, PS

24. no. 1. Any indication of an infection, such as an elevated temperature, is a contraindication for surgery. The decision must be made by the physician. Options no. 3 and no. 4 would occur after calling the physician. C/SPP, IM, E

25. no. 2. This position prevents aspiration of any secretions or blood and helps to keep the airway clear. C/SPP, PL, E

26. no. 2. These are signs of hemorrhage, the major postoperative complication. Options no. 1 and no. 4 are expected and normal responses. Option no. 3 often results from altered sensation after anesthesia and increased output from IV fluids. C/SPP, AN, PS

27. no. 1. Children often regress in the hospital and need support from parents. Quiet holding and rocking prevent crying and facilitate healing. C/SPP, IM, E

28. no. 3. Recovery should be complete in a week. Gargling is contraindicated; delayed hemorrhage occurs between the fifth and tenth postoperative day. C/SPP, PL, PS

29. no. 4. A bulging fontanel is the most significant indication of increased intracranial pressure that would result from cerebral edema secondary to the bacterial infection. Options no. 2 and no. 4 are indicative of dehydration from the vomiting. The

specific gravity is normal. C/SPP, AS, PS

30. no. 2. The definitive test for meningitis is a lumbar puncture to obtain a cerebrospinal fluid specimen for culture. C/SPP, AN, PS

31. no. 1. Administration of potassium in the presence of diminished renal function may lead to hyperkalemia because potassium is excreted through the kidneys. C/SPP, AS, PS

32. no. 4. Children with meningitis are sensitive to sensory stimuli that can precipitate seizures. The activity involved in bathing could cause a seizure and would be unnecessary during the acute stage of the illness. All other options would be followed. C/SPP, PL, E

33. no. 1. Specific antibiotic therapy must be instituted immediately to prevent death and to avert residual disabilities. Isolation is only needed for 24 hours after antibiotics are begun. Support for parents is a secondary goal during this life-threatening situation. Option no. 4 is never appropriate. C/SPP, PL, PS

34. no. 2. Penicillin must be given for the entire course (usually about 10 days). Options no. 1 and no. 4 are contraindicated; option no. 3 is not as important as no. 2. C/SPP, IM, H

35. no. 3. Vision is fully developed by age 7. Option no. 1 is more appropriate for an older child. Option no. 2 is fine from 3 to 7 years, and no. 4 is appropriate for toddlers. C/SPP, IM, H

36. no. 2. Scratching the anal area at night and insomnia are characteristic of pinworm infestation. Option no. 4 also causes itching, but the parasite infects epidermis, not living tissue. Neither no. 1 nor no. 2 causes itching. C/SPP, AN, PS

37. no. 2. The sticky surface of the tape over the anus can pick up ova in less than a minute in the early morning. Option no. 1 is rarely used in young children. Option no. 4 is a test for syphilis. C/SPP, PL, PS

38. no. 1. Children often regress to previous patterns when they are hospitalized; the 4-year-old child sleeps soundly and may sleep right through the urge to urinate. Putting a 4-year-old in diapers in the hospital is not appropriate, since this encourages regression and does not help the child move to the next developmental task. C/SPP, IM, H

39. no. 2. Personnel at both the poison control center and the emergency room will need to know the substance consumed. Observing and waiting for symptoms to develop may use up too much valuable time. C/SPP, IM, PS

40. no. 3. This is an emetic. Tepid water in small amounts increases gastric irritation. Option no. 1 is appropriate for hydrocarbon ingestion. By the time symptoms appear, the substance has been absorbed, and time has been wasted. Option no. 4 is

given *after* an emetic to help absorb many compounds. C/SPP, IM, PS

41. no. 3. She is too young to understand or remember everything that is poisonous. It is the poorest of the four choices. The other options prevent access or condition her to respect medicine. C/SPP, PL, H

42. no. 4. This is the only option that addresses prevention. She has actually followed through on what she learned and provided a safe environment for her toddler. The other options are short term or are aimed at intervention after poisoning has occurred. C/SPP, EV, PS

43. no. 1. This is characteristic of the 24-month-old child. All the other behaviors are characteristic of a younger child. C/SPP, AS, H

44. no. 3. Spastic cerebral palsy results in hypertonicity of muscles and reflexes, leading to scissoring of legs. Mental retardation is not necessarily an associated problem. C/SPP, AS, PS

45. no. 3. Sandy needs assistance with feeding because of her motor impairment. This approach is the safest while providing motor stability to improve feeding. C/SPP, IM, H

46. no. 3. Reflecting the mother's feelings opens communication for further exploration and expression of her specific concerns. C/SPP, IM, H

47. no. 3. This is the only description that is characteristic of second-degree burns. The other options are characteristic of third-degree burns. C/SPP, AS, PS

48. no. 3. Children with orofacial burns are at risk of developing upper airway edema. Option no. 4 would be important information to obtain after the child was stabilized. C/SPP, PL, PS

49. no. 2. Blood volume is reduced from the fluid loss resulting in poor peripheral absorption. Even though the IV route is the fastest, that is not the reason it would be selected for this child. C/SPP, AN, PS

50. no. 4. There is no way to accurately determine fluid loss from wounds. The other options are more accurate measures. C/SPP, EV, PS

51. no. 1. Mafenide acetate (Sulfamylon) is a carbonic anhydrase inhibitor and can lead to impairment of the renal buffering system. The other options are side effects of silver nitrate. C/SPP, AS, PS

52. no. 3. The major cause of death in burn clients is infection, so this is the primary goal. The other options would be important secondary goals. C/SPP, PL, PS

53. no. 4. By 9 months, a child can eat ground or pureed meats. This child needs protein sources that are easily digestible. Option no. 1 contains foods that can cause choking (raisins and hot dogs). Option no. 3 contains egg whites (omelet), which should not be introduced until 1 year of age. C/ SPP, EV, H

54. no. 1. Children with Down syndrome are hypotonic, not spastic. This decreased muscle tone compromises respiratory excursion, making the child more prone to respiratory infections. Hypotonicity may also delay achievement of motor skills, but developmental potential is greatest during infancy. What to expect needs to be reinforced with parents, because they may see their child developing along a somewhat normal developmental curve and thus come to have unrealistic expectations of the final potential. C/SPP, IM, H

55. no. 4. Trisomy 21, or Down syndrome, is caused by the presence of an extra chromosome 21. All other options are true. C/SPP, AN, PS

56. no. 4. Although teaching socially acceptable behaviors is important in "normalizing" the child, mentally retarded children really need consistency and structure in their daily routines to foster learning and promote security. Limiting stimulation will not promote the mentally retarded child's optimal development. Having the same parent always work with the child to learn new skills is unrealistic. C/ SPP, PL, E

57. no. 3. The initial phase of grief is shock and disbelief. C/SPP, AN, PC

58. no. 1. It is very important for Mr. Carlton to have contact with his new baby so he can begin to develop an attachment to her and to see her as a baby first and then as a baby with a health problem. Role-modeling parenting behaviors is helpful for parents who are grieving. C/SPP, IM, PC

59. no. 2. Rupture of the sac can cause leakage of cerebrospinal fluid and lead to central nervous system infection with permanent brain damage. C/ SPP, PL, E

60. no. 2. Although the myelomeningocele requires taking special precautions, these infants can be held. Touch is the most comforting, highly developed sense in infants. The other measures would stimulate the visual and hearing senses, but would not be as comforting as touch. C/SPP, IM, H

61. no. 3. If a dressing is ordered, it must be kept moist to prevent damage to the friable covering of the myelomeningocele. C/SPP, IM, E

62. no. 1. The most common complication following surgical closure of a myelomeningocele is hydrocephalus. Daily measurement of the head circumference is essential for early detection and treatment of this complication. C/SPP, AS, PS

63. no. 3. The number of drops per minute is equal to the number of milliliters per hour when a microdrip is used. C/SPP, IM, PS

64. no. 2. Keeping her hips abducted encourages the hip joints to develop normally, decreasing the prob-

ability of congenital hip dysplasia. C/SPP, PL, PS

65. no. 4. The first priority is to prevent Natalie from injuring herself on the crib rails during the seizure. Tongue blades are never used for seizures. Oxygen would only be given for prolonged apnea after a seizure. C/SPP, IM, PS

66. no. 1. Children tend to eliminate anticonvulsants more readily and therefore are usually given higher doses to achieve desired blood levels of the drug. C/SPP, AN, PS

67. no. 4. Although phenytoin may cause malaise, it does not cause excessive sleepiness in children (as phenobarbital may) and is often selected as the drug of choice for this reason. C/SPP, IM, PS

68. no. 1. A high-pitched cry is one of the key manifestations of increased intracranial pressure in infants. Other signs include bulging fontanel and dilated pupils. Reflexes are not affected. C/SPP, AS, PS

69. no. 3. The shunt may become obstructed with cells or tissue debris. Infection is also a common complication of shunt insertion. C/SPP, AN, PS

70. no. 1. It is essential to maintain patency of the shunt by pumping the valve in order to prevent any increase in intracranial pressure. C/SPP, PL, PS

71. no. 3. Overhydration can cause an increase in intracranial pressure and thus interfere with shunt functioning or cause damage to brain cells. C/SPP, PL, PS

72. no. 3. The major goal of treatment is to prevent neurological damage. This is best evaluated by appraising the child's neurological functioning using cognitive and motor development as indicators. C/ SPP, EV, H

73. no. 2. An aura is a sensory clue that often precedes a generalized tonic-clonic seizure. Absence seizures do not have an aura. C/SPP, AS, PS

74. no. 2. This is the only test listed that is diagnostic of seizure disorders. C/SPP, PL, PS

75. no. 3. Sudden withdrawal of medication can precipitate status epilepticus. All other options are correct. C/SPP, EV, H

76. no. 1. In their shock, numbness, and disbelief immediately after their daughter's death, the Howards will not be able to grasp a detailed explanation and may be overwhelmed by it. All the other options provide support and comfort, which are the priority goals. C/O, IM

77. no. 1. The nurse is reflecting what she perceives the father is saying as a way to help him identify his feelings. Guilt is a normal response to SIDS. Options no. 2 and no. 4 are not helpful. Option no. 3 does not respond to the feelings expressed. C/O, IM, PC

78. no. 2. Involvement in a parents' support group indicates the Howards' willingness to face and deal

openly with their daughter's death. C/O, EV, PC

79. no. 1. Diminished breath sounds occur because of bronchiolitic obstruction. If a cough were present, it would be moist, not dry. Option no. 3 indicates upper respiratory problems. Expirations are long because air is trapped in lower field. C/O, AS, PS

80. no. 3. An infant with very fast respirations barely has a chance to swallow before he must take another breath, thus making aspiration a real possibility. Hydration is a major concern because the infant loses fluid with easy respiration. Options no. 1 and no. 2 are false. C/O, AN, PS

81. no. 1. Accumulation of mucus occurs at the bronchiolar level; therefore suctioning would not be effective. C/O, PL, E

82. no. 2. A semi-Fowler's position facilitates expansion of the lungs. C/O, PL, PS

83. no. 1. Performing chest physical therapy before meals minimizes the possibility of vomiting. Every 8 hours is too long an interval. C/O, PL, PS

84. no. 2. An infant's birth weight should double by 5 to 6 months and triple at 1 year (3.5 kg × 2 = 7 kg [15 pounds 7 ounces]). C/H, AS, H

85. no. 3. Voluntary grasping and improved eye-hand coordination enable the infant to begin picking up finger foods. Options no. 2 and no. 4 would meet his nutritional needs rather than his developmental needs. Egg whites are not given until after 1 year of age. C/H, PL, H

86. no. 2. Rice cereal is hypoallergenic and is easily digested. The other options have a higher propensity for causing allergy. C/H, PL, H

87. no. 4. Tuberculin testing provides systematic screening of the population; it is usually done before the measles, mumps, and rubella vaccination. C/O, PL, PS

88. no. 1. Instillation of several milliliters of sterile saline loosens thick secretions and mechanically stimulates the cough reflex. It has nothing to do with sleep patterns, nor is saline a source for fluid intake. The saline instillation makes suctioning more effective. A/O, AN, PS

89. no. 3. This action provides baseline information regarding the need for and effectiveness of suctioning. Placing him in a chair would be determined by his medical problem rather than the suctioning. A/O, IM, PS

90. no. 3. The act of suctioning mechanically removes oxygen directly from the airway. Presuction oxygenation replaces that oxygen so that the child does not become hypoxic. Oxygen will not directly relax Pedro, but the lack of oxygen will cause him to become agitated. A/O, AN, PS

91. no. 1. The outer cannula is never removed. The inner cannula is cleaned every shift and as needed. Pediatric tracheal tubes are not cuffed in order to prevent tracheal damage. A/O, IM, PS

92. no. 1. Suctioning will improve respiratory exchange; therefore breath sounds will be improved. Options no. 2, no. 3, and no. 4 are evidence of continued respiratory problems. A/O, EV, PS

93. no. 2. Ampicillin destroys the normal flora of the gastrointestinal tract; yogurt will help promote its return. C/O, IM, H

94. no. 4. Cromolyn sodium is an inhalant that can irritate the throat and trachea. It suppresses histamine and is used prophylactically. C/O, AN, PS

95. no. 1. Ten-year-olds can understand some abstract concepts, including math. Options no. 3 and no. 4 are typical of early adolescence, and no. 2 reflects behaviors of the early school-age child. C/H, AS, H

96. no. 3. Medications that interfere with the cough reflex are contraindicated. The priority concern during an acute asthma attack is to promote effective air exchange by loosening secretions, so they can be coughed up and expectorated. C/O, IM, PS

97. no. 4. The 6-year-old is in a stage of concrete operations and needs to test new experiences firsthand. C/H, IM, PL

98. no. 2. The methylxanthines, of which aminophylline is one, are used IV during an acute attack. Initially, as an emergency measure, epinephrine is used as a short-acting bronchodilator. It is only given subcutaneously, never IV. Cromolyn sodium is used prophylactically. Penicillin would be used if a concurrent infection, sensitive to the drug, existed. C/I, PL, PS

99. no. 1. The school-age child's greatest fear is loss of control. This is especially accentuated by frightening experiences such as hospitalization and an acute asthma attack. Option no. 3 would be of lesser priority during recuperation. Options no. 2 and no. 4 are appropriate for younger children. C/O, PL, E

100. no. 2. The risk of having an asthma attack is lessened when the asthmatic child's immunizations are up-to-date and when she has received seasonal flu shots. Her room should be kept as dust free as possible. Option no. 3 is not safe and no. 4 is not necessary. C/O, IM, H

101. no. 2. Hemolytic anemia is present throughout the life of a child with sickle-cell disease; option no. 1 is a condition seen in infants, and answer no. 3 is a clinical sign common in Down syndrome. Pallor precedes jaundice by several days. C/O, AS, PS

102. no. 4. Infections are the major predisposing factor of crisis episodes. Strenuous exertion rather than mild exercise, cold temperatures, dehydration, and environments of low oxygen concentration cause crises. C/O, AS, PS

103. no. 1. Heat increases circulation (and oxygen) to the area that needs it most. Blood transfusions are not used unless the hemoglobin is 4 g or less. Limiting fluids increases problems with sickling. C/O, IM, E

104. no. 3. This test distinguishes between the heterozygous (trait) and homozygous (disease) genetic pattern. Usually a Sickledex is done for mass screening because it shows that the Hb S is present. It does not differentiate between the individual who is heterozygous or homozygous. Option no. 2 is done prenatally to examine amniotic fluid for genetic testing. C/O, AS, H

105. no. 4. Hemarthrosis (bleeding into a joint space) is the classic sign of hemophilia and the manifestation most likely to cause serious or permanent sequelae. C/O, AS, PS

106. no. 4. This allows Darryl to be involved with his peers and also maintain his interest in football. C/O, PL, PC

107. no. 3. Packed cells do not contain factor VIII, the needed coagulation factor. C/O, AN, PS

108. no. 2. Affected joints should be immobilized in a slightly flexed position during the bleeding episode. Aspirin and heat are contraindicated because they may exacerbate the bleeding. C/O, IM, PS

109. no. 4. Hemophilia is a sex-linked recessive disorder transmitted to offspring by female carriers. Darryl's sons will receive a normal sex chromosome from each parent. His daughters will all receive the abnormal "Xr" chromosome from him and thus will be carriers. C/O, AN, PS

110. no. 1. Prevention and control of bleeding episodes is the priority concern. Therefore the fewer the number of bleeding episodes the child has, the more successful the outcomes of treatment. C/O, EV, H

111. no. 1. A normally developing 1-year-old will be cruising and possibly walking. The other behaviors are accomplished in later months. C/H, AS, H

112. no. 3. The PPD skin test is interpreted in terms of induration, not erythema. Induration of 10 mm or more is considered positive. A lesion with 5 to 9 mm of induration is considered doubtful, although it may indicate tuberculosis in a child less than 2 years old. C/SPP, AS, PS

113. no. 2. Isoniaziad (INH) is the major treatment for tuberculosis and is often given with rifampin (RMP). None of the other drugs are given for tuberculosis. C/SPP, PL, H

114. no. 4. The usual course of treatment is at least a year. A sputum specimen, if needed, is only done for diagnostic purposes. The diet should be particularly high in calcium and nitrogen. Children can return to school almost immediately if they are feeling well. C/SPP, EV, H

115. no. 1. In addition to addressing the mother's concerns, the nurse should give Barbara a simple, honest explanation of the basic steps in the cardiac catheterization. Because 4-year-old children are in the preoperational period of cognitive development, they are capable of prelogical reasoning about medical interventions. C/O, IM, PC

116. no. 1. Barbara desperately needs her "security" object to give her a sense of constancy and comfort, especially during the stressful period of hospitalization. C/I, IM, PC

117. no. 3. The best course of action for dealing with a hospitalized toddler going through the protest phase of separation anxiety would be to stay with the child and offer support and comfort. C/I, IM, PC

118. no. 4. A sinus dysrhythmia is a normal physiological phenomenon of childhood. The heart rate increases on inspiration and decreases on expiration. Breath holding causes the rate to remain steady, thus allowing assessment between breaths of any potentially pathological dysrhythmia. C/O, AS, PS

119. no. 3. The left-to-right shunt with a ventricular septal defect causes increased blood flow to the lungs because extra amounts of blood enter the right ventricle and are carried to the lungs through the pulmonary artery. C/O, AN, PS

120. no. 2. Children with cardiac problems are particularly susceptible to recurrent upper respiratory tract infections. This results from pulmonary vascular congestion, since large amounts of blood pool in the lungs. C/O, AN, PS

121. no. 2. Parents of children with congenital heart disease frequently attempt to overprotect their children, because of their fears of overexerting and exposing the child to environmental risks. The child may have had fewer opportunities for coping with frustrations or delayed gratification. C/O, AN, H

122. no. 4. Most children with exercise intolerance rest when they need to do so. Option no. 2 is incorrect because a ventricular septal defect is an acyanotic problem that does not cause anemia. C/O, IM, H

123. no. 1. This is a part of preoperative teaching to decrease the child's fear of the tent after surgery. C/O, PL, PS

124. no. 4. This is an abnormally slow pulse for a 3-year-old, and thus digoxin is contraindicated. C/O, IM, PS

125. no. 2.

$$\frac{.05 \text{ mg}}{1 \text{ ml}} \times \frac{.06 \text{ mg}}{x \text{ ml}}$$

$$.05x = .06 \text{ ml}$$

$$x = 1.2 \text{ ml}$$

$$\frac{1 \text{ ml}}{15 \text{ min}} \times \frac{1.2}{x}$$

$$x = 18 \text{ minims}$$

C/O, IM, PS

126. no. 3. Digoxin slows conduction as a result of decreased cardiac rate. It enhances urinary output by increasing renal perfusion. C/O, AN, PS

127. no. 4. Hypothermia reduces oxygen needs during surgery by decreasing metabolic rate. Too low temperatures can stop cardiac functioning, an undesirable effect. Option no. 1 is unaffected. Respirations are controlled by a mechanical ventilator. C/O, AN, PS

128. no. 4. Two to three chest tubes are placed for drainage or suction, or both, to remove fluid and air that entered the pleural cavity and mediastinal space during surgery. C/O, AN, PS

129. no. 3. A chest drainage system will remove solids, such as fibrin or clotted blood; liquids, such as serous fluids; and gaseous materials. "Milking" the tubes prevents them from becoming plugged with clots or other material. The thoracotomy tube should be immediately clamped if it becomes disconnected to prevent air from entering the pleural cavity and causing a possible tension pneumothorax. C/O, IM, PS

130. no. 2. Placement of the nurse's hands on either side of the operative site (encircling the chest) may reduce the pain associated with the coughing procedure by decreasing movement in the area. A side-lying position would encourage better drainage and may be easier for him to tolerate than sitting up. C/O, IM, PS

131. no. 3. Hospitalization and stress cause regression in toddlers, and regression is best dealt with by accepting the behavior. C/O, IM, PC

132. no. 1. During the convalescent period, it is most appropriate to focus upon management of the child in a manner that will promote a healthy life-style. The child's heart defect is likely to have been associated with parental anxiety and overprotective behavior. Parents must be told to treat a child like Ronald as they would any other child. C/O, PL, H

133. no. 1. Temper tantrums are best handled by ignoring them. Without the attention, toddlers will stop using this behavior. C/O, EV, H

134. no. 3. Use of large muscles, as in throwing, allows for a safe release of energy. C/O, IM, PC

135. no. 4. This syndrome usually describes infants who fail to gain weight as a result of psychosocial factors, such as interference with parent-infant attachment or environmental deprivation. Option no. 1 is a possible cause of *organic* failure to thrive. C/NM, AN, PC

136. no. 4. The infant with failure to thrive avoids eye contact with others, has a flat affect, is withdrawn, and does not exhibit any stranger anxiety. When held, these infants often become very stiff and try to pull away. C/NM, AS, H

137. no. 3. Head control comes at 2 months; rolling over comes at 5 months; sitting without support and transferring objects from one hand to another come at 8 months. Marcus is around 5 to 6 months developmentally. C/NM, AN, E

138. no. 3. The infant with failure to thrive needs to have one primary caregiver per shift so that trust can be established; having many persons pick up the child ad lib does not help promote bonding. A schedule of stimulation geared to the infant's developmental level and given by the primary caregiver would be more helpful. C/NM, PL, E

139. no. 3. Infant and mother must be cared for as a unit. Marcus can be helped most by promoting his mother's feelings of worth and confidence in her mothering role and behaviors. Option no. 2 would be a secondary goal. Once mother feels better about herself, she will be more able to use the information. C/NM, IM, E

140. no. 1. Stacking blocks are appropriate for a toddler who has developed fine motor control. C/NM, IM, H

141. no. 1. Weight gain reflects the nurturance that Marcus is receiving and is the most important measure of improvement with nonorganic failure to thrive. The other options are not valid measures of reversal of failure to thrive. C/NM, AN, H

142. no. 2. The ultimate concern in treating the infant with failure to thrive is restoring physical growth to normal limits for age. Weight gain especially is used as an indicator that the infant is responding to treatment. C/NM, EV, H

143. no. 2. In mild dehydration, the body compensates for fluid loss with increased heart rate and peripheral vasoconstriction, which maintains a normal blood pressure. The peripheral vasoconstriction decreases blood supply to the kidneys, resulting in a decreased urine output with increased specific gravity. Low blood pressure is a finding in severe dehydration when compensatory mechanisms have failed. C/NM, AS, PS

144. no. 3. Because of their egocentrism, magical thinking, and developing superego (conscience), preschool children frequently view hospitalization and invasive procedures as punishment for previous wrongdoings. C/NM, AN, PC

145. no. 1. Potassium is excreted by the kidneys; therefore an adequate urine output is essential to prevent hyperkalemia. C/NM, AS, PS

146. no. 2. Adequate urine output for infants and children is 1 ml/kg/hr. Based on Cassie's weight of 14 kg, her urine output should be at least 14 ml/hr, or 56 ml for 4 hours. Urine output of only 36 ml in 4 hours necessitates immediately notifying the physician. C/NM, IM, PS

147. no. 4. With diarrhea, there is a loss of bicarbonate, which results in metabolic acidosis. Compensation is by the respiratory system with hyperventilation. C/NM, AN, PS

148. no. 2. Temporary lactose intolerance is common with diarrhea because of depletion of lactase from the intestines. Therefore milk and milk products should be added last to Cassie's diet. C/NM, PL, H

149. no. 2. A favorite toy will give her some sense of continuity with home. A doll can be dried off when it becomes wet, yet it does not pose a safety hazard in the croup tent. Options no. 1 and no. 3 require too much energy expenditure in relation to decreased oxygenation. C/NM, IM, E

150. no. 1. Four-year-olds have exaggerated fears that need to be understood in helping them adapt to new procedures, such as a croup tent. By staying with her in the tent, the nurse can facilitate Brooke's adjustment. Neither options no. 2 nor no. 3 will lessen her fear. Option no. 4 is appropriate after her fear is lessened. C/NM, IM, PC

151. no. 2. When using the microdrip, drops/min equals ml/hr; 250 ml ÷ 8 = 31.25. C/NM, IM, PS

152. no. 3. Diarrhea is a side effect of ampicillin and is usually self-limiting. C/NM, IM, PS

153. no. 3. Take axillary temperatures to avoid irritating the anal area or increasing her respiratory distress. C/NM, PL, E

154. no. 3. 40 mg/65 mg = 1 ml/x; 40x = 65; x = 1.62 ml. C/NM, IM, E

155. no. 1. For the most reliable absorption, ampicillin should be administered on an empty stomach. All liquid antibiotics require shaking to mix the suspension adequately. They must be stored in the refrigerator. C/NM, IM, PS

156. no. 2. Nutrition and feeding are priority concerns preoperatively and postoperatively. Postoperatively, nothing can be inserted in the mouth, so using a cup is the best method for oral fluid intake. C/NM, AS, H

157. no. 1. The child under 5 years is most vulnerable and at psychological risk when separated from parents, especially the mother, if she is the primary caregiver. Separation can interrupt emotional development and result in loss of trust in others. The child's initial reaction to separation anxiety is protest. C/I, AN, PC

158. no. 3. Sitting at the bedside and spending time is a way to begin to build a trusting relationship so that Peter will want to come to the nurse. C/NM, IM, PC

159. no. 1. Prone position facilitates drainage of secretions, which may be copious following cleft palate surgery. C/NM, PL, PS

160. no. 2. Elbow restraints will prevent Peter from getting his hands or fingers into his mouth. Exercise his arms one at a time at least q2h. The Logan bow is used following cleft lip repair to prevent tension on the suture line. C/NM, IM, E

161. no. 1. Listening to a story is appropriate in terms of Peter's energy level postoperatively, and it promotes security through interaction with someone. Peter cannot use his arms because of the elbow restraints. C/NM, IM, E

162. no. 2. Regression and inactivity are behaviors of despair when the primary caregiver, the mother, is lost. The child feels mother really is not coming back and begins to grieve. C/I, AN, PC

163. no. 3. To survive, the child must repress feelings about the lost mother and bond to caregivers who are present. C/I, AN, PC

164. no. 2. With vomiting, there is loss of hydrochloric acid from the stomach, which results in metabolic *alkalosis*. Infants with pyloric stenosis are usually dehydrated with weight loss and progressive constipation. Peristaltic waves are typically visualized after a feeding as the stomach contracts in an attempt to force its contents through the narrowed pyloric lumen into the small intestines. A sausage-shaped mass is characteristic of intussusception, not pyloric stenosis. C/NM, AS, PS

165. no. 2. Placing the infant in a semi-Fowler's position on his right side would be the best position anatomically to facilitate flow of formula from stomach to duodenum. C/NM, PL, E

166. no. 3. In diabetic ketoacidosis, there is a lack of insulin, which results in *high* blood glucose and glycosuria. Because glucose is unable to enter the cells, fats are broken down into ketones and eventually excreted in the urine. The accumulation of ketone acids in the blood causes metabolic acidosis. C/NM, AN, PS

167. no. 3. The classic signs of insulin-dependent diabetes are (1) polyuria (increased urine output resulting from osmotic diuresis from hyperglycemia), (2) polydipsia (increased thirst as a result of fluid loss from increased urine output), (3) polyphagia (increased appetite in an attempt to provide starving cells with energy), and (4) weight loss (the result of fluid loss in combination with fat and protein breakdown). C/NM, AN, PS

168. no. 3. Glucagon stimulates the release of stored glycogen from the liver, which increases blood glucose. C/NM, AN, PS

169. no. 4. During exercise, there is increased use of glucose, which may precipitate a hypoglycemic reaction. In order to prevent low blood glucose, extra calories should be provided before exercise. C/NM, PL, H

170. no. 1. Thirst is a symptom of hyperglycemia. In hypoglycemia, there is hunger and release of catecholamines in an attempt to increase blood glu-

cose. This often results in diaphoresis and tremors. C/NM, AN, PS

171. no. 3. Peer acceptance is extremely important for school-age children. Because of the special dietary and health practices necessary for diabetics, these children often feel they are different and fear rejection by their peer group. C/NM, AN, PC

172. no. 3. Children should never have completely negative urinary glucose because urine tests do not diagnose blood levels below 180 mg/dl. Children are advised to maintain urinary glucose levels of at least 1+. Options no. 1 and no. 3 indicate a potential for diabetic ketoacidosis. The effects of NPH do not occur for 10 to 12 hours. Hypoglycemic episodes have a quick onset; hyperglycemia occurs insidiously. C/NM, AS, PS

173. no. 2. This is evidence that Angela can assume responsibility for her care and has accepted that she has the disease. C/NM, PL, H

174. no. 2. Eight-year-olds can ride a bike; activities in options no. 1 and no. 4 occur at earlier ages; option no. 3 is characteristic of adolescence. C/H, AS, H

175. no. 2. This type of stool (steatorrhea) results from the undigested fat in the gastrointestinal tract. Most children with cystic fibrosis have good appetites. C/NM, AS, PS

176. no. 3. Enzymes must be given with every meal and snack to help digest the food. Pancrease comes in capsules that can be opened and sprinkled on food such as applesauce or ice cream. They are never placed on hot food, because heat will destroy the enzyme. C/NM, IM, H

177. no. 3. Because of the particular exocrine glands involved, large amounts of salt are lost and must be replaced, especially in hot weather. Fluids should never be restricted. The diet should be low in fat content because of malabsorption. C/NM, IM, H

178. no. 4. Respiratory changes leading to progressive pulmonary involvement pose the most serious threat to life. C/NM, PL, H

179. no. 4. Because of decreased glomerular filtration, there is a resulting increased circulatory congestion that leads to an elevated blood pressure. Options no. 1 and no. 2 are typical of nephrotic syndrome. Weight gain, rather than loss, would result from any edema that develops. C/E, AS, PS

180. no. 1. Diuresis is the priority goal. Once diuresis occurs, the child feels better and the blood pressure will decrease. Options no. 2 and no. 3 are appropriate for nephrotic syndrome. Option no. 4 is applicable after diuresis occurs. C/E, AN, PS

181. no. 4. Acute glomerulonephritis is an inflammatory process in the glomeruli that is caused by a reaction to a streptococcal infection. This test measures streptococcal antibody levels, which would be elevated after a streptococcal infection. Options no. 2, no. 3 and no. 4 are not affected by the diagnosis. ADH would be elevated with nephrotic syndrome. C/I, PL, PS

182. no. 2. Initial actions should be designed to orient the client and family to the hospital, offer information about immediate procedures of care, and build a trusting relationship. C/E, IM, E

183. no. 2. Cindy's history is strongly suggestive of a ruptured appendix. Often there is sudden relief from pain after perforation, then a subsequent increase in pain when peritonitis occurs. If the appendix has perforated, Cindy will need surgery, so she should have nothing by mouth. The white blood cell count is often elevated with appendicitis, so a complete blood count would be a useful diagnostic tool. C/E, PL, PS

184. no. 4. Frequent dressing changes are essential to prevent skin excoriation and infection from drainage and to permit inspection of the incision. A ruptured appendix releases many organisms into the peritoneal cavity; thus broad-spectrum antibiotics are needed in order to prevent infection. Positioning the child in a semi-Fowler's position or on the right side facilitates drainage and helps prevent formation of a subdiaphragmatic abscess. C/E, IM, PS

185. no. 3. The use of a rectal tube is directed toward removing the cause of her discomfort. C/E, IM, PS

186. no. 3. A soft, flat abdomen indicates that flatus has been reduced. The other symptoms would indicate pain relief, but that would be accomplished by relieving the distension. C/E, EV, PS

187. no. 4. Because of the lack of distal colonic peristalsis, the infant is frequently unable to pass stools. When stool and flatus accumulate in the colon, the abdomen becomes distended, and the infant refuses fluids. C/E, AS, PS

188. no. 4. Steatorrhea (fat in the stool) indicates a problem with fat metabolism but is not a problem in Hirschsprung's disease. The infant may not want to eat because of the elimination problem. Constipation and vomiting are due to the "backup" of stools and flatus in the colon. Diarrhea may result when liquid stool seeps around the stationary hard stool. C/E, AS, PS

189. no. 1. A high-residue diet would aggravate the problem by increasing the stool mass. Clear liquids would not provide adequate nutrition. This infant does not have a problem with sodium or potassium so option no. 4 has no purpose. C/E, PL, PS

190. no. 1. Although options no. 2, no. 3, and no. 4 are a part of the complete health history, the bowel habits pertain to this disease process. C/E, AS, PS

191. no. 1. The colostomy is usually temporary and will be closed when the surgical repair of the colon is completely healed and the bowel functions normally. This usually takes from a few months to a year. C/E, IM, E

192. no. 3. Since the proximal end receives the stool, only mucus should be in the distal portion of the colon. C/E, EV, PS

193. no. 1. As with any bowel surgery, the client is given nothing by mouth until bowel function returns. C/E, IM, PS

194. no. 1. Jams and preserves contain portions of the fruit that provide residue (e.g., tiny seeds, skins). C/E, IM, PS

195. no. 2. Preadolescent and young adolescent girls are at highest risk for developing scoliosis. C/M, AS, H

196. no. 3. The child bending forward at the waist with head and arms hanging freely allows the nurse to most easily detect any flank asymmetry or rib hump. C/M, AS, PS

197. no. 3. Change in body image and loss of control are the major fears of adolescence. C/M, AN, PC

198. no. 2. Mood swings are common in adolescence. C/M, AN, PC

199. no. 2. The other options are incorrect and would lead to inadequate bracing or skin breakdown. C/M, IM, E

200. no. 3. During early adolescence, girls are about 2 years ahead of their male counterparts in physical development. C/M, AS, PS

201. no. 4. Mary will be susceptible to infection because of neutropenia. Clients in options no. 1, no. 2, and no. 3 might have an infectious process associated with their conditions and are, therefore, not suitable roommates. C/CA, PL, PS

202. no. 4. The developmental task of adolescence consists of developing a strong sense of identity; body image is an integral part of an adolescent's identity. This would be the same for any 13-year-old and is not specific to her problem. C/H, AN, H

203. no. 4. Coping with cancer and the medical regimen can best be facilitated by expressing feelings. The procedures never become routine, and each carries some risk. Parents can often be most helpful if they are out of the room during procedures but are available afterwards for comfort. C/CA, EV, PC

204. no. 2. Hemolysis will occur if dextrose is used; salt-poor albumin and fresh frozen plasma are never used to flush an IV line. C/O, IM, PS

205. no. 3. Hypotension; fever; pain in back, legs, or chest; and apprehension are all indicative of a reaction. C/CA, AS PS

206. no. 3. The immediate responsibility is to stop the transfusion, keep the line open with saline, obtain vital signs, and stay with the child while someone notifies the physician. C/CA, IM, E

207. no. 1. Semi- or high-Fowler's positions prevent choking or aspiration of blood. This position also lessens the pressure in the vessels to the head. Option no. 4 would increase bleeding; no. 3 is a later action. C/CA, IM, PS

208. no. 3. Aspirin is contraindicated in clients with bleeding problems because it increases bleeding time. C/CA, IM, PS

209. no. 2. Adolescents have increased anxiety about death and worry that they will die before they have a chance to live. C/I, AS, H

210. no. 4. Peeling skin is a side effect of radiation therapy. Options no. 1, no. 2, and no. 3 are effects of chemotherapy. C/CA, AS, PS

211. no. 3. Vitamins with folic acid will interfere with the cytotoxic action of methotrexate since it is a folic acid antagonist. C/CA, AN, PS

212. no. 4. Uric acid is released during cell destruction and can accumulate in the renal tubules, resulting in uremia. Allopurinol interferes with the metabolic breakdown of xanthine oxidase to uric acid; therefore uric acid production is inhibited. C/CA, AN, PS

213. no. 1. Encouraging oral fluids ensures adequate excretion of the end products of metabolism. C/CA, PL, PS

214. no. 2. Immunizations are contraindicated with clients receiving immunosuppressive drugs. C/CA, AN, PS

215. no. 3. Children with leukemia are sensitive to touch because of osseous invasion by leukemic cells. C/CA, AN, PS

216. no. 4. Vincristine can be neurotoxic; numbness, tingling, jaw pain, and ataxia are manifestations of vincristine toxicity. C/CA, IM, PS

217. no. 2. The peak incidence for Wilms' tumor is 3 to 4 years. C/CA, AN, PS

218. no. 1. This is the most common sign. The child appears healthy except for increased abdominal size. Decreased output is seen only if the renal collecting system is involved in bilateral tumors. Hypertension is seen in children when there is pressure of the tumor on the renal artery (about 25% of the time). C/CA, AS, PS

219. no. 1. Dolls and puppets are familiar objects that the young child can actively manipulate, and thus they are good ways for the young child to learn. C/I, IM, H

220. no. 3. The abdomen is not palpated unless absolutely necessary to prevent the spread of cancer cells into the surrounding abdominal areas. C/CA, PL, PS

221. no. 4. Although the other options may be objectives, the overall goal is to return the child to a normal life-style so that growth and development may continue along their normal course. C/CA, PL, H

222. no. 1. Including the parents in planning and implementation of care makes them feel useful, knowledgeable, and that they have an important role in the child's recovery. This increases compliance in the treatment regimen. Literature is a good teaching reinforcement but second in importance. Discharge planning begins with admission. Free time is important but not the sole factor for teaching objectives. C/CA, IM, H

Sample Tests

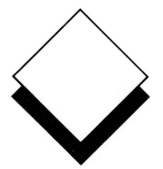

Sample Tests

The questions and answers in this section have been organized to simulate two separate NCLEX-RN exams.

Each test has been divided into four books of 95 questions each. Each book tests your nursing knowledge regarding care of the adult, the child, the childbearing family, and the client with psychosocial/psychiatric problems.

INSTRUCTIONS FOR TAKING THE TEST

1. Review the information in Section One, *Preparing for the NCLEX-RN*.
2. Time yourself, allowing 1½ hours per book (6 hours per test).
3. Read each question carefully and select *one* best answer to each question.
4. Do not leave questions blank, because you will not be penalized for random answers on the NCLEX-RN.
5. Score your exam using the answer key. Count any questions left unanswered as incorrect.
6. Review the questions you answered incorrectly and restudy that specific material. Ask yourself two questions:
   a. Did I miss the question because I overlooked a key word, a key timeframe, or a critical piece of data? If you answer "yes," then focus on stress reduction techniques before answering more test questions. You may be suffering from a high level of test anxiety.
   b. Did I miss the question because I was unfamiliar with the content? If you answer "yes," then look up and review this content in the *AJN/Mosby Nursing Boards Review*, your school textbooks, or other resources. You probably have a need to refresh your content knowledge.
7. Good luck!

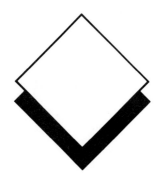

Test 1, Book I

QUESTIONS

Stella Garcia, age 66, is brought to the hospital by ambulance after having suffered a fainting spell while Christmas shopping. She is accompanied by her sister, who tells the admitting physician that Mrs. Garcia recently learned she has diabetes mellitus. After a blood sample for sugar has been drawn, she is admitted for further evaluation with the diagnosis of hyperglycemia.

1. Before approaching Mrs. Garcia, what other information would be important to obtain from her sister?
   - [ ] 1. Is Mrs. Garcia a U.S. citizen?
   - [ ] 2. Does Mrs. Garcia speak or understand English?
   - [ ] 3. Was the sister present when Mrs. Garcia had her fainting spell?
   - [ ] 4. Does Mrs. Garcia have any medical insurance?
2. What information is most important to obtain during her admission process?
   - [ ] 1. Mental status.
   - [ ] 2. Respiratory status.
   - [ ] 3. Blood pressure.
   - [ ] 4. Heart rate.
3. Mrs. Garcia's understanding of the English language is limited. What would be the best means of communicating with her?
   - [ ] 1. Through a hospital interpreter.
   - [ ] 2. Through a close family member.
   - [ ] 3. Through a health practitioner fluent in both English and Spanish.
   - [ ] 4. Through anyone who is available who speaks both languages.
4. Which of the following is an *inappropriate* goal in the care of Mrs. Garcia?
   - [ ] 1. The client will learn dietary principles and the role of diet.
   - [ ] 2. The client will be able to adapt her own cultural diet to meet diabetic requirements.
   - [ ] 3. The client will safely administer the prescribed hypoglycemic agents.
   - [ ] 4. The client will be able to adequately teach another newly diagnosed diabetic client in Spanish.

Ellen Evenson is a 20-year-old woman admitted to the psychiatric hospital after attempting to kill her 16-year-old sister, Tanya, by pushing her out of a second-story window. Her only explanation was, "She got in my way." She displays no remorse, nor any attachment to her family, and she has a history of truancy and inability to retain employment. Both parents work full time and have been unable to provide close supervision.

5. Soon after Miss Evenson has been admitted to the unit, she shows interest in a young male nurse who is assigned to her. She is charming and cooperative and frequently says to him, "I'm so glad you're my nurse. You're the best nurse on the unit." Which of the following statements provides the best interpretation of Miss Evenson's behavior?
   - [ ] 1. She has finally found someone for whom she feels a real attachment.
   - [ ] 2. She recognizes the superior ability of this particular nurse.
   - [ ] 3. She is proficient at getting her way at the expense of others.
   - [ ] 4. She is demonstrating a willingness to change, so that a personal relationship with this nurse would be possible.
6. Which of the following statements most accurately describes factors that probably contributed to the character of Miss Evenson?
   - [ ] 1. There was ample opportunity for involvement with appropriate role models, but she chose to avoid close relationships.
   - [ ] 2. Early needs for security and love were met, but later associations with parents were distant.
   - [ ] 3. Impaired superego development occurred because she did not internalize positive identifications.

4. Much of her lifelong pattern of difficulty is a result of below-average intelligence.

7. When working with Miss Evenson, the nurse would primarily use which of the following strategies?
   1. Allow the client to prepare as much of her own treatment plan as possible.
   2. Offer as many opportunities as possible for recreational and occupational therapies.
   3. Use interdisciplinary team planning to determine and enforce appropriate limits for behavior on the unit.
   4. Repeatedly provide sympathy and support for the client in her attempts to avoid anxiety.

8. One day Miss Evenson's sister comes to visit her. Miss Evenson says, "She can come in if she wants to. I really don't care." This best demonstrates what combination of responses common to the antisocial personality?
   1. Low self-esteem and poor impulse control.
   2. Suspicion and aloofness.
   3. Guilt and depression.
   4. Self-centeredness and lack of consideration for others' feelings.

9. Miss Evenson participates in family therapy with her parents. The parents frequently blame her for their difficulties and complain about the expense at the hospital. They also persist in requesting passes for her to go home and for an early discharge. Which of the following statements best describes the parents' beliefs or feelings?
   1. They believe she has improved enough to function efficiently outside the hospital.
   2. They believe she has been punished enough for her previous behavior.
   3. They have ambivalent feelings about her.
   4. They feel guilty about causing their daughter's antisocial behavior.

10. After having been on the unit for several months, Miss Evenson shows signs of depression and feelings of guilt and remorse. What evaluation of her progress would be most appropriate?
    1. She has acquired a dysthymic disorder in addition to her antisocial personality.
    2. She has experienced a major depression in addition to her antisocial personality.
    3. She is gaining insight into the effect her behavior has had on others, and this resulted in depression.
    4. She is gaining insight into her problems, and this has made her realize that she has a poor prognosis.

11. One day in occupational therapy, Miss Evenson is observed briefly assisting a depressed client with a project. She is helpful but not superior in her attitude. Which of the following statements best describes her behavior?

1. She is trying to impress the staff by her good behavior.
2. She cares about the other client's completing the project.
3. She is showing improvement by demonstrating more appropriate relationships with others.
4. She is demonstrating apathy by doing no more than what she feels is expected of her.

Peggy Smythe excitedly shares with the nurse that she thinks she is pregnant. She wants to know how soon after she has missed her period she can expect laboratory test results to confirm her hopes.

12. The nurse's response to Mrs. Smythe is based on knowledge of the hormonal changes of pregnancy. Which hormone is necessary for a positive pregnancy test?
    1. Placental estrogen.
    2. Human chorionic gonadotropin.
    3. Human placental lactogen.
    4. Chorionic progesterone.

13. In response to Mrs. Smythe's question, how soon after the first missed menstrual period will latex agglutination tests such as Gravidex and Prognosticon detect pregnancy?
    1. 1 to 2 days.
    2. 7 days.
    3. 14 days.
    4. 21 days.

14. The nurse explains to Mrs. Smythe that a teratogen is any factor that has an adverse effect on the developing child in utero and that the timing of exposure to such a factor is significant. The most critical period for disruption of fetal development by teratogen exposure exists during which period?
    1. From conception to the twelfth week, during organogenesis.
    2. After 16 weeks, when the fetus begins swallowing amniotic fluid.
    3. Beginning at 20 weeks, when the fetus is capable of producing antibodies.
    4. During the eighth to ninth month, which is a period of very rapid growth.

15. Fetal circulation differs from the circulatory pattern after birth. One special structure, the ductus arteriosus, allows the majority of fetal blood to bypass which major organ system?
    1. Heart.
    2. Liver.
    3. Lungs.
    4. Spleen.

16. Which of the following is a function of the placenta?
    1. Produces oxytocin in increasing amounts throughout the pregnancy.

☐ 2. Allows exchange by osmosis across a semiper-meable membrane.

☐ 3. Protects the fetus from viral infections during the first 3 months.

☐ 4. Permits maternal and fetal blood to mix freely.

Sam Weston, age 21, was brought to the emergency unit for acute abdominal pain. His condition was diagnosed as acute appendicitis. He is currently in the emergency unit waiting to go to surgery.

17. In the limited time available, the nurse recognizes the need to include which of the following in the preoperative teaching?

☐ 1. Leg exercises to prevent venous stasis.

☐ 2. Abdominal splinting for coughing and deep breathing.

☐ 3. Explanation of the nasogastric tube that he can expect postoperatively.

☐ 4. Explanation of drainage on his dressing.

18. Before administering Mr. Weston's preoperative medication, which of the following nursing actions is most essential?

☐ 1. Report to the physician the elevated white blood cell count.

☐ 2. Check to ensure that the laboratory has completed the urinalysis.

☐ 3. Ensure that the surgical consent form has been signed.

☐ 4. Provide a quiet environment.

19. Mr. Weston is taken to the operating room, and preparation for surgery begins. The circulating nurse's primary goal when positioning Mr. Weston on the operating room table is to achieve

☐ 1. A comfortable position for the client.

☐ 2. A position that is acceptable to the surgeon.

☐ 3. A position that prevents exposure and promotes privacy.

☐ 4. A position that avoids circulatory impairment and protects nerve function.

20. Mr. Weston receives a general anesthetic in the operating room. In order to suppress pain, general anesthesia must depress which part of the brain?

☐ 1. Medulla.

☐ 2. Thalamus.

☐ 3. Cerebellum.

☐ 4. Cortex.

21. Mr. Weston is admitted to the postanesthesia room. The nurse obtains admitting vital signs of blood pressure 90/60 mm Hg, pulse 100, and respirations 18. Which of the following actions would the nurse take?

☐ 1. Recheck the vital signs in 5 minutes.

☐ 2. Increase the rate of the IV slightly.

☐ 3. Place him flat and elevate his feet.

☐ 4. Cover him with a warm blanket.

22. It is now 7 hours after Mr. Weston's surgery. He complains of being unable to void, even though he has the urge. Which nursing action is most appropriate?

☐ 1. Obtain an order to catheterize him.

☐ 2. Help him to stand at the bedside to void.

☐ 3. Wait one more hour before taking any action.

☐ 4. Explain to him that this is a common sensation postoperatively.

23. Retained secretions in the lungs, especially postoperatively, most often result in which of the following?

☐ 1. Pulmonary edema.

☐ 2. Fluid imbalance.

☐ 3. Atelectasis and pneumonia.

☐ 4. CO_2 retention.

Five-year-old Marianne has varicella (chickenpox). Her fever is 102.5° F (39.2° C).

24. Which clinical sign would *not* be related to her diagnosis?

☐ 1. Pruritus.

☐ 2. Lesions in four stages.

☐ 3. Lymphadenopathy.

☐ 4. Strawberry tongue.

25. Marianne has two younger brothers. Marianne's mother would be advised to institute which type of isolation precautions at home?

☐ 1. Respiratory isolation.

☐ 2. Universal precautions.

☐ 3. Wound and skin isolation.

☐ 4. Enteric precautions.

26. It is also imperative to advise Marianne's mother to do which of the following?

☐ 1. Dim the light in Marianne's room.

☐ 2. Keep Marianne's fingernails short and clean.

☐ 3. Apply cool compresses to Marianne's lesions.

☐ 4. Avoid giving Marianne acidic foods or fluids.

27. Marianne's fever has subsided and she is very bored. Which activity is most appropriate for her as she convalesces?

☐ 1. Watching cartoons on television.

☐ 2. Talking on the telephone with her friends.

☐ 3. Painting with watercolors.

☐ 4. Reading a book of riddles.

28. Marianne's mother asks when Marianne can return to school. What would be the best response?

☐ 1. "When she no longer has a fever."

☐ 2. "In 2 weeks."

☐ 3. "When all her lesions have dried."

☐ 4. "When no new lesions have appeared for 24 hours."

Charles Arden, age 25, the victim of an automobile accident, is admitted to the emergency room with a deep laceration on the right side of his head and a

bleeding abrasion on his face. He is drowsy but able to respond to verbal stimuli. His vital signs are blood pressure 110/70 mm Hg, pulse 100, respirations 28. Dexamethasone (Decadron) is ordered, and he is admitted to the intensive care unit for further observation.

29. The nurse knows that injury to the right side of the brain will *not* include problems in which of the following?
 □ 1. Speech.
 □ 2. Perception.
 □ 3. Coordination.
 □ 4. Personality.

30. Which of the following would be *inappropriate* as an assessment priority for Mr. Arden?
 □ 1. Level of consciousness.
 □ 2. Vital signs.
 □ 3. Bladder fullness.
 □ 4. Motor reflexes.

31. Why is dexamethasone (Decadron) the corticosteroid drug of choice in this situation?
 □ 1. It is an antiinflammatory drug.
 □ 2. It decreases the amount of spinal fluid secreted.
 □ 3. It crosses the blood-brain barrier.
 □ 4. It causes fewer side effects than any of the other corticosteroids.

Mr. Arden becomes confused during the night and falls quietly asleep. The nurse takes his vital signs and finds his blood pressure is 155/60 mm Hg, his pulse is 64, and his respirations are 18. The physician suspects increased intracranial pressure (ICP).

32. Which of the following nursing actions would be first?
 □ 1. Institute seizure precautions.
 □ 2. Start an IV infusion.
 □ 3. Order a suction machine.
 □ 4. Start oxygen by cannula at 6 L.

33. Several hours later, Mr. Arden has a seizure. Which of the following nursing actions would be *inappropriate*?
 □ 1. Protect his head.
 □ 2. Restrain him.
 □ 3. Turn his head or body to the side.
 □ 4. Time the seizure.

34. It is determined that Mr. Arden's seizures are the result of increased ICP. Which of the following would be included in the initial treatment?
 □ 1. Craniectomy.
 □ 2. Induced barbiturate coma.
 □ 3. Osmotic diuretics, corticosteroids, and hyperventilation.
 □ 4. Phenobarbital (Luminal) and phenytoin sodium (Dilantin).

35. Which drug is most likely to have a "rebound" effect in the treatment of cerebral edema?
 □ 1. Dexamethasone (Decadron).
 □ 2. Diazepam (Valium).
 □ 3. Mannitol.
 □ 4. Prednisone.

36. Two weeks later, Mr. Arden's condition has stabilized. He is restless, talks incessantly, and asks repetitive questions. These behaviors are most indicative of
 □ 1. Depression.
 □ 2. Anxiety.
 □ 3. Anger.
 □ 4. Denial.

37. Which of the following is probably not the underlying cause of his behavior?
 □ 1. Powerlessness.
 □ 2. Fear of dying.
 □ 3. Decreased self-esteem.
 □ 4. Role acceptance.

38. The most therapeutic independent nursing approach at this time is to do which of the following?
 □ 1. Administer diazepam (Valium).
 □ 2. Use active-listening skills.
 □ 3. Obtain psychiatric consultation.
 □ 4. Schedule a team conference.

Sixteen-year-old Scott Metzger is admitted to the hospital with severe injuries following a car accident in which his best friend had been driving. Both boys had been drinking, and his friend was driving at high speeds and in an erratic manner. When the police attempted to stop them, his friend tried to outrun the police. After speeds exceeding 80 mph, his friend lost control of the car and crashed into a telegraph pole. Scott suffered multiple fractures and a severely burned left foot. Extensive skin grafting and antibiotic therapy were instituted. Amputation of the foot remains a possibility. His friend suffered lacerations and bruises but was not hospitalized.

39. A week after admission, when his physical condition is well stabilized, Scott becomes extremely demanding of the nursing staff, putting on his call light constantly and yelling for the nurse if the light is not answered immediately. Scott's behavior is most likely related to which of the following?
 □ 1. Withdrawal from alcohol.
 □ 2. Boredom.
 □ 3. Psychotic depression.
 □ 4. Reactive depression.

40. What is the most therapeutic nursing approach to Scott's behavior?
 □ 1. Rotate the nurse assigned to his care on a daily basis.
 □ 2. Ignore his inappropriate demands.

☐ 3. Consider that he is frightened and angry and fulfill as many of his demands as possible.

☐ 4. Let him know that his inappropriate demands will be refused.

41. One morning Scott tells the nurse that he is feeling better because he has spent the night planning a way to "get even" with his friend. The nurse responds by saying, "Sounds like you are feeling angry." This is an example of which of the following therapeutic communication techniques?

☐ 1. Accepting what the client says.

☐ 2. Reflecting what the client says.

☐ 3. Verbalizing inferred thoughts and feelings.

☐ 4. Encouraging the client to express private thoughts.

42. The physician writes an order that Scott may be out of bed on crutches only to use the bathroom in his room. The nurse finds Scott in another young client's room watching a football game. When the nurse confronts him about this, he responds, "What does it matter? I'm going to lose my foot anyway." Which is the most therapeutically correct response?

☐ 1. "Who told you that?"

☐ 2. "You probably will if you keep up this behavior."

☐ 3. "You seem worried about losing your foot."

☐ 4. "I'll get a wheelchair and take you back to your room."

43. One evening as the nurse is helping Scott, he asks her for a date to go dancing after he is discharged. What explanation best fits his behavior?

☐ 1. He is acting out sexual feelings.

☐ 2. He wants to embarrass the nurse.

☐ 3. He wants to be reassured that his foot will heal normally with unimpaired functioning.

☐ 4. His comments are normal, given the situation.

44. Which of the following would be the most therapeutic response from the nurse?

☐ 1. "I don't go out with patients."

☐ 2. "Are you worried that you'll never be able to dance again?"

☐ 3. "Don't you have a girlfriend?"

☐ 4. "I'm your nurse, not your friend."

Helen Jenkins, age 8, is admitted to the pediatric unit with a diagnosis of acute bronchial asthma. She has had a bad cold for several days before the attack and would awaken during the night with coughing and shortness of breath.

45. Which of the following is most characteristic of asthma?

☐ 1. Inspiratory stridor.

☐ 2. Expiratory wheezing.

☐ 3. Prolonged inspiration.

☐ 4. Hoarse voice.

46. Helen's physician has ordered epinephrine (Adrenalin) 0.03 ml stat, to be repeated in 20 minutes if no relief is obtained. What is the most common route of administration for epinephrine?

☐ 1. Intramuscular.

☐ 2. Subcutaneous.

☐ 3. Intravenous.

☐ 4. Sublingual.

47. Which of the following actions is expected of epinephrine?

☐ 1. Relax bronchial spasms.

☐ 2. Liquefy respiratory secretions.

☐ 3. Increase antibody formation.

☐ 4. Reduce airway diameter.

48. Following the administration of epinephrine, the nurse would monitor Helen for which sign of epinephrine toxicity?

☐ 1. Tinnitus.

☐ 2. Coryza.

☐ 3. Tachycardia.

☐ 4. Dyspnea.

49. Helen begins to show signs of increasing respiratory distress. These include all of the following *except*

☐ 1. Cyanosis and tachypnea.

☐ 2. Intercostal retractions.

☐ 3. Increased restlessness.

☐ 4. Irregular respirations.

50. Helen is receiving a continuous IV drip of aminophylline. Which observation by the nurse indicates aminophylline toxicity?

☐ 1. Lethargy.

☐ 2. Hypertension.

☐ 3. Diarrhea.

☐ 4. Tachycardia.

51. Which of the following nursing actions would be most appropriate for Helen?

☐ 1. Position Helen in a supine position.

☐ 2. Limit oral fluids in order to decrease secretions.

☐ 3. Monitor intake and output and specific gravity.

☐ 4. Turn, cough, and deep-breathe q2h.

52. Helen begins to receive hydrocortisone (Solu-Cortef) IV q12h. Prolonged use of steroids in children can lead to

☐ 1. Laryngeal edema.

☐ 2. Growth suppression.

☐ 3. Grand mal seizures.

☐ 4. Chronic osteoarthritis.

53. What is the rationale for administering hydrocortisone (Solu-Cortef)?

☐ 1. It reduces anxiety.

☐ 2. It diminishes inflammation.

☐ 3. It mobilizes secretions.

☐ 4. It relieves bronchospasms.

54. Helen's mother asks if a pet would help her recovery after discharge. Which of the following pets would be most appropriate for Helen?

☐ 1. Parakeet.

☐ 2. Dog.
☐ 3. Cat.
☐ 4. Fish.

Armand and Julia Cirrone have been married 8 years. The first 2 pregnancies resulted in spontaneous abortions. This pregnancy has been healthy, and in the seventh month they decide upon delivery in a birthing center. The nurse conducts a tour of the suite and describes the adaptations common to such a birth.

55. As the nurse discusses the birth process with the couple, which statement best indicates they understand all options?
☐ 1. "We know that the midwife will call the physician if needed."
☐ 2. "If Julia needs pain medication, we know it is available."
☐ 3. "Armand and I will be together with our new baby for the first hours."
☐ 4. All the above statements indicate understanding.

56. Mrs. Cirrone's labor begins while her husband is on a business trip. She is very upset that he cannot be with her at this time because they had prepared together for active participation in the birth. What approach can the nurse take to meet the client's needs at this time?
☐ 1. Ask if there is another individual she would like as support person.
☐ 2. Assure her that a member of the nursing staff will be with her at all times.
☐ 3. Tell her you will continue to try to locate her husband.
☐ 4. Reinforce Mrs. Cirrone's confidence in her own abilities to cope and maintain a sense of control.

57. In assessing Mrs. Cirrone's progress during labor, which of the following observations best indicates imminent delivery?
☐ 1. Spontaneous rupture of membranes.
☐ 2. 100% effacement.
☐ 3. Bulging perineum.
☐ 4. Strong contractions lasting 60 to 70 seconds.

58. A healthy daughter is delivered and Mrs. Cirrone initiates breastfeeding. In accordance with policies, mother and baby will be discharged in 8 hours, to be visited the following day by the nurse-midwife. Which of the following aspects of postpartal teaching is of highest priority with an early discharge?
☐ 1. Demonstrate correct breastfeeding techniques.
☐ 2. Teach Mrs. Cirrone palpation and massage of the fundus.
☐ 3. Give a demonstration of infant bathing techniques.
☐ 4. Answer all questions of both parents.

59. Which of the following is a priority goal for mother and infant during the first postpartum day?

☐ 1. Promote health during the perinatal period.
☐ 2. Teach developmental needs of the first 12 months.
☐ 3. Support maternal and neonatal thermoregulation.
☐ 4. Promote attachment.

Barbara Case's myasthenia gravis (MG) was diagnosed 4 years ago. The initial onset of symptoms occurred during a pregnancy. Her disease was well controlled with medication until she contracted an upper respiratory tract infection recently.

60. Mrs. Case asks why this had to happen to her even though she is very careful to always take her pyridostigmine (Mestinon) on time, 3 times every day. What explanation would be most appropriate to give Mrs. Case?
☐ 1. "You have become resistant to pyridostigmine (Mestinon), but there are other medications that work just as well."
☐ 2. "Symptoms of MG are often exacerbated by any kind of stress, such as infection."
☐ 3. "You need to increase your medicine to 6 times a day."
☐ 4. "Surgical excision of the thymus gland (thymectomy) often promotes better control of symptoms."

61. Which of the following would *not* be a typical finding in the physical assessment of Mrs. Case?
☐ 1. Bilateral ptosis of the eyelids.
☐ 2. Difficulty swallowing and chewing.
☐ 3. Muscle rigidity and tremors at rest.
☐ 4. Inability to raise her arms over her head.

62. To prevent aspiration, what would the nurse do before offering food or fluids to Mrs. Case?
☐ 1. Check to see if she is NPO for a Tensilon test.
☐ 2. Question her about muscarinic effects of the pyridostigmine (Mestinon) (nausea, abdominal cramping, and diarrhea).
☐ 3. Assess cranial nerves III (oculomotor), IV (trochlear), and VI (abducens) for weakness.
☐ 4. Assess cranial nerves IX (glossopharyngeal) and X (vagus) for weakness.

63. Mrs. Case is conscientiously taking her medication on time. What would the nurse teach her about her medication regimen at discharge?
☐ 1. Never use atropine sulfate as an antidote for muscarinic effects.
☐ 2. Edrophonium (Tensilon) probably will be given with the pyridostigmine (Mestinon) until her infection is completely resolved.
☐ 3. Take pyridostigmine (Mestinon) on an empty stomach, 1 hour before meals.
☐ 4. Take pyridostigmine (Mestinon) with or immediately following meals.

64. To facilitate the management of MG, which is the

most important information to discuss with Mrs. Case?

□ 1. No over-the-counter medications are known to affect the action of anticholinesterase medications used in the treatment of MG.

□ 2. Observe for symptoms of thyroid disease because clients with MG also experience thyroid dysfunction.

□ 3. Planned rest periods throughout the day will maximize strength.

□ 4. Good body mechanics will prevent deformities.

65. Mrs. Case asks whether getting pregnant again will have any effect on her MG. What would be the nurse's best response?

□ 1. "Pregnancy has no effect on MG."

□ 2. "Pregnancy is considered to be a precipitating or aggravating event in MG."

□ 3. "What do you think?"

□ 4. "As long as you take your medication, you have nothing to worry about."

66. Mrs. Case asks, "Just what is MG?" What is the pathophysiological principle upon which the nurse would base a response?

□ 1. It is an autoimmune process affecting nerves and muscles.

□ 2. It is an autoimmune process affecting the myoneural junction.

□ 3. It is a genetic defect that destroys myelin.

□ 4. It is a "slow" viral infection that attacks skeletal muscle.

67. The physician considers corticosteroid therapy for Mrs. Case. Which of the following can often result from long-term corticosteroid therapy?

□ 1. Adrenal gland hypertrophy.

□ 2. Adrenal insufficiency in response to excess stress.

□ 3. Elevated levels of corticotropin-releasing factor.

□ 4. Atrophy of the posterior pituitary gland.

68. Why must corticosteroid drugs always be stopped gradually?

□ 1. ACTH and corticotropin-releasing factor levels are diminished from the supplemental steroids, so no cortisol would be available with abrupt withdrawal.

□ 2. ACTH and melanocyte-stimulating hormone (MSH) levels are elevated because the negative feedback loop has been lost.

□ 3. Ectopic ACTH syndrome could result with rapid withdrawal.

□ 4. Poor wound healing will occur with rapid withdrawal, along with sodium retention and edema.

Deborah Smolins, gravida 1 para 0, is 32 years old and classified as a class II cardiac client.

69. Careful assessments are particularly essential from 28 to 32 weeks of gestation because of the risk of which of the following?

□ 1. Premature delivery.

□ 2. Cardiac decompression.

□ 3. Fluid retention.

□ 4. Fetal circulatory problems.

70. Teaching Mrs. Smolins the symptoms associated with congestive heart failure is very important. Which of the following statements best indicates that she understands what has been taught?

□ 1. "The doctor will be able to listen to my heart and lungs at my weekly visits and see how I am doing."

□ 2. "If there is swelling of my feet and hands, I should reduce the amount of salt that I eat."

□ 3. "When I have inadequate rest, I will have palpitations."

□ 4. "If I have a cough or get tired more easily, I should see the doctor immediately."

71. Mrs. Smolins may need drugs during the antepartal period because of her cardiac status. Which one of the following is the most accurate statement about the use of drugs for cardiac conditions during pregnancy?

□ 1. Penicillin cannot be used prophylactically to prevent infections.

□ 2. Heparin is a safe anticoagulant because it does not cross the placenta.

□ 3. Digitalis is safe because it is not teratogenic.

□ 4. No drugs should be used because they all cause damage to the fetus.

72. Mr. Smolins is concerned about the type of delivery that his wife might have. What is the nurse's most appropriate response when explaining the nature of the delivery?

□ 1. "A cesarean delivery would cause the least exertion because your wife will not have to go through labor and delivery."

□ 2. "A forceps delivery will reduce the strain caused by pushing."

□ 3. "A spontaneous delivery is probable because no surgical intervention should be used."

□ 4. "What is important is that a regional anesthetic is used. The type of delivery is not relevant."

73. What position will Mrs. Smolins need to assume in labor to allow for maximum functioning of her heart?

□ 1. Supine.

□ 2. Sims' position.

□ 3. Dorsal recumbent.

□ 4. Semi-Fowler's.

74. Which of the following aspects of care would be most appropriate regarding Mrs. Smolins' interaction with her infant?

□ 1. If the labor, delivery, and postpartum recovery is uneventful, breastfeeding is appropriate, if desired.

☐ 2. Rooming-in will be possible, and Mrs. Smolins will be encouraged to care for herself and her baby.

☐ 3. A regular schedule will have to be arranged for Mrs. Smolins to visit the nursery and interact with her infant.

☐ 4. Caring for the baby will be too great a strain on Mrs. Smolins for at least 6 weeks, so provisions will need to be made for someone to help during this time.

Vera Thompson, a 40-year-old woman, is brought to the emergency room by her sister. During the assessment, the nurse finds out that Mrs. Thompson's husband moved out that morning rather unexpectedly and into an apartment with his 24-year-old secretary. He has asked for a divorce. Mrs. Thompson has two girls, age 12 and 14. She has a high school diploma and has not worked outside her home in 18 years. The nurse noted a pulse of 120, blood pressure 130/70 mm Hg, tearfulness, narrowed perception, decreased attention span, and fidgeting.

75. Mrs. Thompson is most likely experiencing which of the following?

☐ 1. Situational crisis.

☐ 2. Depression.

☐ 3. Psychosis.

☐ 4. Paranoid state.

76. Which of the following is an important characteristic of crisis intervention?

☐ 1. It is necessary to determine the cause before a solution to the problem can be found.

☐ 2. It will not be of lasting value unless the client achieves insight and increased self-knowledge.

☐ 3. The client is passive because of a decreased ability to function, so appropriate solutions are presented by the therapist.

☐ 4. It deals only with helping an individual or family cope with the immediate presenting problem.

77. Factors that need to be assessed by the nurse when evaluating a client like Mrs. Thompson include which of the following?

☐ 1. Precipitating events, coping styles, and support systems.

☐ 2. Hallucinations, delusions, and tensions.

☐ 3. Anxiety, suspicious behavior, and irrational thoughts.

☐ 4. Eating habits, sleeping habits, affect, and elimination difficulties.

78. What is the nurse's first priority with Mrs. Thompson?

☐ 1. Reassure her that all crises are time limited.

☐ 2. Determine the extent of the immediate problems and how significant she perceives them to be.

☐ 3. Advise her to contact an attorney and make an appointment for her to return the next day.

☐ 4. Contact her husband and notify him of the situation.

79. Mrs. Thompson begins to cry. Select the correct nursing response.

☐ 1. Provide her with privacy.

☐ 2. "Everything will be all right in a day or so."

☐ 3. Administer antianxiety medicine.

☐ 4. "Tell me what's upsetting you, Mrs. Thompson."

80. Which setting would be the most appropriate referral for the emergency room nurse to make for Mrs. Thompson?

☐ 1. Day treatment center.

☐ 2. Community mental health center.

☐ 3. Self-help groups.

☐ 4. Inpatient psychiatric setting.

81. In planning crisis intervention with Mrs. Thompson, which of the following schedules would the nurse recommend?

☐ 1. Every day for a week.

☐ 2. Two times a week for 2 weeks.

☐ 3. Three times a week for 3 weeks.

☐ 4. Once a week for 6 weeks.

82. At the end of 6 weeks, Mrs. Thompson reports that she has begun working as a teachers' assistant at her daughters' school, has seen an attorney, and is receiving child support. Based on this information, at what level is Mrs. Thompson functioning?

☐ 1. At the same level, since she has been unaffected by the crisis.

☐ 2. At a lower level, because of all the trauma she has experienced.

☐ 3. At a higher level, because of her personal growth.

☐ 4. At the same level. Despite the changes in her life, she is still the same person she was 6 weeks ago.

Tommy Miller is a 15-year-old with lymphosarcoma. During the terminal phase of his illness, he is hospitalized with nausea, edema, and pruritus. His mouth is ulcerated with some infected areas visible. His parents refuse to leave him. He is becoming very restless.

83. During the terminal stages of Tommy's illness, the nurse needs to support Mr. and Mrs. Miller. Which of the following is *not* considered supportive nursing action?

☐ 1. Call their religious advisor if they request.

☐ 2. Arrange an opportunity for them to talk with the physician.

☐ 3. Allow them to stay with Tommy and give them privacy.

☐ 4. Wait to be asked before providing help.

84. When giving mouth care to Tommy, what would the nurse use?

☐ 1. A toothbrush.

☐ 2. Peroxide solution.

☐ 3. A mild mouthwash solution.

☐ 4. Nothing; it will only annoy him.

85. Skin care for Tommy would include

☐ 1. Keeping his fingernails short.

☐ 2. A daily tub bath.

☐ 3. A shower as desired.

☐ 4. A scrub with pHisoHex.

86. Mrs. Miller is overheard telling another visitor that Tommy will be going home soon and will be able to return to high school. Mrs. Miller is exhibiting behavior typical of which stage of loss?

☐ 1. Denial.

☐ 2. Acceptance.

☐ 3. Restitution.

☐ 4. Guilt.

87. Tommy has an order for meperidine (Demerol), 50 mg with hydroxyzine (Vistaril), 25 mg IM q3h to q4h prn for pain. Which of the following is *not* an action of hydroxyzine?

☐ 1. Antiemetic.

☐ 2. Antihistaminic.

☐ 3. Central nervous system stimulant.

☐ 4. Opiate and barbiturate potentiator.

88. Tommy requests that the radio be played at night, which is against hospital rules. What would be the best course of action for the nurse?

☐ 1. Gently refuse and explain the rules.

☐ 2. Let him play the radio, but keep his door shut.

☐ 3. Consider the possibility of obtaining earphones for the radio.

☐ 4. Strictly enforce the rules and set limits.

89. Mr. Miller says to the nurse, "I don't think I can go on living when Tommy is gone." What would be the best response?

☐ 1. "Do you think your life will be over?"

☐ 2. "You will find it difficult to continue your life without Tommy."

☐ 3. "Your wife will need you."

☐ 4. "I can understand how you feel."

Sandra Gibson is admitted to the hospital with a diagnosis of acute bacterial pneumonia.

90. Miss Gibson's initial symptoms are not likely to include which of the following?

☐ 1. Cyanosis.

☐ 2. Dehydration.

☐ 3. Pleuritic pain.

☐ 4. Audible wheezing.

91. In caring for Miss Gibson, why must the nurse be careful to avoid overmedication with sedatives?

☐ 1. They suppress bone marrow function.

☐ 2. They depress the cough reflex and cause accumulation of fluids in the lung.

☐ 3. They increase the risk of superinfection.

☐ 4. They cause hypersensitivity reactions.

92. Which of the following actions is *not* appropriate treatment for Miss Gibson's bacterial pneumonia?

☐ 1. Auscultate the lungs q2h to q4h.

☐ 2. Encourage fluids to 3 L/day.

☐ 3. Give ampicillin if the client is allergic to penicillin.

☐ 4. Encourage the client to cough by splinting her chest.

93. What is the best reason for encouraging Miss Gibson to increase her fluid intake?

☐ 1. To promote bronchial dilatation.

☐ 2. To prevent the need for a nasogastric tube.

☐ 3. To improve antibiotic therapy.

☐ 4. To loosen and thin bronchial secretions.

94. Why is aspiration pneumonia more common in the right lung?

☐ 1. There is an increased amount of lung tissue available for infection on the right side.

☐ 2. There is an absence of ciliated mucosal lining on the right.

☐ 3. The right bronchus is shorter and wider.

☐ 4. There is enhanced conduction through the airways on the right.

95. Which of the following statements best describes why a pleural effusion may be a complication of Miss Gibson's pneumonia?

☐ 1. Excess connective tissue accumulates in the lungs during healing and repair.

☐ 2. Increased hydrostatic pressure or decreased oncotic pressure occurs with movement of fluid out of the capillaries.

☐ 3. Thrombotic occlusion of the pulmonary arterial system occurs.

☐ 4. The pleurae become inflamed.

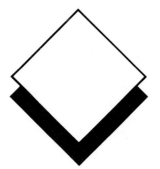

Test 1, Book I

KEY TO ABBREVIATIONS
Section of the Review Book

P = Psychosocial and Mental Health Problems
    T = Therapeutic Use of Self
    L = Loss and Death and Dying
    A = Anxious Behavior
    C = Confused Behavior
    E = Elated-Depressive Behavior
    SM = Socially Maladaptive Behavior
    SS = Suspicious Behavior
    W = Withdrawn Behavior
    SU = Substance Use Disorders
A = Adult
    H = Healthy Adult
    S = Surgery
    O = Oxygenation
    NM = Nutrition and Metabolism
    E = Elimination
    SP = Sensation and Perception
    M = Mobility
    CA = Cellular Aberration
CBF = Childbearing Family
    W = Women's Health Care
    A = Antepartal Care
    I = Intrapartal Care
    P = Postpartal Care
    N = Newborn Care
C = Child
    H = Healthy Child
    I = Ill and Hospitalized Child
    SPP = Sensation, Perception, and Protection
    O = Oxygenation
    NM = Nutrition and Metabolism
    E = Elimination
    M = Mobility
    CA = Cellular Aberration

Nursing Process Category

AS = Assessment
AN = Analysis
PL = Plan
IM = Implementation
EV = Evaluation

Client Need Category

E = Safe, Effective Care Environment
PS = Physiological Integrity
PC = Psychosocial Integrity
H = Health Promotion and Maintenance

1. no. 2. The ability to communicate with the client is essential to the quality of care. A/NM, AS, E
2. no. 2. Respiratory status is always the primary concern, especially with a client who has had an unconscious espisode. Vital signs and mental status would be the next priority. A/NM, AS, PS
3. no. 2. During the admission process, a family member fluent in both languages is the best person to help gather the essential data. In Mrs. Garcia's culture, the family plays an important role in the care of the client and the success of treatment. A/NM, IM, E
4. no. 4. Adjusting to life changes, especially for the older person, is a difficult process. Option no. 4 does not consider this problem of the difficulty of change. A/NM, PL, E
5. no. 3. Manipulation is a dominant characteristic of the client who exhibits antisocial behavior. Clients such as this have difficulty relating to others because of inner feelings of abandonment. Although it is possible that this particular nurse has superior abilities, it is likely that a number of other staff also have superior abilities. Clients such as Miss Evenson are rarely motivated to change. Any genuine changes

that might occur will happen very slowly. P/SM, AN, PC

6. no. 3. Lack of opportunity to identify with appropriate role models, such as parents, results in a poorly developed and unsocialized superego. It is not likely that Miss Evenson had appropriate role models. Clients like this often have developmental histories suggesting that early needs were not met adequately. There is no data suggesting below-average intelligence. P/SM, AS, PC

7. no. 3. The cooperation of all staff is necessary to achieve consistency in setting limits on behavior. Miss Evenson needs firm limits, not freedom of choice or independence. The client is not likely to do well in a group setting, since she has not internalized self-control. The client needs a matter-of-fact attitude and firm limits. She will mistake sympathy for weakness and try to manipulate staff more. P/SM, IM, E

8. no. 4. Clients demonstrating antisocial characteristics have no lasting attachments or sense of loyalty. They attempt to achieve pleasurable ends at the expense of others. Although these clients have low self-esteem and poor impulse control, this example does not demonstrate these traits. Although the client may be suspicious and aloof, her statement best demonstrates option no. 4. P/SM, AN, E

9. no. 3. Ambivalent feelings are exemplified by these opposing behaviors. Ambivalence is demonstrated in behaviors described in the question. Further information is necessary to determine whether guilt is present. Option no. 1 is unlikely. P/SM, AN, PC

10. no. 3. After realizing how inappropriate past behavior was, the client often feels depressed. Depression occurs as a consequence of dealing with difficulties in therapy and an emerging awareness of how her behavior affects others. Dysthymic disorder refers to a neurotic depression. A major depressive episode has psychotic features including severe impairment of reality testing and physiological disturbances. The client may begin to think her prognosis is not good, but such thoughts would not be as likely to occur at this time as option no. 3. P/SM, EV, PC

11. no. 3. More appropriate relationships with others demonstrates a decrease in antisocial behavior. Motivation for impressing the staff is difficult to discern. Her feelings for the other client are not known. The behavior described does not indicate apathy. P/SM, E, PC

12. no. 2. Pregnancy tests are based on the presence of human chorionic gonadotropin (HCG) in the blood or urine of the woman. CBF/A, AS PS

13. no. 3. Latex agglutination tests become positive approximately 10 to 14 days after the first missed menstrual period. A sample of the first morning urine is used for the test because it is generally the most concentrated urine of the day. CBF/A, IM, PS

14. no. 1. Although teratogenic effects may be specific depending on the causative agent, the greatest danger exists during the formation of the organ systems, or organogenesis, which typically is completed by the end of the twelfth week of pregnancy. CBF/A, IM, PS

15. no. 3. The ductus arteriosus allows most of the fetal blood to bypass the fetal lungs. Circulation to the lungs of the fetus is needed only for nutrition of the lungs because oxygen exchange occurs across the placental barrier. The ductus venosus allows fetal blood to bypass the fetal liver. CBF/A, AN PS

16. no. 2. The placenta provides a semipermeable membrane across which exchange occurs by osmosis. In addition, diffusion, facilitated diffusion, active transport, and pinocytosis occur. Oxytocin is produced by the maternal posterior pituitary gland. Viruses readily pass through the placenta. Maternal and fetal blood do not mix unless there is a break in the placental barrier. CBF/A, AN, PS

17. no. 2. The practice of abdominal splinting facilitates postoperative performance of coughing and deep breathing. Practicing leg exercises is inappropriate because they would increase abdominal pain preoperatively. A nasogastric tube is usually not required following a simple appendectomy. There is usually little wound drainage as a result of a simple appendectomy. A/S, PL, PS

18. no. 3. After the client has received preoperative sedation, he is no longer considered competent to sign the operative permit. The other options are true but are unrelated to preoperative medication. A/S, IM, E

19. no. 4. The circulating nurse is responsible for ensuring the safety of the client and preventing any harm from positioning. A/S, PL, E

20. no. 4. The conscious interpretation of pain takes place in the cerebral cortex. A/S, AN, PS

21. no. 1. Movement of the client from the operating room table to the postanesthesia room may cause a transient drop in blood pressure. A/S, IM, PS

22. no. 2. Standing a male client who is experiencing postoperative urinary retention at the bedside may facilitate voiding. Waiting is not appropriate, and explanations will not solve the problem. Catheterization may eventually be necessary but is not the first step. A/S, IM, PS

23. no. 3. When secretions are retained, they block the small alveoli and cause them to collapse. The resultant inflammation often leads to pneumonia. A/S, AN, PS

24. no. 4. Strawberry tongue is characteristic of scarlet fever, an infection by beta-hemolytic streptococci, group A. The other three options are characteristic of chickenpox. C/SPP, AS, PS

25. no. 1. Varicella is an airborne virus, and respiratory isolation procedures should be used to prevent its spread. C/SPP, IM, H

26. no. 2. Keeping Marianne's fingernails short and clean decreases the chance of her acquiring a secondary infection of the pruritic lesions of chickenpox. C/SPP, IM, PS

27. no. 3. Painting with watercolors allows her to use her imagination for expression of feelings and ideas; it also promotes development of fine motor skills, which is important at this age. C/SPP, IM, H

28. no. 3. Once the lesions have dried, chickenpox is no longer communicable, and Marianne can return to school. A fever may be gone by the time the rash appears. Option no. 4 indicates she is still contagious. C/SPP, IM, H

29. no. 1. The speech center is located in the left posterolateral side of the frontal lobe (Broca's center). A/SP, AS, PS

30. no. 3. Bladder fullness is a priority assessment if the client has spinal cord injuries. There is loss of bladder reflex to empty during spinal shock that occurs within 30 minutes of injury. A/SP, AS, PS

31. no. 3. Dexamethasone (Decadron) is the only corticosteroid that crosses the blood-brain barrier. It is the most commonly used steroid in clients with neurological damage because of its antiinflammatory action. A/SP, AN, PS

32. no. 1. All the choices listed are important, but instituting seizure precautions is the priority. A/SP, IM, PS

33. no. 2. During any seizure, restraining the client can create more trauma than the seizure itself. Other options listed are appropriate to protect client safety. A/SP, IM, E

34. no. 3. These measures will decrease cerebral edema, which will reduce the intracranial pressure. A/SP, AN, PS

35. no. 3. Mannitol is an osmotic diuretic. When it is discontinued, there is a temporary increase in fluid retention. A/SP, AN, PS

36. no. 2. These behaviors are signs of anxiety. Depression is usually manifested by withdrawal and lack of interest and energy. Yelling, threats, and demands would indicate anger or agitation. Someone in denial would probably not ask repetitive questions; instead the individual might avoid the issues. P/A, AN, PC

37. no. 4. It is too soon for role acceptance to be a major concern. Options no. 1, no. 2, and no. 3 are current issues that are inherent in the client's condition, given the suddenness of the accident, his age, and severity of injury. P/A, AN, PC

38. no. 2. Active listening allows the gathering of more information and provides an opportunity for psychosocial intervention. Options no. 3 and no. 4 may be appropriate after further assessment. Option

no. 1 is not an independent nursing action. P/A, IM, PC

39. no. 4. Reactive depression is related to precipitating stress and personal loss. In Scott's case, loss of freedom of movement and the possibility of the loss of his foot have caused a reactive depression. A common response is angry and demanding behavior. Withdrawal from alcohol probably would have occurred within 24 to 72 hours after hospitalization. Boredom usually manifests as complaining and restlessness, not yelling and demanding. The current behavioral presentation is not consistent with a psychotic depression; however, one would want to continue monitoring him for a possible delirium syndrome. P/E, AN, PC

40. no. 4. Firmness and consistency will make the client feel more secure and help to alleviate his fear. Minimizing the number of nurses who care for the client facilitates the implementation of a consistent approach. Ignoring or meeting the inappropriate demands only serves to escalate the behavior and does not solve the problem of his fear and insecurity. P/E, IM, PC

41. no. 3. Anger is implied in his desire for revenge. Option no. 1 is not an acceptance of the retaliation theme but an inference of what the client may be feeling or thinking. A reflective statement uses part of what the client has already stated, i.e., "You are going to get even with your friend." Option no. 4 would be the outcome of using any one of the previously stated communication techniques. P/E, IM, PC

42. no. 3. Reflecting is the proper therapeutic technique to use in this situation. It gives the client permission to express his feelings about the loss of his foot. Option no. 1 does not address his fears or concerns and will only provide the nurse with a factual option, not an exploration of feelings. Option no. 2 is a threat which, with an adolescent, will probably precipitate a power struggle. Option no. 4 will be perceived as a punishment and humiliating in front of a peer who could be beneficial in helping the client to verbalize his fears. P/E, IM, PC

43. no. 3. The fact that Scott asked the nurse for a date, to go dancing in particular, is the clue to his concern. Options no. 1 and no. 4 are possibilities; however, the specific activity for the date is dancing, which would require a healthy foot. He is taking a risk with this request, which could embarrass him, not the nurse. P/E, AN, PC

44. no. 2. This option both acknowledges the client's concern and allows him to discuss it if he wishes to do so. Options no. 1 and no. 4 establish a behavioral limit with the client; however, these responses also diminish the chance of the client sharing any feelings with this nurse. Option no. 3 completely misses and avoids the feeling tone of this client's request. P/E, IM, PC

45. no. 2. Expiratory wheezing is the result of air attempting to pass through narrowed bronchial lumens. Option no. 1 characterizes croup and laryngotracheobronchitis; no. 4 relates to croup; expirations in asthma are prolonged. C/O, AS, PS

46. no. 2. Subcutaneous is the preferred route. On occasion, it may be given IM, but the gluteal sites should be avoided. There is no epinephrine preparation suitable for sublingual use. The IV route may be used only if the drug is adequately diluted. C/O, IM, PS

47. no. 1. Epinephrine relieves bronchospasm. It does not liquefy secretions (a subemetic dose of syrup of ipecac does this), nor does it increase antibody formation. The drug increases (not reduces) airway diameter. C/O, AN, PS

48. no. 3. Epinephrine is a beta-adrenergic agent that strengthens myocardial contractions and increases blood pressure, heart rate, and cardiac output. The vasoconstrictive effects predispose the child to tachycardia as well as elevated blood pressure, pallor, weakness, tremors, and nausea. C/O, AS, PS

49. no. 4. Options no. 1, no. 2, and no. 3 are definite signs of respiratory distress. Irregular respirations may occur for many other reasons and are frequently normal in young children. C/O, AS, PS

50. no. 4. Tachycardia is the only manifestation of aminophylline toxicity listed. Other manifestations include headache, hypotension, vomiting, and nervousness. C/O, EV, PS

51. no. 3. Intake and output and specific gravity are good indicators of hydration. Hydration helps to liquefy secretions and enables the child to expel the mucus. Option no. 1 is contraindicated. Position of choice is high-Fowler's position. Option no. 4 is unnecessary. C/O, PL, E

52. no. 2. Adrenocortical steroids interrupt normal linear growth in children when used over a prolonged time. C/O, AN, PS

53. no. 2. Hydrocortisone's (Solu-Cortef) antiinflammatory action relieves airway obstruction by reducing edema. It is administered IV when the usual drugs (e.g., epinephrine) are not effective. Hydrocortisone (Solu-Cortef) does not reduce anxiety, mobilize secretions, or relieve bronchospasms. The other asthma drugs achieve these actions. C/O, AN, PS

54. no. 4. The usual cause of asthma is an allergy or hypersensitivity to a foreign protein. A fish would be the most logical choice of pet for an asthmatic child. C/O, IM, H

55. no. 4. Couples preparing for delivery in a birthing center are well informed about these and other options, such as sibling participation. CBF/I, EV, H

56. no. 1. Allow the client to select another individual to take on the supporting role. If no one is available, it is helpful to assign one nurse. CBF/I, IM, PC

57. no. 3. This indicates that the presenting part of the fetus is at the perineum; delivery will be very soon. CBF/I, AS, PS

58. no. 2. Many clients are now discharged early from the hospital or birthing centers; it is essential to assess uterine firmness frequently and to massage as needed. The other options are important but can be addressed during follow-up visits. CBF/P, IM, H

59. no. 4. Although other goals are appropriate over a longer period, promoting attachment is the best short-term goal. CBF/P, PS, E

60. no. 2. Myasthenia gravis is exacerbated by infection, emotional stress, menses, pregnancy, surgery, or accidental administration of curare, quinine, or quinidine. The other options would not be discussed by the nurse but by the physician. A/SP, IM, PS

61. no. 3. Muscle rigidity and tremors at rest are symptoms of Parkinson's disease. A/SP, AS, PS

62. no. 4. Myasthenia gravis frequently causes weakness in muscles innervated by cranial nerves IX and X, which is associated with difficult swallowing, regurgitation, and aspiration. A/SP, AS, E

63. no. 4. Pyridostigmine (Mestinon) is absorbed too quickly on an empty stomach. However, if the client is having symptoms, she may need to take the medication, or part of it, before a meal to aid chewing and swallowing. A/SP, IM, H

64. no. 3. Weakness becomes worse on exertion and at the end of the day (as opposed to morning). Rest typically increases muscle strength. A/SP, IM, H

65. no. 2. Myasthenia gravis can be aggravated by pregnancy. Medication will need very careful management during pregnancy but may not be able to prevent problems. A/SP, IM, PS

66. no. 2. Myasthenia gravis is caused by an autoimmune process that impairs receptor function at the myoneural junction. A/SP, AN, PS

67. no. 2. Exogenous steroids cause adrenal gland hypofunction. The body may not be able to respond in times of stress. A/SP, AN, PS

68. no. 1. Stopping steroids suddenly would mimic addisonian crisis, the major complication of which is cardiovascular collapse. A/SP, AN, PS

69. no. 2. This is a period of maximum cardiac output, and as a result, cardiac decompensation may occur. CBF/A, AN, PS

70. no. 4. These are the early symptoms of congestive cardiac failure and must be promptly recognized and treated. CBF/A, EV, H

71. no. 2. Heparin is the drug of choice when an anticoagulant is required because its large molecular weight prevents it from crossing the placenta. Penicillin is used prophylactically to prevent subacute

bacterial endocarditis. Digitalis may have teratogenic properties since it does cross the placenta. CBF/A, AN, PS

72. no. 2. Forceps application reduces the stress and exertion of pushing. Vaginal delivery is the preferred method of delivery for cardiac clients. CBF/I, IM, PS

73. no. 4. The semirecumbent, or Fowler's, position allows for maximum functioning of her heart and respiratory system. CBF/I, IM, PS

74. no. 1. Breastfeeding is permissible if there are no cardiac problems during labor and delivery and immediately postpartum. Rooming-in is possible only with assistance and as she desires. A gradual increase in activity during the postpartum period is recommended. CBF/P, PL, PS

75. no. 1. Characteristics of a situational crisis are a precipitating event (divorce) and signs and symptoms of extreme discomfort (e.g., tearfulness, narrowed perception, loss of thinking ability, fidgeting, and increased values in vital signs). Any depressive symptoms would be related to the current situation and loss. Options no. 3 and no. 4 are diagnoses that are not consistent with the clinical situation. P/T, AN, PC

76. no. 4. The scope of crisis intervention is to deal with here-and-now problems and help the client and family to find coping mechanisms effective in dealing with stress in the environment. New coping can be explored without knowing the cause of the problem. Insight and increased self-knowledge are valuable but may not always produce behavioral change. The client in crisis is facing the opportunity to change for the better or regress. The discomfort of the high anxiety provides leverage for the nurse to assist the client in learning how to problem solve and develop more effective coping. Giving advice reinforces the person's sense of helplessness. P/T, AN, PC

77. no. 1. Crisis intervention involves assessment of the client's support systems, current and previous coping mechanisms, and the precipitating event. Options no. 2, no. 3, and no. 4 can be behavioral manifestations of someone experiencing a crisis state; however, they are more indicative of chronic psychopathological behavior. The crisis intervention framework focuses on the here-and-now and not chronic problems. P/T, AS, PC

78. no. 2. Initially, it is necessary to determine immediate problems and how they are viewed by the client. Reassurance at this time seldom lowers anxiety and tends to make the client feel misunderstood. Advice given before the problem is identified and feelings are explored is usually not taken because the client's anxiety is too high to make use of the suggestion. It is preferable to help the client come up with her own solutions after the distorted perceptions have been corrected and her anxiety lowered. Rather than contacting the husband, explore with the client who her support system is, and encourage her to contact someone with whom she will feel comfortable. P/T, IM, E

79. no. 4. When dealing with Mrs. Thompson's crying, reflect the feeling and ask for more information. Some clients will want privacy, but this should be clarified with the client before the nurse automatically leaves a client alone to cry. False reassurance blocks communication. Although antianxiety medications are commonly used to help clients be less nervous and gain control over themselves, crying is a healthy, emotional outlet and should be permitted and supported rather than circumvented with medication. P/T, IM, E

80. no. 3. The emergency room nurse can refer clients such as Mrs. Thompson to community mental health centers for crisis intervention and for continued therapy or necessary referrals. Mrs. Thompson's condition does not warrant inpatient psychiatric treatment or day care. Professional evaluation would be indicated first before any referral to a self-help group. P/T, IM, PC

81. no. 4. Crises are time-limited and are usually resolved within 6 weeks. Once a week is sufficient and allows time for the client to implement new coping behaviors and be supported during the entire time of the crisis. P/T, PL, PC

82. no. 3. The information given suggests she has experienced personal growth. The goal of crisis intervention is to prevent hospitalization and regression to a permanently maladaptive state. This has been achieved. Even though the client has been traumatized and is the same person she was 6 weeks ago, her coping has become adaptive and enhances her life, so she is functioning at a higher level. P/T, EV, PC

83. no. 4. Do not avoid Tommy and his parents; they may be unable to ask for the help that they need (a common problem for persons in crisis). Provide both privacy and emotional support. C/CA, PL, PC

84. no. 3. The toothbrush and peroxide solution might further damage Tommy's ulcerated and infected mouth. Doing nothing is not an appropriate measure because discomfort will be increased. C/CA, IM, PS

85. no. 1. Fingernails should be kept short to prevent scratching and injury to skin with pruritus. The other answers are inappropriate for a terminally ill client. C/CA, IM, PS

86. no. 1. According to Kübler-Ross, Mrs. Miller is denying the consequences of the terminal phase of Tommy's illness. C/CA, AN, PC

87. no. 3. Hydroxyzine causes sedation and does not

stimulate the central nervous system. C/CA, AN, PS

88. no. 3. This provides sound control for the other clients' benefit and allows Tommy to have his request. Music with earphones is also helpful for pain control and relaxation. C/CA, IM, E

89. no. 2. The nurse is paraphrasing what the client said to encourage feedback. Option no. 1 is a direct question that limits clarification of feelings. Option no. 3 does not respond to the expressed concern and no. 4 is a meaningless statement when the client has not had an opportunity to fully express his feelings. C/CA, IM, PC

90. no. 4. Findings on physical examination of the chest may include dullness to percussion, diminished breath sounds, crackles, and a pleural friction rub. Audible wheezing is a symptom of narrowed bronchioles in hyperinflated lungs such as those found in clients with asthma. A/O, AS, PS

91. no. 2. Sedatives can have this effect. Antineoplastic drugs usually suppress bone marrow. Antibiotics may increase the risk of superinfections. Penicillin-type drugs more commonly cause hypersensitivity reactions. A/O, AN, PS

92. no. 3. Ampicillin is in the penicillin family and should not be given to someone who is allergic to penicillin. A/O, IM, PS

93. no. 4. Fluid intake of at least 3 L/day facilitates the expectoration of bronchial secretions. A/O, PL, PS

94. no. 3. The right and left mainstem bronchi are not symmetrical; the right bronchus is shorter and wider and continues from the trachea in a vertical course. This anatomical difference facilitates aspiration into the right lung. A/O, AN, PS

95. no. 2. Pleural effusions result from the movement of fluid out of the capillaries by an increased hydrostatic pressure or decreased oncotic pressure. A/O, AN, PS

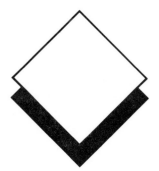

Test 1, Book II

QUESTIONS

Sheila Vogel is admitted to the labor room. Her gestation is estimated to be at 35 weeks, but she is having contractions. Attempts are made to stop labor.

1. Which of the following nursing actions is appropriate when caring for Mrs. Vogel?
   - ☐ 1. Prepare for an oxytocin challenge test to determine fetal status.
   - ☐ 2. Prepare for the application of an internal monitor.
   - ☐ 3. Evaluate cervical dilatation frequently.
   - ☐ 4. Discuss the potential problems and the preparations being made for the infant.

2. Bed rest is prescribed for Mrs. Vogel primarily because it will do which of the following?
   - ☐ 1. Keep the pressure of the fetus off the cervix and enhance uterine perfusion.
   - ☐ 2. Decrease maternal metabolic demands and lower oxygen needs.
   - ☐ 3. Promote comfort and reduce anxiety.
   - ☐ 4. Reduce fetal activity and strengthen the fetal heartbeat.

3. A tocolytic agent is administered to Mrs. Vogel to suppress her labor. Which of the following nursing actions would be most appropriate in preventing side effects from tocolytic therapy?
   - ☐ 1. Maintain Mrs. Vogel in a side-lying position, and monitor for maternal pulse greater than 140 beats/min.
   - ☐ 2. Reduce extraneous stimuli, and record daily weights.
   - ☐ 3. Use side rails, and frequently monitor uterine contractions greater than 50 mm Hg.
   - ☐ 4. Frequently monitor maternal reflexes, and encourage fluid intake of 3000 ml or more.

4. Which of the following drugs is considered a tocolytic agent?
   - ☐ 1. Levallorphan tartrate (Lorfan).
   - ☐ 2. Terbutaline sulfate (Brethine).
   - ☐ 3. Phenobarbital.
   - ☐ 4. Betamethasone phosphate (Celestone).

5. Attempts to stop labor are unsuccessful, and Baby Boy Vogel is born weighing 4 pounds 2 ounces. Which of the following observations of Baby Vogel suggest a gestational age of less than 40 weeks?
   - ☐ 1. Small amounts of lanugo and vernix, testes descended, and palmar and plantar creases.
   - ☐ 2. Parchmentlike skin, no lanugo, and full areolas in breasts.
   - ☐ 3. Upper pinna of ear well curved with instant recoil, small amounts of lanugo, and pink in color.
   - ☐ 4. Dark-red skin, testes undescended with few rugations, and abundant lanugo.

6. The nurse carries out necessary precautions in the delivery room to meet the special needs of the premature infant. Which of the following is an important difference between a premature and term infant?
   - ☐ 1. A premature infant will have a more efficient metabolic rate for heat production and maintenance because of its smaller size.
   - ☐ 2. The premature infant will have more lanugo and more vernix than a full-term infant.
   - ☐ 3. Stools may be infrequent, resulting in abdominal distension because gastrointestinal motility is decreased in the preterm infant.
   - ☐ 4. Heat production is low in the premature infant because of the greater body surface related to weight and lack of subcutaneous fat.

7. Which of the following assessments would most likely indicate respiratory distress in the neonate?
   - ☐ 1. Abdominal breathing and acrocyanosis.
   - ☐ 2. Irregular, shallow respirations.
   - ☐ 3. Respiratory rate of 30 to 60/min.
   - ☐ 4. Nasal flaring.

8. Baby Vogel's hospital stay is uneventful. Which aspect of Baby Vogel's care will have the greatest permanent effect on emotional development?
   - ☐ 1. The position in which he is placed in the crib.
   - ☐ 2. The way in which he is held and touched.
   - ☐ 3. The extent to which a quiet environment is provided for him.

□ 4. The number of caretakers who provide care for him.

9. Provisions are made for Mrs. Vogel to spend time in the premature nursery. Which of the following is the most important reason for doing this?

□ 1. To provide her with written instructions concerning feeding and bathing the infant.

□ 2. To provide a demonstration of feeding and bathing for her.

□ 3. To provide her with the opportunity to handle and care for the infant in a supportive atmosphere.

□ 4. To provide her with an opportunity to ask questions she may have concerning the infant's growth and development.

Henry Nims, age 58, is admitted with a diagnosis of chronic obstructive pulmonary disease (COPD). His orders include antibiotics and respiratory therapy, including intermittent positive pressure breathing (IPPB), chest physical therapy, and ultrasonic nebulizer.

10. Mr. Nims' tidal volume is 250 cc. This is commonly considered

□ 1. High.

□ 2. Low.

□ 3. Normal.

□ 4. High for his age group.

11. Mr. Nims' dead-space volume is most likely to be

□ 1. 150 ml.

□ 2. Above 150 ml.

□ 3. 100 to 150 ml.

□ 4. Below 100 ml.

12. Mr. Nims' vital capacity will be the greatest in which of the following positions?

□ 1. Supine position.

□ 2. Prone position.

□ 3. Fowler's position.

□ 4. Sims' position.

13. Mr. Nims' arterial blood gases on admission were: pH 7.40, P_{O_2} 60 mm Hg, P_{CO_2} 60 mm Hg, HCO_3 30 mEq/L. These values are most indicative of which of the following conditions?

□ 1. Respiratory acidosis.

□ 2. Compensated respiratory acidosis.

□ 3. Respiratory alkalosis.

□ 4. Compensated respiratory alkalosis.

14. Mr. Nims' blood gases could best be considered which of the following?

□ 1. Normal.

□ 2. Normal for a COPD client.

□ 3. Abnormal.

□ 4. Abnormal for a COPD client.

15. Mr. Nims has most likely become adjusted to which of the following?

□ 1. Elevated P_{CO_2} and P_{O_2} levels.

□ 2. Lowered P_{CO_2} and elevated P_{O_2} levels.

□ 3. Elevated P_{CO_2} and lowered P_{O_2} levels.

□ 4. Lowered P_{CO_2} and P_{O_2} levels.

16. Mr. Nims has copious amounts of thick, tenacious yellow mucus, which he cannot expectorate. He requires suctioning, and the nurse becomes concerned that he might have a cardiopulmonary arrest during this procedure. Which of the following would not precipitate a cardiac arrest during suctioning?

□ 1. Depletion of oxygen to the brain.

□ 2. Depletion of oxygen to the heart.

□ 3. Vagal nerve stimulation.

□ 4. Electrolyte imbalance.

17. What is the primary purpose of intermittent positive pressure breathing (IPPB) for this client?

□ 1. Open clogged airways.

□ 2. Loosen accumulated secretions.

□ 3. Promote dilatation of smooth muscle bands around airways.

□ 4. Provide adequate ventilation.

18. Mr. Nims begins to exhibit restlessness, combativeness, and tachycardia, but he is not acyanotic. The nurse would expect to find his arterial P_{O_2} to be which of the following?

□ 1. 48 to 52 mm Hg.

□ 2. 30 to 40 mm Hg.

□ 3. 60 to 70 mm Hg.

□ 4. Greater than 70 mm Hg.

19. Which rate of oxygen flow per cannula would most likely be ordered for Mr. Nims?

□ 1. Rate of 2 to 3 L/min.

□ 2. Rate of 4 to 6 L/min.

□ 3. Rate of 6 to 8 L/min.

□ 4. Rate of 8 to 10 L/min.

20. Which is the *least* reliable sign of adequate ventilation?

□ 1. Patent airway.

□ 2. Chest or abdominal movement with each respiration.

□ 3. Airflow at mouth or nose.

□ 4. Skin color.

While riding his skateboard, 14-year-old Dennis falls and fractures his elbow.

21. Which of the following is a severe complication of this injury?

□ 1. Fluid loss.

□ 2. Pain.

□ 3. Compartment syndrome.

□ 4. Infection.

22. Dennis' fracture is being treated with skeletal traction. Which nursing action would be included in caring for the traction?

□ 1. Remove the counterweights for relief of pain.

□ 2. Change bed position to prevent stasis.

☐ 3. Check pin sites for bleeding, inflammation, and infection.

☐ 4. Encourage active range of motion for the elbow to prevent contractures.

23. What physiological effect of immobility is Dennis likely to experience?

☐ 1. Positive nitrogen balance.

☐ 2. Increased metabolic rate.

☐ 3. Hypercalcemia.

☐ 4. Increased vital capacity.

24. The nurse institutes pin care while Dennis is in traction. Which sign would alert the nurse that a complication may be developing?

☐ 1. The pin moves freely through the bone.

☐ 2. The skin around the pin is dry and pink.

☐ 3. Dennis has an oral temperature of 37° C.

☐ 4. The traction is pulling on the pin.

25. Dennis will be in traction for several weeks. Which diversional activity would best meet his developmental needs?

☐ 1. Reading school books.

☐ 2. Watching educational television.

☐ 3. Receiving visits from friends.

☐ 4. Building model airplanes.

Calvin York is admitted to the coronary care unit with a diagnosis of myocardial infarction.

26. Two days later, Mr. York says to the nurse, "I don't know why they're keeping me here. I can rest at home. I have a lot of things I could be doing. I feel fine." Which of the following defense mechanisms is Mr. York utilizing?

☐ 1. Denial.

☐ 2. Rationalization.

☐ 3. Sublimation.

☐ 4. Compensation.

27. Mr. York has started eating a salt-restricted diet. When his tray is brought to him he shouts at the nurse, "Do you really expect me to eat this? It's not fit for human consumption. It has no taste." Which response by the nurse would be most therapeutic?

☐ 1. "Not fit for human consumption?"

☐ 2. "Mr. York, less salt will decrease the fluid in your body and make it easier for your heart to work."

☐ 3. "I'll arrange for you to see the dietitian."

☐ 4. "You sound angry about the way things are going right now."

Karla Lu, a 25-year-old Chinese woman, is admitted to the hospital with a diagnosis of aplastic anemia.

28. Which of the following is a frequent cause of aplastic anemia?

☐ 1. Vitamin B_{12} malabsorption.

☐ 2. Drugs.

☐ 3. Folic acid deficiency.

☐ 4. Genetic factors.

29. Which diagnostic test will help the physician make the most conclusive diagnosis of aplastic anemia?

☐ 1. Bone marrow aspiration.

☐ 2. Schilling test.

☐ 3. Hemogram.

☐ 4. Differential blood count.

30. When caring for Miss Lu, the most important nursing action is which of the following?

☐ 1. Teach her about her diet.

☐ 2. Balance rest and activity.

☐ 3. Encourage her to have some physical activity.

☐ 4. Maintain her fluid and electrolyte balance.

During the assessment, the nursery nurse finds that newborn Steven Sims has a foot deformity. The deformity is diagnosed as bilateral talipes equinovarus (clubfoot).

31. Which of the following most likely alerted the nurse that Steven has an abnormality?

☐ 1. The feet were in plantar flexion.

☐ 2. The feet deviated from the midline when dorsiflexed.

☐ 3. Manipulation of the feet seemed to induce pain.

☐ 4. The feet were not in alignment with the knees.

32. Plaster casts are applied to both of Steven's feet to reestablish the correct alignment. Cast application is done as soon as possible after diagnosis because

☐ 1. Developmental delays are prevented by early application of casts.

☐ 2. The infant's rapid growth will facilitate the correction.

☐ 3. Clubfoot abnormalities cannot be corrected after the age of 6 months.

☐ 4. The skin of a newborn is less susceptible to breakdown.

33. Steven leaves the hospital with casts and returns to the clinic in 3 weeks for a cast change. What would indicate that the nurse's instructions about cast care had not been adequately understood?

☐ 1. The cast was covered with ink drawings.

☐ 2. The cast had a urine odor.

☐ 3. The cast edges were rough.

☐ 4. The cast was wet from a bath.

34. Correction of Steven's foot abnormality is not achieved by casts alone. Steven is hospitalized at the age of 4 months for corrective surgery. Immediate postoperative care would include

☐ 1. Elevation of the lower extremities to decrease edema.

☐ 2. Elevation of the head to prevent feeding difficulties.

☐ 3. Placement in Bryant's traction.

☐ 4. Positioning on the abdomen.

35. Following several months of postoperative cast-wearing, a brace is ordered to maintain the corrected position of Steven's feet. The nurse discusses important aspects about the brace and about Steven's care with his parents. To determine the parents' understanding of the information provided, the best question for the nurse to ask is which of the following?
    □ 1. "Do you have any questions?"
    □ 2. "Could you explain to me how to apply the brace?"
    □ 3. "Could you show me how to apply the brace?"
    □ 4. "How will you apply Steven's brace?"

Baby Girl Snow is beginning to show signs of respiratory distress.

36. What is one of the major symptoms that would lead the nurse to suspect a tracheoesophageal fistula in Baby Girl Snow?
    □ 1. Barrel chest.
    □ 2. Snorting respirations.
    □ 3. Refusal of food.
    □ 4. Persistent drooling.
37. A diagnosis of tracheoesophageal fistula is made. The postoperative nursing care of an infant with a repaired tracheoesophageal fistula would *not* include which of the following?
    □ 1. Careful monitoring of IV solutions.
    □ 2. Vigorous nasotracheal suctioning.
    □ 3. Elevation of the head and thorax 30°.
    □ 4. Good skin care of gastrostomy site.
38. In collecting data about Baby Girl Snow, which finding is the nurse most likely to see in Mrs. Snow's perinatal records?
    □ 1. Exposure to rubella in the first trimester.
    □ 2. Active herpes lesions at delivery.
    □ 3. Polyhydramnios in the third trimester.
    □ 4. Prolonged active stage of labor.

Ann Perry, a 45-year-old woman, is admitted to the nursing unit with the diagnosis of hyperthyroidism.

39. The initial assessment would include physical findings that support this diagnosis. What are they?
    □ 1. Elevated vital signs, nervousness, and weight gain.
    □ 2. Elevated vital signs, nervousness, and weight loss.
    □ 3. Decreased vital signs, lethargy, and weight gain.
    □ 4. Decreased vital signs, nervousness, and weight loss.
40. The nurse would monitor Mrs. Perry for which of the following signs and symptoms of complications?
    □ 1. Cold intolerance.
    □ 2. Sensitivity to narcotics.
    □ 3. Increased tachycardia.

□ 4. Increased lethargy.
41. Mrs. Perry's nursing diagnosis of sleep pattern disturbance could be aided by
    □ 1. Restricting fluid intake.
    □ 2. Administering liotrix (Thyrolar).
    □ 3. Using a private room.
    □ 4. Providing a warm environment.
42. Mrs. Perry will require which of the following dietary modifications?
    □ 1. Six meals per day of a regular diet.
    □ 2. Low-fat, low-sodium, low-calorie diet.
    □ 3. High-protein, high-carbohydrate, high-calorie diet.
    □ 4. Low-carbohydrate, high-protein diet.
43. Mrs. Perry is discharged on a levothyroxine (Synthroid) regimen following an uncomplicated, subtotal thyroidectomy. During her clinic visit several months later, Mrs. Perry complains of tiredness and of feeling cold. What content area would be most emphasized if the nursing diagnosis of knowledge deficit regarding self-management is made?
    □ 1. The lack of thyroid hormones produced by the body requires daily intake of thyroid medication.
    □ 2. Symptoms arise from taking too much thyroid-replacement medication, so the dose needs adjusting.
    □ 3. The parathyroids will grow and will be able to meet the body's needs for the hormones.
    □ 4. The parathyroids are overactive from having been disturbed during surgery, but symptoms should disappear soon.

Rachel Rosen has been given a diagnosis of cancer of the colon. Her physician has told her that the disease has progressed to the point that it cannot be treated and that her life expectancy is less than a year. Mrs. Rosen is 47 years old, married, and has two adult children.

44. After the physician and Mr. Rosen have left, the nurse enters the room to see how the client is feeling. Mrs. Rosen says, "That doctor must be crazy. He thinks I'm dying, but I'm not really that sick." What is the best interpretation of this remark?
    □ 1. It indicates a common response to what she has just been told.
    □ 2. It implies she is unable to cope with her problem.
    □ 3. It is an aberrant reaction.
    □ 4. It requires further data for interpretation.
45. What is the most therapeutic response to Mrs. Rosen's remark?
    □ 1. Remain silent and allow her to continue talking.
    □ 2. Notify her physician, and request appropriate orders.
    □ 3. Ask her to say more about what she means.
    □ 4. Reassure her.

46. What is the first goal in working with Mrs. Rosen?
□ 1. The client will begin to deal with impending death.
□ 2. The client will accept her impending death.
□ 3. The client will be able to say goodbye to relatives and friends.
□ 4. The client will verbalize an understanding of the disease process.

47. Which of the following would be included in planning for Mrs. Rosen's care?
□ 1. Help the client to identify the destructiveness of denial.
□ 2. Avoid questions about death and dying until later stages of the process.
□ 3. Stimulate expressions of anger and rage.
□ 4. Offer regular opportunities for the client to talk.

48. One day, Mrs. Rosen says, "I'll be so glad when this is all over and I can go back to work." How would the nurse respond?
□ 1. "Your work is really important to you."
□ 2. "I'm afraid you won't be going back to work."
□ 3. "It must be hard for you right now."
□ 4. "Tell me more about what you mean."

49. After about 3 weeks, Mrs. Rosen has not changed much in her responses to her diagnosis. One morning, she asks the nurse, "Do you think I'm going to die?" What is the best response for the nurse to make?
□ 1. "That is the diagnosis your doctor has given you."
□ 2. "Do you think you're going to die?"
□ 3. "What made you ask that question?"
□ 4. "This seems to be bothering you."

50. A few days later, the nurse enters the room to give Mrs. Rosen her bath. Mrs. Rosen says to the nurse, "Leave me alone. You're all like vultures hovering over me. Get out and don't come back!" What is the best nurse response?
□ 1. "Why are you so mad at me?"
□ 2. "You sound like you're pretty upset right now. Let's talk about it."
□ 3. "We may seem like vultures, but we're trying to help you."
□ 4. "I'll come back later when you've calmed down."

51. After Mrs. Rosen has spent more than 2 months in the hospital, Mr. and Mrs. Rosen express a desire to have Mrs. Rosen at home for the remaining time she has to live. What is the most appropriate nursing approach?
□ 1. Encourage them to reconsider this idea.
□ 2. Leave it up to them to work out with the physician.
□ 3. Help them to discuss the denial of the seriousness of Mrs. Rosen's illness.
□ 4. Help them to make realistic arrangements.

52. Which statement indicates that the goal for Mrs. Rosen was met?
□ 1. Mrs. Rosen moves through the stages of the dying process and experiences a dignified death.
□ 2. Mrs. Rosen discontinues denial and expresses anger appropriately.
□ 3. Mrs. Rosen resumes a life-style comparable to that before her diagnosis.
□ 4. Mrs. Rosen becomes as independent as possible for her remaining life.

Four-and-a-half-year-old Erik is being prepared for correction of a mild pulmonary stenosis. He is not sure why he has to stay in the hospital.

53. Which assessment factor is most important in deciding how much information to give him?
□ 1. Developmental age.
□ 2. Desire to learn.
□ 3. Previous hospitalization history.
□ 4. Attitudes of his parents about hospitalization.

54. Erik's parents ask about his cardiac problem. The nursing response is based on knowledge that pulmonary stenosis most often includes which of the following cardiac pathological conditions?
□ 1. Left-to-right shunting of blood.
□ 2. Left ventricular hypertrophy.
□ 3. Right ventricular hypertrophy.
□ 4. Aortic insufficiency.

55. Preoperatively, which of the following nursing approaches is most important for Erik?
□ 1. Allow him to play with other children.
□ 2. Encourage him to express his feelings through play.
□ 3. Keep him isolated to prevent exposure to infection.
□ 4. Suggest vigorous exercise to build up his strength.

56. After surgery, the nurse prepares Erik and his parents for his return home. Which of the following suggestions by the nurse is most appropriate for the time when the recovery period is over?
□ 1. Limit his physical activity in the future.
□ 2. Provide for a tutor to decrease risk of infection from classmates.
□ 3. Help Erik understand that he will have special needs.
□ 4. Treat Erik like a normal child.

57. As a goodbye gift for the nurse, Erik draws a multicolor picture that has as its focus a figure consisting of two circles (head and body), two stick arms, and one stick leg. What is the best response for the nurse to make?
□ 1. "Oh, what a nice picture!"
□ 2. "Tell me about your drawing."
□ 3. "What is it?"

☐ 4. "Is that your doctor?"

58. As Erik prepares to leave the hospital, which of the following motor skills would the nurse be *least* likely to see him perform?

☐ 1. Riding a tricycle.

☐ 2. Using scissors to cut out a favorite picture.

☐ 3. Tying a bow.

☐ 4. Climbing stairs like an adult.

Steve Ray is admitted to the emergency room with a stiff neck and temperature of 102° F (38.8° C). He has had an earache for 1 week, but has not sought treatment for it.

59. Nuchal rigidity will *not* be seen in which of the following?

☐ 1. Meningitis.

☐ 2. Intracranial mass with herniation.

☐ 3. Intracranial hematoma.

☐ 4. Cerebral concussion.

60. Which of the following is a *contraindication* to lumbar puncture?

☐ 1. Unequal pupils.

☐ 2. Lack of lateralization.

☐ 3. Suspicion of meningitis.

☐ 4. Nuchal rigidity.

61. In addition to a brief explanation of the lumbar puncture procedure, which of the following is also the responsibility of the nurse?

☐ 1. Administer a narcotic to the client.

☐ 2. Position the client safely and properly in a lateral recumbent position with his knees flexed.

☐ 3. Administer procaine hydrochloride (Novocain).

☐ 4. Prepare a suture set so that it will be ready after the procedure.

62. Bacterial meningitis is confirmed by the cerebrospinal fluid culture. Mr. Ray has been transferred to a dimly lit private room. Why?

☐ 1. Increased stimulation such as bright lights may precipitate a seizure.

☐ 2. Inappropriate secretion of antidiuretic hormone (ADH) can be minimized.

☐ 3. It is easier to check his pupils in a darkened room.

☐ 4. Most clients with meningitis have photophobia.

63. Mr. Ray is placed on a hypothermia blanket. Twenty minutes following the start of hypothermia treatments, what response would the nurse most likely expect to find?

☐ 1. Lowered vital signs.

☐ 2. Elevated vital signs.

☐ 3. Unchanged vital signs.

☐ 4. Complaints of hot and cold flashes.

64. A serious complication associated with hypothermic therapy is which of the following?

☐ 1. Sunburn.

☐ 2. Burns.

☐ 3. Frostbite.

☐ 4. Heat exhaustion.

65. Hypothermia treatment will most likely put Mr. Ray at risk for the development of which of the following?

☐ 1. Emboli.

☐ 2. Respiratory alkalosis.

☐ 3. Metabolic alkalosis.

☐ 4. Excess ADH secretion.

66. As Mr. Ray's temperature begins to drop, the nurse will most likely observe which of the following?

☐ 1. Loss of corneal response.

☐ 2. Loss of gag reflex.

☐ 3. IM medications taking effect quickly.

☐ 4. Fading of sensorium, including hearing.

67. Nursing measures for Mr. Ray would include which of the following?

☐ 1. Turning frequently.

☐ 2. Applying a thin coating of lotion to his skin, following this with talcum powder, which is washed off and reapplied q8h.

☐ 3. Encouraging passive range-of-motion exercises.

☐ 4. All the above nursing measures.

68. The most desirable method of rewarming Mr. Ray following induced hypothermia is which of the following?

☐ 1. Surface rewarming.

☐ 2. Natural rewarming.

☐ 3. Bloodstream rewarming.

☐ 4. Artificial rewarming.

69. A common complication to watch for during the rewarming process is which of the following?

☐ 1. Acidosis.

☐ 2. Oliguria.

☐ 3. Shock.

☐ 4. Cardiac irregularity.

70. Mr. Ray continues on bed rest. During morning care, how would the nurse assist him with preventing joint and muscle complications?

☐ 1. Active range of motion to all extremities.

☐ 2. Passive range of motion to all extremities.

☐ 3. Exercises to augment motor function as it returns.

☐ 4. Nerve stimulation.

Twenty-two-year-old Al Welch is admitted to the hospital with a diagnosis of manic-depressive illness, manic phase (bipolar disorder). He is bizarrely dressed with a colorful scarf tied around one arm and another tied around his leg. He wears a large gold earring in one ear and a beaded headband to hold back his long, flowing hair. He is obviously agitated and tells the nurse that he is Jesus Christ and has come to save the world. He is accompanied by his parents, who report that Mr. Welch has not slept for at least 24 hours and only at 1- to 2-hour intervals for the past week.

71. Which of the following would *not* be an appropriate goal for Mr. Welch at this time?
    - ☐ 1. Client will participate in quiet activities.
    - ☐ 2. Client will remain free of injury.
    - ☐ 3. Client will experience increased sensory stimuli.
    - ☐ 4. Client will perform self-care and personal hygiene measures.

72. After admission procedures are completed, the most effective nursing measure would be which of the following?
    - ☐ 1. Take him on a tour of the unit to acquaint him with the other clients and staff.
    - ☐ 2. Suggest that he go to his room and get some sleep.
    - ☐ 3. Send him to the recreation room with several other young clients to develop his social skills.
    - ☐ 4. Accompany him to his room, sit, and talk quietly with him.

73. After assessing Mr. Welch, an additional action would be which of the following?
    - ☐ 1. Treat physical problems that may result from hyperactive, manic state.
    - ☐ 2. Promote increased physical activity.
    - ☐ 3. Increase sensory stimuli.
    - ☐ 4. Work with client regarding his low self-esteem.

74. Mr. Welch's physician orders lithium carbonate, 300 mg qid, to control the symptoms. Why is lithium considered a potentially dangerous drug?
    - ☐ 1. The amount of the drug that is therapeutic is only slightly less than the amount that produces toxicity.
    - ☐ 2. The drug is potentially addicting.
    - ☐ 3. The drug has severe sedative effects.
    - ☐ 4. Lithium causes tardive dyskinesia with long-term use.

75. Lithium is often used in combination with an antipsychotic drug for initial treatment of acute manic episodes. Which of the following statements best explains the rationale for this?
    - ☐ 1. Antipsychotic drugs increase the beneficial effects of lithium.
    - ☐ 2. Manic-depressive clients are also usually schizophrenic.
    - ☐ 3. There is an initial lag period between administration of lithium and symptom reduction.
    - ☐ 4. Antipsychotic drugs reduce lithium toxicity.

76. Clients in the acute manic phase of manic-depressive illness often resist taking lithium. Which of the following is *not* likely to be the reason for their refusal?
    - ☐ 1. Lithium therapy might result in weight gain.
    - ☐ 2. The client often finds the manic periods are pleasurable or "rewarding" in some manner.
    - ☐ 3. Lithium therapy causes severe and permanent side effects.
    - ☐ 4. The client fears or dislikes the mood change from elation to a more normal state or depression.

77. Mr. Welch loudly demands to be discharged so that he can go to South America. The nurse observes that he is agitated and is wearing bizarre clothing. Which of the following approaches would be most appropriate at this time?
    - ☐ 1. Call the physician for a discharge order.
    - ☐ 2. Recognize that underneath his demands, the client is feeling dependent, unable to cope, and overwhelmed.
    - ☐ 3. Assess the client's abilities realistically.
    - ☐ 4. Involve the client in planning activities of daily living.

78. Mr. Welch has angry outbursts, calms down quickly, and is easily provoked a short time later. Which of the following actions would be most appropriate for this problem?
    - ☐ 1. Use measures to prevent overt aggression such as distraction and reduction of environmental stimuli.
    - ☐ 2. Encourage him to release his aggression by participating in competitive games.
    - ☐ 3. Set up a debate in the client-government group, so that he can practice stating his feelings.
    - ☐ 4. Distract him by taking him to the exercise yard whenever he appears angry.

79. Mr. Welch stays up all night, pacing the halls in his pajamas, and approaching male staff and clients in an aggressively sexual way. He states, "You are all frozen and impotent. You don't know how to live." Which of the following would be the *least* helpful approach?
    - ☐ 1. Avoid becoming defensive.
    - ☐ 2. Hold staff conferences to develop a plan for countering his aggressive sexual behavior.
    - ☐ 3. Confront him with his sexual behavior and inform him of his need to embarrass others.
    - ☐ 4. Involve the client in planning and participating in quiet, adaptive activities for nighttime.

80. Which of the following behaviors would *not* be an indication to anticipate client discharge?
    - ☐ 1. The client makes requests in a quiet voice.
    - ☐ 2. The client identifies and expresses feelings of depression.
    - ☐ 3. The client accepts limits on manipulative and acting out behaviors.
    - ☐ 4. The client is cheerful, is the life of the party, and denies depression.

Allan Miller, 4 years old, is admitted to the pediatric unit with a diagnosis of sickle-cell crisis. Mrs. Miller is expecting her second child in 4 months.

81. Mrs. Miller is concerned that her next child will have sickle-cell disease. What is the nurse's best response to this concern?

1. "Sickle-cell disease affects every other child in a family."
2. "The child will have either the trait or the disease."
3. "There is a 25% chance the baby will have the disease."
4. "There is no risk of developing sickle-cell disease."

82. Mrs. Miller remarks that Allan never had any problems with sickle-cell disease until about 1 year of age. Which of the following responses best addresses Mrs. Miller's concern?
    1. "Infections are not a problem until 1 year of age."
    2. "Fetal hemoglobin levels remain high during infancy."
    3. "Maternal antibodies protected Allan during the first year."
    4. "Breastfeeding provides passive immunity for the infant."

83. What is the most common cause of sickle-cell crisis?
    1. Acute infection.
    2. Emotional stress.
    3. Strenuous activity.
    4. Environmental change.

84. Which of the following actions would receive the highest priority while caring for Allan?
    1. Hydration.
    2. Elimination.
    3. Mobility.
    4. Oxygenation.

85. Allan is to receive meperidine (Demerol), 20 mg IM q3h to q4h prn for pain. The vial reads "Demerol 50 mg/ml." How much will the nurse administer?
    1. 0.2 ml.
    2. 0.3 ml.
    3. 0.4 ml.
    4. 0.5 ml.

86. Which of the following behaviors indicate that the Demerol has been effective?
    1. Increased restlessness.
    2. Respirations of 38.
    3. Decreased attention span.
    4. Apical heart rate of 90.

87. A transfusion is ordered for Allan. Infusing the blood components too rapidly may lead to which of the following problems?
    1. Hypostatic pneumonia.
    2. Cardiac failure.
    3. Hemolytic anemia.
    4. Stress ulcer.

88. Thirty minutes after the transfusion begins, Allan's cheeks are flushed and he has hives on his abdomen and lower extremities. What would the nurse do first?

1. Continue to monitor Allan for any increase in the symptoms.
2. Stop the transfusion and begin an IV infusion of normal saline.
3. Check Allan's vital signs and notify the physician immediately.
4. Contact the blood bank to double-check Allan's blood type.

Julie Warner is a 28-year-old admitted on the nurse's shift with a fever of 102° F (38.9° C). Her complaints indicate dysuria, frequency, and malaise. Acute pyelonephritis is suspected.

89. Which of the following diagnostic findings would be *least* likely to be found in acute pyelonephritis?
    1. Cloudy, foul-smelling urine.
    2. Bacteria and pus in the urine.
    3. Low WBC count.
    4. Hematuria.

90. What is the most important nursing action when caring for Mrs. Warner?
    1. Encourage ambulation.
    2. Force fluids up to 3000 ml/day.
    3. Restrict protein in the diet.
    4. Keep urine acid.

91. Phenazopyridine hydrochloride (Pyridium) is ordered for Mrs. Warner. This drug has which of the following actions?
    1. Antibiotic.
    2. Narcotic.
    3. Analgesic.
    4. Antipyretic.

92. Long-term management for Mrs. Warner includes preventing reinfection. Which of the following nursing instructions would be included in teaching?
    1. Void at least every 6 hours.
    2. Use vaginal sprays to mask the odor.
    3. Empty her bladder before and after intercourse.
    4. Discontinue antibiotics when pain disappears.

93. Before administering the initial dose of phenazopyridine hydrochloride (Pyridium), what would the nurse tell Mrs. Warner about this drug?
    1. This drug causes transient nausea.
    2. Food interferes with absorption.
    3. It colors the urine red or orange.
    4. Bladder spasms are a side effect.

94. Sulfamethoxazole-trimethoprim (Bactrim DS) is a common antimicrobial agent ordered in combination with phenazopyridine hydrochloride (Pyridium). What does "DS" stand for?
    1. "Dose specific."
    2. "Decreased symptoms."

☐ 3. "Double strength."

☐ 4. "Deficient strain."

95. Methenamine mandelate (Mandelamine) is also prescribed for Mrs. Warner's urinary tract infection. Which of the following conditions is necessary to increase the effectiveness of this drug?

☐ 1. Crystalluria.

☐ 2. Leukocytosis.

☐ 3. Alkaline urine.

☐ 4. Acid urine.

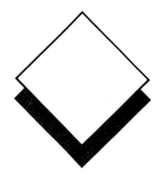

Test 1, Book II

ANSWERS WITH RATIONALES

KEY TO ABBREVIATIONS
Section of the Review Book

P = Psychosocial and Mental Health Problems
  T = Therapeutic Use of Self
  L = Loss and Death and Dying
  A = Anxious Behavior
  C = Confused Behavior
  E = Elated-Depressive Behavior
  SM = Socially Maladaptive Behavior
  SS = Suspicious Behavior
  W = Withdrawn Behavior
  SU = Substance Use Disorders
A = Adult
  H = Healthy Adult
  S = Surgery
  O = Oxygenation
  NM = Nutrition and Metabolism
  E = Elimination
  SP = Sensation and Perception
  M = Mobility
  CA = Cellular Aberration
CBF = Childbearing Family
  W = Women's Health Care
  A = Antepartal Care
  I = Intrapartal Care
  P = Postpartal Care
  N = Newborn Care
C = Child
  H = Healthy Child
  I = Ill and Hospitalized Child
  SPP = Sensation, Perception, and Protection
  O = Oxygenation
  NM = Nutrition and Metabolism
  E = Elimination
  M = Mobility
  CA = Cellular Aberration

Nursing Process Category

AS = Assessment
AN = Analysis
PL = Plan
IM = Implementation
EV = Evaluation

Client Need Category

E = Safe, Effective Care Environment
PS = Physiological Integrity
PC = Psychosocial Integrity
H = Health Promotion and Maintenance

1. no. 4. Information should be given to the client. Oxytocin challenge testing would be contraindicated for a client experiencing the possibility of premature labor. An internal monitor cannot be applied unless membranes are ruptured. Vaginal examinations are kept to a minimum. CBF/I, IM, E
2. no. 1. This is the best description of the beneficial effects of bed rest for the client in premature labor. CBF/I, AN, PS
3. no. 1. Tocolytic drugs stimulate type II beta-receptors, resulting in vasodilatation and hypotension. To compensate, the maternal heart rate increases even to the point of cardiac failure. For this reason, tocolytic drugs are usually discontinued if the pulse rate exceeds 140 beats/min. CBF/I, IM, PS
4. no. 2. Levallorphan tartrate is a narcotic antagonist. Phenobarbital does not have tocolytic properties. Betamethasone is a glucocorticoid given to the mother to accelerate fetal lung maturity. CBF/I, AN, PS
5. no. 4. These signs are all indicative of a gestational age of less than 40 weeks. Lanugo and vernix are shed in utero as the fetus matures. Palmar and plantar creases increase with age. Development in the ears,

breast tissue, and scrotum occurs with age. Testes begin descent at approximately 36 weeks of gestation. Dark-red skin in the premature infant is reflective of lack of subcutaneous fat. Parchmentlike skin is typical of the postterm infant. CBF/N, AS, PS

6. no. 4. The premature infant is at greater risk for heat loss than the full-term infant. The nurse must keep this in mind while carrying out routine delivery-room procedures. Drying the infant is important to prevent heat loss by evaporation. CBF/N, AN, PS

7. no. 4. Nasal flaring is the only indication of respiratory distress listed. The nares flare to take in more oxygen to compensate for hypoxia. CBF/N, AS, PS

8. no. 2. Research and observations of infants who have not been touched have shown that there are differences in the behavior of these babies when they are compared with babies who have received normal mothering. CBF/N, AN, H

9. no. 3. It is desirable for parents to take an active role as care providers for their infants. This will promote attachment as well as help to develop their comfort and confidence in caring for the infant at home. CBF/N, PL, PC

10. no. 2. Normal tidal volume is about 500 cc. A/O, AN, PS

11. no. 2. The amount of dead space in the lung increases with chronic obstructive pulmonary disease. Usual dead space is 100 to 150 ml. A/O, AS, PS

12. no. 3. Fowler's position increases the expansibility of the lungs. A/O, IM, PS

13. no. 2. The high P_{CO_2} is balanced by an increased bicarbonate, resulting in a pH of 7.40. The pH is within normal range (7.35-7.45); thus, he is compensated. If the pH is abnormal, then the client is said to be in a decompensated state. A/O, AN, PS

14. no. 2. The normal state of a client with chronic obstructive pulmonary disease is compensated respiratory acidosis. A/O, AN, PS

15. no. 3. A client with chronic obstructive pulmonary disease adjusts to an increased P_{CO_2} and a decreased P_{O_2}. A/O, AN, PS

16. no. 4. This client's electrolyte levels will not be affected by suctioning him. A/O, AN, PS

17. no. 2. Emphysema produces bronchiolar and alveolar changes that cannot be reversed. Treatment is aimed at relieving symptoms. A/O, AN, PS

18. no. 1. Mr. Nims is slightly hypoxemic, but not cyanotic. This means his P_{O_2} is around 50 mm Hg. A/O, AS, PS

19. no. 1. For clients with chronic obstructive pulmonary disease, the breathing stimulus is based on a low P_{O_2}. Administration of more than 2 to 3 L of oxygen impairs the respiratory drive. A/O, IM, PS

20. no. 4. Skin color is affected by many things other than oxygenation, including circulation, hot or cold environment, and trauma. A/O, AS, PS

21. no. 3. Compartment syndrome is possible because this type of fracture is frequently caused by substantial force that produces neurovascular disruption. Fluid loss is not a major problem. Infection (osteomyelitis) is a potential complication of any bone trauma and not specific to elbow fracture. Severe pain is associated with compartment syndrome but is a symptom of the complication and not a complication in itself. C/M, AN, PS

22. no. 3. Skeletal traction involves pull directly to a bone by a pin inserted through the bone distal to the fracture. The pin sites should be checked each shift for potential problems. Only skin traction can be periodically removed for rewrapping if pull to the part is maintained. The other options counteract the treatment regimen. C/M, PL, PS

23. no. 1. Hypercalcemia results from osteoclastic activity occurring more rapidly than does osteoblastic activity when weightbearing is diminished. Calcium is released into the bloodstream, leading to osteoporosis. The other options occur with normal mobility. C/M, AN, PS

24. no. 1. The pin should be secure and immobile in the bone. Options no. 2, no. 3, and no. 4 are normal. C/M, EV, PS

25. no. 3. Peer contact is most important for the adolescent. Removal from school and normal physical activities make it necessary that peer contacts are maintained. The other options could be healthy diversions, but they are of secondary importance. C/H, AN, PC

26. no. 1. The denial is evident. He is not yet able to consciously face the seriousness of his situation. Rationalization is an unconscious mechanism whereby a person creates a logical, socially acceptable explanation for a thought, feeling, or behavior. Sublimation is the conscious or unconscious channeling of unacceptable drives into acceptable activities. Compensation is a mechanism by which the individual attempts to make up for real or imagined deficiencies. P/L, AN, PC

27. no. 4. This response indicates to the client that the anger he is expressing was heard and offers the opportunity to deal with those feelings. Restating the most provocative part of his complaint will further escalate his anger. Option no. 2 is an excellent explanation of why he needs a low-sodium diet, but only after he has had an opportunity to verbalize his anger and feel understood will he be able to listen to it. Option no. 3 avoids the feeling tone of his complaint. He will only have numerous other complaints because the real issue has been circumvented. P/L, IM, PC

28. no. 2. Many drugs can cause suppression of the bone marrow and aplastic anemia. A/O, AN, PS

29. no. 1. A bone marrow sample will allow evaluation of the marrow condition and number of erythrocytes, leukocytes, and thrombocytes. A/O, AN, PS

30. no. 2. When providing nursing care to a client who has a low hemoglobin, conserve the client's energy. With low hemoglobin, less oxygen will be carried and available to the cells. Maintenance of fluid and electrolyte balance is important for any client but is not specific to someone with a diagnosis of aplastic anemia. A/O, PL, E

31. no. 2. This is the physical finding that would indicate clubfoot. Pain is not associated with clubfoot. Newborns usually have bowed legs, and frequently the foot is not aligned with the knee. C/M, AS, PS

32. no. 2. This is the basis for the treatment regimen. Temporary developmental delay may actually be caused by treatment. After the age of 6 months, clubfoot can be corrected but requires longer and more invasive treatment than if it were detected at birth. A newborn's skin is thin and fragile and has potential for breakdown. C/M, AN, PS

33. no. 4. A plaster cast should not be allowed to become wet because it will soften and lose its effectiveness. Cleaning should be done with a nonchlorine cleanser. Rough edges can occur but only present a problem if the skin underneath becomes excoriated. With an infant in a cast, urine soiling cannot be completely prevented. C/M, EV, E

34. no. 1. Elevation is critical to decrease edema and resulting circulatory compromise. Feeding difficulties have no relationship to the foot problem. Infants having casts with plaster foot molds should be turned with legs supported on pillows or blankets to avoid pressure on the toes. Option no. 3 is used for hip deformities. C/M, PL, PS

35. no. 3. This is the only question leading to a measurable outcome. The only true measurement of successful teaching is if the parents can apply the brace. C/M, EV, H

36. no. 4. The most common form of tracheoesophageal fistula is one in which the proximal esophageal segment terminates in a blind pouch. When the child swallows saliva, water, milk or formula, it accumulates in the blind pouch, resulting in excessive salivation or aspiration. CBF/N, AS, PS

37. no. 2. Vigorous nasotracheal suctioning may easily disrupt the integrity of the suture line, so it is contraindicated. Gentle oropharyngeal suctioning would be indicated if the infant cannot handle oral secretions. IV fluids will be necessary until the infant can be fed through a gastrostomy tube. Elevation of the head of the bed at 30° promotes pooling of secretions at the catheter tip if an indwelling nasal catheter is

in use. Skin care will prevent skin breakdown and infection. CBF/N, IM, PS

38. no. 3. Amniotic fluid is continually produced by the mother. A normal fetus swallows and excretes the amniotic fluid while in utero. If there is a gastrointestinal obstruction or neurological problem that interferes with swallowing in the fetus, then the amniotic fluid accumulates and results in hydramnios. CBF/N, AS, PS

39. no. 2. The thyroid (being the regulator for the metabolic rate) produces and releases more thyroid hormones in hyperthyroidism, which increases the metabolic rate. The increased metabolic rate leads to elevated vital signs, nervousness, and weight loss, because of increased activity in and demands on all body systems. A/NM, AS, PS

40. no. 3. Tachycardia is usual in hyperthyroidism, and a further increase in cardiac rate indicates thyroid crisis, a more toxic state. Cold intolerance, sensitivity to narcotics, and lethargy are symptoms of hypothyroidism. A/NM, AS, PS

41. no. 3. Assigning the client to a private room may promote rest by decreasing stimulation. A/NM, PL, E

42. no. 3. The client would have increased hunger as a result of the increased metabolic rate and would require a high-protein, high-calorie intake. A/NM, PL, PS

43. no. 1. These symptoms are characteristic of hypothyroidism. The client will need lifelong daily replacement of thyroid hormones. A/NM, AN, H

44. no. 1. The first stage in dealing with a terminal illness is denial, and the client's comment is a typical expression of denial. There is insufficient data to conclude that Mrs. Rosen may not be able to cope with her problem or that her behavior is unusual. P/L, AN, PC

45. no. 3. Respond to expressions of denial with statements that encourage exploration of feelings and thoughts, in order to help the client proceed through later stages. The client may interpret silence as agreement by the nurse and she may not continue talking. Reassurance would be false and nontherapeutic and suggests anxiety on nurse's part. P/L, IM, PC

46. no. 1. Since the client is in the first stage of dealing with a loss, the first priority is to help her to begin dealing with her diagnosis. The client must begin to deal with impending death before initiating goals no. 2 and no. 3. Option no. 4 is not the first or more important goal, and it would not necessarily help her face death. P/L, PL, PC

47. no. 4. The client needs opportunities to talk and to proceed at her own pace. She must not be abandoned or pushed into other stages. Deal with questions about death as they arise. Denial may be adaptive

and normal up to a point. If the client verbally denies the seriousness of the health threat but complies with treatment, denial can be adaptive. P/L, PL, E

48. no. 3. Respond to remarks indicating denial with realistic and empathic statements about the client's feelings. Do not encourage denial or try to interrupt it abruptly. Responding to the client's work, rather than feelings, is an avoidance remark by the nurse. Option no. 2 is too confronting at this point and would cause a high anxiety level. Option no. 4 would encourage the client's denial. P/L, IM, PC

49. no. 2. The client should be encouraged to express her own feelings about death. A willingness to talk about it should be met with encouragement to do so. Option no. 1 is unfeeling and cuts off further exploration of the client's concerns. Option no. 3 avoids the issue of death, which the client is willing to talk about. Option no. 4 assumes the client is bothered, rather than exploring her feelings about accepting her prognosis. P/L, IM, PC

50. no. 2. Anger is a normal stage in the dying process. Although it may be directed at nurses, it is usually displaced anger. The nurse should respond in a way that indicates acceptance of the client while encouraging her to talk about the underlying feelings. Option no. 1 indicates that the nurse has interpreted the client's anger as personal. Option no. 3 is a defensive remark that avoids the client's feelings and may increase her guilt. Option no. 4 is a withdrawal reaction and may be helpful to the nurse, but it leaves the client with unresolved feelings. P/L, IM, PC

51. no. 4. This is a reasonable request that should be pursued in order to determine whether or not it is possible. If so, the nurse can assist the client in making arrangements. Option no. 1 is not helpful because they need further information about this possibility. Discharge planning falls within the purview of nursing, and it is appropriate for the nurse to discuss this with the family. No data suggest denial of seriousness at this time. P/L, IM, PC

52. no. 1. This indicates the realization of the most comprehensive and realistic goals for the client. Anger is not the end stage of the grief process; the expectation is for her to move beyond this phase. Option no. 3 is not realistic. Independence is an important achievement, but dealing with the emotional impact of impending death is more important. P/L, EV, PC

53. no. 1. This determines a child's ability to handle information. Options no. 2, no. 3, and no. 4 are factors for consideration but are not as important as no. 1. C/I, AS, H

54. no. 3. This is the result of a backup of blood in the right ventricle, which enlarges to accommodate the extra volume. C/O, AN, PS

55. no. 2. It is most important to determine his understanding and allow him to express his feelings. Op-

tion no. 4 is contraindicated; option no. 3 is too severe a measure. C/O, PL, E

56. no. 4. Since his defect was mild, repair should be complete. He should not be encouraged to develop a chronically ill, dependent personality. C/O, PL, H

57. no. 2. Use an open-ended comment to encourage the child's own expressions. The other options are judgmental or discourage sharing of comments by the child. C/I, IM, PC

58. no. 3. This skill comes at age 6. He should be able to do the other skills listed. C/O, AS, H

59. no. 4. Nuchal rigidity (the neck becomes rigid when flexion is attempted) results from meningeal irritation. This does not usually occur with concussions. A/SP, AN, PS

60. no. 1. Unequal pupils indicate possible increased intracranial pressure, which makes a lumbar puncture very dangerous. A/SP, AS, PS

61. no. 2. Maintenance of proper positioning for a lumbar puncture is very important. Narcotics are avoided in clients with neurological problems; they can mask symptoms and change pupil responses. Procaine hydrochloride (Novocain) is given as a local anesthetic, if used at all. A/SP, IM, E

62. no. 4. Meningitis is often accompanied by photophobia, a visual intolerance to light; therefore the client will be more comfortable in a dark room. A/SP, AN, PS

63. no. 2. The body will attempt to compensate for hypothermia, and the vital signs will initially become elevated; later, they decrease. A/SP, AS, PS

64. no. 3. During hypothermic therapy the client's skin must be protected from frostbite, most commonly caused by skin contact with the hypothermic blanket. A/SP, AS, PS

65. no. 1. Circulation slows at low temperatures, predisposing the client to the formation of emboli. A/SP, AN, PS

66. no. 4. The gag and corneal reflexes are not lost until the client is completely comatose; an earlier sign is a fading of the senses. A/SP, EV, PS

67. no. 4. All the options will help prevent vascular pooling without greatly increasing oxygen demand. A/SP, IM, E

68. no. 2. Natural rewarming is the least invasive and safest method of regaining the normal body temperature following induced hypothermia. A/SP, PL, PS

69. no. 4. Cardiac irregularity is the most common complication of rewarming. A/SP, AS, PS

70. no. 2. During the acute phase, complete bed rest and passive range of motion will help to conserve energy, yet maintain good joint mobility. A/SP, PL, PS

71. no. 3. Mr. Welch needs decreased, not increased,

sensory stimuli at this time. With sleep deprivation, the client may have impaired judgment, so protecting this client from self-injury would be important. Although the client is delusional, he should be able to care for his personal hygiene. P/E, PL, E

72. no. 4. It is important to decrease environmental (sensory) stimulation for these clients and, at the same time, to keep them under close observation. Taking him on a tour of the unit may be too stimulating. He may not be able to sleep at this time because of being in a new environment. Developing social skills while in a delusional state is impossible and his bizarre dress might scare off others and not benefit the client. P/E, IM, PC

73. no. 1. Initial actions with the hypermanic client would focus on physical problems such as poor nutrition, hygiene, and sleep and rest problems. Promoting increased physical activity would promote exhaustion. Increased sensory stimuli would overload him. Working on low self-esteem is not appropriate during a hypomanic state because he would not be able to pay attention. P/E, IM, PC

74. no. 1. Lithium has a very narrow therapeutic index. Therefore clients must be closely observed for signs of lithium toxicity. Lithium is not addicting, nor does it have sedative side effects. Lithium does not cause tardive dyskinesia, but it is often given with antipsychotic agents, which do. P/E, AN, PS

75. no. 3. Once a therapeutic serum level is attained, it takes 7 to 10 days for a clinical response from lithium. Therefore antipsychotic drugs that have a therapeutic-response time that can be measured in minutes are used to alleviate the acute symptoms of mania until lithium begins to take effect. Manic-depressive clients are not usually schizophrenics, but both have psychotic features. Antipsychotic drugs do not reduce lithium toxicity or increase the beneficial effects. P/E, AN, PS

76. no. 3. There is no evidence to date that lithium therapy causes irreversible side effects with long-term use. Lithium therapy does produce mild discomfort such as nausea, vomiting, dizziness, headache, impaired vision, and diarrhea, among other symptoms. Manic clients often report liking the euphoric feeling, and once the lithium takes effect, clients fear having to face their underlying depression. P/E, AN, PS

77. no. 2. Manic-depressive clients cover their dependency needs and confusion by acting independent, controlling, and bossy. Calling the physician for discharge orders would not be appropriate when the client is agitated and shows bizarre grooming. Distraction only works temporarily and may only increase his irritation when the real issue is not addressed. P/E, IM, PC

78. no. 1. Competitive games, group debates, and phys-

ical movement serve to escalate manic behavior and should be avoided. P/E, IM, PC

79. no. 3. Confronting this client is not helpful and serves to escalate his manic, anxious behaviors. A staff conference would help to reduce defensiveness of the staff and define consistent, helpful strategies to promote adaptive activities for nighttime. P/E, IM, PC

80. no. 4. This option describes hypermanic behavior and would not be an indication for discharge. Option no. 1 indicates the client is in good control of his feelings. Option no. 2 indicates the client has an awareness of his underlying feelings of depression. Option no. 3 indicates the client will not use his hostility to threaten others into doing what he wants. P/E, EV, PC

81. no. 3. Sickle-cell disease is an autosomal-recessive disease. Both parents are carriers; therefore, with each pregnancy, Mrs. Miller has a 25% chance of having a child with the disease, a 50% chance of having a child with the trait, and a 25% chance of having a child without the disease or the trait. C/O, IM, H

82. no. 2. The presence of fetal hemoglobin prevents sickling; it begins to decrease around 4 to 6 months of age, and the child eventually develops symptoms of the disease. C/O, IM, PS

83. no. 1. Children with sickle-cell disease have an increased susceptibility to infections. The exact cause is unknown, but supporting data suggest that many organisms thrive in a state of diminished oxygen and that phagocytosis is reduced in a hypoxic state. C/O, AN, PS

84. no. 1. Hydration promotes hemodilution, which in turn decreases blood viscosity and prevents further sickling; hydration also interferes with the cycle of stasis, thrombosis, and ischemia. C/O, PL, PS

85. no. 3.

$$\frac{50 \text{ mg}}{1 \text{ ml}} = \frac{20 \text{ mg}}{x \text{ ml}}$$
$$50x = 20 = \frac{20}{50} = 0.4 \text{ ml}$$

C/I, IM, PS

86. no. 4. The normal heart rate for a 4-year-old is approximately 100 beats/min; a heart rate of 90 beats/min would indicate that the child is resting comfortably. C/I, EV, PS

87. no. 2. Infusion of blood too rapidly may lead to hypervolemia, which in turn may lead to heart failure. C/O, AN, PS

88. no. 2. The child is experiencing an allergic reaction. The transfusion should be stopped immediately, but the patency of the IV line is maintained as a route for emergency drugs, if they become necessary. C/O, IM, PS

89. no. 3. Leukocytosis (an elevated white blood cell

count) is present with a bacterial infection. All other options are indicative of acute pyelonephritis. A/E, AS, PS

90. no. 2. Increased fluids will help treat the symptoms of infection (i.e., elevated temperature, dysuria). A/E, PL, PS

91. no. 3. Phenazopyridine hydrochloride (Pyridium) is a urinary analgesic. A/E, AN, PS

92. no. 3. The female urethra is short, and its proximity to the vagina predisposes the client to infection. Bacterial contamination can result from sexual intercourse, and emptying the bladder before and after intercourse reduces this risk. A/E, IM, H

93. no. 3. The azo dye in phenazopyridine hydrochloride (Pyridium) stains the urine reddish-orange. It is important to inform the client, when the initial dose is given, so that she does not think something is wrong when she voids. A/E, IM, PS

94. no. 3. The "DS" product denotes double strength. A/E, AN, PS

95. no. 4. Methenamine decomposes to formaldehyde and ammonia. The urine should be maintained at a pH of 5.5 or less for effective treatment. A/E, AN, PS

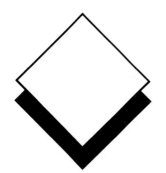

Test 1, Book III

QUESTIONS

Joan Plum, a 35-year-old physicist, trips and falls while walking to work. The next day she finds her lower extremities to be "very weak." She can stand only with assistance. She is admitted to the hospital with complaints of back pain. A motor assessment reveals flaccid paralysis in the lower extremities. She states that her hands feel numb. A brief health history reveals that Miss Plum has been healthy, never sick. She did have a slight upper respiratory infection 2 weeks ago. A diagnosis of polyneuritis (Guillain-Barré syndrome) is made after cerebrospinal fluid (CSF) reports have been returned showing a negative culture, increased protein, and normal pressure and cell count.

1. When planning care, why must respiratory-assistance equipment be kept immediately available?
   ☐ 1. The pattern of the paralysis is ascending, and respiratory failure can occur if intercostal muscles are affected.
   ☐ 2. Intracranial pressure can exert pressure on the medulla and cause respiratory arrest.
   ☐ 3. High fever associated with this syndrome often disrupts the normal respiratory patterns.
   ☐ 4. The particular bacteria or viruses (or both) in the cerebrospinal fluid have a special affinity for the nerves that control respiration.

2. Cranial nerves can be affected by Guillain-Barré syndrome. The facial nerve is most frequently involved. A baseline has been established, and the cranial nerves are being assessed at frequent intervals. What would the nurse most likely observe if the motor nucleus of the facial nerve becomes dysfunctional?
   ☐ 1. Decreased ability to distinguish tastes in the anterior two thirds of the tongue.
   ☐ 2. Pain in the distribution of the affected nerve.
   ☐ 3. Inability to wrinkle the forehead and smile.
   ☐ 4. Inequality of pupils and sluggish response to light.

3. What is the primary role of the nurse in caring for Miss Plum during this acute phase?

☐ 1. To make accurate assessments and prevent complications.
☐ 2. To give medications on time and control blood pressure.
☐ 3. To provide nutrition and control of temperature.
☐ 4. To prevent contractures and suction the respiratory tract.

4. When Miss Plum asks whether or not she has a fatal disease, which of the following would be the nurse's best reply?
   ☐ 1. "The great majority of people with Guillain-Barré syndrome recover completely, so your chances of recovery are good."
   ☐ 2. "You never know what can happen when something goes wrong with your nervous system."
   ☐ 3. "You should have checked with your doctor when you fell down yesterday."
   ☐ 4. "Most clients have remissions, but eventually an exacerbation is apt to occur, because this disease has a long, progressive course."

5. As Miss Plum's recovery begins, the nurse notes that neurological return is taking place in a descending order. However, she still retains some paresthesia in her right hand, even though she is ambulatory. During discharge planning, what would the nurse emphasize most to Miss Plum considering this sensory impairment?
   ☐ 1. Maintain bed rest for several months to prevent fatigue and exacerbation of the disease.
   ☐ 2. Test bath water with a bath thermometer as a safety precaution in order to avoid burns.
   ☐ 3. Avoid contact with others until the first clinic visit, so she will not contract a viral infection.
   ☐ 4. Surgery may be required to correct the paresthesia.

Daphne Runyon is admitted to the psychiatric hospital with a diagnosis of conversion disorder. She is a 21-year-old college student who was functioning ade-

234

quately until yesterday, when she suddenly lost the use of her right arm. She was taken to the emergency room, where no physical reason could be found for the paralysis. She was then transferred to the psychiatric unit.

6. What is most important for the nurse to know concerning Miss Runyon's symptoms?
   - ☐ 1. They are caused by a demonstrable physical lesion.
   - ☐ 2. They follow motor-nerve paths.
   - ☐ 3. There is no primary gain as a result of the symptoms.
   - ☐ 4. They represent symbolic dysfunction.

7. The cause of Miss Runyon's symptoms can best be explained as tension resulting from which of the following?
   - ☐ 1. A fixation at the anal stage of development, producing feelings that are converted into the symptom.
   - ☐ 2. Repression of feelings converted into a symptom that has special meaning to the person.
   - ☐ 3. Suppression of feelings converted into the presenting symptom.
   - ☐ 4. Sublimation of feelings converted into the presenting symptom.

8. When meeting the rest of the clients on the unit, Miss Runyon describes her difficulties blandly, with no apparent distress. Miss Runyon is demonstrating which of the following?
   - ☐ 1. Ambivalence.
   - ☐ 2. Lability.
   - ☐ 3. *La belle indifférence.*
   - ☐ 4. Narcissism.

9. When Miss Runyon's parents come to visit, they are very concerned about their daughter's condition. Which of the following will most likely apply to Miss Runyon?
   - ☐ 1. She might receive secondary gain of increased attention from her family because of her symptoms.
   - ☐ 2. She might have her dependency needs met and have fewer school responsibilities as long as she has symptoms.
   - ☐ 3. She may assume a chronic illness role over time as a result of symptoms.
   - ☐ 4. All of the above are likely to apply.

10. One of the most important aspects of Miss Runyon's care will be which of the following?
    - ☐ 1. Confrontation to help her become aware of her feelings.
    - ☐ 2. Supportive measures so that she will have increased feelings of acceptance.
    - ☐ 3. Diversion from the sick role to other more productive behaviors.
    - ☐ 4. Antipsychotic medication to keep her comfortable until her symptoms are gone.

Three-year-old Mark Elliot has just been admitted to the pediatric unit. Upon entering his room to begin the initial admission assessment, the nurse finds Mark sitting upright in bed, leaning forward with his mouth open. He is drooling and complaining of a sore throat.

11. The nurse would realize that Mark's problem most likely is which of the following?
    - ☐ 1. Spasmodic croup.
    - ☐ 2. Infectious laryngitis.
    - ☐ 3. Laryngotracheobronchitis.
    - ☐ 4. Acute epiglottitis.

12. In developing a nursing care plan for Mark, which of the following would receive the highest priority?
    - ☐ 1. Airway.
    - ☐ 2. Hydration.
    - ☐ 3. Mobility.
    - ☐ 4. Elimination.

13. Which of the following manifestations would best indicate that Mark's respiratory distress is increasing?
    - ☐ 1. Progressive hoarseness.
    - ☐ 2. Productive cough.
    - ☐ 3. Change in heart rate.
    - ☐ 4. Expiratory wheeze.

14. Mark has been placed on a regimen of ampicillin, 450 mg IV q6h. Which of the following nursing actions would receive the highest priority?
    - ☐ 1. Check for hypersensitivity.
    - ☐ 2. Monitor patency of the IV line.
    - ☐ 3. Check client's name band.
    - ☐ 4. Administer correct dose of medications.

15. Mark is placed in a Croupette with cool mist. What is the best rationale for this action?
    - ☐ 1. To restrict his activity.
    - ☐ 2. To control his elevated fever.
    - ☐ 3. To stimulate the cough reflex.
    - ☐ 4. To reduce mucosal edema.

16. While Mark is in the Croupette, three of the following nursing actions would be appropriate. Which one would *not* be appropriate?
    - ☐ 1. Periodically change Mark's linen and pajamas.
    - ☐ 2. Frequently monitor Mark's vital signs.
    - ☐ 3. Loosely tuck the tent edges around the mattress.
    - ☐ 4. Encourage Mark's mother to stay with him if possible.

17. Which one of the following lab reports would give the nurse the most information about Mark's hydration status?
    - ☐ 1. White blood cell count of 12,500.
    - ☐ 2. Urine specific gravity of 1.005.
    - ☐ 3. Blood P_{O_2} of 85 mm Hg.
    - ☐ 4. Serum potassium of 3.8 mEq/L.

18. Mrs. Elliot states that Mark says he has an imaginary friend who plays with him. She is obviously concerned. The nurse's response would include which of the following?

☐ 1. Suggest she discuss this with her pediatrician.

☐ 2. Tell her that imaginary friends are normal for this age group.

☐ 3. Encourage her to spend more time with Mark.

☐ 4. Discuss preschool or day care experience with her.

19. Developmentally, Mark would be expected to perform which of the following activities?

☐ 1. Tie his shoelaces.

☐ 2. Hop in place.

☐ 3. Jump rope.

☐ 4. Walk backward.

Ernest Washo has had diabetes mellitus for 20 years. He is admitted to the hospital with dry gangrene of the right great toe.

20. When assessing Mr. Washo's gangrenous condition, the nurse will *least* likely expect which of the following?

☐ 1. Intense pain in the affected area.

☐ 2. Extension of the metatarsal-phalangeal joints.

☐ 3. Changes in skin temperature of both feet.

☐ 4. Tissue destruction.

21. When the nurse is working with Mr. Washo, what information is most important to ascertain?

☐ 1. His age when diabetes mellitus developed.

☐ 2. His understanding of hygienic skin measures.

☐ 3. His technique in administering insulin.

☐ 4. His willingness to look at, touch, or talk about his gangrenous foot.

22. Bed rest is prescribed for Mr. Washo. Which nursing care measure would be *least* therapeutic for this client?

☐ 1. Heel protectors.

☐ 2. Footboard.

☐ 3. Foot cradle.

☐ 4. Sheep skin or foam pad.

23. To prevent complications of the bed rest imposed on Mr. Washo, which nursing action would be *contraindicated*?

☐ 1. Inspect Mr. Washo's feet.

☐ 2. Teach about appropriate foot care.

☐ 3. Restrict fluid intake.

☐ 4. Exercise joints and muscles.

24. The nurse would perform which of the following when providing care to the skin surrounding the lesion?

☐ 1. Apply an occlusive dressing.

☐ 2. Dry the skin thoroughly.

☐ 3. Put lotion on the healthy tissue.

☐ 4. Soak the foot.

25. The physician orders sodium hypochlorite and boric acid (Dakin's solution) for the lesion and petroleum jelly for the adjoining healthy skin. Which of the following best describes their actions?

☐ 1. Dakin's solution is an antiinflammatory agent; petroleum jelly is an antiabsorbent agent.

☐ 2. Dakin's solution debrides the wound; petroleum jelly protects the healthy tissue.

☐ 3. Dakin's solution dries out the lesion; petroleum jelly lubricates the surrounding tissue.

☐ 4. Dakin's solution cleanses the wound; petroleum jelly moisturizes the skin.

26. If an infection develops, which effect is this most likely to have on Mr. Washo's need for insulin?

☐ 1. Undeterminable.

☐ 2. No effect.

☐ 3. Increase the need.

☐ 4. Decrease the need.

27. Mr. Washo asks if his toe will be amputated. Which of the following approaches is the most therapeutic?

☐ 1. Discuss the meaning this would have for him.

☐ 2. Explain the different types of medical management.

☐ 3. Help him value the importance of his health.

☐ 4. Refer the question to his physician.

Sean O'Connor has become increasingly depressed and is brought to the emergency room after slashing his wrists with a razor blade. He is conscious and crying uncontrollably.

28. Which of the following actions by the emergency room nurse would have the highest priority?

☐ 1. Examine the extent of his wounds.

☐ 2. Check his pulse, respiration, and blood pressure.

☐ 3. Sit quietly with him until he is calmer.

☐ 4. Talk with him about the problems he has been experiencing.

29. Mr. O'Connor's condition stabilizes, and he is admitted to the psychiatric unit. He states dejectedly, "I don't know why they saved me. As soon as I can, I will try it again. Nothing in my life is ever going to get better." What would be the best response by the nurse?

☐ 1. "You'll feel differently after you've been here awhile."

☐ 2. "You're feeling things are pretty hopeless right now."

☐ 3. "You're quite angry at the people who saved you."

☐ 4. "It sounds as if you've already made up your mind."

30. In assessing the suicide potential as reflected in Mr. O'Connor's statement, what other information would be the most useful for the nurse to have?

☐ 1. Does he have a workable plan?

☐ 2. Is there a family history of suicide?

☐ 3. Have there been suicide attempts before this one?

☐ 4. What precipitated this attack?

31. What would be the best placement for the client at this time?
 - ☐ 1. A single room on a locked psychiatric unit.
 - ☐ 2. A single room on an open psychiatric unit.
 - ☐ 3. A double room on either type of unit.
 - ☐ 4. Any room where he can be closely observed.

32. Mr. O'Connor has been taking amitriptyline (Elavil) for 7 days. He continues to appear depressed and expresses a desire to commit suicide. What is the most likely explanation for this?
 - ☐ 1. Amitriptyline is not effective for Mr. O'Connor.
 - ☐ 2. This is a side effect of amitriptyline.
 - ☐ 3. Tolerance to amitriptyline has developed.
 - ☐ 4. Amitriptyline may take 4 weeks to take effect.

Cheryl Fick is seen in the obstetrical clinic in her third month of pregnancy. She complains of an intermittent, brownish-red discharge and excessive nausea and vomiting. Abdominal palpation reveals the uterus to be at the level of the umbilicus. Fetal heart tones are absent. A preliminary diagnosis of a hydatidiform mole is made.

33. Additional symptoms characteristic of molar pregnancy that Mrs. Fick might have include which of the following?
 - ☐ 1. Hyperkalemia and polycythemia.
 - ☐ 2. Decreased HCG levels and bradycardia.
 - ☐ 3. Hypertension and anemia.
 - ☐ 4. Constipation and petechiae.

34. In order to confirm the diagnosis, further assessment is carried out. Which of the following would best confirm the above diagnosis?
 - ☐ 1. Dilatation and curettage.
 - ☐ 2. Ultrasound.
 - ☐ 3. Laparoscopy.
 - ☐ 4. Serum estriol levels.

35. Which of the following would *not* be used to treat the hydatidiform mole?
 - ☐ 1. Dilatation and curettage.
 - ☐ 2. Prostaglandin and oxytocin induction.
 - ☐ 3. Hysterectomy.
 - ☐ 4. Laser treatments.

36. Following the removal of the hydatidiform mole, which of the following complications would be of greatest concern for Mrs. Fick?
 - ☐ 1. Ectopic pregnancy.
 - ☐ 2. Choriocarcinoma.
 - ☐ 3. Pelvic inflammatory disease.
 - ☐ 4. Incompetent cervix.

37. Mrs. Fick indicates she is very disappointed that this pregnancy did not have a successful outcome. She wonders how soon she can plan to become pregnant again. In response to Mrs. Fick's question, the nurse indicates that the recommended waiting period before the next pregnancy is
 - ☐ 1. As soon as possible.
 - ☐ 2. After 6 months.
 - ☐ 3. After 1 year.
 - ☐ 4. After 2 years.

38. Which of the following responses would best indicate to the nurse that Mrs. Fick has understood discharge instructions?
 - ☐ 1. She maintains a diet high in calcium.
 - ☐ 2. She avoids the use of tampons.
 - ☐ 3. She is taking oral contraceptives.
 - ☐ 4. She avoids heavy lifting for 6 weeks.

Ralph Damian is a 60-year-old client admitted to the surgical unit with complaints of left lumbosacral pain that occasionally radiates down to his groin. He reports that, a year ago, his physician told him that he had kidney stones. He also has a long history of recurrent gout. Medication for pain is listed on his admitting orders.

39. In Mr. Damian's case, the renal stones are most likely caused by which of the following?
 - ☐ 1. Urinary stasis.
 - ☐ 2. Increased excretion of calcium.
 - ☐ 3. Increased uric acid in the urine.
 - ☐ 4. Urinary infection and large intake of milk.

40. Untreated kidney stones can dislodge, obstructing the ureter. In turn, this obstruction is the primary cause of which of the following?
 - ☐ 1. Kidney abscess.
 - ☐ 2. Hydronephrosis.
 - ☐ 3. Glomerulonephritis.
 - ☐ 4. Nephrosis.

41. One evening while in bed, Mr. Damian complains of severe pain in the left posterior lumbar region radiating down to his groin. The first nursing responsibility would be to do which of the following?
 - ☐ 1. Strain his urine.
 - ☐ 2. Give an analgesic (e.g., morphine) as ordered.
 - ☐ 3. Encourage movement about to facilitate excretion of the stone.
 - ☐ 4. Encourage large fluid intake.

42. A urea-splitting organism such as streptococcus favors the growth of inorganic renal calculi by causing the urine to become which of the following?
 - ☐ 1. Alkaline.
 - ☐ 2. Acidic.
 - ☐ 3. Neutral.
 - ☐ 4. Concentrated with sediments.

43. If the client's urine has a pH of 7.8, which of the following would most likely be given?
 - ☐ 1. Methenamine mandelate (Mandelamine).
 - ☐ 2. Vitamin C.
 - ☐ 3. Sodium bicarbonate.
 - ☐ 4. Sodium phosphate.

44. The use of bethanechol (Urecholine) in the treatment of temporary postoperative urinary retention is suggested because of its action as which of the following?
   - ☐ 1. An anticholinergic.
   - ☐ 2. A cholinergic.
   - ☐ 3. An anesthetic.
   - ☐ 4. A urinary antispasmodic.

45. Decompression drainage of the bladder is used specifically to do which of the following?
   - ☐ 1. Alleviate discomfort by providing continuous drainage.
   - ☐ 2. Prevent increased intraabdominal pressure by avoiding bladder distension.
   - ☐ 3. Provide a means of constant irrigation of the bladder.
   - ☐ 4. Help the muscles of the bladder to maintain their tone.

Three-and-a-half-year-old Courtney has been hospitalized with nephrosis.

46. Which of the following manifestations would most likely be observed?
   - ☐ 1. Ascites.
   - ☐ 2. Elevated blood pressure.
   - ☐ 3. Low urine specific gravity.
   - ☐ 4. Hematuria.

47. Because of their work commitments, Courtney's parents are not able to stay with him in the hospital. In addition to the stress created by his separation from his parents, Courtney will most likely be fearful of which of the following?
   - ☐ 1. Intrusive procedures.
   - ☐ 2. Unfamiliar caretakers.
   - ☐ 3. Dying.
   - ☐ 4. Monsters.

48. When planning Courtney's nursing care, the nurse would include activities that promote a sense of
   - ☐ 1. Trust.
   - ☐ 2. Industry.
   - ☐ 3. Esteem.
   - ☐ 4. Initiative.

49. Courtney is receiving prednisone by mouth. Which of the following actions is *not* indicated?
   - ☐ 1. Give the prednisone after meals.
   - ☐ 2. Withhold the prednisone if Courtney's blood pressure becomes elevated.
   - ☐ 3. Observe Courtney closely for signs of infection.
   - ☐ 4. Provide foods high in potassium in Courtney's diet.

50. During the acute phase of his illness, which position is best for Courtney to be placed in?
   - ☐ 1. On his left side.
   - ☐ 2. On his back.
   - ☐ 3. On his abdomen.
   - ☐ 4. Semi-Fowler's position.

51. Which of the following snacks would be the best choice for Courtney?
   - ☐ 1. 1 ounce processed cheese spread, celery sticks, and Kool-Aid.
   - ☐ 2. 1/2 cup vanilla pudding and grape juice.
   - ☐ 3. 1/2 peanut butter sandwich, apple slices, and 1/2 cup hot cocoa.
   - ☐ 4. 1/2 cup corn flakes, milk, and raisins.

52. Which activity would be most appropriate for Courtney while he is hospitalized?
   - ☐ 1. Playing with other children in the playroom.
   - ☐ 2. Riding a push-pull toy in the hall.
   - ☐ 3. Having a volunteer read him a story about a child in the hospital.
   - ☐ 4. Playing with housekeeping toys in his room.

James Lee is a 23-year-old graduate student who has just been admitted to the unit with behaviors of withdrawal, flat affect, disregard of hygiene and grooming, and associative looseness. His diagnosis is paranoid schizophrenia.

53. Which of the following is usually *not* characteristic of the client with paranoid schizophrenia?
   - ☐ 1. Delusions.
   - ☐ 2. Hallucinations.
   - ☐ 3. Decreased sensitivity.
   - ☐ 4. Ideas of reference.

54. Which defense mechanism is most characteristic of the client with paranoid schizophrenia?
   - ☐ 1. Undoing.
   - ☐ 2. Projection.
   - ☐ 3. Rationalization.
   - ☐ 4. Suppression.

55. Which of the following would *not* be an appropriate goal when working with a client with paranoid hallucinations?
   - ☐ 1. The client will learn to define and test reality.
   - ☐ 2. The client will devalue internal voices and hallucinations.
   - ☐ 3. The client will discuss feelings with the primary nurse.
   - ☐ 4. The client will act out fantasies in group therapy.

56. Which of the following would *not* be appropriate if the goal was "client will develop a relationship with a staff member"?
   - ☐ 1. Allow client to set the pace of the relationship.
   - ☐ 2. Suggest solitary activities for the suspicious client.
   - ☐ 3. Allow ample time for response if the client is very regressed.
   - ☐ 4. If the client withdraws from social interactions, allow the client to be alone.

57. Which of the following actions would *not* be helpful when dealing with paranoid hallucinations?
   - ☐ 1. Help the client relate with real persons.
   - ☐ 2. Avoid giving attention to the content of halluci-

nations or delusions after an initial investigation of them.

□ 3. Acknowledge the client's belief in the perception, but also indicate that it is not shared by others.

□ 4. Listen carefully to the content of hallucinations and delusions, and encourage the client to describe them.

58. Which of the following would be most helpful to meet the goal "client will demonstrate improved hygiene and grooming"?

□ 1. Identify specific client needs for assistance.

□ 2. Ignore messy clothes and lack of hygiene.

□ 3. Insist that the client participate in a good-grooming group.

□ 4. Encourage the client by doing hygiene and grooming for him.

59. Mr. Lee approaches a staff member with hostile comments about another client who is "out to get me." In responding to Mr. Lee, which of the following would *not* be appropriate?

□ 1. Help Mr. Lee acknowledge and name feelings.

□ 2. Explore appropriate outlets for hostility, such as physical activities, exercise, and sports.

□ 3. Confront Mr. Lee with his hostility.

□ 4. Explore the source of the hostility with Mr. Lee.

60. Thioridazine (Mellaril), an antipsychotic, is usually effective in treating all but one of the following symptoms of schizophrenia. Which symptom will not be affected by this drug?

□ 1. Agitation.

□ 2. Hallucinations.

□ 3. Delusions.

□ 4. Ambivalence.

61. Which of the following is *not* a common side effect of thioridazine (Mellaril) therapy?

□ 1. Dry mouth.

□ 2. Constipation.

□ 3. Urinary hesitancy.

□ 4. Addiction.

Ten-year-old Jackie is admitted to the hospital with a medical diagnosis of rheumatic fever. She relates a history of "a sore throat about a month ago." Bed rest with bathroom privileges is prescribed.

62. Which of the following nursing assessments would be given highest priority when assessing Jackie's condition?

□ 1. Jackie's response to being hospitalized.

□ 2. The presence of a macular rash on her trunk.

□ 3. Her sleeping or resting apical pulse.

□ 4. The presence of polyarthritis and pain in her joints.

63. Jackie exhibits manifestations of Sydenham's chorea. Which of the following is *not* a manifestation of this condition?

□ 1. Intellectual impairment.

□ 2. Muscle weakness.

□ 3. Purposeless tremors.

□ 4. Emotional lability.

64. Which of the following nursing plans would receive the highest priority during Jackie's hospitalization?

□ 1. Minimize cardiac damage by limiting Jackie to bed rest.

□ 2. Relieve pain by administering prescribed analgesics.

□ 3. Help Jackie cope with hospitalization by providing age-appropriate activities.

□ 4. Prevent injury by padding the bed's side rails.

65. Which activity is most appropriate for Jackie during the acute phase of her illness?

□ 1. Playing Nerf basketball.

□ 2. Visiting other children on the unit.

□ 3. Keeping a written diary.

□ 4. Listening to records of her favorite singing groups.

66. Three of the following laboratory results are crucial indicators of Jackie's progress. Which one is *not*?

□ 1. Antistreptolysin-O titer.

□ 2. C-reactive protein.

□ 3. Urine protein.

□ 4. Erythrocyte sedimentation rate.

67. Jackie is discharged after 3 weeks of hospitalization. Which of the following statements best indicates that Jackie's parents have understood discharge teaching?

□ 1. "Jackie should lead a sedentary life-style for at least a year."

□ 2. "Jackie must take daily antibiotics for an extended time to prevent a recurrence of rheumatic fever."

□ 3. "Jackie should not return to her fifth-grade classroom but should have a home teacher the rest of the year."

□ 4. "Jackie may have permanent neurological sequelae as a result of the Sydenham's chorea."

Aurelio Juarez is admitted to the emergency room with an abdominal gunshot wound.

68. Which of the following descriptions of the bleeding is best for the nurse's notes?

□ 1. A moderate-to-large amount of sanguinous drainage noted from abdominal wound.

□ 2. Severe bleeding from wound.

□ 3. Copious amounts of blood coming from abdomen.

□ 4. Sanguinous drainage from abdominal wound soaked 2 towels and 6 abdominal pads in 10 minutes.

69. Towels can be used to pack the gunshot wound because

☐ 1. The injury is usually fatal.
☐ 2. The wound is already grossly contaminated.
☐ 3. Towels absorb more than ABD pads.
☐ 4. The client is probably bleeding minimally.

70. Mr. Juarez also has a knife protruding from his chest. The best nursing action is to do which of the following?
☐ 1. Immediately remove the knife.
☐ 2. Leave the knife in until an operative setup is arranged.
☐ 3. Clean the exposed knife blade with povidone-iodine solution.
☐ 4. Cover area with a sterile towel soaked in saline.

71. Select the most correct statement about subcutaneous emphysema.
☐ 1. It is caused by air sucked into the chest wall from a superficial wound.
☐ 2. It is caused by internal injury.
☐ 3. It can always be noted easily.
☐ 4. It is not exacerbated by coughing.

72. Mr. Juarez is unable to void. A catheterization yields a small amount of bloody urine. This is most likely an indication of which of the following?
☐ 1. Urethral tear.
☐ 2. Urethritis.
☐ 3. Ruptured bladder.
☐ 4. Prostatitis.

73. Several blood transfusions are ordered. When administering a blood transfusion, what is a mandatory nursing function requiring two nurses?
☐ 1. Check the type and crossmatch data, numbers on the lab slips, and the information on the blood with that on the client's blood band.
☐ 2. Check the type and crossmatch data, numbers on the lab slips, and the information on the blood with that on the client's chart.
☐ 3. Check for the best possible vein to ensure correct infusion.
☐ 4. Ensure that Mr. Juarez is rational in order to establish a baseline of behavior.

74. Mr. Juarez's girlfriend volunteered to donate blood for him. What information is necessary to ascertain if she can be a donor?
☐ 1. History of gonorrhea within the last year.
☐ 2. History of bacterial endocarditis within the last 4 years.
☐ 3. History of hepatitis within the last 5 years.
☐ 4. History of upper respiratory tract infection within the last 6 months.

75. When assembling the equipment to start the blood transfusion, which of the following solutions is used to start the IV?
☐ 1. Sterile water.
☐ 2. Normal saline.
☐ 3. 10% dextrose in water.
☐ 4. Lactated Ringer's solution.

76. The nurse must remain at the bedside for 15 minutes after the blood is started to assess for any transfusion reaction. Which of the following is *not* found during a transfusion reaction?
☐ 1. Chills, fever, and dyspnea.
☐ 2. Decreased blood pressure and increased pulse rate.
☐ 3. Bleeding under the skin at the IV site.
☐ 4. Hives and itching.

77. Which one of the following nursing actions must be taken immediately if a transfusion reaction occurs?
☐ 1. Notify the physician.
☐ 2. Check the vital signs, and take a urine sample.
☐ 3. Stop the blood transfusion, and infuse normal saline.
☐ 4. Slow down the rate of blood flow and continue the assessment.

Aretha Benson is admitted to the labor room for induction. She is 20 days past her estimated date of delivery. Her cervix is 50% effaced and fingertip dilated.

78. Before the induction, Mrs. Benson has an oxytocin challenge test. What does this test demonstrate?
☐ 1. Lung maturity of the fetus.
☐ 2. The response of the fetal heart rate to fetal activity.
☐ 3. The degree of well-being of the feto-placental-maternal unit.
☐ 4. The ability of the fetus to tolerate the stress of uterine contractions.

79. An infusion of oxytocin (Pitocin) is administered to Mrs. Benson, and labor is initiated. Which of the following observations would be most critical at this time?
☐ 1. Fetal heart rate and uterine contractions.
☐ 2. Vaginal discharge and vital signs.
☐ 3. Fetal heart rate and maternal blood pressure.
☐ 4. Uterine contractions and maternal emotional responses.

80. In evaluating the action of the oxytocin, which of the following would be most indicative of an adverse reaction to the drug?
☐ 1. A contraction lasting over 120 seconds.
☐ 2. Deep-tendon reflexes of 2 + .
☐ 3. Urinary output of 100 ml/hr.
☐ 4. Increasing intensity of contractions.

81. Mrs. Benson, now in active labor, expresses concern about her ability to maintain control of her behavior during the remainder of labor. Which of these nursing actions would be most supportive?
☐ 1. Reassure her of the nursing staff's competency.
☐ 2. Reassure her that medication is available.
☐ 3. Instruct her in relaxation and breathing exercises.
☐ 4. Reassure her that she will be accepted regardless of her behavior.

82. An external monitor has been applied to Mrs. Benson. A fetal heart deceleration of uniform shape is detected, beginning just as the contraction is underway and returning to the baseline at the end of the contraction. Which of the following nursing actions is most appropriate?
 □ 1. Administer O_2.
 □ 2. Turn the client on her left side.
 □ 3. Notify the physician.
 □ 4. No action is necessary.

83. The fetal monitor begins to show late decelerations. Which of the following would the nurse do first?
 □ 1. Continue to assess the monitor strip for 15 more minutes.
 □ 2. Put her in Trendelenburg's position.
 □ 3. Turn her on her left side.
 □ 4. Inform the attending physician.

84. Mrs. Benson delivers a 7-pound 8-ounce boy. Which of the following descriptions would best describe a postmature infant?
 □ 1. "Wide-eyed" with downy hair.
 □ 2. Long finger nails and increased subcutaneous fat.
 □ 3. Long, coarse hair and meconium-stained skin.
 □ 4. Parchmentlike skin and a thick coating of vernix.

85. The nurse administers methylergonovine (Methergine), 0.2 mg, parenterally to Mrs. Benson after completion of the third stage of labor. Which of the following would indicate that this drug has produced its desired effect?
 □ 1. A firm fundus.
 □ 2. Increased duration and frequency of contractions.
 □ 3. A rise in blood pressure.
 □ 4. An increase in the respiratory rate.

86. Thirty minutes after the client's delivery, the nurse makes the following assessment: fundus firm, 1 inch below the umbilicus; lochia rubra; complains of thirst; slight tremors of lower extremities. Analysis of these data is most suggestive of which of the following?
 □ 1. Impending shock.
 □ 2. Circulatory overload.
 □ 3. Subinvolution.
 □ 4. Normal postpartum adjustment.

87. One hour after delivery, Mrs. Benson complains of severe perineal pain. Which nursing action would take highest priority?
 □ 1. Administer prescribed pain medication.
 □ 2. Administer a sitz bath immediately.
 □ 3. Inspect the perineum.
 □ 4. Instruct client in perineal muscle exercises.

88. Which of the following indicates bladder distension after Mrs. Benson's normal vaginal delivery?
 □ 1. Poor abdominal muscle tone.
 □ 2. Increased lochia rubra with clots.
 □ 3. Uterus contracted below umbilicus.
 □ 4. Uterus soft to the right of midline.

Gina Venters is a 21-year-old college student who has just learned that she contracted genital herpes from her sexual partner.

89. After completing the initial history and assessment for Miss Venters, the nurse will have data concerning areas pertinent to the disease. Which of the following would be *unnecessary* to include at this point?
 □ 1. Voiding patterns.
 □ 2. Characteristics of lesions.
 □ 3. Vaginal discharge.
 □ 4. Prior history of varicella.

90. Which of the following nursing diagnoses would most likely apply to Miss Venters as she copes with this disease?
 □ 1. Altered sexuality patterns.
 □ 2. Impaired physical mobility.
 □ 3. Diversional activity deficit.
 □ 4. Disturbance in self-concept: personal identity.

91. Miss Venters questions the reason why sexually transmitted diseases have reached epidemic proportions lately. Which of the following is the best explanation of the increased incidence?
 □ 1. Sexual permissiveness and promiscuity have increased.
 □ 2. Use of birth control pills has decreased because of better public education about their side effects.
 □ 3. The incidence of these diseases has increased because prostitutes transmit them.
 □ 4. Few people have information about how diseases are spread.

92. Miss Venters requests a shot of penicillin to cure her and promises to continue taking medication faithfully at home. How would the nurse best respond?
 □ 1. "I'll prepare the shot for you as long as you continue the oral medication for 10 days."
 □ 2. "You will need to return for more penicillin if a lesion appears."
 □ 3. "Unfortunately, genital herpes is a lifelong disease, which at present has no cure."
 □ 4. "Tetracycline is the drug of choice for genital herpes."

93. Which of the following techniques would *not* aid in preventing the spread of genital herpes to others?
 □ 1. Refrain from sexual intercourse while lesions are present.
 □ 2. Restrict sexual contact to others already exposed to herpes.
 □ 3. Have sexual intercourse only in a darkened environment.
 □ 4. Use condoms during intercourse.

94. Why is it particularly difficult to assess females for gonorrhea?
 □ 1. They rarely have early distressing symptoms of the disease.
 □ 2. They are less likely to seek medical attention for diseases.

☐ 3. Cultures from the cervix cannot be used for diagnostic purposes.

☐ 4. They have a lower incidence of cystitis than do males.

95. Syphilis may often go undetected without a thorough sexual history. Why is this so?

☐ 1. The disease is usually asymptomatic.

☐ 2. Symptoms disappear after some months, even if syphilis is not treated.

☐ 3. Symptoms appear the day after sexual contact.

☐ 4. The disease first attacks internal organs.

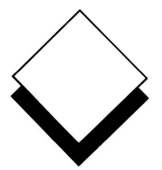

Test 1, Book III

ANSWERS WITH RATIONALES

KEY TO ABBREVIATIONS
Section of the Review Book

P = Psychosocial and Mental Health Problems
   T = Therapeutic Use of Self
   L = Loss and Death and Dying
   A = Anxious Behavior
   C = Confused Behavior
   E = Elated-Depressive Behavior
   SM = Socially Maladaptive Behavior
   SS = Suspicious Behavior
   W = Withdrawn Behavior
   SU = Substance Use Disorders
A = Adult
   H = Healthy Adult
   S = Surgery
   O = Oxygenation
   NM = Nutrition and Metabolism
   E = Elimination
   SP = Sensation and Perception
   M = Mobility
   CA = Cellular Aberration
CBF = Childbearing Family
   W = Women's Health Care
   A = Antepartal Care
   I = Intrapartal Care
   P = Postpartal Care
   N = Newborn Care
C = Child
   H = Healthy Child
   I = Ill and Hospitalized Child
   SPP = Sensation, Perception, and Protection
   O = Oxygenation
   NM = Nutrition and Metabolism
   E = Elimination
   M = Mobility
   CA = Cellular Aberration

Nursing Process Category

AS = Assessment
AN = Analysis
PL = Plan
IM = Implementation
EV = Evaluation

Client Need Category

E = Safe, Effective Care Environment
PS = Physiological Integrity
PC = Psychosocial Integrity
H = Health Promotion and Maintenance

1. no. 1. The medulla may also be affected, along with cranial nerves, but respiratory symptoms generally are not the result of increased intracranial pressure. A/M, AN, PS

2. no. 3. The motor division of cranial nerve VII is specific; it controls the musculature of the face. A/M, AS, PS

3. no. 1. Treatment is symptomatic and supportive. The primary role of the nurse with these clients is careful observation and prevention of complications. A/M, PL, E

4. no. 1. Ninety percent of people with this diagnosis make a complete recovery. The other options are inappropriate or inaccurate. A/M, IM, PC

5. no. 2. The client may burn or injure an extremity if sensory alteration is present. Special care to avoid injury is needed. A/M, IM, H

6. no. 4. Conversion reaction is the loss or alteration of physical function that is not explained by any physical disorder or pathophysiological mechanism. It is postulated that the behavior is reinforced by the gain it represents to the client by repressing some unacceptable feeling or desire. P/A, AN, PC

7. no. 2. Repression of feeling keeps anxiety controlled. The tension generated is converted into the

presenting symptom, which is symbolic. A fixation at the anal stage of development produces defense mechanisms of sublimation and displacement, not conversion. Suppression of feelings is a conscious effort to eliminate feelings of discomfort. Conversion is an unconscious, intrapsychic conflict. Sublimation is a diversion of consciously unacceptable instinctual drives into personally and socially acceptable areas. P/A, AN, PC

8. no. 3. In a conversion disorder, the client displays a level of concern disproportionate to the symptoms exhibited known as *la belle indifférence*. Ambivalence connotes simultaneous conflicting feelings or attitudes. Lability connotes mood swings. Narcissism, which is an abnormal interest in oneself, is not described here. P/A, AS, PC

9. no. 4. In addition to the primary gain of keeping anxiety out of her awareness, all the statements represent possible secondary gains. P/A, AN, PC

10. no. 3. It is important to minimize the physical complaints and stress the positive aspects of her behavior to avoid reinforcement of the sick role. Confrontation will increase defensiveness and will meet resistance because of the client's need for denial. Supportive measures may provide secondary gain and increase dependency. The client is not psychotic; therefore such medication is not indicated. P/A, IM, PC

11. no. 4. Sitting upright, leaning forward with mouth open, drooling, and dysphagia are classic signs of epiglottitis. C/O, AN, PS

12. no. 1. An adequate airway is the primary objective in treating epiglottitis because this child is in imminent danger of complete airway blockage. C/O, PS, PS

13. no. 3. A change in heart rate (i.e., increasing heart rate) is an early sign of hypoxia. Options no. 2 and no. 4 are signs of lower airway involvement; no. 1 is characteristic of spasmodic croup. C/O, AS, PS

14. no. 1. Determine Mark's hypersensitivity to the medication. Penicillin products are at high risk for causing allergic (and life-threatening) reactions. C/O, IM, E

15. no. 4. The Croupette concentrates the cool mist. This facilitates the heavy, cool water droplets reaching deeper into the respiratory tract to reduce edema and soothe irritated mucous membranes. Although the Croupette will also accomplish options no. 1, no. 2, and no. 3 to some extent, they are not the primary goals. C/O, PL, PS

16. no. 3. Loosely tucking the tent edges will allow oxygen to escape; edges should be firmly tucked around the mattress. All other options are necessary because of his age and his problem. C/O, IM, E

17. no. 2. A specific gravity of 1.005 indicates adequate hydration status. The other options measure parameters that do not influence hydration. C/O, AS, PS

18. no. 2. Imaginary friends are normal for this age group. Because this is normal behavior, the other options are not warranted. C/H, IM, PC

19. no. 2. Tying shoelaces, jumping rope, and walking backward are activities performed by a 5-year-old. C/H, AS, H

20. no. 1. Levels of pain will vary in the foot and leg. However, as the gangrenous area develops, pain decreases because of the nerve destruction that occurs. Despite the occurrence of gangrene, infection, or inflammation, pain may be totally absent in the client with advanced neuropathy. A/NM, AS, PS

21. no. 4. An immediate priority for the nurse is to determine the client's psychological response to the physiological happening: in this case, the death of a part of his body. Three ways of assessing this response are included in this option. A/NM, AS, PS

22. no. 2. A footboard is not used for the same reasons that ambulation is not allowed. The nursing actions are directed at promoting circulation by preventing pressure areas from developing in dependent areas. A/NM, PL, E

23. no. 3. When bed rest is prescribed for a client, fluids are increased, not decreased, in order to prevent urinary stasis. A/NM, PL, E

24. no. 2. Keeping the area dry prevents moisture from promoting the growth of infection and macerating the skin. The other options would interfere with this. A/NM, PL, PS

25. no. 2. The correct actions are stated in this option. Dakin's solution is used to debride the area, and petroleum jelly is a precautionary and preventive measure to protect the healthy tissue. A/NM, AN, PS

26. no. 3. Infection will increase the blood glucose level; thus the need for insulin increases. A/NM, AN, PS

27. no. 1. It is important to determine the person's perception of the condition before any teaching takes place. Remember, assessment occurs before planning or implementing nursing care. A/NM, IM, PC

28. no. 1. Maintenance of physiological integrity takes precedence. Determining the extent of the wounds and bleeding provides the most important information about the initial physical status. In an emergency situation, a nurse must provide a calm atmosphere yet attend to the client's safety and physiological needs first. Option no. 4 is a strategy that will be used eventually. P/E, IM, E

29. no. 2. This response allows the client to express the unstated feelings of hopelessness. Though anger may be present, his affect suggests hopelessness. The probability of his discussing or even recognizing anger at this time is minimal. Option no. 1 is a form of reassurance, which is rarely therapeutic. The

nurse cannot presume to know what the client will be experiencing later. Option no. 4 would reinforce the client's determination to attempt suicide and reinforce feelings of hopelessness rather than instill a sense of hopefulness that something could be different. P/E, IM, PC

30. no. 1. Though all choices provide useful information to assess suicide potential, the presence of a plan that is workable greatly increases the risk. Although some attempt at connecting here-and-now events with the current situation is necessary, it is not particularly helpful in deciding suicide potential. P/E, IM, E

31. no. 4. Close observation is imperative in suicide prevention. Although observation may be easier on a closed unit, an open unit is satisfactory as long as the client can be watched closely. A locked psychiatric unit does not imply that the client is being closely watched. A double room would assist the client only during the time that another client was in contact with him. However, other clients cannot bear the responsibility of supervision. P/E, IM, E

32. no. 4. Amitriptyline may take 4 weeks to become effective. It is premature to conclude the drug is not effective. The side effects of amitriptyline are autonomic because of the anticholinergic properties; therefore continued depression would not be a side effect. Tolerance implies that increasing amounts of the substance (drug) must be used in order to achieve desired results. Since the desired results have yet to be achieved, tolerance is not a factor yet. P/E, AS, PS

33. no. 3. These findings are consistent with a diagnosis of a hydatidiform mole. Since preeclampsia is usually a disease of late pregnancy, if symptoms occur in early pregnancy a hydatidiform mole should be suspected. Anemia occurs as a result of blood loss. CBF/A, AS, PS

34. no. 2. Ultrasound is the most useful tool in diagnosing a molar pregnancy; no fetal skeleton is revealed. A dilatation and curettage may be used to treat the condition. A laparoscopy is used to examine the interior of the abdomen. CBF/A, AS, PS

35. no. 4. The current methods of removing a molar pregnancy are dilatation and curettage, prostaglandin/oxytocin induction, or hysterectomy. CBF/A, AN, PS

36. no. 2. Choriocarcinoma, a neoplastic process that often follows a hydatidiform mole, has a tendency to undergo rapid, widespread metastasis. The client's human chorionic gonadotropin levels will be monitored for at least 1 year. Molar pregnancies do not place the client at higher risk for the remaining options. CBF/A, AN, PS

37. no. 3. Because of the concern about choriocarcinoma, it is generally recommended that pregnancy be avoided for 1 year following a molar pregnancy. CBF/A, IM, PS

38. no. 3. Oral contraceptive use is advocated to prevent another pregnancy for at least 1 year following a hydatidiform mole. CBF/A, EV, H

39. no. 3. Gout is a disease of faulty purine metabolism and is characterized by increased amounts of uric acid, which forms stones. The other options are all associated with calcium stones but not indicated by the client's history. A/E, AN, PS

40. no. 2. Hydronephrosis is caused when the ureter is obstructed and urine backs up and distends the kidney. A/E, AN, PS

41. no. 2. Unless the pain is controlled, there is little chance the stone will be safely passed. All of the other choices would be actions to take after pain is controlled. A/E, IM, PS

42. no. 1. Inorganic calcium stones occur in alkaline urine and often follow a urinary tract infection. A/E, AN, PS

43. no. 2. Vitamin C, when given in large (1 g) daily doses, is excreted through the urine, acidifying it. A/E, AN, PS

44. no. 2. Bethanechol (Urecholine) is a cholinergic drug, which increases bladder tone and promotes urination. A/E, AN, PS

45. no. 4. All options may occur, but the specific reason is to prevent loss of bladder tone. A/E, AN, PS

46. no. 1. The child with nephrosis usually exhibits generalized edema, ascites, an elevated urine specific gravity, and normal blood pressure. C/E, AS, PS

47. no. 1. Older toddlers and preschoolers are especially fearful of procedures that threaten their body integrity, such as rectal temperatures and injections. C/I, AN, PC

48. no. 4. The preschooler is involved in mastering a sense of initiative vs. guilt. C/H, AN, H

49. no. 2. Prednisone should never be withheld, but tapered gradually, because sudden withdrawal may precipitate an adrenal crisis. C/E, IM, PS

50. no. 4. Semi-Fowler's position relieves the respiratory difficulties that often occur with ascites. C/E, PL, E

51. no. 3. This snack is highest in potassium and protein and low in sodium. C/E, IM, PS

52. no. 3. This activity requires little energy expenditure while Courtney is acutely ill and also increases his sense of control and security by allowing him to project his own feelings into the story. C/I, IM, H

53. no. 3. The client with paranoid schizophrenia has increased sensitivity. Options no. 1, no. 2, and no. 4 are all characteristic manifestations of paranoid schizophrenia. P/W, AS, PC

54. no. 2. The client with paranoid schizophrenia projects his fantasy world and emotions on others, while undoing, rationalization, and suppression might be used by a paranoid schizophrenic but are not characteristically present. P/W, AS, PC

55. no. 4. Acting out fantasy life in group therapy would give positive reinforcement to fantasy and would not teach the client to cope in the world of reality. Options no. 1, no. 2, and no. 3 are all appropriate goals that are achievable and will incorporate the individual into the "real world." P/W, PL, E

56. no. 4. Mutual withdrawal is a common staff problem when clients withdraw from staff; isolation should be avoided when treating schizophrenic clients. Options no. 1, no. 2, and no. 3 will assist the client by allowing some control over how quickly he establishes a relationship with a staff member. P/W, IM, PC

57. no. 4. This option would give positive reinforcement to the client's unhealthy behaviors. It is more helpful to work with the client's healthy and adaptive behaviors. Options no. 1 and no. 2 will assist the client in focusing on reality and avoiding retreat and withdrawal. It is necessary to initially assess the content of the hallucinations to determine if the voices are directing the individual to harm himself or others. P/W, IM, PC

58. no. 1. Identifying client needs for assistance is the first step in assisting a client to be self-directing with hygiene and grooming. Group work is difficult for a schizophrenic client, and doing hygiene for him makes the client more dependent. Ignoring lack of hygiene is counterproductive to the goal. P/W, IM, PC

59. no. 3. Confronting and arguing with a paranoid client tends to increase the hostility, paranoia, mistrust, and more intense defense of delusions. The other options are beneficial for managing hostile behavior. P/W, IM, PC

60. no. 4. Ambivalence is not treatable with a drug. Agitation, hallucinations, and delusions are the "target" symptoms that antipsychotic agents are specifically prescribed to diminish or alleviate. P/W, AN, PS

61. no. 4. Thioridazine and the other antipsychotic medications are not addictive, and there is no tolerance to their antipsychotic effect. Dry mouth, constipation, and urinary hesitancy are characteristic side effects of thioridazine because of its anticholinergic properties. P/W, AS, PS

62. no. 3. The only permanent damage that may result from rheumatic fever is cardiac damage. Therefore close monitoring of cardiac status is imperative. C/O, AS, PS

63. no. 1. Sydenham's chorea does not impair intellectual functioning. Because of the symptoms, the chief problem is one of safety for the child. C/O, AS, PS

64. no. 1. This goal must have priority because permanent cardiac valvular damage may result from rheumatic fever. C/O, PL, E

65. no. 4. Bed rest is prescribed, so Jackie cannot visit other children on the unit. Because of the chorea, she is unable to play Nerf basketball or write in a diary. Therefore listening to records is the best activity at this time. C/O, IM, PS

66. no. 3. Rheumatic fever does not cause albuminuria. Nephrosis and nephritis cause large amounts of protein loss. C/O, AS, PS

67. no. 2. Long-term antibiotic therapy with penicillin or erythromycin is necessary to prevent serious cardiac damage or a recurrence of rheumatic fever. C/O, EV, H

68. no. 4. Nursing notes should be clear, specific descriptions. A/O, AS, PS

69. no. 2. A gunshot wound is grossly contaminated, and an abdominal wound would bleed profusely; any clean towels would be appropriate. A/O, AN, PS

70. no. 2. Removing or disturbing the knife in a chest wound can cause severe damage or massive hemorrhage. The knife acts as a tamponade to the affected sites. A/O, IM, PS

71. no. 2. Internal injury leads to an air leak within the tissues, thereby causing subcutaneous emphysema. A/O, AN, PS

72. no. 3. A ruptured bladder causes the sensation of needing to void, but urine actually is collecting in the peritoneal cavity. A/O, AN, PS

73. no. 1. This procedure is essential to prevent the administration of incompatible blood, which could result in the client's death. It is essential to check the client's blood band on his arm. Just checking the chart does not ensure that the client receives the correct blood. Options no. 3 and no. 4 are important but do not require two nurses. A/O, IM, E

74. no. 3. A history of hepatitis disqualifies a potential blood donor for life. The other options do not disqualify a person. A/O, AS, PS

75. no. 2. Normal saline is used because it is an isotonic solution. A/O, AN, PS

76. no. 3. Bleeding under the skin at the IV site indicates infiltration or leaking around the site. All the other options given are signs of a transfusion reaction. A/O, AS, PS

77. no. 3. It is imperative that the blood be stopped and the IV needle be left in place and kept patent to administer fluids and medications to counteract the reaction. Option no. 2 is a second action, and no. 1 is a third action. A/O, IM, E

78. no. 4. The purpose of an oxytocin challenge test is to observe fetal heart rate response to uterine contractions. CBF/I, AN, PS

79. no. 1. Risks with the administration of oxytocin are related to uterine tetany and late decelerations. CBF/I, AS, PS

80. no. 1. If contractions exceed 90 seconds in duration, there is a danger of a ruptured uterus as well as interference with placental perfusion. The remaining

options are normal or expected findings with oxytocin induction. CBF/I, EV, PS

81. no. 4. Acceptance is needed in time of stress. As labor progresses the client may have difficulty maintaining control. The client will require acceptance during a time of stress and assurance that she will be accepted regardless of her behavior. The nurse's competency, administration of medication, and instruction may be ineffective in controlling the client's behavior. CBF/I, IM, PC

82. no. 4. This is a normal occurrence called an early deceleration. It is most likely a result of head compression, and it requires no action. CBF/I, IM, PS

83. no. 3. Late decelerations are most likely a result of uteroplacental insufficiency and require prompt action. Turning the client on the left side to relieve pressure on the vena cava by the gravida uterus may correct the problem. The physician should be notified if the heart rate is not corrected by nursing actions. Trendelenburg's position is not appropriate for the pregnant woman because it interferes with respirations. CBF/I, IM, PS

84. no. 3. This best describes the postmature infant. Because of prolonged gestation, these infants are more alert, have decreased vernix, dry and peeling skin, and long fingernails. They exhibit varying degrees of wasting and thus have decreased subcutaneous fat. Meconium staining results from intrauterine hypoxia. CBF/N, AS, PS

85. no. 1. Methylergonovine (Methergine) is an oxytoxic drug given to contract the uterus after a placental delivery. CBF/P, EV, PS

86. no. 4. These are normal observations in the immediate postpartum period. CBF/P, AN, PS

87. no. 3. Such pain may be associated with the development of a hematoma. Assessment is necessary before selecting an appropriate nursing action. CBF/P, IM, PS

88. no. 4. A full bladder displaces the uterus and prevents contraction. CBF/P, AS, PS

89. no. 4. The other three options list common reasons for which clients with herpes seek care. C/SPP, AS, PS

90. no. 1. Having herpes leads to an alteration or limitation in sexual relationships as well as alterations in achieving perceived or desired sex roles. Other nursing diagnoses listed are not applicable. C/SPP, AN, PS

91. no. 1. The idea underlying these social changes is that with the advent of antibiotics and the contraceptive pill, people began to lose fear of untreated disease and pregnancy, leading to increased exposure to infection. The other three options listed are not true statements. C/SPP, AN, PS

92. no. 3. Treatment for genital herpes is most often symptomatic since there is no known cure for the disease at present. C/SPP, IM, PS

93. no. 3. Before sexual intercourse, partners should examine themselves and each other for evidence of disease. A darkened environment is not conducive to this. C/SPP, PL, PS

94. no. 1. Early symptoms of gonorrhea include a slight purulent discharge, a vague feeling of fullness in the pelvis, and discomfort in the abdomen. Many women disregard these vague symptoms (if they are present) and do not seek treatment. C/SPP, AN, PS

95. no. 2. Although the symptoms of syphilis are similar to those of a host of other diseases, they disappear without treatment, providing false reassurance to the client that nothing is really wrong. C/SPP, AN, PS

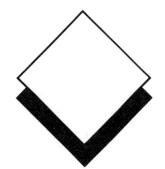

Test 1, Book IV

QUESTIONS

Ann Martin, a 47-year-old retired government employee, is admitted to the psychiatric inpatient service, accompanied by her daughter. Her admission diagnosis is a major depressive episode. She is delusional and has vegetative signs of depression.

1. Oftentimes, depression is accompanied by guilt. The multidisciplinary mental health team develops a care plan that includes "help client to express guilty feelings." The primary nurse realizes that some clients are not aware of their guilt feelings. To implement this goal, it would be best for the nurse to have Mrs. Martin do which of the following?
   □ 1. Attend group therapy.
   □ 2. Explore feelings of resentment and anger.
   □ 3. Examine situations where she may push others away out of fear of rejection.
   □ 4. Participate in planning activities of daily living.

2. In which type of depression would delusions be most likely to occur?
   □ 1. Transitory.
   □ 2. Reactive.
   □ 3. Psychotic.
   □ 4. Neurotic.

3. Which of the following are specific indicators of a serious clinical depression?
   □ 1. Crying and withdrawal.
   □ 2. Constipation, anorexia, and hypersomnolence or hyposomnolence.
   □ 3. Weakness and fatigability.
   □ 4. Negative view of the self and the future.

4. Which of the following statements indicates most clearly that the client is suffering from a depression?
   □ 1. "I don't feel that I have any chance of a good relationship with anyone. I am not very attractive or likable."
   □ 2. "I'm a very private person and don't call my friends when I feel bad."
   □ 3. "I don't have any appetite sometimes, I'm constipated, and I sleep too much."
   □ 4. "I feel weak and tired all the time."

5. Which of the following is *not* considered a sign of depression?
   □ 1. Anorexia.
   □ 2. Early morning awakening.
   □ 3. Morning-evening variations of mood.
   □ 4. Ataxia.

6. Which of the following are considered signs of a retarded depression?
   □ 1. Restlessness, pacing, and anxiety.
   □ 2. Talkativeness and increased motor activity.
   □ 3. Haggard appearance, slow movements and thinking, and great difficulty making decisions.
   □ 4. Argumentative and bosses staff.

7. The largest number of psychiatric hospitalizations are accounted for by which of the following?
   □ 1. Schizophrenia.
   □ 2. Phobic reactions.
   □ 3. Autism.
   □ 4. Depression.

8. Mrs. Martin frequently seeks out a nurse whom she resembles in height, weight, and appearance. In this nurse's presence, Mrs. Martin imitates her mannerisms and supportive ways. This defense mechanism by the client can best be described as which of the following?
   □ 1. Idealization.
   □ 2. Introjection.
   □ 3. Identification.
   □ 4. Substitution.

9. During the course of her treatment, Mrs. Martin's psychiatrist orders amitriptyline (Elavil), 20 mg tid po. Which of the following side effects is usually *not* expected to occur?
   □ 1. Sedation.
   □ 2. Dry mouth.
   □ 3. Hypertension.
   □ 4. Blurred vision.

10. The psychiatrist also orders isocarboxazid (Marplan), 30 mg po daily. When recording these medication orders, the nurse would do which of the following?

☐ 1. Order and administer the medications.

☐ 2. Measure the client's blood pressure and withhold both medications if blood pressure is below 90 mm Hg (systolic) and 60 mm Hg (diastolic).

☐ 3. Inquire first whether the client has had any dizziness or nausea, since both of these medications could worsen these symptoms.

☐ 4. Call the psychiatrist and question the administration of these medications together.

11. Antidepressants may cause a number of side effects. Which of the following antidepressants may lead to hypertensive crisis and possibly a cerebrovascular accident if taken with aged foods, such as cheeses, or alcoholic beverages, such as beer and wine?

☐ 1. Amitriptyline (Elavil).

☐ 2. Imipramine (Tofranil).

☐ 3. Lithium carbonate.

☐ 4. Isocarboxazid (Marplan).

12. All of the following assessments would be included for Mrs. Martin. Which one would be carried out first?

☐ 1. Degree of neglect of physical needs (e.g., fluid intake, nutrition, and elimination).

☐ 2. Possibility of self-harm.

☐ 3. Willingness to attend group therapy.

☐ 4. Response to medications.

13. Which of these suicide methods has a lower rate of lethality than the others?

☐ 1. Ingestion of barbiturates and any sedatives.

☐ 2. Setting herself on fire.

☐ 3. Scratching her wrists.

☐ 4. Cutting the jugular vein.

14. Of the following, which group has the lowest suicide risk?

☐ 1. Alcoholics.

☐ 2. Depressed persons.

☐ 3. Adolescents.

☐ 4. Married men.

Tang Phong is a 3-week-old boy brought into the emergency room by his parents. Mr. and Mrs. Phong say his vomiting has become progressively worse over the past 5 days. It is now projectile.

15. While obtaining a nursing history, which question would be *least* appropriate to ask the Phongs in order to rule out pyloric stenosis?

☐ 1. "Has Tang had a recent immunization?"

☐ 2. "Is anyone else sick at home?"

☐ 3. "Does Tang appear hungry after vomiting?"

☐ 4. "How much did Tang weigh at his last exam?"

16. Tang's condition is diagnosed as pyloric stenosis, and he is transferred to a pediatric unit. What would be the most *unexpected* finding in an infant with this condition?

☐ 1. A palpable, olive-shaped mass in the right upper quadrant.

☐ 2. Visible left-to-right peristaltic waves.

☐ 3. Stringy, frequent stools.

☐ 4. Lethargy.

17. Tang is admitted to the infant unit. Which of the following nursing actions would be implemented?

☐ 1. Prepare Tang and his parents for immediate surgery.

☐ 2. Monitor intravenous hydration.

☐ 3. Give diazepam (Valium) as ordered, to relax the pyloric sphincter.

☐ 4. Give small, frequent feedings.

18. What is the most common metabolic disturbance seen in infants who have pyloric stenosis?

☐ 1. Metabolic acidosis.

☐ 2. Metabolic alkalosis.

☐ 3. Respiratory alkalosis.

☐ 4. Hyperkalemia.

19. Tang has an IV of 5% dextrose in 0.45% saline hanging. The physician has ordered potassium chloride (KCl) to be added to the IV. What important nursing action is carried out before adding KCl to the IV?

☐ 1. Check the time of last voiding.

☐ 2. Look up the last serum chloride level.

☐ 3. Ensure that the IV is infusing through a large-bore needle.

☐ 4. Check skin turgor.

20. Tang is extremely restless and his repeated movements cause two IVs to infiltrate. Cloth extremity-restraints are applied to prevent recurrent infiltration. Which of the following measures is most important to ensure the safety of a restrained infant?

☐ 1. Avoid placing padding under the restraints, since it will only increase pressure and the chance of injury.

☐ 2. Fasten the restraint ties securely to the crib rails.

☐ 3. Secure all four extremities since one loose extremity can cause the child to become entangled in the restraints.

☐ 4. Frequently check how the restraints are applied and the circulation in the extremities.

21. Tang has had his pyloric stenosis surgically repaired. Which would *not* be considered when planning his postoperative nursing care?

☐ 1. Include parents in giving his feedings.

☐ 2. Oral feedings will be started a few hours after surgery.

☐ 3. Tang will be NPO for days after surgery; thus sucking needs should be satisfied in other ways.

☐ 4. Monitor Tang for signs of hypoglycemia.

22. After surgical repair of the pyloric stenosis, Tang would be placed in which position?

☐ 1. High-Fowler's position.

☐ 2. Prone.

☐ 3. Right side-lying.

☐ 4. Left side-lying.

23. Which of the following postoperative responses to feedings would Tang optimally exhibit?

☐ 1. Immediate tolerance of oral fluids because of release of the hypertrophied muscle.

☐ 2. No vomiting, since the infant is NPO and is on a regimen of IVs for the first 2 to 3 days.

☐ 3. Tolerance for clear fluids, but frequent vomiting of formula or breast milk.

☐ 4. Intermittent vomiting of oral fluids that diminishes over the first 24 to 48 hours.

24. Which nursing observation indicates that Tang's parents are fully prepared for his discharge?

☐ 1. Tang recovers fully from surgery, and his parents express happiness.

☐ 2. He retains his formula after his parents feed him.

☐ 3. His parents demonstrate the correct feeding technique.

☐ 4. Tang gains weight appropriate for his age.

Paul Connelly, a 38-year-old bookkeeper, has suffered from chronic renal failure for 3 years. He has been maintained on outpatient hemodialysis 3 times a week while awaiting transplantation.

25. Donor-recipient compatibility must be assessed before renal transplant. Mr. Connelly asks the nurse to explain tissue typing. Which of the following statements is an *incorrect* response?

☐ 1. Blood typing is the initial step in determining compatibility.

☐ 2. Any natural sibling of the recipient is an ideal donor.

☐ 3. Two human leukocyte antigens (HLA) are inherited from each parent.

☐ 4. A mixed lymphocyte culture (MLC) requires 5 to 7 days to perform.

26. A suitable donor is located, and Mr. Connelly's transplantation is scheduled. He will receive the immunosuppressive drug azathioprine (Imuran) before surgery and following the transplant. What would the nurse teach him about this medication?

☐ 1. Avoid crowds and contact with obviously ill people.

☐ 2. The drug stimulates kidney output.

☐ 3. Frequent monitoring of blood pressure will be required.

☐ 4. An increase in the number of circulating antibodies can be anticipated.

27. The nurse plans to observe Mr. Connelly closely following surgery for signs of rejection of the graft. Which observation is *not* associated with tissue rejection?

☐ 1. Weight gain.

☐ 2. Decreased urine output.

☐ 3. Swelling at the operative site.

☐ 4. Rising white blood cell count.

28. Early postoperative care for Mr. Connelly will *not* include which of the following?

☐ 1. Irrigate the Foley catheter frequently.

☐ 2. Maintain reverse isolation.

☐ 3. Frequent turning and repositioning.

☐ 4. Monitor the stool for blood.

29. Mr. Connelly's niece, Sally Burnside, age 15, is very interested in donating her kidneys for transplant should she die unexpectedly. She asks if she can carry a donor card. Based on the Uniform Anatomical Gift Act, what can the nurse tell her?

☐ 1. She must wait until she is 18, because she is a minor.

☐ 2. All she needs to do is sign a card.

☐ 3. She may carry a donor card, provided her parents have cosigned the card in the presence of witnesses.

☐ 4. A donor card is not necessary, because her parents could give permission if the need arises.

30. Mr. Connelly returns for a follow-up visit 1 year after his transplant. He tells the nurse he feels so well he has decided to stop taking his prednisone. The nurse is concerned because he may experience which of the following?

☐ 1. Infection.

☐ 2. Organ rejection.

☐ 3. Psychosis.

☐ 4. Anemia.

Rachael Carrier seeks treatment in the infertility clinic.

31. The nurse instructs Mrs. Carrier how to take her basal body temperature to identify the time of ovulation. This event can be identified by which of the following?

☐ 1. A slight drop in temperature followed by a rise of 0.5° F to 0.7° F under the influence of progesterone.

☐ 2. An increase in temperature of 2° F under the influence of progesterone.

☐ 3. A substantial drop in temperature followed by a 0.5° F to 0.7° F rise under the influence of estrogen.

☐ 4. An increase in the temperature of 2° F under the influence of estrogen.

32. At the time of ovulation, the blood level of which of the following is high?

☐ 1. Luteinizing hormone.

☐ 2. Follicle-stimulating hormone-releasing factors.

☐ 3. Progesterone.

☐ 4. Human chorionic gonadotropin.

33. After diagnostic testing, clomiphene (Clomid) is prescribed for Mrs. Carrier. Which of the following best describes how this drug works?

☐ 1. Increases the estrogen-progesterone level to cause ovulation.

☐ 2. Increases the amount of gonadotropin secretion to stimulate maturation of the ovarian follicles.

☐ 3. Changes the pH of vaginal secretions to support sperm viability.

☐ 4. Stimulates the development of the endometrium to support pregnancy.

Sean Collins, age 52, experiences retrosternal chest pain that radiates down his left arm when he is engaged in strenuous physical activity. A resting electrocardiagram (ECG) is normal, but a stress ECG shows ST depression.

34. As the nurse takes a history, which of the following questions is most relevant?

☐ 1. "Can you describe the pain and the events that led up to it?"

☐ 2. "Are you taking any medications for chest pain?"

☐ 3. "How many packs of cigarettes do you smoke daily?"

☐ 4. "Did the pain radiate to your jaw or neck?"

35. An ECG primarily gives information about which of the following?

☐ 1. Excitation of the myocardium.

☐ 2. Perfusion of the myocardium.

☐ 3. Contractile force of the myocardium.

☐ 4. Integrity of the myocardium.

36. Cardiac isoenzymes are drawn. Why were they ordered?

☐ 1. To identify the causative organism.

☐ 2. To determine how well the blood is being oxygenated.

☐ 3. To rule out gas or indigestion.

☐ 4. To determine the presence of tissue damage.

37. Based on Mr. Collins' clinical symptoms and laboratory reports, the physician makes a diagnosis of angina pectoris. Anginal pain can involve the left arm and jaw, in addition to the chest, because these areas are all supplied by which of the following parts of the nervous system?

☐ 1. Cranial nerve (vagus).

☐ 2. Spinal nerves.

☐ 3. Autonomic nervous system.

☐ 4. Spinal cord segment.

38. Anginal pain is caused by coronary insufficiency. The coronary arteries fill with blood when which of the following occurs?

☐ 1. The left ventricle contracts, and the aortic valve is closed.

☐ 2. The left ventricle contracts, and the aortic valve is open.

☐ 3. The left ventricle relaxes, and the aortic valve is closed.

☐ 4. The left ventricle relaxes, and the aortic valve is open.

39. Mr. Collins is given nitroglycerin, 0.4 mg, to take sublingually during his angina attacks. Mr. Collins' dosage of 0.4 mg is equivalent to how many grains?

☐ 1. 1/250 grain.

☐ 2. 1/200 grain.

☐ 3. 1/150 grain.

☐ 4. 1/100 grain.

40. Nitroglycerin will produce dilatation of the coronary arteries in 1 to 2 minutes after being put under the tongue. Which of these statements correctly describes the procedure for administering nitroglycerin when one tablet does not relieve the pain?

☐ 1. Administer one tablet q2min for five doses.

☐ 2. Administer one tablet q5min for ten doses.

☐ 3. Administer one tablet q5min for three doses.

☐ 4. Administer one tablet q10min for five doses.

41. Mr. Collins would be observed for common side effects of nitroglycerin therapy. What are they?

☐ 1. Headache, hypotension, and dizziness.

☐ 2. Hypertension, flushing, and loss of consciousness.

☐ 3. Hypotension, shock, and convulsions.

☐ 4. Headache, hypertension, and convulsions.

42. What information would the nurse give to Mr. Collins about nitroglycerin?

☐ 1. "Take the tablets with meals."

☐ 2. "Take the tablets only for severe pain."

☐ 3. "A burning sensation under the tongue is normal."

☐ 4. "Call your doctor if you have a headache or flushing."

43. Which of the following would be most appropriate to teach Mr. Collins in terms of what to report immediately?

☐ 1. The occurrence of pain after a business meeting.

☐ 2. A change in the pattern of pain.

☐ 3. Pain that occurs with eating.

☐ 4. The fact that nitroglycerin does not cause a tingling sensation under the tongue.

44. Mr. Collins is also placed on a regimen of propranolol (Inderal) to control his angina. Propranolol will be contraindicated if Mr. Collins develops which of the following?

☐ 1. Myocardial infarction.

☐ 2. Asthma.

☐ 3. Cerebrovascular accident.

☐ 4. Thrombophlebitis.

45. When administering a beta-blocking agent such as propranolol (Inderal), the nurse would *not* do which of the following?

☐ 1. Teach the client to change positions slowly.

☐ 2. Monitor for occult blood in the stool and urine.

☐ 3. Monitor the blood pressure.

☐ 4. Monitor for dyspnea and respiratory dysfunction.

46. The nurse begins diet teaching with Mr. Collins.

Which of the following is inappropriate for the teaching plan?

☐ 1. Eat smaller meals.

☐ 2. Eat snacks of cheese.

☐ 3. Include more fish and chicken.

☐ 4. Eliminate caffeine intake.

47. Mr. Collins is discharged and referred to the outpatient clinic for a stress test and cardiac catheterization. What is the rationale for the cardiac catheterization?

☐ 1. To dilate the coronary blood vessels.

☐ 2. To confirm a diagnosis of heart disease.

☐ 3. To force oxygen under pressure to the myocardium.

☐ 4. To bypass the diseased coronary artery.

48. Mr. Collins wants to join a class on primary health care habits to prevent cardiovascular and respiratory disease, but he tells the nurse he does not plan to quit smoking. What would be the best response to Mr. Collins?

☐ 1. He cannot join unless he stops smoking.

☐ 2. He can join but cannot smoke in class.

☐ 3. He can join and can smoke in class.

☐ 4. He can join but should not attend classes on smoking cessation.

Four-year-old Sean White was admitted to the hospital with burns received while playing with matches. His legs and lower abdomen are burned.

49. In assessing Sean's hydration status, which of the following indicates less-than-adequate fluid replacement?

☐ 1. Decreasing hematocrit and increasing urine volume.

☐ 2. Falling hematocrit and decreasing urine volume.

☐ 3. Rising hematocrit and decreasing urine volume.

☐ 4. Stable hematocrit and increasing urine volume.

50. Which symptoms indicate overhydration after the first 24 hours?

☐ 1. Diuresis.

☐ 2. Drowsiness and lethargy.

☐ 3. Dyspnea, moist rales.

☐ 4. Warmth and redness around the intravenous site.

51. Sean's burns are to be treated by the "open method." In planning his care, which of the following is *least* appropriate?

☐ 1. Place Sean in reverse isolation.

☐ 2. Prevent him from having visitors from outside the hospital.

☐ 3. Encourage Sean to participate in his care.

☐ 4. Place him in a room near the nurse's station.

52. Sean's output through his Foley catheter is 10 ml/hr. What would be the first nursing action?

☐ 1. Check the catheter to see if it is plugged.

☐ 2. Call the physician immediately.

☐ 3. Record the information on the chart.

☐ 4. Increase the intravenous fluids.

53. When Sean starts oral feedings, it is particularly important that his diet have a high amount of which of the following?

☐ 1. Fats and carbohydrates.

☐ 2. Minerals and vitamins.

☐ 3. Fluids and vitamins.

☐ 4. Proteins and carbohydrates.

54. What would be the best diversional activity for Sean while he is in reverse isolation?

☐ 1. Lace leather wallets.

☐ 2. Watch television.

☐ 3. Play with puppets.

☐ 4. Use computer word games.

Robert Benson, a middle-aged business executive, is admitted to the psychiatric unit. He tells the nurse that he came to the hospital because he needs a few days of relief from the constant harassment of FBI agents, who have been following him for years. He believes the FBI wants to steal his plans for world peace.

55. Mr. Benson's diagnosis is paranoid disorder. Which of the following is *not* characteristic of paranoia?

☐ 1. Suspiciousness.

☐ 2. Superiority.

☐ 3. Hostility.

☐ 4. Intellectual impairment.

56. Mr. Benson's behavior is most characteristic of which of the following?

☐ 1. A fixed delusional system.

☐ 2. Hallucinations.

☐ 3. Acting out.

☐ 4. Manipulation.

57. In order to help Mr. Benson, it is most important for the nurse to do which of the following?

☐ 1. Gather more details about his problems with the FBI.

☐ 2. Point out to him that his story is not logical.

☐ 3. Acknowledge his feelings without agreeing with them.

☐ 4. Explain to him that he will have to learn to live with the existing situation.

58. Mr. Benson screams at the nurse that a spy is after him. The best nursing response at this time is which of the following?

☐ 1. "You are upset, Mr. Benson. I understand how you feel."

☐ 2. Ignore his comment.

☐ 3. "I am Miss Smith, a nurse on the unit."

☐ 4. "Mr. Benson, you are in the hospital now. I'm sure there are no spies here."

59. Later, Mr. Benson refuses to eat his dinner. He says he is hungry, but that his wife is trying to poison him. Taking note that Mr. Benson said he was hun-

gry, which of the following is the best nursing action?

- ☐ 1. Explain that his wife did not prepare the food.
- ☐ 2. Offer to taste his food before he eats it.
- ☐ 3. Call for another tray and eat with Mr. Benson.
- ☐ 4. Arrange to have food in sealed containers served to Mr. Benson.

60. Mr. Benson has been placed on a regimen of chlorpromazine (Thorazine). One side effect usually *not* expected is

- ☐ 1. Agranulocytosis.
- ☐ 2. Photophobia.
- ☐ 3. Postural hypotension.
- ☐ 4. Dermatitis.

Betty Spaulding, age 17, has begun to show early signs of pregnancy-induced hypertension (PIH).

61. Which of the following assessments by the nurse would most likely indicate that Betty may have PIH?

- ☐ 1. A blood pressure change from 110/80 mm Hg to 120/88 mm Hg.
- ☐ 2. Complaints of swelling of fingers and eyelids.
- ☐ 3. Weight gain of 4 pounds during the eighth month.
- ☐ 4. Presence of 1+ glucose in the urine.

62. Which of the following statements best describes the pathophysiological changes that occur in PIH?

- ☐ 1. There is an increase in both plasma proteins and glomerular filtration.
- ☐ 2. There is a decrease in aldosterone production and an increase in fluid retention.
- ☐ 3. There is an increase in circulating blood volume and a decrease in cardiac output.
- ☐ 4. There is a decrease in renal and uterine circulation because of vascular constriction.

63. The most likely goal of treatment for Betty, as for any mother with PIH, is to do which of the following?

- ☐ 1. Stabilize her vital signs.
- ☐ 2. Reduce the number and severity of headaches.
- ☐ 3. Increase urinary output.
- ☐ 4. Prevent convulsions.

64. Betty's symptoms worsen, and she is admitted to the hospital. The physician orders an IV of 200 ml magnesium sulfate diluted in 10% dextrose in water. Which of the following findings would most likely lead the nurse to withhold magnesium sulfate and notify the physician?

- ☐ 1. An apical pulse of 75/min.
- ☐ 2. A hyperactive knee-jerk reflex.
- ☐ 3. A respiratory rate of less than 12/min.
- ☐ 4. A urinary output of 50 ml/hr.

65. Magnesium sulfate is often used in cases of severe PIH because it acts as which of the following?

- ☐ 1. Central nervous system depressant.
- ☐ 2. Antihypertensive.

- ☐ 3. Diuretic.
- ☐ 4. Analgesic.

66. Betty's labor is to be induced with 10 units of oxytocin (Pitocin). After the oxytocin is started, Betty becomes very uncomfortable during contractions and states, "I don't think I'll be able to stand this pain." Vaginal examination indicates the cervix is dilated 2 cm. What would be the most appropriate initial nursing action?

- ☐ 1. Call the physician.
- ☐ 2. Give an analgesic.
- ☐ 3. Help her try some breathing exercises.
- ☐ 4. Increase the rate of the IV.

67. Betty's cervix is fully dilated. The physician makes the determination that the fetus will need to be delivered with the help of forceps. Because of the need for forceps, the nurse can expect which type of anesthestic will be used with Betty?

- ☐ 1. Saddle block.
- ☐ 2. Paracervical block.
- ☐ 3. Pudendal block.
- ☐ 4. Local.

68. Betty delivers a healthy infant at 38 weeks of gestation. On Betty's first postpartum day, the nurse finds that her fundus is boggy. What is the first action the nurse would take?

- ☐ 1. Lower the head of the bed.
- ☐ 2. Firmly massage the fundus.
- ☐ 3. Give 1 ampule of oxytocin (Pitocin) intramuscularly.
- ☐ 4. Take Betty's vital signs.

Charles Woodward, a 57-year-old salesman, is admitted to the hospital with suspected cancer of the colon.

69. Mr. Woodward provides the nurse with pertinent information during the nursing history. From the data collected, which of the following factors has been implicated in the development of colorectal cancer?

- ☐ 1. Exposure to x-rays.
- ☐ 2. Low-fiber diet.
- ☐ 3. High intake of smoked fish.
- ☐ 4. A long history of alcohol abuse.

70. Mr. Woodward is scheduled for a lower GI tract study. Which would be *inappropriate* to include in his care for this test?

- ☐ 1. Clear tea and Jell-O for breakfast the day before the test.
- ☐ 2. Castor oil or an enema, or both, before the test.
- ☐ 3. Low-cholesterol, low-fat diet the day of the test.
- ☐ 4. Tap-water enemas until clear on the morning of the test.

71. A malignant rectal tumor is diagnosed and Mr. Woodward is scheduled for surgery. Which of the following would *not* be included in Mr. Woodward's preoperative bowel preparation?

☐ 1. Antibiotics.
☐ 2. Gastrointestinal decompression.
☐ 3. Sodium polystyrene sulfonate (Kayexalate) enemas.
☐ 4. Clear liquids for the 2 days before the surgery.

72. Mr. Woodward has an abdominoperineal resection and returns to the unit with a single-barreled sigmoid colostomy. Which of the following would the nurse expect following this surgical procedure?
☐ 1. Continuous liquid stool until the client is discharged from the hospital.
☐ 2. Regulation of the colostomy.
☐ 3. Sanguinous drainage from the stoma mixed with feces.
☐ 4. Reconnection of the bowel after a short time.

73. The nurse inspects the colostomy stoma as part of a postoperative assessment and finds the tissue is moist with a slight bluish color. This would best be interpreted as which of the following?
☐ 1. Early sign of necrosis.
☐ 2. Normal tissue (postoperative trauma).
☐ 3. Infection.
☐ 4. Internal hemorrhage.

74. During the first postoperative day, nursing assessments of Mr. Woodward include which of the following?
☐ 1. Taking rectal temperatures.
☐ 2. Noting passage of flatus.
☐ 3. Noting tolerance of oral intake.
☐ 4. Doing urine sugar and acetone test.

75. As Mr. Woodward recuperates, he begins instruction on colostomy irrigation. Which of the following would be included in the teaching?
☐ 1. Irrigate well when diarrhea is present.
☐ 2. Irrigate with 1500 ml to 2000 ml water.
☐ 3. Lubricate the catheter tip with antibiotic ointment.
☐ 4. Insert the catheter tip gently 3 to 4 inches into the stoma.

76. Which of the following would be included in the teaching plan regarding common problems for the ostomate?
☐ 1. If diarrhea occurs, eat small, high-calorie meals until normal motility returns.
☐ 2. Prevent hard stools by taking a laxative such as milk of magnesia up to 3 times per week.
☐ 3. Colostomy odor can be reduced by taking charcoal and bismuth subcarbonate orally.
☐ 4. Abdominal cramping can be relieved by taking small sips of ginger ale.

77. The effectiveness of diet teaching is evaluated as Mr. Woodward prepares for discharge. Mr. Woodward demonstrates his understanding of foods *least* likely to cause intestinal gas. Which list does he select?

☐ 1. Canned peaches, red beets, and squash.
☐ 2. Milk, lima beans, and cheese.
☐ 3. Steak with onions, peas, and corn.
☐ 4. Yogurt, cola, and cheese.

Five-year-old Tommy is scheduled for surgery to correct hypospadias.

78. In hypospadias, where is the urethral opening usually located?
☐ 1. Anywhere along the ventral surface of the penis.
☐ 2. On the dorsal surface of the penis.
☐ 3. In the scrotal sac.
☐ 4. In the abdominal cavity.

79. Which of the following signs and symptoms usually alerts the nurse to suspect hypospadias?
☐ 1. Nausea and vomiting.
☐ 2. Urinary retention.
☐ 3. Abnormal urinary stream direction.
☐ 4. Ambiguous genitalia.

80. When obtaining a health history for the child with hypospadias, it is most important to include which of the following?
☐ 1. Family history.
☐ 2. History of childhood illnesses.
☐ 3. History of immunizations.
☐ 4. History of toilet-training techniques.

81. What is *not* necessary to include in the preoperative teaching?
☐ 1. Explanation to parents about the surgical procedure.
☐ 2. Explanation of the expected cosmetic results.
☐ 3. Explanation to the child about the procedure.
☐ 4. Explanation about a nephrostomy tube.

82. Tommy's fears would most likely *not* include fear of which of the following?
☐ 1. Mutilation.
☐ 2. Punishment for misdeeds.
☐ 3. Strange hospital environment.
☐ 4. Loss of sexuality.

83. Which postoperative nursing measure would be *incorrect*?
☐ 1. Change the surgical site dressing frequently.
☐ 2. Provide for quiet play.
☐ 3. Record intake and output.
☐ 4. Encourage fluids.

84. Postoperatively, Tommy develops a temperature of 101.5° F (38.6° C). What would be the priority nursing action?
☐ 1. Notify the physician.
☐ 2. Call Tommy's parents.
☐ 3. Provide a cool environment.
☐ 4. Start oral penicillin.

85. Following surgical correction of hypospadias, which

of the following information is *least* pertinent 3 months postoperatively?

☐ 1. The child is able to void in a standing position.
☐ 2. Genitalia appear normal or near-normal.
☐ 3. The child is comfortable with his body.
☐ 4. Urinary tract infections are decreased.

Rose Potts, age 24, has just delivered an 8-pound 4-ounce boy.

86. When determining Baby Boy Potts' Apgar score, the nurse assesses five aspects of the newborn, including which of the following?

☐ 1. Sole creasing.
☐ 2. Amount of vernix.
☐ 3. Degree of head lag.
☐ 4. Color.

87. Mrs. Potts is transferred to the recovery room, and the nurse brings the baby in order to initiate breastfeeding. How can the nurse best assist Mrs. Potts?

☐ 1. Stay with her through the first feeding as needed.
☐ 2. Leave her and the baby alone.
☐ 3. Ask her if she has any questions.
☐ 4. Give her a pamphlet on breastfeeding.

88. Mrs. Potts wants to know what benefits her baby derives from breastfeeding before the onset of milk production. What would be the nurse's best response?

☐ 1. "This is good practice time for the two of you."
☐ 2. "There are no particular benefits."
☐ 3. "The baby ingests colostrum, which contains antibodies, for the first 2 to 4 days."
☐ 4. "Early breastfeeding allows us to assess the infant's neurological status."

89. What would be the best short-term goal of a teaching plan for Mrs. Potts?

☐ 1. Client will demonstrate confidence and relaxation during breastfeeding.
☐ 2. Infant will achieve a regular schedule (every 4 hours) for breastfeeding.
☐ 3. Client will supplement breastfeeding with formula.
☐ 4. Infant will nurse as long as he wishes for the first week.

90. Because of the trauma and edema resulting from vaginal delivery, Mrs. Potts is at risk to develop postpartum cystitis. All of the following nursing actions may aid in the prevention of postpartum cystitis. Which would be the *least* likely to do so?

☐ 1. Encourage voiding.
☐ 2. Ensure the first voiding after delivery is adequate.
☐ 3. Give perineal care following each urination.
☐ 4. Provide a nutritional diet.

91. To determine whether Mrs. Potts is completely emp-

tying her bladder, the nurse would do which of the following?

☐ 1. Judge fundal height, and percuss the bladder.
☐ 2. Catheterize her after each voiding.
☐ 3. Ask the mother whether she feels back pressure.
☐ 4. Ask the mother to record each voiding.

Gabriel Pacetti, a 25-year-old construction worker, is injured when his foot and ankle are crushed by a heavy, jagged tool. The foot becomes cold and dark, and the pedal pulses are absent. He is scheduled for a below-the-knee amputation.

92. What instruction would the nurse give Mr. Pacetti if he is to be taught quadriceps-setting exercises preoperatively?

☐ 1. Alternately pinch the buttocks together and then relax them.
☐ 2. Lift the buttocks off the bed while lying flat.
☐ 3. Move the buttocks and both legs in order to place the feet in plantar flexion.
☐ 4. Move the patellas proximally, and press the popliteal spaces against the bed.

93. Which of the following would best be included in the plan of care for Mr. Pacetti during the first 24 hours postoperatively?

☐ 1. Apply a heating pad to the stump to relieve discomfort.
☐ 2. Have a tourniquet in view at the bedside.
☐ 3. Anticipate the need for large doses of narcotic analgesics.
☐ 4. Encourage him to look at the stump.

94. Following surgery, which is the best instruction to give Mr. Pacetti?

☐ 1. Keep the stump elevated on a pillow until the wound is healed.
☐ 2. Keep a pillow between the thighs when in a supine position.
☐ 3. Lie in a prone position for 30 minutes several times a day.
☐ 4. Apply lotion to the stump several times a day after the incision has healed.

95. Mr. Pacetti will be taught to use crutches until he can manage with a prosthesis independently. Which of the following crutch-walking instructions would be *incorrect*?

☐ 1. Extend the arms while holding weights to strengthen the triceps.
☐ 2. The crutches should be 16 inches less than the client's total height.
☐ 3. The axillary bars on the crutches should support the client's weight.
☐ 4. Both crutches and the affected leg are moved forward first, followed by the normal leg.

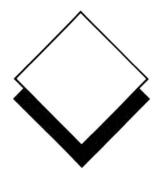

Test 1, Book IV

ANSWERS WITH RATIONALES

KEY TO ABBREVIATIONS
Section of the Review Book

P = Psychosocial and Mental Health Problems
  T = Therapeutic Use of Self
  L = Loss and Death and Dying
  A = Anxious Behavior
  C = Confused Behavior
  E = Elated-Depressive Behavior
  SM = Socially Maladaptive Behavior
  SS = Suspicious Behavior
  W = Withdrawn Behavior
  SU = Substance Use Disorders
A = Adult
  H = Healthy Adult
  S = Surgery
  O = Oxygenation
  NM = Nutrition and Metabolism
  E = Elimination
  SP = Sensation and Perception
  M = Mobility
  CA = Cellular Aberration
CBF = Childbearing Family
  W = Women's Health Care
  A = Antepartal Care
  I = Intrapartal Care
  P = Postpartal Care
  N = Newborn Care
C = Child
  H = Healthy Child
  I = Ill and Hospitalized Child
  SPP = Sensation, Perception, and Protection
  O = Oxygenation
  NM = Nutrition and Metabolism
  E = Elimination
  M = Mobility
  CA = Cellular Aberration

Nursing Process Category

AS = Assessment
AN = Analysis
PL = Plan
IM = Implementation
EV = Evaluation

Client Need Category

E = Safe, Effective Care Environment
PS = Physiological Integrity
PC = Psychosocial Integrity
H = Health Promotion and Maintenance

1. no. 2. Anger and resentment often underlie guilt. The depressed client may not be ready to attend group therapy upon admission. When the psychiatrist orders group therapy, the client may or may not deal with her anger and resentment in that setting. Options no. 3 and no. 4 do not facilitate expression of guilty feelings. P/E, IM, PC

2. no. 3. In a psychotic depression, the client loses contact with reality. This may be manifested by a fixed false belief (delusion), such as paranoid ideation that evil forces will destroy the client. Reactive depression is related to grief reactions and usually does not include distortions of thought severe enough to be considered delusions. Delusions are also not characteristic of neurotic and transitory depression. P/E, AN, PC

3. no. 4. Options no. 1 to no. 3 may apply to a number of other health care problems; no. 4 is specific to depression. P/E, AS, PC

4. no. 1. The negative view of the self and the future are indicated by option no. 1. These cognitive changes best indicate depression. Option no. 2 indicates that she at times feels bad; however, she also demonstrates awareness of her mood and her style of coping. This is not an indication of suffering from

depression. Options no. 3 and no. 4 indicate a need for further assessment but do not necessarily indicate depression. P/E, AS, PC

5. no. 4. Options no. 1 through no. 3 are commonly associated with depression. Ataxia, an inability to coordinate voluntary muscular movements, has not been reported in depression. P/E, AS, PC

6. no. 3. The term retarded depression refers to the client who presents with general physical and cognitive slowness, head hanging, looking haggard, and sitting idly. Such clients are usually indecisive and uncooperative, but not argumentative. P/E, AS, PC

7. no. 1. Although depression is the most frequently complained of emotional illness, schizophrenia accounts for the largest number of psychiatric hospitalizations. Phobic reactions do not normally require hospitalization. Autism is not a common condition and occurs usually in childhood. Although depression is a common condition, it frequently does not require hospitalization. P/E, AN, PC

8. no. 3. Identification means that a person takes on certain qualities associated with others. Idealization is the conscious or unconscious overestimation of another's attributes. Introjection refers to the incorporation of the traits of others, internalizing feelings toward others. Substitution refers to unconscious attempts to make up for a deficiency in one area by concentrating efforts in another area that is more attainable. P/E, AS, PS

9. no. 3. Hypotension, rather than hypertension, may occur as a side effect. Options no. 1, no. 2, and no. 4 are commonly reported side effects of amitriptyline (Elavil) and therefore require nurses' consideration. P/E, AS, PS

10. no. 4. Clients who take tricyclic antidepressants such as amitriptyline should not be given MAO inhibitors either simultaneously or immediately following treatment. Isocarboxazid should be withheld until orders are clarified. P/E, AN, PS

11. no. 4. Isocarboxazid (Marplan), as well as phenelzine (Nardil) and tranylcypromine (Parnate) are MAO inhibitors. When these drugs are combined with tyramine-containing foods (e.g., aged cheese and alcoholic beverages), the reaction cited in the question can occur. Side effects of tricyclic antidepressants (amitriptyline and imipramine) are usually associated with hypotension, not hypertension. Side effects of lithium are usually not associated with cardiovascular changes unless toxic levels are reached; then the changes are hypotensive. P/E, IM, PC

12. no. 2. Unless the client is first assessed for self-harm or suicide potential, the staff will not observe the necessary degree of vigilance needed in the client's environment. Although essential, physical needs are not the most critical concern with a depressive client. Though the client may be encouraged to attend group therapy as part of the treatment plan, the client's safety takes precedence. Response to medication takes time and is not an initial concern. P/E, AS, PC

13. no. 3. The nurse must consider the seriousness and the rapidity with which the client may die unless intervention occurs following a suicide attempt. The lethality of the method may give indications about the seriousness of the client's attempt. Following options no. 2 and no. 4, death can occur quickly and is highly likely. Following ingestion of sufficient quantities of barbiturates or sedatives, the client can also die because of central nervous system depression. Scratching one's wrists has a lower lethality than options no. 1, no. 2, and no. 4 and also has a lower lethality than cutting the veins of the wrist. P/E, AN, PC

14. no. 4. Specialists in suicidology have developed profiles of high-risk groups. Generally, persons cited in options no. 1 through no. 3 have a higher risk of suicide than married men. Alcoholics have a high risk associated with lack of impulse control. Women *attempt* suicide more frequently than do men (a 3 to 1 ratio), but men *commit* suicide more often than women by a 3 to 1 ratio. Suicide rates vary according to marital status, with married persons having the lowest rates, followed by the never married. Widowed or divorced persons have the highest rate. P/E, AS, PS

15. no. 1. The immunization schedule recommended by the American Academy of Pediatrics suggests giving the first immunization at 2 months of age. C/NM, AS, PS

16. no. 3. Stools usually become small and infrequent, depending on the amount of food passing through the gastrointestinal tract. Lethargy may be present if the fluid and electrolyte imbalances are significant. C/NM, AS, PS

17. no. 2. An infant with pyloric stenosis often suffers from fluid and electrolyte imbalances, primarily from vomiting. These need to be corrected before surgery; a child in proper acid-base and fluid balance is a much better surgical risk. C/NM, PL, PS

18. no. 2. The obstruction is at the pyloric sphincter. The child becomes dehydrated from vomiting; thus, metabolic alkalosis and hypokalemia are common findings. C/NM, AN, PS

19. no. 1. Potassium is excreted through the kidneys. If the client is not voiding and potassium is infusing, levels rapidly become toxic. C/NM, AS, PS

20. no. 4. Since restraints can severely restrict circulation and injure tissue, they must be checked frequently and regularly. The padding mentioned in

option no. 1 is often helpful. Restraints should never be tied to the side rails. C/NM, IM, E

21. no. 3. Feedings are usually started shortly after surgery. Parents may have become negatively conditioned to preoperative vomiting, so they need to be included in positive postoperative feeding experiences. Hypoglycemia may occur as a result of preoperative depletion of hepatic glycogen. C/NM, PL, PS

22. no. 3. This position facilitates emptying of the stomach by taking advantage of the stomach's normal curvature. C/NM, PL, PS

23. no. 4. The usual response following surgery for pyloric stenosis includes some vomiting up to about 48 hours after surgery. C/NM, AS, PL

24. no. 3. This indicates that parental learning has taken place. C/NM, EV, H

25. no. 2. Perfect matches of all four HLAs are found in monozygotic twins and 25% of natural siblings (born of the same pair of parents). The degree of compatibility of remaining siblings varies. A/E, IM, PS

26. no. 1. Azathioprine (Imuran) is a potent drug that produces immunosuppression by inhibiting purine synthesis in cells. It is used in renal transplants to prevent organ rejection. The client should avoid crowds and infectious individuals since infection is a serious consequence in a client who is immunocompromised. The client is instructed to report chills, fever, sore throat, and fatigue immediately. Azathioprine does not stimulate kidney output or increase the number of circulating antibodies. In fact, leukopenia occurs during therapy. Azathioprine does not significantly alter blood pressure, so frequent monitoring is not required. A/E, IM, PS

27. no. 4. Rejection is the body's reaction to foreign tissue. Symptoms of kidney rejection include a swollen and tender kidney, weight gain, fever, elevated blood pressure, decreased urine output, elevated serum creatinine levels, anorexia, and drowsiness. The white blood cell count does not rise. A/E, AS, PS

28. no. 1. Opening up and irrigating a closed sterile urinary drainage system increases the risk of infection in the immunosuppressed client. Reverse isolation will be maintained to protect the client from infection. Frequent turning and repositioning is required to prevent pneumonia. The stools need to be routinely checked for blood because of the high risk of gastrointestinal bleeding with immunosuppressant drug therapy. A/E, PL, E

29. no. 3. A witnessed, cosigned donor card is appropriate for the client who is a minor. A/E, IM, H

30. no. 2. Prednisone is prescribed for its immunosuppressive effects. Withdrawal of the drug makes it more likely that the body will reject the transplanted tissue. Increased risk of infection and psychosis are

two side effects of prednisone. Anemia will not occur if prednisone is stopped. A/E, AN, PS

31. no. 1. Ovulation is believed to occur just before, at, or just after the temperature drop. Progesterone has a thermogenic effect, causing a rise in temperature. CBF/A, AS, H

32. no. 1. Ovulation occurs 24 to 30 hours after the appearance of luteinizing hormone. CBF/A, AS, PS

33. no. 2. Increased amounts of gonadotropins (follicle-stimulating hormone and luteinizing hormone) stimulate the maturation of the ovarian follicle, followed by ovulation and, later, development of the functioning corpus luteum. CBF/A, AN, PS

34. no. 1. To correctly evaluate chest pain, it is essential to obtain an accurate description. Also, this question can elicit the client's knowledge about heart attacks. This will provide a basis for the discharge teaching plan. Option no. 4 is closed-ended, only giving a partial description and closing off other descriptions of the pain. Option no. 2 is important, but it is not the most relevant choice. Option no. 3 assumes that the client smokes cigarettes. A/O, IM, PS

35. no. 1. An electrocardiogram reflects the electrochemical activity of the heart (i.e., the transmission of the cardiac impulse through the heart muscle). Information about heart perfusion, contraction, and integrity is inferred from this information but not measured directly. A/O, AN, PS

36. no. 4. When an organ such as the heart is damaged, it releases specific enzymes into the bloodstream. Options no. 1, no. 2, and no. 3 are incorrect. A culture and sensitivity is used to detect causative organisms. Arterial blood gas studies determine how well the blood is oxygenated. A/O, AN, PS

37. no. 2. Options no. 1, no. 3, and no. 4 do not relate to chest pain in any way. A/O, AN, PS

38. no. 3. The coronary arteries fill, and the aortic and pulmonary valves close during ventricular diastole. A/O, AN, PS

39. no. 3. 1/150 grain = 0.4 mg. A/O, AN, PS

40. no. 3. Sublingual nitroglycerin appears in the bloodstream in about 2 minutes and peaks in 4 minutes; the effect begins to disappear in 10 minutes. The sublingual form should be taken at the onset of chest pain and every 5 minutes until the pain is relieved for a maximum of three doses. The client should notify the physician if the pain is not relieved after three doses. A/O, IM, PS

41. no. 1. Because of its dilating effect, nitroglycerin may cause headache, hypotension, and dizziness. Other side effects of nitroglycerin include flushing, increased heart rate, and nausea. Shock, convulsions, hypertension, and loss of consciousness are not side effects of nitroglycerin. A/O, AS, PS

42. no. 3. Fresh nitroglycerin tablets cause a burning, tingling sensation. Sublingual nitroglycerin should

be taken at the onset of chest pain. The client should not wait until the pain is severe. Sublingual nitroglycerin is not taken with meals. Headache and flushing are normal side effects so the physician does not need to be notified. A/O, IM, H

43. no. 2. Pain patterns of angina vary from individual to individual but usually are the same in one individual. A change may indicate new ischemic areas. Anginal pain frequently occurs with stress or after eating a heavy meal. The client needs to purchase a fresh supply of nitroglycerin if the current medication does not cause a tingling sensation under the tongue. A/O, IM, H

44. no. 2. Propranolol (Inderal) is a beta-adrenergic-blocking agent. As such, it blocks the bronchodilator effect of sympathetic (adrenergic) stimulation and is contraindicated for all chronic obstructive lung conditions. It is also contraindicated in cardiac failure, cardiac shock, and second- or third-degree A-V heart block. It is not contraindicated for MI, CVA, or thrombophlebitis. A/O, AN, PS

45. no. 2. There is no indication that propranolol causes GI bleeding, so there is no need to check stools for occult blood during propranolol therapy. Propranolol does cause bradycardia and hypotension, so the blood pressure should be closely monitored, and the client should be instructed to change positions slowly. Propranolol can cause bronchospasms, so the client should be assessed for dyspnea and respiratory difficulties. A/O, IM, PS

46. no. 2. Cheese is high in fat and sodium content, which makes it unsuitable for a cardiac client. Eating smaller meals is important because of the increased incidence of angina after eating a heavy meal. In addition, exercise should be avoided after eating because it increases demand on the heart. Fat consumption should be reduced. Fish and chicken are appropriate low-fat, high-protein foods. Caffeine should be eliminated because it may increase the heart rate. A/O, PL, H

47. no. 2. A cardiac catheterization is done to confirm heart disease, determine the extent of heart disease, obtain pressures, measure oxygen in the blood, and inject contrast medium for angiography. A cardiac catheterization does not dilate coronary blood vessels, force oxygen to the myocardium, or bypass the blocked coronary artery. A/O, AN, PS

48. no. 2. The client is responsible for his own health care and has a right to choose his own habits. The nurse has a right to insist on a model of health behavior in class. A/O, PL, H

49. no. 3. This is indicative of decreased total blood volume, since hematocrit is a measure of packed red blood cells per deciliter of blood volume. C/SPP, AS, H

50. no. 3. These symptoms are indicative of fluid overload resulting in congestive heart failure. C/SPP, AS, PS

51. no. 2. Restriction of visitors is unnecessary if they are healthy and are instructed in proper isolation technique. C/SPP, PL, E

52. no. 1. A urinary output of 10 ml/hr is abnormally low. However, the first measure is always to see if the catheter is patent. If it is, the next step would be to notify the physician. C/SPP, IM, PS

53. no. 4. Proteins and carbohydrates are needed for wound healing and tissue replacement. The other options do not achieve these goals primarily. C/SPP, PL, PS

54. no. 3. Fantasy, play therapy that allows expression of emotions, is best for preschoolers. C/I, IM, E

55. no. 4. In areas outside their delusional system, these clients are in good contact with reality with no impairment of intellectual functioning. Suspicious behavior, superiority, and hostility are characteristics of paranoia and cause others to withdraw from such a client. P/S, AS, PC

56. no. 1. A fixed delusional system is characterized by a belief system that is rigid and inaccessible to reason and modification, although the basic premise on which the system is based is illogical. An hallucination is an imagined sensory perception that occurs without an external stimulus. Acting-out and manipulative behaviors occur in clients with manic-depressive disorder, borderline personality disorder, and substance abuse disorders. P/S, AN, PC

57. no. 3. Trying to reason with the client, correct his beliefs, or delve into the content will cause the client to work harder at defending the delusion, thereby reinforcing it and making it more entrenched. The nurse should acknowledge to Mr. Benson that it must be upsetting to feel as he does. This will promote trust by providing empathy. Thus the nurse begins to build the relationship with the client. If the nurse focuses on the content and details of the delusion or acknowledges the delusion as reality, she gives it credibility, which reinforces it. P/S, IM, PC

58. no. 3. Presenting reality is the best response. Tell the client who you are concisely and specifically. Communication should avoid reinforcing the client's delusion. In option no. 1, the nurse does not understand how the client feels and the response could be interpreted as a reinforcement of his delusional system. Ignoring his comment can cause his anxiety to rise, or he may interpret the nurse's silence as agreement. Rational explanations will only make the client adhere more firmly to the delusion. P/S, IM, PC

59. no. 4. The nurse cannot talk the client out of his suspicions. Serving foods in sealed containers may diminish the client's anxiety. It is also possible that the action may not, but it allows him some control

about whether to eat. Option no. 2 may lead the client to conclude that the nurse believes there may be some reality to his delusion *or* is refuting his belief. This is a "no-win" option. After the nurse tastes it, he can reply that the poison will be slow to kill. He may believe that both he and the nurse are going to die from poisoned food. P/S, IM, PC

60. no. 2. Photosensitivity, not photophobia, is a side effect of chlorpromazine. Abrupt onset of sore throat, fever, malaise, and sores in the mouth may mean that agranulocytosis has occurred. A complete blood count should be done immediately to see if leukopenia is present. Postural hypotension usually occurs early in the course of treatment and disappears 1 or 2 weeks after the dose is stabilized. Pruritic maculopapular rash (dermatitis) is a common allergic response. Contact dermatitis can also occur from contact with the liquid concentrate or tablets. P/S, AS, PS

61. no. 2. Swelling in the upper part of the body is more significant than dependent edema of the lower extremities. The blood pressure rise in option no. 1 is not significant enough to indicate a problem. Protein in the urine, not glucose, would be a significant finding. CBF/A, AS, PS

62. no. 4. The primary problem is a generalized vasospasm leading to uterine insufficiency. There is a decrease in plasma proteins as a result of protein loss through damaged kidneys into the urine, and there is a decrease in glomerular filtration as a result of vasoconstriction. Sodium and water retention is augmented by an increase in aldosterone. Cardiac output falls as the result of hypovolemia. CBF/A, AN, PS

63. no. 4. There is no cure for PIH except delivery of the child. The aim of all treatment is to prevent progression of the disease to eclampsia. CBF/A, PL, E

64. no. 3. A decreased respiratory rate indicates central nervous system depression from the magnesium sulfate. The pulse rate and urinary output listed are within normal limits. The drug produces hypoactive reflexes. CBF/A, AS, PS

65. no. 1. Magnesium sulfate is used to depress the central nervous system. It also reduces blood pressure and produces diuresis, but this is not its main action. CBF/A, AN, PS

66. no. 3. When the client seems to be losing control, the first action should be to help the client cope with the contractions through breathing and relaxation. Analgesia should not be used in early labor. CBF/I, IM, PC

67. no. 1. A saddle block is an intradural anesthetic that affects the sensory and motor pathways. The client therefore does not have the involuntary urge to push during the second stage of labor. This is desirable if forceps are indicated. That ability is not lost with the other types of anesthetic listed. CBF/I, AN, PS

68. no. 2. Firmly massaging the fundus is always the first action to take with a boggy uterus. If that is ineffective, oxytocin may need to be ordered. These measures will contract the uterus, preventing hemorrhage. CBF/P, IM, PS

69. no. 2. A low-fiber diet has been associated with an increased risk of colorectal cancer, possibly by promoting a slow stool transit time and fecal stasis, which gives potential carcinogens more contact time with the intestinal lining. X-ray exposure is associated with leukemia. A high intake of smoked foods is associated with gastric cancer. Alcohol abuse has been linked to laryngeal cancer. A/E, AS, H

70. no. 3. The lower GI series (barium enema) requires a very specific dietary and bowel-cleansing protocol before the exam. The day before the exam the client is restricted to clear liquids for lunch and supper. The client is then NPO after midnight. The bowel is cleansed with magnesium citrate and bisacodyl (Dulcolax) the day before the exam and suppositories or enemas the day of the exam. The rationale is that the bowel must be free of fecal debris for the barium to outline the intestinal surfaces. Any solid food the day of the exam is contraindicated. Options no. 1, no. 2, and no. 4 are appropriate preprocedural interventions. A/E, IM, PS

71. no. 3. Sodium polystyrene sulfonate (Kayexalate) enemas reduce serum potassium levels. Cleansing enemas reduce bacteria, old blood, and fecal matter in the bowel; antibiotics reduce gastrointestinal flora. The client is restricted to clear liquids for 2 or 3 days before the surgery to control fecal accumulation. Gastrointestinal decompression may be required during the preoperative period if the client has a total or partial bowel obstruction from the tumor. A/E, PL, PS

72. no. 2. A single-barreled colostomy is always permanent. When the sigmoid colon has been preserved, regulation of bowel evacuation is possible, because stools are more formed here. Some such ostomates will be able to go without a colostomy bag. Others may find varying need for one, depending on their diet and success with irrigation. Sanguinous drainage from the stoma is abnormal and should be reported to the physician. A/E, AN, PS

73. no. 1. The bluish color is a sign of decreased vascularity of the tissue. The stoma should appear reddish-pink (immediate postoperative phase) and moist. A/E, AN, PS

74. no. 2. The passage of flatus signals the return of gastrointestinal motility. (Flatus may also appear as air in the colostomy bag.) Rectal temperatures are contraindicated; the rectum was removed and the anal area was sutured or packed with a dressing following an abdominoperineal resection. Oral intake is not usually begun for several days. Sugar and acetone tests are rarely done. If the client is a diabetic or is receiving hyperalimentation, serum glucose levels, such as Accuchecks, are done. A/E, PL, PS

75. no. 4. The irrigation catheter may be inserted up to 4 inches. Use 1000 ml of water or less to irrigate; more may produce abdominal cramping. To prevent further electrolyte imbalance do not irrigate if diarrhea is present. The catheter tip should be lubricated, but antibiotic preparations are not necessary. A/E, IM, E

76. no. 3. Ostomates sometimes find odor is reduced by taking charcoal or bismuth subcarbonate, with the physician's approval. Clear liquids such as tea and water are advised during diarrhea, and the physician should be notifed in order to monitor electrolyte imbalances. Stool softeners such as docusate sodium (Colace) can help prevent hard stools, but laxatives are not advised. Carbonated beverages can exacerbate cramping. A/E, IM, H

77. no. 1. These are the only foods listed that are not known gas producers. Legumes, onions, peas, cabbage, carbonated beverages, nuts, and chewing gum often cause gas. Milk can cause gas in clients with a lactose intolerance. Foods that caused gas before the surgery will continue to cause a problem. A/E, EV, H

78. no. 1. Hypospadias is located anywhere along the ventral surface of the penile shaft. In mild cases, the opening is just off center of the glans; in the most severe cases, it is on the perineum. C/E, AS, PS

79. no. 3. Nausea and vomiting are unrelated to hypospadias. Urinary retention is due to obstruction of flow and is not the case with hypospadias. Ambiguous genitalia may be seen in conjunction with hypospadias in severe cases, but it is not the norm. The abnormal stream direction is often the first indication. C/E, AS, PS

80. no. 1. Family history is important because certain genitourinary anomalies are familial. Childhood illness, immunizations, and toilet-training do not have significance for embryonic development (and detection) of these anomalies. C/E, AS, PS

81. no. 4. Diversion of urinary flow is usually accomplished with a urethral-bladder catheter. A nephrostomy tube is uncommon because the kidneys are not usually involved. Explanations to the child and parents are important along with an explanation of the expected outcome so that there are no surprises. C/E, PL, PS

82. no. 4. The 5-year-old has not developmentally defined completely his sexuality although fear of mutilation is common to this age group. Also, fear of

punishment for misdeeds is common in the preschool child. C/E, AN, PC

83. no. 1. Dressings are usually not changed for several days to allow the plastic surgery repair to heal. Too much activity can damage the surgical site. Fluids are needed to encourage urinary output. C/E, PL, PS

84. no. 1. Notifying the physician is most appropriate. Medications are ordered by the physician and then given by the physician or nurse. Option no. 3 may help to decrease fluid loss but should be a secondary action. Parents can be called after the physician is notified. C/E, EV, PS

85. no. 4. Urinary tract infections are not a primary concern. The other data indicate the male child can function within the physical and psychosocial habits of the male sex. C/E, EV, PS

86. no. 4. Color, along with heart rate, reflex irritability, muscle tone, and respirations, is evaluated as part of the Apgar score. C/N, AS, PS

87. no. 1. An experienced nurse should be available to mothers who are beginning breastfeeding to provide explanation and reinforcement. Written material may be helpful but is no substitute for one-on-one teaching. CBF/P, IM, E

88. no. 3. Colostrum is secreted for 2 to 3 days after birth and is rich in antibodies. Early breastfeeding not only allows for practice but stimulates the production of breast milk. Neurological status is best assessed through observation of Moro's reflex. CBF/P, IM, PS

89. no. 1. The let-down reflex can be influenced profoundly by the mother's emotions. An immediate short-term goal would be that the client is able to confidently initiate the process of breastfeeding. Breastfeeding is generally done on demand. Supplements are discouraged until breastfeeding is successfully established. The time the infant breastfeeds is controlled initially to prevent nipple breakdown. CBF/P, PL, E

90. no. 4. The postpartum client is vulnerable to the development of cystitis. The diet would be least likely to prevent this condition. Keeping the bladder empty will prevent urinary stasis, a common cause of cystitis. Perineal care will reduce microorganisms that may ascend into the urinary tract. CBF/P, IM, PS

91. no. 1. When the bladder is not emptied, it may push the uterus upward and to the side of the abdomen. On percussion, a full bladder emits a dull sound. CBF/P, IM, PS

92. no. 4. This motion is the only one listed that uses the quadriceps muscles to perform. Thus it increases their strength. A/M, IM, PS

93. no. 2. Hemorrhage has very serious consequences. The first postoperative day is too early for the client

to accept his loss (option no. 4), and temperature sense in the stump is too impaired to risk a hot pad. The pain after amputation is almost always quite mild. A/M, IM, PS

94. no. 3. This position prevents hip contracture. Lotion is contraindicated for the stump; it keeps the skin soft, with increased risk of skin breakdown. Elevating the stump after the first 24 hours results in flexion contractures, and a pillow between the thighs promotes abduction fixation. Both of these result in difficulty walking with the prosthesis. A/M, IM, PS

95. no. 3. The weight of the client should be carried on the wrists and palms, not on the axilla because this can damage the radial nerve and cause paralysis of the elbow and wrist extensor muscles. The axillary bar should be 1-2 inches below the axilla. Crutches should be 16 inches shorter than the client for best fit. The elbow should be fully extended when a step is taken. In the three-point gait (the most common crutch-walking gait) both crutches are moved forward first, then the involved leg, then the unaffected leg. A/M, IM, PS

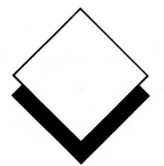

Test 2, Book I

QUESTIONS

Twenty-six-month-old Crystal visits the well-child clinic for a checkup.

1. When assessing Crystal's development, the nurse would expect her to exhibit which one of the following abilities?
   - [ ] 1. Dressing herself unassisted.
   - [ ] 2. Pointing to parts of her body when asked.
   - [ ] 3. Drawing a person with 3 to 6 parts.
   - [ ] 4. Speaking in four- to five-word sentences.

2. During the otoscopic examination, Crystal cries loudly and tries to pull away. What is the best approach?
   - [ ] 1. Explain to Crystal why you must look into her ears.
   - [ ] 2. Postpone the ear exam until Crystal's next visit when she will be older.
   - [ ] 3. Say to her, "I thought you were a big girl, Crystal."
   - [ ] 4. Get someone to restrain Crystal, and proceed with the exam.

3. Crystal's mother mentions that she and her husband have been trying to toilet train Crystal because she seems interested. Which of the following would *not* facilitate this process?
   - [ ] 1. Give Crystal a toy to play with while she sits on the potty.
   - [ ] 2. Dress her in clothing with Velcro fasteners.
   - [ ] 3. Provide her with her own potty chair.
   - [ ] 4. Respond matter-of-factly when Crystal has an "accident."

4. Crystal's mother tells you, "Crystal just doesn't seem to eat enough; I don't know where she gets all her energy." After assessing the child's condition and finding no evidence of nutritional deficiency, the nurse's best response is which of the following?
   - [ ] 1. "You may want to increase her milk intake to be sure she gets enough calories."
   - [ ] 2. "Why don't you double her daily vitamin and mineral dose for your peace of mind?"
   - [ ] 3. "Try giving her small portions of a variety of foods, and allow her to decide which of those foods she will eat."
   - [ ] 4. "It's best at this age to insist that she take at least two bites of the foods you offer her to be sure she is getting enough to eat."

Andrew Goll, a 56-year-old rancher, is admitted for an episode of acute pancreatitis. This is Mr. Goll's eighth admission for this disorder over the past 3 years.

5. Pancreatitis can best be described as which of the following?
   - [ ] 1. Infectious disease of the pancreas primarily seen in the black population.
   - [ ] 2. Inherited disease affecting the pancreas that is primarily seen in the black population.
   - [ ] 3. Inflammation of the pancreas resulting in obstruction and edema.
   - [ ] 4. Outpouching of the pancreas.

6. The nurse knows that the pancreas is responsible for secreting which of the following?
   - [ ] 1. Sucrase, dipeptidase, lipase, and amylase.
   - [ ] 2. Amylase, lactase, trypsin, and chymotrypsin.
   - [ ] 3. Amylase, lipase, pepsin, and maltase.
   - [ ] 4. Amylase, lipase, trypsin, and chymotrypsin.

7. Which of the following would be an unlikely finding with chronic pancreatitis?
   - [ ] 1. Hypoglycemia.
   - [ ] 2. Extreme epigastric pain.
   - [ ] 3. Elevated serum amylase and lipase.
   - [ ] 4. Abdominal distension.

8. Mr. Goll's laboratory values show hypocalcemia as a result of the inadequate metabolism of which of the following?
   - [ ] 1. Fat.
   - [ ] 2. Protein.

☐ 3. Starch.

☐ 4. Glucose.

9. In planning for adequate nutrition for Mr. Goll, which of the following would be considered *inappropriate*?

☐ 1. Administer cholinergic drugs.

☐ 2. Supplement nutrition with IV fluids.

☐ 3. Give clear liquids after inflammation subsides.

☐ 4. Include a bland, low-fat diet in the teaching plan.

10. Mr. Goll is complaining of severe pain. The physician has ordered meperidine (Demerol) and morphine. The nurse chooses meperidine. The best reason for selecting meperidine is that

☐ 1. Meperidine depresses respirations less than morphine.

☐ 2. Meperidine exerts its effects on striated muscles.

☐ 3. Morphine has a tendency to produce spasms of the sphincter of Oddi.

☐ 4. Morphine has less effect on smooth muscle.

Tim Lampert, a 52-year-old alcoholic, has been drinking excessively for 20 years. He drinks 2 pints of whiskey daily. For the last 2 days, he has cut his drinking back to 1 pint per day. Although he plans to stop drinking, he has decided to keep drinking 1 pint a day to avoid withdrawal symptoms.

11. Mr. Lampert comes to the emergency room of his community hospital with an elevated blood pressure, tremors, and "nervousness." He tells the nurse his drinking history and how he cut back, but did not stop, drinking. The nurse needs to be most alert for which of the following?

☐ 1. Increased withdrawal symptoms.

☐ 2. Possible stroke.

☐ 3. Cardiac arrest.

☐ 4. Increased anxiety reactions.

12. While in the hospital, Mr. Lampert is believed to be in the early stages of Korsakoff's syndrome. Which of the following symptoms is most common with this disease?

☐ 1. Chronic gastritis.

☐ 2. Excessive perspiration.

☐ 3. Confabulation.

☐ 4. Fatty liver.

13. Mr. Lampert tells the nurse that the effects of alcohol on his body frighten him. He wants to quit but is afraid he cannot do it. Which of the following nursing actions would be most helpful at this point in the treatment program?

☐ 1. Discuss coping mechanisms he might use under stress other than alcohol.

☐ 2. Discuss ways to decrease the number of his social contacts.

☐ 3. Find ways he can decrease the amount of emotional support he needs from others.

☐ 4. Recommend psychoanalysis as part of discharge planning.

14. Mr. Lampert starts his disulfiram (Antabuse) regimen while in the hospital. The nurse, when teaching him what may occur if he ingests alcohol, will tell him to be aware of which of the following?

☐ 1. Increased blood pressure, pulse, and respirations.

☐ 2. Headache, pallor, and vomiting.

☐ 3. Nausea and vomiting, flushed face, and decreased blood pressure.

☐ 4. Ataxia, muscle contractions, and dilated pupils.

15. Mr. Lampert and his family have agreed to start family therapy. The nurse would tell them to expect that the focus of the therapy would primarily be on which of the following?

☐ 1. Mr. Lampert's drinking problem.

☐ 2. Mrs. Lampert and the ways in which her behavior may cause her husband to drink.

☐ 3. Increasing communication among the family members.

☐ 4. Teaching the family members to be more like each other.

Annie Daugherty is a 28-year-old multigravida admitted to the labor room in active labor. The nurse admitting Mrs. Daugherty determines that her cervix is 90% effaced, and the fetus is in left occiput posterior position with a fetal heart rate of 136. The cervix is 4 cm dilated, and the fetus is at −1 station.

16. Which type of breathing and relaxation techniques would be appropriate for Mrs. Daugherty to use at this time?

☐ 1. Panting.

☐ 2. Candle blowing.

☐ 3. Accelerated.

☐ 4. Slow abdominal.

17. Fetal heart rate is being evaluated by using a fetoscope. When is the most appropriate time to listen to fetal heart sounds?

☐ 1. During uterine contractions.

☐ 2. Sixty seconds after uterine contractions.

☐ 3. During and immediately following uterine contractions.

☐ 4. Immediately following uterine contractions.

18. Mrs. Daugherty complains of severe back pain. Which nursing action would be best?

☐ 1. Apply a warm pad to the sacral area.

☐ 2. Encourage her to bear down.

☐ 3. Keep her flat with a pillow under her head.

☐ 4. Turn her on her side, and apply sacral pressure.

19. Mrs. Daugherty's membranes rupture spontaneously. In addition to assessing the color of the fluid, what is the most important nursing action at that time?

☐ 1. Call the physician.

☐ 2. Take the fetal heart rate.

☐ 3. Time the contractions.

☐ 4. Transfer Mrs. Daugherty to the delivery room.

20. Which of the following most likely indicates that the third stage of labor is coming to an end?
   □ 1. The episiotomy is being performed.
   □ 2. Dilatation and effacement are complete.
   □ 3. The birth of the baby is completed.
   □ 4. There is a gush of blood from the vagina and a lengthening of the cord.

Jennifer Theil, a 60-year-old homemaker, is admitted to the orthopedic unit and is scheduled for a left total hip replacement in 3 days. She states that she has had severe pain in the hip for several years and takes large doses of aspirin. She says she has no other health problems.

21. Which of the following would normally *not* be included as part of her preoperative lab work?
   □ 1. Blood type and crossmatch.
   □ 2. Prothrombin time.
   □ 3. Sedimentation rate.
   □ 4. Bence Jones protein.
22. Which of the following would be *inappropriate* to include in Mrs. Theil's plan of care preoperatively?
   □ 1. Teach her to use the trapeze.
   □ 2. Measure her for antiembolic hose.
   □ 3. Restrict her to bed rest until discharge.
   □ 4. Avoid extreme flexion and adduction of the hip.
23. Mrs. Theil is at risk of an infection developing in the operative site. Which of the following measures will *not* prevent this complication?
   □ 1. Scrub the leg bid before surgery with a bacteriostatic soap.
   □ 2. Caution the client not to shave any part of the body.
   □ 3. Use reverse isolation for 3 days preoperatively.
   □ 4. Restrict in-and-out traffic in the surgical suite during the operation.
24. Which of the following nursing measures would be *inappropriate* for Mrs. Theil postoperatively?
   □ 1. Schedule active range of motion to both ankles.
   □ 2. Remind her to keep her toes pointed outward.
   □ 3. Help her to pivot on the unaffected foot.
   □ 4. Remind her not to cross her legs.
25. Which of the following assessment findings indicates an abnormality in Mrs. Theil's cardiovascular status?
   □ 1. Capillary refill: 10 seconds.
   □ 2. Apical pulse rate: 74/min.
   □ 3. Absence of pitting edema.
   □ 4. Feet warm and pink; nonpalpable posterior tibial pulse.
26. Mrs. Theil has a wound drain connected to suction. During the first 8 hours, there was 100 ml of bright bloody drainage. She is alert, and her vital signs are stable. Which of the following nursing actions would be most appropriate?
   □ 1. Notify the physician.
   □ 2. Apply a pressure dressing to the wound.
   □ 3. Continue to observe and record the amount of drainage.
   □ 4. Anticipate a stat order for a transfusion by ordering a unit of blood.
27. Which of the following is a common sequela of a total hip replacement within the first postoperative week?
   □ 1. Urinary retention.
   □ 2. Contractures.
   □ 3. Weight loss.
   □ 4. Incontinence, especially with coughing.
28. A serious complication of a total hip replacement is displacement of the prosthesis. What is the primary sign of displacement?
   □ 1. Pain on movement and weight bearing.
   □ 2. Hemorrhage.
   □ 3. The affected leg will be 1 to 2 inches longer.
   □ 4. Edema in the area of the incision.
29. Mrs. Theil has an abductor splint in place. What is the best guide to the placement of the splint?
   □ 1. Fasten the splint firmly in place.
   □ 2. Position the splint so that it does not interfere with the use of the bedpan.
   □ 3. Position the strap so that it is not directly over the peroneal nerve.
   □ 4. Position the proximal strap just above the knee.
30. The nurse evaluates the client's readiness for discharge. Mrs. Theil identifies which of the following as being *incorrect* behavior?
   □ 1. Use a rocking chair or reclining chair when sitting for an extended time.
   □ 2. Continue to sleep with a pillow between the knees.
   □ 3. Take antibiotics prophylactically when dental work is being done.
   □ 4. Hyperextend the affected leg while flexing the other one when retrieving objects from the floor.

Gerald Schmidt, a 36-year-old veteran of the Vietnam War, comes to the Veterans Administration Hospital saying he cannot go on "like this" and requests admission. He states he has not slept in days and that his wife has left him. He has been unable to work for 2 weeks. The admitting physician diagnoses posttraumatic stress disorder.

31. During Mr. Schmidt's admission interview, three of the following symptoms are noted. Which one would the nurse *not* likely assess?
   □ 1. Recurrent nightmares reliving various Vietnam experiences.
   □ 2. Feelings of numbness toward previously enjoyed experiences.
   □ 3. Active hallucinations of insects crawling on his legs.
   □ 4. Difficulty concentrating on current activities.
32. Mr. Schmidt is admitted to the crisis unit. He is assigned to a primary nurse who establishes a re-

lationship with him. In helping Mr. Schmidt to establish a therapeutic relationship, the nurse would first do which of the following?
1. Provide support to help him believe that the nurse is understanding and cares about him.
2. Explore the coping behaviors that he used in the past that were not successful, and decide on new coping techniques.
3. Teach him relaxation techniques to help reduce his anxiety.
4. Arrange a meeting between Mr. Schmidt and his wife to establish a support system.

33. The nurse needs to use a variety of creative techniques in assisting Mr. Schmidt to cope with his stress. Which of the following nursing actions would be *least* helpful?
1. Encourage him to describe his experiences in Vietnam.
2. Encourage him to express the relationship between his experiences in Vietnam and his present life.
3. Encourage expression of the anger and rage he feels toward society for sending him to Vietnam.
4. Communicate confidence that the nurse will assist him in finding solutions to his problems.

34. Mr. Schmidt and the nurse develop a plan to be implemented after he is discharged. Which one of the following would be most helpful for Mr. Schmidt to use to reduce stress after discharge?
1. Move back with his wife.
2. Attend a support group of Vietnam veterans.
3. Take diazepam (Valium) as needed.
4. Begin a job-training program.

Four-year-old Steffan is admitted for a tonsillectomy.

35. When preparing Steffan for surgery, it is most important for the nurse to check his chart for which of the following laboratory values?
1. Hematocrit and hemoglobin.
2. Urinalysis.
3. Bleeding and clotting times.
4. White blood cell count.

36. When preparing a child for surgery, it is especially important to check for loose teeth in which age group?
1. Older infant.
2. Toddler-preschool.
3. School-age.
4. Adolescent.

37. Which of the following best describes the nursing rationale for providing Steffan with role playing as part of his preoperative preparation?
1. To ensure compliant behavior.
2. To minimize Steffan's need to express his feelings verbally.

3. As a means of permitting physical expression of feelings that Steffan cannot express verbally.
4. As a teaching strategy and to decrease anxiety.

38. What would be *least* effective in getting Steffan ready for the operating room?
1. Allow Steffan to kiss the nursing staff before leaving the unit.
2. Allow Steffan to take his stuffed tiger with him.
3. Allow Steffan to wear his underwear to surgery.
4. Have a familiar nurse stay with Steffan in the operating room until he is asleep.

39. Twelve hours following Steffan's surgery, the nurse would be most concerned about observing which one of the following signs or symptoms?
1. Fever of 100° F (37.8° C).
2. Respirations 24/min and shallow.
3. Frequent swallowing.
4. Complaint of a sore throat.

40. The nurse would implement which of the following nursing measures to promote Steffan's comfort postoperatively?
1. Apply an ice collar.
2. Administer 5 grains of aspirin orally.
3. Have Steffan gargle with normal saline.
4. Encourage Steffan to drink some hot chocolate.

41. The nurse is aware that certain factors may lead children to deny the existence of actual pain. Which of the following is *not* one of these factors?
1. Fear of an injection.
2. Better tolerance for pain than adults.
3. Lack of understanding of what "pain" means.
4. Attempts to meet expectations of others.

42. Which of the following is most helpful to the nurse in evaluating a young child's pain status?
1. A verbal statement of pain.
2. Physiological changes.
3. Behavioral changes.
4. Parental comments.

Gordon Isaac has cancer of the bladder. He has been admitted for a cystectomy and urinary diversion.

43. Most clients are curious about the appearance and placement of the stoma of their urinary diversion. What area of the abdomen is usually used?
1. Right side, 1 to 2 inches below the waist.
2. Superior, anterior region of the iliac crest.
3. Left side, just above the waist.
4. Area near the umbilicus.

44. During this critical period immediately after surgery, the nurse would be especially observant of the client's general condition. What is the most critical sign or symptom Mr. Isaac could exhibit?
1. Absence of urinary output over a period of 1 to 2 hours.
2. Pain along the incision site.

☐ 3. Increased pulse rate to 100/min.

☐ 4. Serous drainage from the incision line.

45. Mr. Isaac has a collecting appliance fastened around the ileal conduit stoma. Select the most common problem that the nurse is trying to prevent with the use of this bag.

☐ 1. Infection of the stoma.

☐ 2. Skin excoriation.

☐ 3. Stricture of the ileal stoma.

☐ 4. Ammonia odor from the stoma.

46. What is the most important reason for attaching the ileostomy bag to gravity drainage at night?

☐ 1. To prevent infection of the stoma resulting from urinary stasis in the bag.

☐ 2. To prevent leakage of urine around the bag on the skin that can be caused by overdistension of the bag.

☐ 3. To facilitate the normal urinary method of excretion.

☐ 4. To prevent reflux of urine into the renal pelvis.

47. Mr. Isaac needs adequate teaching before his discharge. In doing discharge teaching, which complication needs to be emphasized?

☐ 1. Recurrent bladder infection.

☐ 2. Frequent emptying of the colon.

☐ 3. Ileal stoma dilatation.

☐ 4. Inflammation and infection of the kidney.

Maria Cordobas, a 26-year-old woman in computer sales, is raped on her way home from work one evening. The rape occurs in the parking lot where she is employed. A passerby finds her lying on the ground. She tells him, in a very calm voice, that she has been raped. He brings her to an emergency room. Although she is in physical pain, her condition is not serious.

48. Which of the following actions is the most important for the emergency room nurse to take?

☐ 1. Call the police.

☐ 2. Call a psychiatrist.

☐ 3. Provide emotional support.

☐ 4. Offer protection from pregnancy.

49. The nurse in the emergency room can provide the best emotional support to Miss Cordobas by doing which of the following?

☐ 1. Asking her questions to help her talk about the rape.

☐ 2. Telling her it is very important that she discuss the rape now while it is still fresh in her mind.

☐ 3. Telling her that at some point she may feel angry, afraid, or sad, and that these feelings are normal.

☐ 4. Explaining that since her initial reaction is different from other victims, she probably will not have problems coping.

50. A co-worker tells the nurse, "Miss Cordobas is so calm, I bet she wasn't even raped." The source of the co-worker's response is probably reflected in which of the following statements?

☐ 1. She knows the client personally and knows she may be lying.

☐ 2. She may know the rapist and is trying to protect him.

☐ 3. The client's rape reminds her that she is also vulnerable to rape.

☐ 4. She correctly knows that rape victims are hysterical after a rape, not calm.

51. After the physical exam is finished, Miss Cordobas quietly and calmly asks the nurse if she can see the psychiatric clinical specialist. The clinical specialist provides crisis intervention. This type of therapy is most appropriate for which of the following reasons?

☐ 1. It will help the client gain insightful understanding about her feelings.

☐ 2. It will help her to understand childhood conflicts brought into awareness by this trauma.

☐ 3. It provides the long-term therapy needed for an event this serious.

☐ 4. It may prevent serious psychiatric symptoms.

52. The clinical specialist assesses Miss Cordobas. Which of the following will *not* necessarily be important for Miss Cordobas at this stage?

☐ 1. An identified support system.

☐ 2. A positive response to the significant others who come to pick her up at the hospital.

☐ 3. An ability to maintain some level of control over her care.

☐ 4. An awareness of how she might prevent a rape in the future.

53. When the clinical specialist tries to talk with Miss Cordobas, the client angrily tells her, "You certainly took long enough. No one cares enough here to provide decent support." The clinical specialist knows that the staff had dealt with Miss Cordobas gently and supportively. Which of the following statements most accurately describes the source of Miss Cordobas's anger?

☐ 1. She is displacing her anger about the rapist on to the hospital staff.

☐ 2. She is angry at the staff for hurting her during the examination.

☐ 3. She may have been raped as a child, and this rape brings up memories.

☐ 4. She is angry because it happened to her and not someone else.

54. Which of the following is the best response the clinical specialist could make to Miss Cordobas's angry remark?

☐ 1. "I think you're angry at something else and not myself or the staff."

☐ 2. "You sound angry."

☐ 3. "I'd rather talk with you about the rape."

☐ 4. "It is not productive being angry with me and the staff."

55. According to the community mental health model, Miss Cordobas's rape would be considered a crisis if which of the following conditions occurred?

☐ 1. Her supports were excessive and overpowered the stress of the event.

☐ 2. Her defense mechanisms were not adequate for the situation.

☐ 3. The stress caused by the rape was great, and she could not contain it unless she stayed with a friend.

☐ 4. The stress generated was much greater than her support systems could handle.

56. Crisis-intervention therapy is considered to be which of the following?

☐ 1. Secondary prevention.

☐ 2. Tertiary prevention.

☐ 3. Insight-oriented therapy.

☐ 4. Long-term therapy.

57. Primary prevention for the community problem of rape would best be achieved by which of the following?

☐ 1. Emergency care after the rape.

☐ 2. A class by policewomen on how to avoid rape.

☐ 3. Hospitalization for the rape victim.

☐ 4. A long jail sentence for the rapist.

Flora Robinson has missed two menstrual periods and has experienced some nausea in the mornings. She comes to the health clinic to confirm her suspicion that she might be pregnant.

58. Mrs. Robinson's urine specimen was positive for human chorionic gonadotropin. Which of the following physical signs might be observed on the initial examination?

☐ 1. The outline of the fetus is palpated by the clinician.

☐ 2. Softening of the lower uterine segment is demonstrated on bimanual examination.

☐ 3. Fetal movement is reported by Mrs. Robinson.

☐ 4. Effacement of the cervix is noted on vaginal examination.

59. While the nurse is taking a history, Mrs. Robinson tells the nurse that she has four children at home, that this baby will be her fifth child, and that, in addition, she has had two miscarriages, both at 8 weeks' gestation. Based upon this information, what would the nurse record?

☐ 1. Gravida 4, para 2.

☐ 2. Gravida 7, para 5.

☐ 3. Gravida 5, para 2.

☐ 4. Gravida 7, para 4.

60. Mrs. Robinson asks what she can do to eliminate her nausea. Which of the following would the nurse suggest?

☐ 1. "Avoid foods that are high in fiber."

☐ 2. "Drink a glass of water before going to bed."

☐ 3. "Eat some dry toast before getting up."

☐ 4. "Eliminate breakfast, and eat a large lunch."

61. During the eighth month of pregnancy, Mrs. Robinson returns for a prenatal visit. As part of her assessment, the nurse performs Leopold's maneuver. What is the best explanation the nurse can give Mrs. Robinson about this procedure?

☐ 1. Helps push the fetus into the pelvis.

☐ 2. Helps to turn the baby around.

☐ 3. Helps to determine fetal abnormalities.

☐ 4. Helps to determine the baby's position.

62. Mrs. Robinson tells the nurse that she has been having painless uterine contractions for the last week. They occur at irregular intervals and are relieved by walking. Based on this information, what would the nurse best conclude?

☐ 1. This is a pathological sign.

☐ 2. This is a sign of true labor.

☐ 3. These are Braxton Hicks' contractions.

☐ 4. This is a sign of impending fetal distress.

63. During this visit, the nurse listens to the fetal heart tones and determines that the rate is 96 beats/min and the heart sound is strong. In view of these findings, what would the nurse's next action be?

☐ 1. Record this rate in the mother's chart.

☐ 2. Take the mother's blood pressure.

☐ 3. Take the mother's pulse.

☐ 4. Notify the physician immediately.

64. Mrs. Robinson is scheduled for a nonstress test when she is 36 weeks pregnant. Which of the following is true regarding a nonstress test?

☐ 1. An IV of oxytocin is started to stimulate mild contractions.

☐ 2. The test determines the gestational age of the fetus.

☐ 3. Late decelerations in relation to contractions are monitored.

☐ 4. The test evaluates fetal heart rates in relation to fetal movement.

Three-month-old Heather has cystic fibrosis. As a neonate, she had surgery for meconium ileus.

65. Heather's parents were told that meconium ileus was related to cystic fibrosis, but they state that they do not understand why. Which of the following explanations is most accurate?

☐ 1. The bile ducts become obstructed with tenacious mucus.

☐ 2. The intestinal cilia are blunted and prevent meconium from passing through the intestinal tract.

3. The small intestine is constricted, resulting in meconium impaction.

4. The pancreas is unable to secrete the enzymes necessary for digestion.

66. Heather's parents also ask what test was used to diagnose Heather's condition. Which one of the following tests is used initially to diagnose cystic fibrosis?

1. Stool exam for trypsin, amylase, and lipase.
2. Sweat chloride test.
3. Chest x-ray.
4. Stool exam for fat content.

67. Heather is hospitalized with pneumonia in the right lower lobe. Which of the following nursing orders concerning Heather's chest physical therapy is indicated?

1. To right lower lobe qh.
2. To right lung q2h.
3. To all lobes q2h to q4h.
4. To all lobes once each shift.

68. Ampicillin, 100 mg IV q6h, has been prescribed for Heather. The ampicillin vial contains 250 mg/1.2 ml when reconstituted. How much would be administered?

1. 0.25 ml.
2. 0.48 ml.
3. 0.75 ml.
4. 2.5 ml.

69. A developmental assessment indicates that Heather is developing at an age-appropriate level. Which of the following actions will best promote her continued development?

1. Provide bright-colored objects within reach.
2. Provide space for her to practice crawling.
3. Offer her small objects to improve her pincer grasp.
4. Teach her to play pat-a-cake.

70. Heather is receiving pancreatic enzymes to aid digestion. Her parents would be instructed to administer the enzymes in which of the following ways?

1. Add it to her formula.
2. Put it in a small amount of pureed applesauce.
3. Mix it with an ounce of orange juice.
4. Mix it with water in a syringe.

71. Which one of the following is the best indicator of a successful outcome of Heather's treatment plan?

1. Growth rate within normal limits.
2. Achievement of developmental milestones.
3. Ability to digest a variety of foods.
4. Decrease in incidence of respiratory infections.

72. Heather's mother asks what the risk is of having another child with cystic fibrosis, since she and her husband are "thinking about having another baby some day." Which of the following is the best nursing response?

1. "It's probably best if you don't have any more children."
2. "Your next child may be a carrier but won't have the disease."
3. "You can have an amniocentesis in early pregnancy to detect whether the baby has cystic fibrosis and, if so, you may choose to have a therapeutic abortion."
4. "I'd like to refer you to the genetic counselor on our staff, who can discuss with you the probability of your second child having cystic fibrosis."

Joseph Fenter, a 55-year-old black man, is admitted to the hospital with a diagnosis of hypertension. While taking his history, the nurse learns that he is employed as a sales manager for a large video business. His hypertension was discovered on a routine visit to the medical department at work.

73. On admission, Mr. Fenter would most likely be expected to make which of these statements?

1. "I don't know why I am here. There is nothing wrong with me."
2. "I have been having numerous episodes of nausea and vomiting."
3. "I have been experiencing shortness of breath."
4. "I am here because I have hypertension."

74. Which of these findings would constitute a significant index of hypertension?

1. A pulse pressure of 10 mm Hg.
2. A regular pulse of 90 beats/min.
3. A sustained diastolic pressure greater than 90 mm Hg.
4. A systolic pressure fluctuating between 135 and 140 mm Hg.

75. Mr. Fenter is to receive a diet low in fat, sodium, and cholesterol. His knowledge of foods lowest in these elements would be good if he selected which of these menus?

1. Beans, ham, rye bread, and a carrot.
2. Cold baked chicken, tomatoes, and applesauce.
3. Cold cuts, salad with blue cheese dressing, and custard pie.
4. Cheese sandwich, cream of mushroom soup, and chocolate pie.

76. When teaching Mr. Fenter about his diet, the nurse would include which of these instructions?

1. Season food with lemon juice.
2. Limit salt to 3 to 4 teaspoons/day.
3. Eat a lot of canned foods.
4. Restrict green vegetable intake.

77. Mr. Fenter is taking the medication isosorbide dinitrate (Isordil) for symptoms of angina. Discharge teaching about isosorbide dinitrate (Isordil) would

include information that this drug is which of the following?

☐ 1. A nonnitrite preparation that will not cause dilatation of peripheral vessels.

☐ 2. A nitrite preparation that will constrict both small and large vessels.

☐ 3. A vasodilator that will cause an increase in vascular resistance.

☐ 4. A nitrite preparation that will dilate both large and small vessels.

78. Mr. Fenter has a prescription for metoprolol (Lopressor) to control his hypertension. This drug reduces blood pressure by which of the following mechanisms?

☐ 1. Decreases cardiac output and suppresses renin activity.

☐ 2. Increases cardiac output and suppresses aldosterone activity.

☐ 3. Depletes norepinephrine from the heart and peripheral organs.

☐ 4. Suppresses norepinephrine secretion from the medulla of the brain.

79. Which one of the following types of adrenergic-blocking agents is particularly useful in producing vasodilatation?

☐ 1. Alpha-blocking agents.

☐ 2. Beta-blocking agents.

☐ 3. Adrenergic neuron-blocking agents.

☐ 4. Gamma-blocking agents.

Gladys Stein is admitted to the postpartal unit following delivery of her second child.

80. Which of the following mothers on the postpartum unit is at greatest risk for a postpartal infection?

☐ 1. A woman who delivered vaginally with marginal placenta previa.

☐ 2. A primipara who had rupture of membranes 36 hours before delivery.

☐ 3. A mother who had an elective cesarean delivery because of cephalopelvic disproportion.

☐ 4. A multigravida who delivered twins after a 10-hour labor.

81. While caring for Mrs. Stein on the second postpartal day following a normal spontaneous delivery, the nurse notes that each of the following is on the chart. Which of the following requires prompt notification of the physician?

☐ 1. White blood cell count of 11,000.

☐ 2. Oral temperature of 101° F (38.3° C).

☐ 3. Slight diaphoresis.

☐ 4. Urinating large quantities.

82. Cervical culture indicates a streptococcal infection; a diagnosis of endometritis is confirmed. Isolation precautions are initiated, and the infant is separated from the mother. Mrs. Stein is upset about this and

promises to wash her hands carefully if she can be allowed to be with the infant. What action would best meet her needs at this time?

☐ 1. Remind her that the isolation is required by the health department.

☐ 2. Suggest she get a second opinion from another physician.

☐ 3. Encourage her to verbalize her feelings about the separation.

☐ 4. Offer her opportunities for diversional activities at the bedside.

83. Ampicillin, 1 g, is to be administered in 50 ml of 5% dextrose in water every 6 hours. The drop factor of the infusion set is 10 drops per ml. The medication is to infuse over 30 minutes. What is the rate of infusion?

☐ 1. 6 drops per minute.

☐ 2. 60 drops per minute.

☐ 3. 16 drops per minute.

☐ 4. 1.6 drops per minute.

The school nurse is asked to teach the school staff about inspecting the children for head lice. This infestation has recently become prevalent in the community.

84. Head lice and dandruff look very similar. How can the school nurse best determine that a child has lice instead of dandruff?

☐ 1. Preadolescents rarely have dandruff.

☐ 2. Areas of alopecia on the nape of the neck indicate lice.

☐ 3. Children scratch more with lice than with dandruff.

☐ 4. Nits will not fall off the hair shaft when it is moved.

85. In addition to explaining how to look for the ova (nits) on the hair shafts, the nurse would instruct the staff to assess for which one of the following?

☐ 1. Honey-colored vesicles.

☐ 2. Enlarged cervical lymph nodes.

☐ 3. Alopecia.

☐ 4. Ringlike lesions.

86. Several cases of head lice are discovered in the school. The nurse telephones the children's parents to inform them. Each of the infested children is treated with Kwell shampoo. What is the most important information to give their parents?

☐ 1. Follow shampoo directions explicitly.

☐ 2. Cut the children's hair short.

☐ 3. Prevent the children from scratching their heads.

☐ 4. Launder or disinfect the children's clothing and bedding.

87. One of the mothers states she prides herself on keeping a spotlessly clean house and cannot imagine how her daughter got the lice. Knowing how lice are

transmitted, the nurse identifies which of the following as the most likely source?
- [ ] 1. Letting her cat sleep on her bed.
- [ ] 2. Walking to school with someone who has lice.
- [ ] 3. Sharing her friend's pretty new hat.
- [ ] 4. Playing with the neighbor's dog.

88. One child's parents ask when the child can return to school. What would be the nurse's response?
- [ ] 1. "After she has been shampooed three times with Kwell."
- [ ] 2. "When all the nits are gone, after shampooing with Kwell."
- [ ] 3. "After you cut her hair short all over."
- [ ] 4. "In 2 weeks."

Fernando Cruz, 21 years old, sustained a compound, comminuted fracture in the distal portion of the left femur while learning to ride his new motorcycle. He was placed in skeletal traction with a Thomas splint and a Pearson attachment with a 20-pound weight. A Steinman pin was inserted into the femur distal to the fracture.

89. Which of the following is a definition of a compound, comminuted fracture?
- [ ] 1. The fracture is associated with injury to surrounding tissue and structures.
- [ ] 2. Bone fragments are forcibly driven into one another.
- [ ] 3. The bone is splintered into fragments that extend through the skin.
- [ ] 4. The line of the fracture forms a spiral that encircles the bone.

90. Mr. Cruz is admitted to the orthopedic unit. The nursing care plan would include which of the following?
- [ ] 1. Ensure that the sole of the affected foot is supported against the foot of the bed.
- [ ] 2. Instruct the client to move about in bed as little as possible.
- [ ] 3. Position the Thomas splint around the upper thigh without putting pressure on the groin.

- [ ] 4. Place and remove the bedpan from the affected side.

91. Which of the following statements made by Mrs. Cruz indicates a need for further teaching or discussion?
- [ ] 1. "A diet high in roughage and fiber will prevent constipation."
- [ ] 2. "Maintaining a positive nitrogen balance is important."
- [ ] 3. "Mr. Cruz needs an increased calcium intake."
- [ ] 4. "The 2700-calorie diet should provide nutrients that promote healing."

92. To maintain traction, there must be countertraction. How is countertraction best applied to Mr. Cruz's leg?
- [ ] 1. By raising the head of the bed to a 45° angle.
- [ ] 2. By elevating the foot of the bed on 6-inch shock blocks.
- [ ] 3. By using 20 pounds of weight supported by the Steinman pin.
- [ ] 4. By keeping the Thomas splint in an inclined position.

93. Because a Steinman pin has been inserted, Mr. Cruz is at risk of acquiring which of the following?
- [ ] 1. Flexion contracture of the knee.
- [ ] 2. Impaired skin sensations.
- [ ] 3. Addiction to pain medication.
- [ ] 4. Osteomyelitis.

94. Mr. Cruz complains that the ropes hurt his thigh. Which of the following would be the most appropriate nursing action?
- [ ] 1. Replace the spreader bar with a wider one.
- [ ] 2. Place padding between the thigh and the rope.
- [ ] 3. Employ distraction techniques.
- [ ] 4. Medicate with a mild analgesic.

95. What is the purpose of the Pearson attachment on Mr. Cruz's traction?
- [ ] 1. To support the lower part of the leg.
- [ ] 2. To support the upper part of the leg.
- [ ] 3. To provide traction to the fracture.
- [ ] 4. To prevent flexion contracture of the ankle.

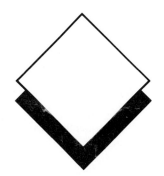

Test 2, Book I

ANSWERS WITH RATIONALES

KEY TO ABBREVIATIONS
Section of the Review Book

P = Psychosocial and Mental Health Problems
    T = Therapeutic Use of Self
    L = Loss and Death and Dying
    A = Anxious Behavior
    C = Confused Behavior
    E = Elated-Depressive Behavior
    SM = Socially Maladaptive Behavior
    SS = Suspicious Behavior
    W = Withdrawn Behavior
    SU = Substance Use Disorders
A = Adult
    H = Healthy Adult
    S = Surgery
    O = Oxygenation
    NM = Nutrition and Metabolism
    E = Elimination
    SP = Sensation and Perception
    M = Mobility
    CA = Cellular Aberration
CBF = Childbearing Family
    W = Women's Health Care
    A = Antepartal Care
    I = Intrapartal Care
    P = Postpartal Care
    N = Newborn Care
C = Child
    H = Healthy Child
    I = Ill and Hospitalized Child
    SPP = Sensation, Perception, and Protection
    O = Oxygenation
    NM = Nutrition and Metabolism
    E = Elimination
    M = Mobility
    CA = Cellular Aberration

Nursing Process Category

AS = Assessment
AN = Analysis
PL = Plan
IM = Implementation
EV = Evaluation

Client Need Category

E = Safe, Effective Care Environment
PS = Physiological Integrity
PC = Psychosocial Integrity
H = Health Promotion and Maintenance

1. no. 2. Most toddlers are able to point to their body parts by 15 to 18 months of age. All other options are too advanced for a toddler. C/H, AS, H

2. no. 4. Toddlers will resist invasive procedures, so it is best to proceed confidently. Obtain assistance to restrain the child and be matter-of-fact so the child does not feel that what is happening is a punishment or the result of being "bad." The child is too young to benefit from options no. 1 and no. 3. Deferring the exam is not appropriate. C/H, IM, PC

3. no. 1. Playing with a toy will divert Crystal's attention from the task of learning independent toileting skills. C/H, IM, H

4. no. 3. The toddler often has physiological anorexia and is more likely to accept small portions of a variety of foods. This approach also allows the toddler to exert autonomy by making choices. C/H, IM, H

5. no. 3. Pancreatitis is an inflammation of the pancreas, which leads to pancreatic tissue change, edema, swelling, ductal obstruction, necrosis, and hemorrhage. Autodigestion of the pancreas by the pancreatic enzymes has been suggested as a possible cause of the disease. The two major causes are high alcohol consumption and gallstones. There appears

to be no relationship between race and incidence of pancreatitis. A/NM, AN, PS

6. no. 4. The exocrine portion of the pancreas secretes more than 500 ml of pancreatic juice daily that contains water, bicarbonate, electrolytes, and enzymes. The primary enzymes are amylase, lipase, chymotrypsinogen (converts to chymotrypsin), and trypsinogen (converts to trypsin). The enzyme pepsin is secreted by the stomach. Sucrase, lactase, dipeptidase, and maltase are enzymes secreted by the intestine. A/NM, AN, PS

7. no. 1. Chronic pancreatitis causes degeneration of the islet cells, thereby decreasing production and secretion of insulin, which elevates the blood glucose level. Severe, steady, boring abdominal pain is a hallmark of pancreatitis. Serum amylase and lipase will be elevated. The abdomen will be distended related to intestinal hypomotility and chemical peritonitis. A/NM, AS, PS

8. no. 1. Fats are incompletely metabolized, and calcium ions are bound to fats; thus calcium ions are not absorbed in normal amounts. A/NM, AN, PS

9. no. 1. Clients with pancreatitis are given anticholinergic drugs to decrease secretions and relax spasms. The client will be kept NPO initially to rest the GI tract and then will be started on clear liquids once the acute phase has passed. IV fluids will be given to maintain fluid and electrolyte balance. Once the clear liquids are tolerated, the client will be placed on a bland, low-fat diet with no alcohol or caffeine in order to decrease stimulation of the pancreas. A/NM, PL, PS

10. no. 3. Meperidine is preferred for the treatment of the pain of pancreatitis because it produces less spasm of the sphincter of Oddi. A/NM, AN, PS

11. no. 1. Withdrawal can occur if the client cuts back the amount of alcohol consumed as well as if drinking is stopped altogether. Emergency room nurses must always evaluate cardiovascular status; however, Mr. Lampert's history and presenting clinical picture are more consistent with withdrawal. Increased anxiety is only one symptom of alcohol withdrawal. P/SU, AS, PS

12. no. 3. Since Korsakoff's syndrome causes gaps in the client's memory, confabulation is used to fill in these gaps with relevant, but untrue, pieces of information. Alcoholics often suffer from chronic gastritis and fatty liver; however, Korsakoff's syndrome is an organic brain syndrome. Excessive perspiration is often experienced in alcohol detoxification but is usually noted about 72 hours after cessation of drinking. P/SU, AS, PS

13. no. 1. Working with the client to find new ways of handling difficult situations without alcohol is a long-term goal of treatment. Short-term goals would include learning to handle specific situations. Mr. Lampert needs the support from his friends and family and increased emotional support to assist him through this difficult time. Psychoanalysis has not been found to be very effective in treating alcoholism. P/SU, IM, PC

14. no. 3. Although disulfiram (Antabuse) does cause tachycardia, it also causes a drop, not an increase, in blood pressure and respiratory depression. A pulsating headache (from dilatation of peripheral blood vessels) and vomiting do occur; however, a generalized flushing becomes apparent rather than pallor. Although ataxia and blurred vision do occur, dry skin does not since the person experiences profuse sweating. P/SU, IM, PS

15. no. 3. Family therapy looks upon the presenting problem as a family problem. Family therapy does not focus on any one individual; instead, it aims at getting a better understanding of the relationship between the alcoholic and family members. Its goal is to help the family members communicate more effectively in order to find healthy ways to meet their needs. The family therapy sessions would not be centered on getting Mr. Lampert to stop drinking, but on having the members express themselves clearly on important matters, including the drinking issue, and on helping the members to listen carefully to what each member is saying. P/SU, PL, PC

16. no. 4. A slow breathing pattern is desirable in early labor to ensure adequate oxygenation to the fetus. Candle blowing and accelerated breathing are useful in active labor. Panting is carried out when the client has the desire to push when it is not indicated. CBF/I, IM, PS

17. no. 3. Decelerations can be detected early only if fetal heart tones are evaluated during and soon after contractions, because they occur at this time. CBF/I, AN, PS

18. no. 4. The fetus is in a posterior presentation, resulting in fetal pressure on the mother's back. This can be relieved by side-lying, tailor-sitting, or having the client crouch on her hands and knees. Sacral pressure can also be an effective comfort measure. CBF/I, IM, PS

19. no. 2. The fetal heart rate should be checked every 5 minutes for 15 minutes after rupture of the membranes, because of the possibility of cord prolapse, an emergency that can be detected by a changed fetal heart rate pattern. CBF/I, IM, PS

20. no. 4. These signs are indicative of delivery of the placenta, which signals the end of the third stage. Other signs of placental separation include a firmly contracting uterus, a change in its shape from discoid to globular, and a lengthening of the umbilical cord. CBF/I, AN, PS

21. no. 4. The Bence Jones protein is a test for multiple myeloma. A type and crossmatch would be done because of anticipated blood loss, which is substantial in bone or joint surgery. The prothrombin time is required because she has been taking large doses of aspirin. A sedimentation rate can rule out the possibility of infection. A/SP, AS, PS

22. no. 3. The client will be maintained on bed rest for only 2 to 5 days, depending on the surgeon. Early ambulation is encouraged to decrease the risk of postoperative complications. An overhead frame and trapeze are placed on the bed to prevent flexion of the hip when the client lifts up for back care and linen changes. Extreme flexion and adduction of the hip should be avoided because this can cause dislocation. If hip dislocation occurs the client may require further surgery, traction, or a hip spica cast. Antiembolic hose or a sequential compression device will be used to promote venous return. A/SP, PL, E

23. no. 3. Reverse isolation is not used, but the other interventions listed are done in an effort to prevent infection. A/SP, PL, E

24. no. 2. The client should keep her toes pointed toward the ceiling to prevent adduction or external rotation. Plantar and dorsiflexion of both ankles should be encouraged to promote venous return. Legs should not be crossed because this abducts the hip. The client will pivot on the unaffected leg until full weight bearing is allowed. A/SP, PL, PS

25. no. 1. Normal capillary refill occurs within 2 seconds. A delay of over 5 seconds is considered abnormal. An apical pulse rate of 74 is within normal limits. Pitting edema is an abnormality that indicates accumulation of excess fluid in the body tissues. A posterior tibial pulse is frequently nonpalpable; this absence is considered a normal variation if skin color and temperature are normal. A/SP, AN, PS

26. no. 3. Wound drainage of 100 ml after hip replacement over an 8-hour period is not unusual. The nurse should continue to monitor the amount of drainage. It should diminish over the first 2 postoperative days. If not, the physician will need to be notified. A/SP, AS, PS

27. no. 1. Urinary retention is a common problem after a total hip replacement because of the recumbent position. In the elderly male client, prostatic enlargement can also be a contributing factor. Incontinence with coughing is called *stress incontinence* and is not related to hip replacement. Weight loss and contractures normally do not occur if appropriate positioning is done and nutritional supplements are provided. A/SP, AN, PS

28. no. 1. Pain on movement and weight bearing indicates pressure on the nerves and/or muscles caused by the dislocation. Other symptoms of dislocation include inability to bear weight and a shortening of the affected leg. Edema is not a primary sign of displacement. A/SP, AS, PS

29. no. 3. Pressure on the peroneal nerve places the client at risk for foot drop. The other three options are appropriate interventions for the use and placement of abductor splints. A/SP, IM, PS

30. no. 1. Rocking chairs and recliners are difficult to get out of and cause the hip to be flexed beyond the safe limits. A/SP, EV, H

31. no. 3. This client is experiencing severe anxiety and stress. Recurrent nightmares, feelings of numbness, and difficulty in concentration are all symptoms commonly found in posttraumatic stress disorder. Hallucinations that involve insects are generally a part of toxic reactions such as alcohol withdrawal. P/A, AS, PC

32. no. 1. The client experiencing posttraumatic stress disorder has a sense of isolation and believes he is alone and that no one understands his pain. In establishing a relationship, the nurse must demonstrate that he or she is on the client's side and will be a helping person. It is important to identify past coping behaviors and to teach the client relaxation techniques; however, this will prove easier after a therapeutic relationship has been established. Until the client and his wife gain insight into the cause of their difficulties, their relationship will probably not be a source of support for the client. P/A, IM, H

33. no. 3. Although encouraged ventilation of feelings might include crying or an angry outburst, the continued expression of anger and rage can lead the client to lose self-control or to experience increased tension and anxiety rather than help to reduce it. Encourage the client to describe his thoughts rather than his feelings. He should think through how his Vietnam experiences affect his current relationships in society. Assist him by discussing ways to control anger and gain a perspective on his experiences. As the nurse communicates confidence that he or she will help him find solutions, the client gains a sense of the "normalcy" of his reactions and that his problems are not insurmountable. P/A, IM, PS

34. no. 2. The client will need continued support after he leaves the hospital. Self-help groups are an effective way to decrease feelings of loneliness, integrate past experiences into present life, and explore new coping methods and solutions to problems. Unless both the client and his wife have had an opportunity to explore the reason for their separation, moving back with his wife might cause increased stress for the client. Diazepam might be useful as adjunctive therapy for reduction of anxiety, but it is not the best long-term solution for the client. Since the client's job is probably not what has caused the increase in his anxiety, a job-training program might

not be necessary after the client's emotional state is stabilized. P/A, EV, E

35. no. 3. Hemorrhage is the most common complication following tonsillectomy. Bleeding and clotting times are necessary to determine whether the child is at risk for hemorrhage and to serve as a baseline value postoperatively. C/SPP, AS, E

36. no. 3. During the school-age period, most children lose their primary teeth and develop their permanent teeth. By adolescence, all deciduous teeth should be gone. Options no. 1 and no. 2 are periods when deciduous teeth are erupting. C/SPP, AN, PC

37. no. 4. The use of play to prepare a child for surgery is an effective teaching strategy and helps to decrease anxiety. Although there is some truth to option no. 3, option no. 4 describes a wider application of play. C/I, PL, PC

38. no. 1. Minimizing the risk of a respiratory infection carried by others would be important preoperatively. C/I, IM, PS

39. no. 3. Frequent swallowing is often an early sign of bleeding from the operative site after a tonsillectomy. The other options are normal following a tonsillectomy. C/SPP, AS, PS

40. no. 1. An ice collar decreases the risk of hemorrhage and provides soothing relief from throat discomfort as well. The other measures increase the risk of bleeding. C/I, IM, PS

41. no. 2. This statement is a myth. C/I, AN, PS

42. no. 3. Behavioral manifestations are most frequently noted in children experiencing pain. This is especially true of young children who may not have the vocabulary to communicate pain and in children who fear injections for pain relief. C/I, EV, PS

43. no. 1. This is the best position both anatomically (near the terminal ileum) and for the client. It will be visible for self-care but will not interfere with clothing. Inappropriate placement can make appliance management very difficult for the client. The stoma should be placed on a flat surface of the abdomen, away from scars, incisions, bony prominences, indentations, skin folds, the umbilicus, and inguinal creases. The stoma should not be placed at a client's belt line. A/E, AN, PS

44. no. 1. Urine output of at least 30 ml per hour is vital to show adequate renal perfusion. Because there is no bladder, urine output becomes evident immediately. Pain and serous drainage at the incision line are expected findings. Changes in pulse rate are important to monitor; however, this is not the most critical sign. A/E, AS, PS

45. no. 2. Skin excoriation is caused when urine remains in contact with the skin, and the appliance prevents this contact. A/E, AN, PS

46. no. 4. Although leakage could occur, the most important reason is to prevent reflux, which predisposes the client to pyelonephritis. A/E, AN, PS

47. no. 4. This is the most common long-term problem other than skin excoriation. A cystectomy involves removal of the bladder, so recurrent bladder infections are not a possibility. Because the urine does not drain into the functioning GI tract, frequent emptying of the colon does not occur; this is a complication with a ureterosigmoidostomy. Ileal stomal dilatation is not a complication. A/E, PL, H

48. no. 3. Of the options provided, no. 3 is most crucial. In high-stress situations, it is important for the nurse to provide emotional support as a key part of the care. Notifying the police is important, but of a lower priority. The client may or may not need a psychiatrist. Crisis intervention includes emotional support and is part of the emergency room nurse's or clinical specialist's role. Pregnancy concerns can be dealt with later. P/SM, IM, PC

49. no. 3. It is important to give the client an opportunity to talk if she wishes. If she does not want to talk, then a statement or two preparing her for some of the feelings she may experience later may help her. Offering a telephone number she may call for help if she wishes is another way to provide support. Multiple questions are inappropriate and tire a client. It is not important that the client discuss the rape at this time unless she wishes to do so. Not all rape victims want to discuss the rape. How a client copes does not depend on what her initial reaction is like. P/SM, IM, PC

50. no. 3. Staff will sometimes minimize or deny the seriousness of a traumatic event to decrease their own anxiety that it may also happen to them. Sometimes staff will look for ways in which the client did something to "cause" the rape. This, too, helps them feel that they have control over such a traumatic event. However, it is much better for a nurse to accept that people are vulnerable and to be aware of the emotional pain that awareness can cause. This self-awareness can increase the nurses' effectiveness in providing emotional support. Options no. 1 and no. 2 are not likely; people rarely lie about being raped. Responses to rape vary and include both high-anxiety behavior and a seemingly calm external demeanor. P/SM, AN, PC

51. no. 4. The purpose of crisis-intervention therapy is to return clients to a level of functioning equal to or better than that before the crisis. Crisis intervention can be effective whether or not the client develops insightful understanding about her feelings. It deals with the immediate event and does not aim at understanding earlier conflicts. Should a better understanding occur, it is incidental rather than directly intended. Crisis intervention is brief; the focus is on the present; treatment is short term and time limited. P/SM, PL, PC

52. no. 4. The early phase of a crisis is a time when here-and-now issues are dealt with by the client. The client becomes very focused on the present. Options no. 1, no. 2, and no. 3 are all important and necessary components of the assessment. Successful weathering of a crisis is most dependent upon the client's ability to cope with the situation. The support of significant others helps a client cope better. P/SM, AS, PC

53. no. 1. Clients may find the crisis situation too difficult to examine and misdirect their anger at staff, family, or friends. There are no data to suggest that the staff hurt her. The present situation is generating the client's anger at this time. There are no data to suggest that she is angry because the rape did not happen to someone else. An early response may be "Why me?" but does not usually include "Why not someone else?" P/SM, AN, PC

54. no. 2. This option allows the client to focus on her feelings without judging her or pushing her to discuss issues she is not comfortable talking about. It will not be therapeutic to push the client to identify a particular person and may make her feel defensive and ashamed. Such an approach could stifle her anger or even enrage her. Option no. 3 avoids dealing with the client's anger and is not therapeutic. Option no. 4 tries to talk the client out of her anger rather than permitting and encouraging her to express angry feelings. P/SM, IM, PC

55. no. 4. Rape is not a crisis situation for every victim, as defined by the community mental health model. Sometimes the victim may have adequate coping mechanisms and social supports to handle the trauma. Option no. 1 describes conditions that lessen the potential for crisis. Defense mechanism is a term from freudian theory. Coping mechanisms and social supports are terms used in crisis theory. If the client stayed with a friend and was able to contain the stress, a crisis would not occur. P/SM, AN, PC

56. no. 1. Secondary prevention refers to early treatment to prevent long-term illness. Crisis-intervention therapy helps the client during the acute phase of the problem. Tertiary prevention refers to treatment of chronic, long-term problems. Crisis intervention does not aim for insight, although insights may occur. Crisis intervention is a kind of brief psychotherapy. P/SM, AN, PC

57. no. 2. Preventing a rape would be primary prevention. Emergency care after the rape is an example of secondary prevention. Hospitalization is considered to be tertiary prevention. Option no. 4 is a legal action and not a type of prevention. P/SM, AN, H

58. no. 2. About the sixth week of pregnancy, the lower uterine segment becomes much softer than the cervix (Hegar's sign). Palpation of the fetal outline is possible at approximately 26 weeks. Quickening occurs between 16 and 20 weeks' gestation. Effacement occurs at or near term. CBF/A, AS, PS

59. no. 4. The term gravida refers to the number of a woman's pregnancies regardless of their duration. The term para refers to the number of past pregnancies that have produced an infant of viable age, whether the infant is alive or dead at birth. CBF/A, AN, PS

60. no. 3. Eating dry carbohydrates such as crackers or dry toast before getting out of bed in the morning may decrease nausea. CBF/A, IM, PS

61. no. 4. In the second half of pregnancy, palpation of the uterus using Leopold's maneuver determines the position of the fetus. CBF/A, IM, PS

62. no. 3. Contractions that occur at irregular intervals and are relieved by walking are Braxton Hicks' contractions. CBF/A, AN, PS

63. no. 3. This rate is too slow to be a fetal heart rate. The nurse is most likely hearing a uterine souffle as blood rushes through the placenta. This rate is the same as the mother's pulse. If the mother's pulse rate is not 96, further assessment would be required. CBF/A, AN, PS

64. no. 4. The oxytocin challenge test uses medication to assess fetal response to maternal contractions. Ultrasound is used to determine gestational age. CBF/A, AN, PS

65. no. 4. Pancreatic ducts are clogged with mucus, and thus enzymes needed for digestion are not secreted into the small intestine. C/NM, IM, PS

66. no. 2. An elevated sweat chloride level is the definitive diagnostic test for cystic fibrosis. Trypsin from duodenal secretions is sometimes measured if the sweat chloride results are questionable. C/NM, AS, PS

67. no. 3. Chest physical therapy should be done q4h prophylactically for the child with cystic fibrosis and more frequently when the child has a respiratory infection. Percuss and drain all lobes of both lungs. C/NM, PL, PS

68. no. 2.

$$\frac{250 \text{ mg}}{1.2 \text{ ml}} = \frac{100 \text{ mg}}{x \text{ ml}} \quad \frac{100(1.2)}{250} = 0.48 \text{ ml}$$

C/NM, IM, PS

69. no. 1. A 3-month-old is able to focus the eyes on objects, likes bright colors, and is ready to begin practicing reaching for objects. C/NM, PL, H

70. no. 2. Applesauce helps disguise the taste of the enzymes; also, the cellulose in the applesauce retards the otherwise instant action of the enzymes. C/NM, IM, PS

71. no. 4. Pulmonary involvement is the leading cause of illness and death in children with cystic fibrosis. The major goal is to decrease the incidence of pulmonary infections in order to promote adequate

oxygenation and increase life expectancy. C/NM, EV, H

72. no. 4. Refer families with children who have inherited disorders such as cystic fibrosis for genetic counseling. New screening tests are being developed for the prenatal detection of cystic fibrosis. C/NM, IM, H

73. no. 1. Denial of illness and fear of losing control are predominant when clients discover they have a chronic disease. Uncomplicated hypertension is usually asymptomatic so many clients are unaware that they have a chronic illness. If symptoms do occur, they include headache, dizziness, fainting, epistaxis, and tinnitus. As the disease progresses, symptoms are related to target organ damage. Nausea and vomiting and shortness of breath occur with inadequate cardiac perfusion. A/O, AS, PC

74. no. 3. Normal blood pressure ranges from 115 to 120 mm Hg systolic over 75 to 80 mm Hg diastolic. A sustained diastolic pressure of greater than 90 mm Hg is defined as hypertension by the American Heart Association. A pulse pressure of 10 mm Hg is abnormally low (normal is 30 to 40 mm Hg). A narrowed pulse pressure may be seen in shock, pericardial effusion, aortic stenosis, and constrictive pericarditis. A widened pulse pressure is seen in hypertension. A resting pulse rate over 100 beats/min is considered abnormal in adults. A systolic blood pressure greater than 140 is considered elevated. Systolic hypertension is frequently seen in elderly clients who have atherosclerosis. A/O, AS, PS

75. no. 2. Foods low in fat, sodium, and cholesterol include baked chicken (fowl), raw vegetables, and raw fruits. Ham, cold cuts, and chocolate pie are all high in sodium. Cheese, cream-based soups, and blue-cheese dressing are all high in cholesterol and saturated fat as well as sodium. A/O, EV, H

76. no. 1. Lemon juice and vinegar are acceptable to season foods when no added salt is allowed in the diet. Canned foods are very high in sodium. Fruits and vegetables should be encouraged because they are low in sodium, fat, and cholesterol. One teaspoon of salt alone has 2400 mg sodium. Total sodium intake on a low-sodium diet should be below 3000 mg. A/O, IM, E

77. no. 4. Isosorbide dinitrate (Isordil), a nitrite preparation, dilates small and large blood vessels. A/O, IM, PS

78. no. 1. Metoprolol (Lopressor) is a beta-adrenergic blocking agent that reduces blood pressure by its action on the beta receptors in the heart. A/O, AN, PS

79. no. 1. Alpha-blocking agents are nonspecific and produce significant vasodilatation. A/O, AN, PS

80. no. 2. Both mother and neonate are at risk because

of prolonged labor after membrane rupture. Because of the high risk of amnionitis following early rupture of membranes, labor is induced within 72 hours if it does not occur spontaneously. CBF/P, AS, PS

81. no. 2. All other assessments are normal in the postpartal period. A temperature elevated above 100.4° F (38° C) indicates sepsis. Leukocytosis normally occurs after delivery and may be related to the stress of labor and delivery. A process of diuresis begins 2 to 4 days after delivery. The client eliminates excess fluid through the skin and urinary tract in an attempt to return to normal water metabolism. CBF/P, AS, PS

82. no. 3. Although isolation is required, the client needs an opportunity to talk about her feelings at this time. CBF/P, IM, PC

83. no. 3.

$$\frac{\text{Amount to be infused} \times \text{gtt factor}}{\text{total time in minutes}}$$
$$= \frac{50 \text{ ml} \times 10 \text{ gtt/ml}}{30 \text{ minutes}} = 16$$

S, IM, PS

84. no. 4. Lice nits attach firmly to the hair shaft; dandruff flakes off easily. Lice do not cause areas of alopecia (ringworm does). Itching can occur with lice or dandruff. C/SPP, AS, PS

85. no. 2. Enlarged lymph nodes often accompany head lice. Honey-colored vesicles are characteristic of impetigo. Alopecia and ringlike lesions are characteristic of ringworm (tinea). C/SPP, AS, PS

86. no. 1. Kwell shampoo can cause neurotoxicity if used more often than prescribed. The shampoo directions explicitly state not to shampoo more frequently than once a week. Laundering, but not disinfecting, clothing is helpful as a secondary activity. C/SPP, IM, E

87. no. 3. Lice are most often spread by sharing personal articles (e.g., comb or hat). C/SPP, AN, PS

88. no. 2. A single shampoo with Kwell kills the ova in nearly all cases. If observable nits are no longer present, the nurse and parent can safely assume the child's condition is no longer communicable. C/SPP, IM, H

89. no. 3. Option no. 1 describes a closed fracture; no. 2, an impacted fracture; no. 4, a spiral fracture. A/SP, AN, PS

90. no. 3. The splint tends to dig into the groin, causing irritation. The foot plate is attached to the Pearson splint. Immobility is not likely to be a problem because balanced traction allows a great deal of freedom to move. Bedpan use is easier from the unaffected side. A/SP, PL, E

91. no. 3. Calcium is lost from the bone following a fracture. Serum calcium levels are increased, and the potential for renal calculi is increased. Thus a

normal or decreased calcium intake is indicated along with sufficient fluids. The U.S. Recommended Caloric Intake for an average healthy male is 2600 cal. Nutritional needs will be met if the diet is well-balanced with foods from all four basic food groups. A positive nitrogen balance is important in wound healing. Roughage and fiber are very important in preventing constipation when bed rest is prescribed for the client. A/SP, EV, H

92. no. 2. Raising the foot of the bed enables the client's body weight to oppose the traction. The body weight is the countertraction. A/SP, PL, PS

93. no. 4. The pin enters the bone, providing an opening for bacteria. The pin does not inhibit knee-joint movement or cause nerve damage. A/SP, AN, PS

94. no. 1. A narrow spreader bar allows the ropes to rub against the outer aspect of the thigh. Placing padding would still result in pressure on the skin. Options no. 3 and no. 4 are inappropriate because if the ropes are correctly positioned, the client will not be uncomfortable. A/SP, IM, E

95. no. 1. The skeletal traction and Thomas splint provide traction and support of the upper leg. A/SP, AN, PS

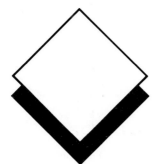

Test 2, Book II

Questions

Marsha Hanover is admitted to rule out cholecystitis. She is 40 years old, 5 feet 2 inches, 215 pounds. She is a homemaker with two teenage children.

1. Which of the following statements is *incorrect* about obesity and its treatment?
   ☐ 1. Exercise is the most practical method of weight control.
   ☐ 2. Obesity tends to run in families because of eating habits.
   ☐ 3. Food can become an individual's major source of gratification.
   ☐ 4. Obese children tend to become obese adults.

2. Mrs. Hanover is scheduled for an upper gastrointestinal series. Which of the following will be used to prepare her?
   ☐ 1. Clear liquids for breakfast the day of the exam.
   ☐ 2. A cleansing enema the morning of the exam.
   ☐ 3. Food and fluids withheld 10 to 12 hours before the exam.
   ☐ 4. Radiopaque tablets given the evening before the exam.

3. The physician schedules Mrs. Hanover for a gastric analysis with a nasogastric tube. Which of the following nursing actions would be essential when preparing a client for gastric analysis?
   ☐ 1. Force fluids for 24 hours preceding the test.
   ☐ 2. Administer enemas on the preceding evening.
   ☐ 3. Withhold food the morning of the analysis.
   ☐ 4. Record the pulse rate when beginning the test.

4. Which of the following findings from gastric analysis would best support the diagnosis of a peptic ulcer?
   ☐ 1. Absence of gastric secretion.
   ☐ 2. Increased hydrochloric acid.
   ☐ 3. Lack of intrinsic factor.
   ☐ 4. Decreased gastric motility.

5. A tubeless gastric analysis test is used to determine which of the following?

   ☐ 1. The presence or absence of hydrochloric acid in the stomach.
   ☐ 2. The presence of gastric ulcers.
   ☐ 3. The ability of the stomach to empty solids and liquids.
   ☐ 4. The amount of free acid in the stomach.

6. Mrs. Hanover's test results indicate a duodenal ulcer. She is discharged with a prescription for a 1500-calorie diet with no coffee or hot spices and ranitidine (Zantac), 150 mg bid po. What is the therapeutic effect of this drug?
   ☐ 1. Neutralizes gastric acid.
   ☐ 2. Inhibits gastric secretions.
   ☐ 3. Slows digestion.
   ☐ 4. Reduces gastric motility.

7. In spite of conservative treatment, Mrs. Hanover's ulcer perforates and an emergency vagotomy and pyloroplasty are performed. What is the expected outcome following the vagotomy?
   ☐ 1. An increase in the blood supply to the stomach.
   ☐ 2. A decrease in gastric secretions and motility.
   ☐ 3. A decrease in the epigastric pain postoperatively.
   ☐ 4. An increase in gastric emptying and motility.

8. Mrs. Hanover returns to her room with an IV and a nasogastric tube attached to suction. That evening she is ambulated to the bathroom and returned to bed. Suddenly she begins to gag and has dry heaves. What is the nurse's initial action?
   ☐ 1. Notify the physician.
   ☐ 2. Check her abdomen to see if an evisceration has occurred.
   ☐ 3. Check the nasogastric tube and suction equipment for kinks or malfunction.
   ☐ 4. Irrigate the nasogastric tube with 50 ml of normal saline.

Mary Washington, a 34-year-old unemployed secretary, has been admitted to the psychiatric unit with a diagnosis of hypochondriasis. She was brought in by her sister who states that Miss Washington has a history of severe headaches for which she has sought help in many hospitals and clinics.

9. What is the best definition of hypochondriasis?
☐ 1. A morbid concern with one's physical health.
☐ 2. A morbid concern with one's mental health.
☐ 3. An organic loss of physical functioning.
☐ 4. A category of psychosis characterized by sensory or motor disturbances.

10. Which ego-defense mechanism is most frequently demonstrated in this disorder?
☐ 1. Substitution resulting in adaptation.
☐ 2. Suppression resulting in physical symptoms.
☐ 3. Rationalization resulting in justification of behavior.
☐ 4. Displacement producing symptoms in an effort to manage anxieties.

11. The best action to use in caring for Miss Washington would be which of the following?
☐ 1. Allow her to talk about her headaches since ventilation is therapeutic.
☐ 2. Minimize the care given for physical symptoms so that her attention to them will be decreased.
☐ 3. Avoid discussion of physical symptoms since additional information may encourage her to develop further symptoms.
☐ 4. Allow her to discuss her feelings and concerns without focusing on physical symptoms.

Su-Jen Chang delivered her first child, a boy, 24 hours ago. She had a normal vaginal delivery with a midline episiotomy and is breastfeeding her baby.

12. Which one of the following assessments on the first postpartal day would most likely indicate normal postpartal adjustment?
☐ 1. Fundus two finger-breadths above the umbilicus.
☐ 2. Breasts tender and engorged.
☐ 3. Moderate, steady flow of lochia serosa.
☐ 4. Lack of bowel movement since delivery.

13. Instructions to Mrs. Chang regarding care of the perineal area would include which of the following?
☐ 1. Separate the labia while cleansing.
☐ 2. Cleanse the perineum after each elimination.
☐ 3. Use sterile water to cleanse the perineum.
☐ 4. Perform perineal care only if an episiotomy was performed.

14. Which one of the following behaviors indicates Mrs. Chang has correctly understood the nurse's instructions for preventing cracked nipples while breastfeeding?
☐ 1. She uses an alcohol swab to cleanse her nipples before feeding.
☐ 2. She air-dries her nipples 15 minutes after feeding.

☐ 3. She cleanses her nipples daily with soap and water.
☐ 4. She allows the baby to nurse 15 minutes on each breast on her first postpartum day.

15. Which of the following behaviors would indicate that Mrs. Chang is in the taking-hold phase of the postpartum period?
☐ 1. Talking about the details of her labor and delivery experience.
☐ 2. Questioning the nurse about lochia flow.
☐ 3. Requesting the nurse to return the baby to the nursery immediately after feeding.
☐ 4. Asking to do a return demonstration of cord and circumcision care for her baby.

16. Mrs. Chang asks the nurse when it is safe to resume sexual intercourse after delivery. In response to Mrs. Chang's question, the nurse replies that intercourse can safely be resumed at which of the following times?
☐ 1. As soon as Mrs. Chang returns home.
☐ 2. When the physician gives approval.
☐ 3. Once lochia flow has stopped.
☐ 4. After the 6-week postpartum check-up.

17. Mrs. Chang is 2 days postpartum. In addition to an elevated temperature and chills, which assessment finding would most likely suggest Mrs. Chang has acquired postpartal endometritis?
☐ 1. Complaint of increased thirst.
☐ 2. Lochia change from rubra to serosa.
☐ 3. Uterus very tender when palpated abdominally.
☐ 4. Diastasis recti detected on abdominal inspection.

Erma Olin, an 86-year-old widow, is brought to the emergency room by ambulance after suffering a fall at home. She is accompanied by a neighbor who tells the admitting nurse that Mrs. Olin is active in church and several senior-citizen groups. She is self-sufficient and financially secure. She has a history of heart problems and is taking medication.

18. When approaching Mrs. Olin, what would be the nurse's first action?
☐ 1. Explain the emergency room procedures.
☐ 2. Tell her that a physician will be in to examine her shortly.
☐ 3. Introduce himself or herself.
☐ 4. Apply electrode patches to monitor her cardiac activity.

19. When applying electrode patches to monitor Mrs. Olin's cardiac activity, which of the following assessments will the nurse *not* be able to make?
☐ 1. Level of consciousness and orientation.
☐ 2. Skin color and temperature.
☐ 3. Muscle tension and motor activity.
☐ 4. Cardiac output.

20. A complete 12-lead ECG applied to Mrs. Olin shows that she has a heart rate of 48 beats per minute. She

is given a diagnosis of sinus bradycardia. The most common cause of this condition is which of the following?

- ☐ 1. Stress and excitement.
- ☐ 2. Severe pain.
- ☐ 3. Digitalis toxicity.
- ☐ 4. Hyperthyroidism.

21. When planning care for Mrs. Olin, what would the primary goal be at this stage of her illness?

- ☐ 1. The client will be free from further damage to her myocardium.
- ☐ 2. The client will maintain optimum cardiac output.
- ☐ 3. The client will experience a decrease in environmental and emotional stimuli.
- ☐ 4. The client will maintain close communication with her significant others.

22. The laboratory report indicates that the causes of Mrs. Olin's condition are digitalis toxicity and an acceleration of cardiac atherosclerosis. She is to receive a permanent pacemaker in the left side of her chest. The nurse assigned to prepare Mrs. Olin would remember which of the following?

- ☐ 1. A planned, systematic approach to teaching a client to live with a pacemaker is a vital part of nursing care.
- ☐ 2. Mrs. Olin will easily adjust to a pacemaker because she has had a heart problem for 20 years.
- ☐ 3. Mrs. Olin probably already has some information about pacemakers from discussion in the media.
- ☐ 4. It is the physician's responsibility to teach Mrs. Olin about her pacemaker.

23. Which of the following interventions would *not* be appropriate for Mrs. Olin in the immediate post-operative period?

- ☐ 1. Assess the incision q30min for bleeding.
- ☐ 2. Monitor for dizziness, light-headedness, and chest pain.
- ☐ 3. Monitor the ECG for pacing spikes or pacing artifacts.
- ☐ 4. Use active and passive ROM exercises of the left arm and shoulder.

24. Discharge planning for Mrs. Olin would *not* include which of the following?

- ☐ 1. Activity and exercise.
- ☐ 2. Awareness of environmental hazards that might interfere with the function of the pacemaker.
- ☐ 3. How to take a radial pulse daily.
- ☐ 4. How to care for a permanently implanted pacemaker.

Two siblings, Bobby, age 5, and Tina, age 2, are admitted to the hospital with a diagnosis of chronic lead poisoning.

25. Which of the following is the most important assessment of Bobby and Tina?

- ☐ 1. Cardiovascular status.
- ☐ 2. Urinary output.
- ☐ 3. Dietary habits.
- ☐ 4. Neurological status.

26. To best promote Bobby and Tina's adaptation to being in the hospital, which nursing action would be implemented?

- ☐ 1. Insist that one of their parents stay with them.
- ☐ 2. Give each of them a new stuffed animal.
- ☐ 3. Take them to the playroom to get acquainted with the other children.
- ☐ 4. Place them together in the same hospital room.

27. Both children are receiving injections of EDTA and dimercaprol (BAL). Which of the following observations indicate a toxic response to these drugs?

- ☐ 1. Seizures.
- ☐ 2. Long-bone pain.
- ☐ 3. Oliguria.
- ☐ 4. Anemia.

28. The nurse would prepare to administer Tina's injection in which of the following sites?

- ☐ 1. The gluteus medius muscle.
- ☐ 2. The deltoid muscle.
- ☐ 3. The vastus lateralis muscle.
- ☐ 4. The subcutaneous tissue of the abdomen.

29. As the nurse prepares to administer Bobby's injections, he begins to cry and kick. What is the best nursing response to Bobby?

- ☐ 1. "Bobby, Tina is going to get an injection, too."
- ☐ 2. "Bobby, you can cry as much as you want, but you must hold still."
- ☐ 3. "Be a big boy now, Bobby, and this will be over in a minute."
- ☐ 4. "Bobby, this will just feel like a little stick in your leg."

30. What would be *least* important to assess as possible sources of the lead poisoning?

- ☐ 1. The type of home the family lives in.
- ☐ 2. The children's eating habits.
- ☐ 3. The family's income level.
- ☐ 4. How closely the children are supervised.

31. Which of the following menus is most appropriate to serve Bobby and Tina?

- ☐ 1. Hamburger and bun, peas, milk, and orange slices.
- ☐ 2. Spaghetti, lettuce, grape juice, and gelatin with bananas.
- ☐ 3. Peanut butter sandwich, raw carrots, apple juice, and vanilla pudding.
- ☐ 4. Liver, broccoli, bread and butter, milk, and a cookie.

32. Bobby and Tina are discharged but will return to the clinic in 2 weeks. When they come to clinic, which of the following laboratory tests is *not* likely to be ordered?

☐ 1. Blood lead level.
☐ 2. Hematocrit and hemoglobin.
☐ 3. Urinalysis.
☐ 4. Clotting and bleeding times.

33. Which of the following outcomes is the best long-term indicator of successful treatment of Bobby and Tina?
☐ 1. Physical growth within normal limits.
☐ 2. Adequate dietary intake of essential nutrients.
☐ 3. Age-appropriate achievement of developmental milestones.
☐ 4. Normal sleep patterns.

Esteban Caliente, age 71, is brought to the psychiatric unit by his son. The police found him wandering along the highway a mile from home. This is the fourth time Mr. Caliente has wandered away. His son states that his father is becoming increasingly confused and un-kempt, and he says that he is no longer able to care for his father at home.

34. Which factor is most relevant concerning the behavior that Mr. Caliente is likely to exhibit in the hospital?
☐ 1. The amount of alcohol he has ingested in the last 50 years.
☐ 2. The amount of brain damage he shows.
☐ 3. The degree of orientation he shows at the time of admission.
☐ 4. His specific personality traits.

35. In checking Mr. Caliente's orientation, the nurse will most likely find that he knows which of the following?
☐ 1. What day it is.
☐ 2. Where he is.
☐ 3. Who he is.
☐ 4. How old he is.

36. In planning for Mr. Caliente's care, what will be most helpful?
☐ 1. Schedule him for as many activities as possible so that he will not have time to miss his family.
☐ 2. Ensure that he meets everyone on the ward right away so he will feel more at home.
☐ 3. Vary his schedule every day to prevent boredom.
☐ 4. Adhere to the same schedule every day to provide structure and security.

37. The information Mr. Caliente gives about his past varies from day to day. Filling in the gaps caused by memory loss is known as which of the following?
☐ 1. Amnesia.
☐ 2. Confabulation.
☐ 3. Flashbacks.
☐ 4. Free association.

38. Mr. Caliente's son and daughter-in-law come to visit. He does not recognize them. Which response by the nurse would be most appropriate?

☐ 1. "He is disoriented because of his new surroundings. He will know who you are tomorrow."
☐ 2. "There is no need for you to visit very often, since he probably won't recognize you most of the time."
☐ 3. "I know this is difficult for you. I hope you will continue to visit as often as possible."
☐ 4. "Perhaps you could send other family members to visit. He might recognize them."

39. One evening as the nurse is helping him prepare for bed, Mr. Caliente says, "Why didn't I get my supper?" The nurse knows he received his meal and that this client is exhibiting which of the following?
☐ 1. Circumstantiality.
☐ 2. Manipulation.
☐ 3. Memory loss for recent events.
☐ 4. Retardation of thought.

40. One day the nurse finds Mr. Caliente standing in the doorway of his room. He has soiled his clothing. Which is the best response for the nurse to make?
☐ 1. "Why didn't you let me know you had to go to the bathroom, Mr. Caliente?"
☐ 2. "How can we keep this from happening, Mr. Caliente?"
☐ 3. "Go in and change your clothes, Mr. Caliente."
☐ 4. "Let me help you change, Mr. Caliente. I know this upsets you."

41. Mr. Caliente says to the nurse, "I have to meet a client in an hour." Which response shows the best understanding of his condition on the part of the nurse?
☐ 1. "Your client just called and said he was sick today, Mr. Caliente."
☐ 2. "I understand you were a stockbroker, Mr. Caliente. Tell me about that."
☐ 3. "You can't meet a client, Mr. Caliente. You're in the hospital now."
☐ 4. "You don't have to go, Mr. Caliente. Someone else is going to see him."

Jack Reynolds is a 45-year-old, unemployed engineer. He was admitted to the hospital 2 days ago with acute gastrointestinal bleeding. Two years ago, cirrhosis was diagnosed; he has been a heavy drinker for many years. Although Mr. Reynolds stopped drinking several months ago, he has had two recent admissions for bleeding esophageal varices.

42. An emergency endoscopy is performed on Mr. Reynolds. Following this procedure, what would be the nurse's primary concern?
☐ 1. Urinary output.
☐ 2. Respiratory pattern.
☐ 3. Level of consciousness.
☐ 4. Gag reflex.

43. The endoscopy reveals bleeding esophageal varices. A Sengstaken-Blakemore tube was inserted to con-

trol the bleeding. What is most important to remember in caring for a client with this tube?

☐ 1. The esophageal outlet is attached to suction.

☐ 2. Pressure on the gastric balloon can be maintained for no more than 4 hours at a time.

☐ 3. Iced saline lavages can be discontinued after the tube is inserted.

☐ 4. Traction can be discontinued when the bloody drainage is less than 50 ml/hr.

44. Which of the following laboratory tests is most helpful in determining the excretory function of the liver?

☐ 1. Albumin/globulin ratio.

☐ 2. Alkaline phosphatase.

☐ 3. Prothrombin time.

☐ 4. Sulfobromophthalein (Bromsulphlein) test.

45. The nurse assesses Mr. Reynolds' ascites. Which of the following does *not* contribute to the ascites?

☐ 1. Decreased plasma proteins.

☐ 2. Increased portal pressure.

☐ 3. Inability of liver to detoxify aldosterone.

☐ 4. Inability of kidneys to handle the solute load.

46. What is the diuretic of choice for Mr. Reynolds?

☐ 1. Furosemide (Lasix).

☐ 2. Hydrochlorothiazide (HydroDIURIL).

☐ 3. Ethacrynic acid (Edecrin).

☐ 4. Spironolactone (Aldactone).

47. Mr. Reynolds is being considered as a candidate for a portacaval shunt. What is the primary purpose of this operation?

☐ 1. Eliminate the incidence of further bleeding episodes.

☐ 2. Restore hepatic function.

☐ 3. Reduce portal hypertension and congestion.

☐ 4. Decrease further hepatic degeneration.

48. Mr. Reynolds is at high risk for infection. Protecting him is a major nursing goal. To achieve this goal, the nurse would do which of the following?

☐ 1. Discourage ambulating in the corridor.

☐ 2. Initiate cooling measures for any temperature above 100° F (37.6° C).

☐ 3. Discourage visitors from coming to see him at this time.

☐ 4. Change his IV tubing and dressing q24-48h.

49. The nurse caring for Mr. Reynolds assesses that he is slightly confused and has flapping tremors of his hands. The nurse reports this to Mr. Reynolds' physician. The physician will most likely order which of the following?

☐ 1. Increased sodium by way of an IV route.

☐ 2. Diazepam (Valium) to decrease tremors.

☐ 3. Neomycin by mouth.

☐ 4. A CT scan to rule out any neurologic complications.

50. Mr. Reynolds' daughter comes to the nurse saying, "I know Daddy is going to die. If only I'd done more to help him." The nurse might best respond by saying which of the following?

☐ 1. "Why do you think your father is going to die?"

☐ 2. "You must not feel guilty for your actions."

☐ 3. "Have you shared your feelings with your father?"

☐ 4. "I can see that you are upset. Would you like to talk?"

51. It is often difficult for the nurse to help the alcoholic client explore behavioral alternatives. An effective initial step for the nurse is to do which of the following?

☐ 1. Enlist the family's support.

☐ 2. Assess the client's motivation.

☐ 3. Explore his or her own feelings and attitudes about alcohol.

☐ 4. Acquire knowledge about community treatment programs.

Four-month-old Emalee is brought to the clinic for a checkup and immunizations.

52. When assessing Emalee's development, the nurse would be most concerned about which one of the following observations?

☐ 1. Visually follows objects 180°.

☐ 2. Does not attempt to transfer a toy from one hand to the other.

☐ 3. Is unable to roll from back to front.

☐ 4. Does not turn her head to locate sounds.

53. Emalee is scheduled to receive her second diphtheria/pertussis/tetanus and polio immunizations today. She has a slight cough, a runny nose, and a temperature of 100.4° F (38° C). Which of the following nursing actions is most appropriate?

☐ 1. Advise parents of possible side effects of immunizations.

☐ 2. Give the immunizations and recommend use of a mild analgesic as soon as they get home.

☐ 3. Postpone the immunizations.

☐ 4. Advise the parents to notify their physician.

54. Emalee's parents state that she does not like cereal, because she always spits it out when they try to feed it to her. What is the most appropriate nursing response to the parents?

☐ 1. "Discontinue cereal and try fruit instead."

☐ 2. "You may need to position her differently during meals."

☐ 3. "She will outgrow this in a month or so."

☐ 4. "When she is hungry enough she will eat."

55. Emalee's parents have been planning a second honeymoon in Bermuda. They want to leave the baby with an adult relative. At what age will Emalee tolerate this absence with the least amount of emotional trauma?

- ☐ 1. 5 months.
- ☐ 2. 7 months.
- ☐ 3. 9 months.
- ☐ 4. 11 months.

56. In anticipation of Emalee's next stage of development, which of the following toys and games encourage her developmental progress?
- ☐ 1. Let her throw and retrieve objects.
- ☐ 2. Play peek-a-boo.
- ☐ 3. Play a music box.
- ☐ 4. Let her bang on pots and pans.

57. In providing the parents with anticipatory guidance for Emalee, it is important that they know the common causes of mortality and morbidity in her age group. Next to birth defects, which of the following problems results in the highest death rate in infants?
- ☐ 1. Drowning.
- ☐ 2. Accidents.
- ☐ 3. Child abuse and neglect.
- ☐ 4. Communicable disease.

Arnold Hindricks is a 30-year-old college graduate who has been employed as a manager of a print shop for the past 5 years. In the past 9 months, he has gradually become less effective in his performance, demonstrating an inability to communicate clearly and a deterioration in appearance. His wife accompanies him to the unit where he states, "They keep telling me I'm the one who did it." He is admitted with a diagnosis of schizophrenia, paranoid type.

58. When planning for activities and therapy for Mr. Hindricks, the nurse would know that which statement is characteristic of the schizophrenic client?
- ☐ 1. He is very receptive to the attention of others.
- ☐ 2. He will respond very rapidly to hospitalization and psychotropic medications.
- ☐ 3. He is very sensitive to what others are feeling.
- ☐ 4. He will require electroconvulsive therapy to disrupt the pattern of psychosis.

59. Mr. Hindricks is experiencing sensory perceptions without external stimuli. Which of the following does this best describe?
- ☐ 1. A delusion.
- ☐ 2. An illusion.
- ☐ 3. A hallucination.
- ☐ 4. A loose association.

60. Which of the following would be the best response by the nurse to Mr. Hindricks' statement?
- ☐ 1. "I don't hear the voices. What else do they say to you?"
- ☐ 2. "I don't hear any voices but ours, but something seems to be frightening you."
- ☐ 3. "I don't hear the voices. It is time for you to go to occupational therapy now."
- ☐ 4. "I don't hear the voices. They are only in your head."

61. As a result of withdrawing from reality, Mr. Hindricks exhibits preoccupation with ideas and fantasies that have meaning only to him. This is an example of which of the following?
- ☐ 1. Adaptation.
- ☐ 2. Ambivalence.
- ☐ 3. Apathy.
- ☐ 4. Autism.

62. One day while watching TV, Mr. Hindricks suddenly runs over and states to the announcer, "I told you before, I am not a homosexual." This behavior best describes which of the following?
- ☐ 1. An idea of influence.
- ☐ 2. An idea of reference.
- ☐ 3. Introjection.
- ☐ 4. Labeling.

63. Mr. Hindricks is to start taking fluphenazine (Prolixin), 5 mg po bid. Which side effect is he most likely to experience from this drug?
- ☐ 1. Hypotension.
- ☐ 2. Hypothermia.
- ☐ 3. Impotence.
- ☐ 4. Nausea and vomiting.

64. After taking fluphenazine for 1 week, Mr. Hindricks is restless. The nurse notices that he is moving his hands and mouth and pacing in the hallway. What is the term used to describe these side effects of fluphenazine?
- ☐ 1. Akinesia.
- ☐ 2. Akathisia.
- ☐ 3. Catatonia.
- ☐ 4. Waxy flexibility.

65. Which of the following drugs and dose would be most appropriate to alleviate Mr. Hindricks' symptoms?
- ☐ 1. Benztropine mesylate (Cogentin) 1 mg po bid.
- ☐ 2. Trihexyphenidyl (Artane) 15 mg po bid.
- ☐ 3. Chlordiazepoxide (Librium) 25 mg po bid.
- ☐ 4. Diazepam (Valium) 5 mg po tid.

66. Mr. Hindricks will remain on a fluphenazine regimen after discharge. What is the primary advantage of this drug for outpatient use?
- ☐ 1. It is safer than other phenothiazines.
- ☐ 2. It has fewer side effects than other phenothiazines.
- ☐ 3. It is less addicting than other phenothiazines.
- ☐ 4. It is available in a long-acting form.

67. Mr. Hindricks participates in milieu therapy on the unit. Milieu therapy manipulates the hospital environment in order to provide which of the following?
- ☐ 1. Positive living and learning experiences.
- ☐ 2. A safe atmosphere.
- ☐ 3. An opportunity for improvement of socialization skills.
- ☐ 4. The opportunity to learn new skills through adjunctive therapies.

68. Mr. and Mrs. Hindricks plan to go to family therapy. What is the main objective of this therapy?
- ☐ 1. The client will verbalize the cause of the illness.
- ☐ 2. The client will reestablish effective communication patterns.
- ☐ 3. The client will avoid rehospitalization.
- ☐ 4. The client's children will remain free of the symptoms of schizophrenia.

Daniel Jackowitz has just been born. He weighs 8 pounds and appears to be normal. He is being breastfed.

69. Silver nitrate drops are used in Baby Daniel's eyes at birth to prevent which of the following?
- ☐ 1. Retrolental fibroplasia.
- ☐ 2. Ophthalmia neonatorum.
- ☐ 3. *Treponema pallidum.*
- ☐ 4. Chemical conjunctivitis.

70. Five minutes after birth, Baby Daniel's Apgar score was 9 because of acrocyanosis. This condition in newborns is a result of which of the following?
- ☐ 1. Retained amniotic fluid in the lungs.
- ☐ 2. Failure to breathe within the expected amount of time.
- ☐ 3. Sluggish peripheral circulation.
- ☐ 4. Increased estrogen levels in the mother.

71. What would Baby Daniel's stool look like at 1 week of age?
- ☐ 1. Black and tarry.
- ☐ 2. Green and seedy.
- ☐ 3. Light-yellow and mushy.
- ☐ 4. Bright-yellow and formed.

72. When testing a breastfed neonate for phenylketonuria, a false-negative result is most often the result of which condition?
- ☐ 1. Decreased vitamin K level.
- ☐ 2. Inadequate fluid intake.
- ☐ 3. Increased serum bilirubin.
- ☐ 4. Insufficient protein absorption.

73. In order to determine Baby Daniel's gestational age, the admitting nurse would assess which one of the following?
- ☐ 1. Body temperature.
- ☐ 2. Amount of vernix and lanugo.
- ☐ 3. Heart rate.
- ☐ 4. Degree of jaundice.

74. Baby Daniel has a core temperature of 100.4° F (38° C). The temperature of the Isolette reads 98° F (36.6° C). The neonate's elevated temperature is most probably a result of which of the following?
- ☐ 1. An infection.
- ☐ 2. The temperature of the Isolette.
- ☐ 3. A maternal infection.
- ☐ 4. A neonatal abnormality.

75. Baby Daniel is now 2 days old and weighs 7 pounds 9 ounces. He is voiding eight times a day and breastfeeds every 3 to 4 hours around-the-clock. Which nursing action would probably be appropriate at this time?
- ☐ 1. Consult with the physician about adding supplementary formula to his diet.
- ☐ 2. Weigh him before and after breastfeeding.
- ☐ 3. Continue to support his mother's breastfeeding efforts.
- ☐ 4. Observe him for signs of impending dehydration.

76. Baby Daniel is circumcised on the second postpartal day. Care of Baby Daniel within the first 4 hours would include which of the following?
- ☐ 1. Inspect the site every hour for signs of infection.
- ☐ 2. Monitor and record first voiding.
- ☐ 3. Withhold feeding immediately after the procedure.
- ☐ 4. Apply fresh, sterile gauze dressing to the penis with each diaper change.

77. Baby Daniel's bilirubin level rises to 12 mg, and he is placed on phototherapy. Which of the following assessments is the most important after phototherapy is initiated?
- ☐ 1. Appearance of the sclera.
- ☐ 2. Moro's reflex response.
- ☐ 3. Number and type of stools.
- ☐ 4. Daily weight.

Bert Arnold, age 36, is a sales representative for a large computer corporation. Three years ago, he was diagnosed as having an ulcer, and he was advised to find more time for rest and relaxation. He did not comply and, in the last month, has had more epigastric pain.

78. Which of the following would be the most realistic short-term goal to help Mr. Arnold begin to deal with his stress?
- ☐ 1. Express emotions directly.
- ☐ 2. Decrease work load.
- ☐ 3. Use relaxation techniques daily.
- ☐ 4. Decrease social commitments.

79. When Mr. Arnold's ulcer was diagnosed 3 years ago, his physician prescribed cimetidine (Tagamet). However, Mr. Arnold reports that he has not taken it. Which of the following approaches would be *least* effective in helping Mr. Arnold comply?
- ☐ 1. Help him set up a medical-reminder schedule.
- ☐ 2. Educate him about ulcer complications.
- ☐ 3. Suggest he enlist the help of his wife and co-workers.
- ☐ 4. Explain that taking the medication will help decrease his pain.

80. Perforation is a major complication of a duodenal ulcer. When this has occurred, what is the initial nursing priority?

☐ 1. Insert a nasogastric tube.
☐ 2. Start an IV for infusing fluids.
☐ 3. Administer a high dose of an antibiotic.
☐ 4. Teach turning, coughing, and deep-breathing.

81. Mr. Arnold is taught that he should not take any medications before checking with his physician, since there are many drugs that can aggravate his ulcer. An example of one of these drugs is which of the following?
☐ 1. Indomethacin (Indocin).
☐ 2. Magnesium and aluminum hydroxide (Maalox).
☐ 3. Atropine.
☐ 4. Acetaminophen (Tylenol).

Nine-month-old Bradley is admitted to the pediatric unit with vomiting, colicky abdominal pain, and abdominal distension. A tentative diagnosis of intussusception is made.

82. When assessing Bradley, which type of stool indicates a worsening of Bradley's condition?
☐ 1. Fatty, bulky, and foul-smelling.
☐ 2. Dark-red and jellylike.
☐ 3. Ribbonlike and dark-green.
☐ 4. Clay-colored.

83. Bradley is *not* likely to exhibit which of the following behaviors?
☐ 1. Loud crying when his parents leave him.
☐ 2. Fear of strangers.
☐ 3. Searching for hidden objects.
☐ 4. Saying at least three words besides "mama" and "dada."

84. Bradley is scheduled for surgery. His parents are anxious and ask what will be done in surgery. Which explanation would be given?
☐ 1. The sigmoid colon will be resected with a pull-through anastomosis.
☐ 2. The obstruction will be corrected by manual reduction.
☐ 3. The affected portion of the intestine will be resected with an end-to-end anastomosis.
☐ 4. The ileum will be resected and a permanent ileostomy created.

85. Bradley's parents ask what is wrong with his intestines. Which statement best describes Bradley's condition?
☐ 1. A telescoping of one part of the bowel into a more distal part.
☐ 2. Malrotation of the small intestine.
☐ 3. Atresia of the intestinal tract.
☐ 4. Absence of parasympathetic ganglion cells.

86. Preoperatively, the priority nursing goal for Bradley is to do which of the following?
☐ 1. Maintain Bradley's attachment to his parents.
☐ 2. Meet Bradley's needs for sucking and comfort while he is NPO.

☐ 3. Maintain adequate hydration.
☐ 4. Promote adequate rest and sleep.

87. Following surgery, Bradley returns to the unit. He is fussy and seems to be in discomfort. The nurse palpates his abdomen and notes some distension. Which action would be implemented first?
☐ 1. Call the surgeon to report this observation.
☐ 2. Insert a rectal tube.
☐ 3. Sit Bradley upright and pat him on the back.
☐ 4. Check the nasogastric tube for patency.

88. What is potentially the greatest threat to Bradley's continued development while he is hospitalized?
☐ 1. Developing mistrust of the nursing staff.
☐ 2. Separation from his parents.
☐ 3. Restricted mobility.
☐ 4. Disruption in his sleeping and eating routines.

89. Bradley is recovering well, and his IV and nasogastric tube have been discontinued. He is taking half-strength formula feedings. Assuming Bradley's development is average for his age, which toy would be most appropriate for him at this time?
☐ 1. An activity box for his crib.
☐ 2. A fuzzy stuffed animal.
☐ 3. A small toy truck.
☐ 4. A music box.

90. Bradley is ready for discharge. The nurse discusses his nutritional habits with his mother. Bradley has been taking a commercial iron-fortified formula and juices from a bottle, and he also has been eating cereal, strained fruits, and vegetables, which his parents feed him. Which anticipatory instruction is *not* appropriate to give Bradley's mother at this time?
☐ 1. Switch Bradley to whole milk, and give him supplemental vitamins and minerals.
☐ 2. Begin introducing chopped meats, egg yolk, and breads such as zwieback, one at a time, to Bradley's diet.
☐ 3. Introduce a cup for drinking juices and water.
☐ 4. Give Bradley foods that he can feed himself using his fingers or a spoon.

Robert Heil, age 55, is admitted to the hospital with complaints of nausea and vomiting and dull, wavelike abdominal pains. He appears malnourished and has a markedly enlarged abdomen. The physician suspects cirrhosis and has ordered a liver biopsy to make a definitive diagnosis.

91. The nurse charts the following observations of the admitting physical assessment. Which of the following would *not* be a symptom of cirrhosis?
☐ 1. Jaundiced sclera.
☐ 2. Irregular pulse.
☐ 3. Ascites.
☐ 4. Patches of ecchymosis in the extremities.

92. Why does Mr. Heil have a tendency to bleed as manifested by abnormal bruising?

☐ 1. Inadequate vitamin K absorption.

☐ 2. Inadequate vitamin A absorption.

☐ 3. Depressed production of platelets.

☐ 4. Depressed production of red blood cells.

93. What is the most appropriate nursing action for a client undergoing a liver biopsy?

☐ 1. Explain to the client that he may resume his bathroom privileges after the procedure.

☐ 2. Position the client in semi-Fowler's position for the procedure.

☐ 3. Turn the client on his left side following the procedure.

☐ 4. Assess the client for complaints of abdominal pain after the procedure for at least 24 hours.

94. Which of the following diets would the nurse encourage Mr. Heil to select in order to best meet his nutritional needs?

☐ 1. High-protein.

☐ 2. High-fat.

☐ 3. Low-calorie.

☐ 4. High-sodium.

95. What nursing action would best promote adequate respiratory function?

☐ 1. Instruct client to cough and deep-breathe qh.

☐ 2. Ambulate client frequently.

☐ 3. Maintain client in high-Fowler's position in bed.

☐ 4. Provide postural drainage and percussion q2h.

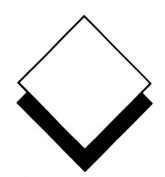

Test 2 Book II

ANSWERS WITH RATIONALES

KEY TO ABBREVIATIONS
Section of the Review Book

P = Psychosocial and Mental Health Problems
    T = Therapeutic Use of Self
    L = Loss and Death and Dying
    A = Anxious Behavior
    C = Confused Behavior
    E = Elated-Depressive Behavior
    SM = Socially Maladaptive Behavior
    SS = Suspicious Behavior
    W = Withdrawn Behavior
    SU = Substance Use Disorders
A = Adult
    H = Healthy Adult
    S = Surgery
    O = Oxygenation
    NM = Nutrition and Metabolism
    E = Elimination
    SP = Sensation and Perception
    M = Mobility
    CA = Cellular Aberration
CBF = Childbearing Family
    W = Women's Health Care
    A = Antepartal Care
    I = Intrapartal Care
    P = Postpartal Care
    N = Newborn Care
C = Child
    H = Healthy Child
    I = Ill and Hospitalized Child
    SPP = Sensation, Perception, and Protection
    O = Oxygenation
    NM = Nutrition and Metabolism
    E = Elimination
    M = Mobility
    CA = Cellular Aberration

Nursing Process Category

AS = Assessment
AN = Analysis
PL = Plan
IM = Implementation
EV = Evaluation

Client Need Category

E = Safe, Effective Care Environment
PS = Physiological Integrity
PC = Psychosocial Integrity
H = Health Promotion and Maintenance

1. no. 1. Obesity is a complex, multidimensional problem with many possible causes. One cause is that there tends to be a familial predisposition; children of obese parents tend to be obese. Food can also become a source of gratification or validation. Eating food often causes a person to feel warm, relaxed, and euphoric. Many people eat to cope with life's stresses. The most comprehensive and effective treatment of obesity combines an eating plan for weight loss, exercise, behavioral change, social support, and cognitive restructuring. Although exercise is a very important component of weight loss, it is not as effective as weight loss that occurs in combination with other therapies. Obesity in children tends to lead to obesity in adulthood because in children there is not only an increase in the size of fat cells, but an increase in their number as well. A/NM, AN, PS

2. no. 3. An upper gastrointestinal series and barium swallow must be done on an empty stomach. Food and fluids are withheld for several hours. Cleansing enemas are given before large-bowel exams. Radiopaque tablets are for gallbladder x-rays. A/NM, PL, PS

3. no. 3. A fasting specimen of hydrochloric acid is

used to obtain baseline data. Eating stimulates acid production. Because this test only assesses the pH of gastric juices, an enema is not required. The test will not cause cardiac alterations, so monitoring the pulse rate is not required. A/NM, PL, PS

4. no. 2. Peptic ulcers are directly related to high levels of hydrochloric acid. Option no. 1 is too vague. Lack of intrinsic factor results in anemia. Decreased motility is not related to ulcers. A/NM, AN, PS

5. no. 1. A tubeless gastric analysis (Diagnex Blue Test) is done to determine the presence or absence of hydrochloric acid in the stomach. It does not indicate the amount of free acid in the stomach. The presence of gastric ulcers is best determined through direct visualization (endoscopy, gastroscopy). The rate of gastric emptying is best determined with a gastric emptying scan. A/NM, AN, PS

6. no. 2. Ranitidine (Zantac) inhibits histamine at the H_2 receptor sites in the parietal cells. This in turn inhibits gastric acid secretion. Antacids (e.g., Maalox) neutralize acids in the stomach. Smooth muscle relaxants decrease motility. A/NM, AN, PS

7. no. 2. A vagotomy is done to eliminate the acid-secreting stimulus of the gastric cells. It has no effect on postoperative pain or stomach perfusion. A/NM, AN, PS

8. no. 3. Nausea and gagging may be due to kinks or a nonpatent tube, which can cause an increased volume of retained gastric secretions and pressure on the anastomosis. The risk of evisceration usually occurs later, once the sutures are removed. Option no. 4 may be a second action if there is an order. A/NM, IM, PS

9. no. 1. There is no attending organic pathological condition or actual loss of function. Clients with hypochondriasis will deny any relationship between their symptoms and their mental health. Hypochondriasis is not a psychotic disorder. P/A, AS, PC

10. no. 4. Anxieties are displaced onto the body in an effort to cope. Although hypochondriasis is a replacement of behavior, it does not produce adaptation. It is not a voluntary exclusion of anxiety from the conscious level as in suppression. Hypochondriacs do not attempt to justify their behavior, nor do they have a conscious understanding about their behavior. P/A, AN, PC

11. no. 4. Symptoms occur as an attempt to cope with stressful situations, and the ability to gain insight may decrease the need for secondary gain. Allowing her to talk about her physical symptoms provides secondary gain and reinforces continuing concern. Physical symptoms must be assessed and treated, not minimized or avoided. P/A, IM, PC

12. no. 4. A spontaneous bowel movement may be delayed until several days after delivery. Within 24

hours following delivery, the fundus should have begun involution and be located below the umbilicus. The breasts should be soft at this time since breast milk does not come in until 2 to 3 days after delivery. Lochia rubra is typical at this time. CBF/P, AS, PS

13. no. 2. The labia should not be separated because this would result in a greater possibility of introducing microorganisms. Clean tap water may be used for perineal care, but sterile water is not necessary. Perineal care is carried out even if an episiotomy was not performed in order to decrease microorganisms. CBF/P, IM, E

14. no. 2. To prevent nipple cracking, air drying after each nursing period is suggested. Soap and alcohol cause drying of the nipples, increasing the chance of skin breakdown. Breastfeeding is begun gradually by starting with 3 minutes on each breast. CBF/P, EV, H

15. no. 4. The mother begins to be the initiator in the taking-hold phase. Her early mothering tasks are especially important to her. This is considered the optimal time for teaching. CBF/P, AS, PC

16. no. 3. It is safe to resume sexual intercourse by the third or fourth week if bleeding has stopped and the episiotomy has healed. Most couples resume intercourse before the 6-week checkup. CBF/P, IM, H

17. no. 3. This is another sign of endometritis. Lochia would have a red-brown color and may be either foul-smelling or odorless. An increase in thirst is most likely a result of dehydration. Diastasis recti is separation of the abdominal muscle as a result of weakened muscles. CBF/P, AS, PS

18. no. 3. This is a basic principle when approaching a client for the first time. It establishes rapport and communicates respect for the individual. The other three options will be done after introductions are made. A/O, IM, PC

19. no. 4. When applying electrodes, an assessment using touch can be done concurrently to determine skin and muscle conditions. Level of consciousness and orientation are assessed when evaluating her response to the explanation of electrode application. Cardiac output is determined by actual monitoring, either noninvasively by blood pressure or invasively by arterial line or central line (e.g., Swan-Ganz). A/O, AS, PS

20. no. 3. Stress, severe pain, and hyperthyroidism are causes of tachycardia. Sinus bradycardia in clients over age 65 is usually a result of medications, especially digoxin. Remember that digitalis toxicity can also result in a heart rate greater than 100 beats per minute. A/O, AN, PS

21. no. 2. Bradycardia results in a decrease in cardiac output; therefore all nursing activity would be directed at maintaining the best possible cardiac output. Options no. 1 and no. 3 are related to this primary goal. Maintaining close contact with significant others is important, but it does not receive priority over maintaining cardiac output. A/O, PL, E

22. no. 1. A planned, systematic approach to client teaching is essential when a major alteration in activities of daily living and life-style will be the outcome of an illness. Options no. 2 and no. 3 are assumptions that cannot be made. Client education is a shared responsibility. A/O, PL, E

23. no. 4. Excess arm movement and arm raising should be avoided for 5 weeks after the insertion of the pacemaker. The incision should be assessed q30min for bleeding. Dizziness, light-headedness, and chest pain are all signs of pacemaker failure and should be monitored. A pacing spike or artifact is a vertical line that appears on the ECG each time the pulse generator fires an impulse. A/O, IM, PS

24. no. 4. Permanently implanted pacemakers require no physical or technical care. Teaching must focus on any adjustments to be made in activities of daily living and of recreation (e.g., no contact sports). A/O, PL, E

25. no. 4. The major and potentially most serious effect of chronic lead poisoning is neurological. Therefore frequent assessment of neurological status is imperative. C/SPP, AS, PS

26. no. 4. Allowing Bobby and Tina to room together will promote security for each of them because they are familiar with each other. C/SPP, IM, PC

27. no. 3. EDTA is potentially toxic to the kidneys and can cause damage that can result in oliguria. C/SPP, AS, PS

28. no. 3. In the toddler, EDTA and BAL should be administered intramuscularly in the anterolateral thigh (vastus lateralis muscle). C/SPP, IM, PS

29. no. 2. This tells Bobby what is expected of him but also gives him an outlet for his fears. The other options either increase fear or belittle him. C/SPP, IM, PC

30. no. 3. The family's income level has no bearing on the risk of lead poisoning. If the family lives in an old house, there may be lead paint chips. Any history of pica is important to ascertain. Also, if the children are not properly supervised in a potentially unsafe environment, the risk of lead poisoning is increased. C/SPP, AS, H

31. no. 1. This menu is highest in vitamin D, calcium, and phosphorus, which are needed to aid in excreting lead from the bones. C/SPP, IM, H

32. no. 4. Lead does not interfere with platelet production or bleeding and clotting mechanisms. C/SPP, AN, PS

33. no. 3. Achievement of age-appropriate developmen-

tal milestones indicates there has been no permanent neurological damage. C/SPP, EV, H

34. no. 4. An exaggeration of personality traits determines the behaviors exhibited in chronic organic brain syndrome. There is no correlation between the amount of brain damage and amount of alcohol ingested to the severity of psychological symptoms. The degree of orientation the client shows at the time of admission may change for the better or worse. P/C, AS, PC

35. no. 3. Deterioration in knowledge of time occurs first, then confusion of place, and finally, confusion of person. P/C, AS, PC

36. no. 4. It is beneficial to reinforce reality by providing structure and order in as many areas of the client's life as possible. In coordinating the client's schedule, it is important to avoid excessive stimulation and variations, which might only serve to confuse the client further. Making numerous introductions may be futile because of the client's loss of memory for recent events. P/C, IM, PC

37. no. 2. Confabulation is a process whereby experiences are imagined to fill in memory blanks. It is a form of protection against anxiety. Amnesia is loss or lack of memory. Flashbacks are a sudden sense of "reliving" past experiences, especially those which were painful or traumatic. Free association is a process whereby the client is encouraged to describe thoughts or feelings as they occur. P/C, IM, PC

38. no. 3. Continued contact is important for both father and son. The client with organic brain syndrome will be aware of a caring person even though he may not always display recognition. Although it is true that Mr. Caliente is probably disoriented by his new surroundings, chances are that he will still not know his son or any other family members tomorrow because of the nature of organic brain syndrome. P/C, IM, H

39. no. 3. Poor memory of recent events is common in this condition. Circumstantiality is a symptom whereby the client introduces into the conversation details which have little if anything to do with the conversation. It is possible that manipulation is part of the client's normal coping skills, but it is more likely that the client is confused rather than manipulative. Retardation of thought refers to a slowing down of thought processes. P/C, AN, PC

40. no. 4. Incontinence may occur frequently in a client with this syndrome. The nurse needs to demonstrate understanding as well as institute nursing measures that will decrease its incidence. Options no. 1, no. 2, and no. 3 convey a lack of understanding of organic brain syndrome, plus an unnecessary annoyance with the client that is nontherapeutic. He will probably be unable to work with the nurse to dis-

cover how to prevent his incontinence or change his clothes and clean up. P/C, IM, PC

41. no. 2. Encouraging clients to reminisce is valuable in maintaining their sense of value. It also helps decrease feelings of isolation and promotes a sense of continuity. Options no. 1, no. 3, and no. 4 reflect his disorientation; the nurse should not "play along" with the client but, rather, reorient him to the present. P/C, IM, PC

42. no. 4. Local anesthesia is used for this procedure; testing for the gag reflex is necessary to prevent aspiration. Although urine output, respiratory patterns, and level of consciousness are always important to monitor, the endoscopy does not directly cause any alterations in these functions. A/NM, PL, E

43. no. 1. The gastric outlet is attached to low intermittent suction to drain blood from the gastrointestinal system. As long as there are bloody returns in the aspirate, iced lavage is continued. Traction is maintained for a time to ensure control of bleeding. It should not be maintained longer than 72 hours, or esophageal necrosis may result. A/NM, PL, E

44. no. 4. Of the options listed, only the sulfobromophthalein test measures liver excretory function. This is a dye-clearance study. Alkaline phosphatase (ALP) is a liver enzyme that is increased in obstructive biliary disease and liver dysfunctions. The albumin-globulin ratio measures the liver's ability to synthesize these proteins. The prothrombin time assesses the liver's ability to synthesize factor VII. A/NM, AS, PS

45. no. 4. Increased hydrostatic pressure from portal hypertension and the diminished synthesis of albumin by the liver result in ascites. The inability of the liver to break down aldosterone also contributes to the process. Thus increased aldosterone levels result in sodium reabsorption. A/NM, AN, PS

46. no. 4. Spironolactone (Aldactone) would be the first choice because its action is to block aldosterone, which the liver cannot detoxify. In addition, spironolactone is potassium sparing. A/NM, AN, PS

47. no. 3. The operation diverts the blood from the portal circulation, thus decreasing some of the portal hypertension. It cannot prevent bleeding, nor does it facilitate liver regeneration. A/NM, AN, PS

48. no. 4. Any opening in the skin is a portal of entry for bacteria. Cooling measures will do nothing to decrease or prevent infection and generally will not be initiated until the temperature has gone above 101° F (38.3° C) or 102° F (38.8° C). Only visitors who are obviously ill with an infectious disorder should be discouraged from visiting. Ambulation will reduce many postoperative complications that can lead to infection. A/NM, IM, E

49. no. 3. In Mr. Reynolds, encephalopathy is likely to develop because of his recent bleeding. Neomycin is given to decrease the ammonia production in the intestines from the breakdown of blood. Increased ammonia levels are believed to bring on symptoms of hepatic encephalopathy. Asterixis (liver flap or liver tremor) and confusion are associated with hepatic encephalopathy. A CT scan is not required because the symptoms indicate a metabolic origin, not structural damage. Sodium should be restricted in clients with liver disease becaue of the risk of ascites. Diazepam (Valium) is contraindicated because it is metabolized by the liver. It will also increase Mr. Reynold's confusion. A/NM, AN, PS

50. no. 4. She needs an opportunity to express feelings and receive some support. Eventually she will need to discuss things with her father. Options no. 1 and no. 2 do not give the daughter an opportunity to express her feelings. A/NM, IM, PC

51. no. 3. Frequently, nurses have been directly or indirectly affected by problems associated with alcohol and are not able to assist the client in a helping manner until they discern their own attitudes. After the nurse is able to explore his or her own feelings about alcoholism, then options no. 1, no. 2, and no. 4 would be appropriate. A/NM, IM, PC

52. no. 4. Turning the head to locate sounds should be present before 4 months of age. All other options are age appropriate. C/H, AS, H

53. no. 3. Immunizations should be postponed if the child has a febrile illness. This is a nursing decision. The child's symptoms do not warrant referral to a physician at this time. C/H, IM, PS

54. no. 3. The extrusion reflex is present until approximately 4 months of age. Although the infant may be hungry, she cannot bring solids to the back of her mouth yet. The child will outgrow this with practice. Altering eating patterns or foods because of this may establish poor feeding habits. C/H, IM, H

55. no. 1. After 7 months of age, stranger anxiety sets in and makes separation from parents very difficult. C/H, AN, H

56. no. 2. This game teaches a sense of object permanence, which gradually develops from 4 to 8 months. The other activities listed are more appropriate for older ages. C/H, PL, H

57. no. 2. Accidents are the second leading cause of death in Emalee's age group. C/H, AN, E

58. no. 3. Even the most withdrawn client is very sensitive to what others are feeling, even though they themselves communicate very little verbally and may be unaware of their feelings. Clients diagnosed with paranoid schizophrenia generally demonstrate social isolation related to impaired ability to trust and are unreceptive to receiving attention from others. Response to treatment is generally slow be-

cause of the client's protectiveness and impaired ability to trust. Electroconvulsive therapy is most successfully used with depressed clients and is usually not effective in disrupting psychosis. P/W, AS, PC

59. no. 3. Auditory hallucinations are the most common. Hallucinations temporarily decrease anxiety by delaying interaction with someone real. Delusion is a fixed, false belief that may be persecutory, grandiose, or somatic in nature and cannot be corrected with reasoning. Illusion is a misinterpretation of a real sensory experience. Loose association is a communication pattern characterized by lack of clarity of connection between one thought and the next. P/W, AN, PC

60. no. 2. This statement points out reality but acknowledges the feelings of the client. The other options reinforce the reality that the nurse does not perceive the voices. No. 1 focuses attention on and gives importance to the voices, no. 3 avoids discussing the client's feelings, and no. 4 will escalate the client's anxiety level and make him more committed to the hallucinations. P/W, IM, PC

61. no. 4. The private reality of the schizophrenic is derived from internal ideas and desires not shared by others. Adaptation is the capability of the body or mind to cope with any type of increased demand made upon it. Ambivalence is having simultaneous conflicting feelings or attitudes toward a person or object. Apathy is a lack of interest and concern. P/W, AN, PC

62. no. 2. An idea of reference is a belief that certain events or statements relate directly to the individual when they do not. Idea of influence refers to an individual's feeling as though he or she has influence over other individuals. Introjection is a type of identification in which the client incorporates qualities or values of another person or group into his or her own ego structure. Labeling is describing or designating something with a label. P/W, AN, PC

63. no. 1. Changes in blood pressure are common with this drug. Instruct clients to rise slowly from a sitting or lying position. The other options are all noted side effects of phenothiazines; however, the most common side effect is orthostatic hypotension resulting from the interference with dopamine reception or synthesis at the neural synapse. P/W, AS, PS

64. no. 2. Akathisia is evidenced by motor restlessness. Akinesia is a lethargic, subjective sense of fatigue and muscle weakness that is a side effect of antipsychotic medication. Catatonia is a state of psychologically induced immobility at times interrupted by episodes of agitation. Dyskinesia is associated with the long-term use of high-dose phenothiazine drugs

and is characterized by involuntary, jerking, and uncoordinated movements. P/W, AN, PS

65. no. 1. Benztropine mesylate (Cogentin) is effective in relieving the symptoms of parkinsonism caused by antipsychotic medications. This is an appropriate dosage and can be given parenterally if indicated. Trihexyphenidyl (Artane) is another good antiparkinson drug; however, the dose is 5 mg bid, not 15 mg. The use of a benzodiazepine (e.g., Librium or Valium) is not appropriate because these drugs do not have a direct effect on the extrapyramidal system. P/W, AN, PS

66. no. 4. Fluphenazine is used parenterally every 7 to 21 days for outpatients. The other statements are false. Fluphenazine has a mild anticholinergic sedating effect and extrapyramidal effect. Tolerance and addiction to antipsychotics are not substantiated in the literature, although mild withdrawal symptoms (e.g., headaches, irritability, and nausea) can occur upon rapid discontinuation. P/W, AN, PS

67. no. 1. Milieu therapy provides the opportunity to improve the physical and emotional condition of the client by providing positive living experiences. The other options are an integral part of milieu therapy but not the overall goal. P/W, PL, E

68. no. 2. Family therapy is helpful to improve communication and acceptance of differences among members. The cause of schizophrenia is unknown. Family therapy in conjunction with drug therapy could prevent rehospitalization. Schizophrenia is not known to be inherited; however, Mr. Hindricks' children could benefit from family therapy. P/W, PL, H

69. no. 2. Ophthalmia neonatorum is an eye disease of infants that causes blindness. It is passed from mother to infant through a birth canal infected with gonorrhea. Silver nitrate or penicillin drops prevent this. CBF/NR, AN, PS

70. no. 3. Acrocyanosis (blue hands and feet) is due to poor peripheral circulation. CBF/NR, AN, PS

71. no. 3. When breastfed, an infant's stool is light-yellow and mushy. Stools go through a transitional process from black meconium in the first 24 hours to a greenish-yellow (transitional) color to a breastfed or bottlefed stool on the fifth day of life. CBF/NR, AS, PS

72. no. 4. Phenylalanine is an amino acid found in milk. Often the mother's breast milk is not sufficiently established at the time of testing to give an accurate result. Therefore it may be necessary to retest the infant later. CBF/NR, AN, PS

73. no. 2. The amount of vernix and lanugo decreases with increasing gestational age. Term infants usually have vernix only in the skin creases, and lanugo tends to be found only over the shoulders. Deter-

mining gestational age by physical examination most often involves the Dubowitz assessment, which provides the correct gestational age within 2 weeks (in 95% of infants). CBF/NR, AS, PS

74. no. 2. An Isolette should be maintained at a temperature of 92° to 94° F (33.3° to 34.4° C). An infection in the neonate, not the mother, may be accompanied by an elevated or subnormal temperature. CBF/NR, AS, PS

75. no. 3. Newborns lose up to 10% of their birth weight in the first few days after birth. Since this is expected weight loss, support the mother in her efforts to breastfeed. The normal neonate will void six to ten times a day. This is indicative of adequate hydration. CBF/NR, IM, PS

76. no. 2. Voiding is monitored to determine if edema from the surgical trauma has closed off the urethra. Feeding the baby who has just been circumcised is comforting and essential, since it is recommended that feedings be withheld for several hours before the procedure. The penis is checked hourly for bleeding; infection would not appear until much later. A sterile petrolatum-jelly dressing rather than dry gauze should be used on the newly circumcised penis to prevent it from sticking to the diaper. CBF/NR, IM, PS

77. no. 3. Phototherapy may result in dehydration. Watery stools are common. Fluid loss is replaced by increasing the fluid volume offered to the neonate by 25%. CBF/NR, AS, PS

78. no. 3. All the other options are appropriate for Mr. Arnold, but immediately using relaxation techniques can be very beneficial. A/NM, PL, PC

79. no. 2. Information about the complications of ulcer may not be helpful. He has not experienced the complications, so he can use denial and choose not to comply. A/NM, IM, PC

80. no. 2. Hypovolemic shock can occur very quickly following a perforation, so fluid replacement must be done first and quickly. Options no. 1, no. 3, and no. 4 are all appropriate once the client is safe and stable. The client initially should be maintained in semi-Fowler's position to localize the gastric contents to one area of the peritoneum. After surgical repair, turning, coughing, and deep-breathing would be appropriate. A/NM, IM, PS

81. no. 1. Indomethacin (Indocin) is very irritating to the stomach and duodenum and can cause or aggravate ulcers. Magnesium and aluminum hydroxide (Maalox) is an antacid that will help, not aggravate, the ulcer. Acetaminophen (Tylenol) is a nonnarcotic, nonsalicylate analgesic that will not aggravate ulcers. Atropine is an anticholinergic drug that decreases gastric secretions. A/NM, AN, PS

82. no. 2. Dark-red, "currant jelly" stools indicate the onset of bowel necrosis from gangrene. C/E, AS, PS

83. no. 4. The average 9-month-old infant may be able to say "mama" or "dada" but has not learned to articulate other words yet. C/H, AS, H

84. no. 3. Only the affected portion of the intestine is resected, and an end-to-end anastomosis of the remaining healthy intestinal segments is done. C/E, IM, E

85. no. 1. Intussusception is the telescoping or invagination of one part of the intestine into a more distal portion. C/E, IM, PS

86. no. 3. Although all these goals are important, Bradley is especially at risk for dehydration and electrolyte imbalance because of vomiting associated with intussusception. C/E, PL, E

87. no. 4. The nasogastric tube may be obstructed, causing the abdominal distension. Inserting a rectal tube is contraindicated because Bradley has had lower intestinal tract surgery. C/E, IM, E

88. no. 2. Separation anxiety begins at about 8 months of age and can cause extreme distress for the infant in this age group. C/E, AN, H

89. no. 1. An activity box will promote continued development of fine motor skills and hand-eye coordination and allow Bradley some activity within the confines of his hospital crib. C/E, IM, H

90. no. 1. Infants should not be switched to whole milk (or 2% low-fat milk) until 1 year of age. C/E, IM, H

91. no. 2. An irregular pulse is characteristic of a disturbance of electrical stimulation or conduction in the heart. This is more commonly found in clients with heart disease. Jaundice occurs when bilirubin accumulates in the skin, sclerae, and other tissues in the body. This relates to obstruction of the bile ducts and liver cells. Edema occurs from decreasing plasma protein levels and increasing portal pressure. In addition, sodium is retained as a result of aldosterone retention. Ecchymosis occurs with vitamin K deficiency from fat malabsorption and defective synthesis of factors II, VII, IX, and X. A/NM, AS, PS

92. no. 1. Clients with liver disease have an increased tendency to bleed. This is caused either by a failure to absorb vitamin K or because the liver is unable to use vitamin K to form prothrombin. If the client's bile duct is obstructed, absorption of vitamin K is reduced. Even if vitamin K is absorbed, damaged liver cells cannot synthesize adequate amounts. A/NM, AN, PS

93. no. 4. A complication of this procedure is accidental penetration of a blood vessel, causing hemorrhage, or penetration of a biliary vessel, causing chemical peritonitis from the leakage of bile into the abdom-

inal cavity. These complications would be manifested as abdominal pain and unstable vital signs. Pressure to the biopsy site can be applied by positioning the client on his right side after the procedure. Strict bed rest is prescribed for the client for 24 hours after the procedure. A/NM, PL, E

94. no. 1. Cellular function in the liver depends upon tissue-building materials supplied by amino acids derived from proteins. Clients with liver disease with no evidence of encephalopathy need high-protein, high-calorie, low-sodium diets. A/NM, PL, PS

95. no. 3. Clients with ascites experience dyspnea, resulting from pressure exerted against the diaphragm. High-Fowler's position reduces this pressure. The client needs rest to reduce metabolic demands on the liver and should keep activities to a minimum by resting quietly in bed most of the day. A/NM, IM, PS

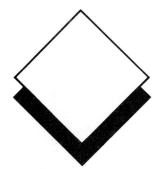

Test 2, Book III

QUESTIONS

Monica Corley enters the labor and delivery unit at 40 weeks' gestation. Her cervix is 2 cm dilated and 80% effaced. Her contractions are 3 to 5 minutes apart and are associated with mild discomfort.

1. Based upon the information presented, the labor room nurse determines that Mrs. Corley is in which phase of labor?
   - ☐ 1. First stage, latent phase.
   - ☐ 2. First stage, active phase.
   - ☐ 3. First stage, deceleration phase.
   - ☐ 4. Second stage of labor.

2. Mrs. Corley is restless and complaining of severe pain. Her cervix is 5 cm dilated and 90% effaced. The vertex is at 0 station. She requests pain medication, and the physician has ordered meperidine (Demerol), 75 mg. Which of the following nursing actions is most appropriate?
   - ☐ 1. Give her the meperidine (Demerol), since it is an optimal time to do so.
   - ☐ 2. Try to have her wait until her cervix is at least 6 cm dilated and the vertex is at 1+ station.
   - ☐ 3. Tell her the meperidine (Demerol) will cause her baby to be "sleepy" when it is born.
   - ☐ 4. Give her one half dose of the medication.

3. The medication contains 100 mg of meperidine/ml. How many milliliters will the nurse administer?
   - ☐ 1. 1.0 ml.
   - ☐ 2. 0.5 ml.
   - ☐ 3. 0.75 ml.
   - ☐ 4. 1.5 ml.

4. Which of the following principles accurately explains the effects on the fetus of analgesics and anesthetics administered to the mother during the intrapartum period?
   - ☐ 1. Medication effects are generally negligible if they are administered 2 or more hours before delivery.
   - ☐ 2. Medication effects are related to the duration of labor.
   - ☐ 3. Medication effects are time, dose, and route related.
   - ☐ 4. Medication effects are related to maternal age and weight.

5. What is the primary rationale for administering an antacid during labor?
   - ☐ 1. To settle the laboring mother's stomach.
   - ☐ 2. To increase digestion during labor.
   - ☐ 3. To prevent pneumonia in case of aspiration during general anesthesia.
   - ☐ 4. To lower the pH of the blood in cases of possible hyperventilation.

6. Mrs. Corley states she heard someone say her baby is "ROP" and asks what that means. What would be the nurse's best response?
   - ☐ 1. "Your baby is fine. Those initials simply refer to the baby's position in the birth canal."
   - ☐ 2. "ROP stands for right occiput posterior. This means your baby is head down, with the back of its head pointing toward your right flank."
   - ☐ 3. "ROP means your baby is bottom down and turned the opposite direction from the way most babies are turned. This does not mean you will not be able to deliver vaginally."
   - ☐ 4. "ROP stands for right orbital presentation. This means your baby's head is extended and will need to flex before delivery can be completed."

7. In planning care for Mrs. Corley, the nurse will need to take into account the typical consequences of fetal malpresentation. Which of the following consequences is most pertinent to the care of Mrs. Corley?
   - ☐ 1. Malpresentation frequently slows the dilatation of the cervix.
   - ☐ 2. Malpresentation does not increase the risk of fetal trauma when the head is the presenting part.

☐ 3. Because labor is more efficient in multiparas, malpresentation does not have a significant impact on the effectiveness of the contractions.

☐ 4. Regardless of presentation, the cardinal movements of labor remain the same.

Mary Smith is brought to the emergency room by a friend. Mrs. Smith is tense, shaking, and pale. When the nurse touches her to guide her to a chair, the nurse notes that Mrs. Smith's skin is cool and clammy. The friend reports that Mrs. Smith is a graduate student at the university and that she has been preparing for her oral examinations for her doctoral degree. When the nurse asks Mrs. Smith how she is feeling, Mrs. Smith says, "How do you think I feel?" She bursts into tears, then says, "I'm sorry. I'm just so scared. I feel like something awful is about to happen to me."

8. What level of anxiety is the client experiencing?
☐ 1. Mild.
☐ 2. Moderate.
☐ 3. Severe.
☐ 4. Panic.

9. What is the most appropriate immediate goal for the nurse to set for the client?
☐ 1. The client will develop a trusting relationship with the nurse.
☐ 2. The client will gain insight into her problems.
☐ 3. The client will demonstrate alternate methods of coping.
☐ 4. The client will reduce anxiety at least one level.

10. Which of the following is appropriate to try with Mrs. Smith in her current state?
☐ 1. Recognize and reflect the feelings the client is experiencing, and indicate that the nurse will be there to help her.
☐ 2. Leave her alone until she feels more like being around other persons.
☐ 3. Reassure her that nothing bad is going to happen to her.
☐ 4. Encourage her to act out anxiety by moving around or to express her feelings verbally.

11. When the physician on duty sees Mrs. Smith, she orders 5 mg of diazepam (Valium) IM and asks the nurse to stay with the client until she becomes less anxious. When the nurse prepares to administer the medication, Mrs. Smith becomes more agitated and says, "You're not going to make a junkie out of me!" Which of the following is the best response?
☐ 1. "The doctor wouldn't have ordered something that was going to hurt you. You need this to calm down."
☐ 2. "It might help you calm down, but I won't give it to you without your permission."
☐ 3. "No one is trying to turn you into a junkie. You are so upset that you are confused."

☐ 4. "You can't become a junkie from just one shot. Please let me give you this shot to help you."

12. When Mrs. Smith's friend urges her to take the medication, she consents to do so. Which of the following would be the best way to begin interviewing Mrs. Smith?
☐ 1. "How do you usually cope with anxiety?"
☐ 2. "You must be really upset about your doctoral work."
☐ 3. "Tell me about what was happening in your life when you started feeling anxious."
☐ 4. "What can I do to help you?"

13. About 30 minutes after the diazepam was administered, Mrs. Smith asks to lie down because she feels dizzy and faint. Which of the following is the most likely cause of these symptoms?
☐ 1. Her level of anxiety.
☐ 2. An allergic response to the drug.
☐ 3. Common side effects of the drug.
☐ 4. Her state of exhaustion.

Jorge Benton is a newborn with a bilateral cleft lip and a cleft palate.

14. Jorge's parents are young but seem very concerned and willing to learn about his care. Which of the following would be *inappropriate* to include in the teaching plan for the parents?
☐ 1. Remove the nipple frequently when feeding Jorge.
☐ 2. Encourage mother to breastfeed.
☐ 3. Jorge's security needs can be met in other ways besides sucking.
☐ 4. Jorge's mental functioning should be normal.

15. When Jorge is 10 weeks old, he is hospitalized for repair of his cleft lip. Preoperatively, which of the following nursing actions is most important for Jorge?
☐ 1. Burp him frequently during feedings.
☐ 2. Offer him small, frequent feedings to avoid tiring him.
☐ 3. Hold him in a low or flat position to facilitate swallowing.
☐ 4. Offer thickened bottle feedings to increase his intake.

16. When Jorge is 13 months old, he is admitted for repair of his cleft palate. What is the best reason for the palate to be repaired at this age?
☐ 1. To give Jorge a chance to develop basic speech patterns.
☐ 2. To prevent damaging tooth buds.
☐ 3. To allow better postoperative cooperation from Jorge.
☐ 4. So Jorge can be weaned from breastfeeding.

17. Jorge's long-range nursing care plans would include

follow-up and referral for several potential problems. Which of the following problems will Jorge's mother be most likely to observe?

☐ 1. Headaches and malocclusion.
☐ 2. Dental caries and emotional problems.
☐ 3. Contractures of the mandible.
☐ 4. Speech problems and otitis media.

Ann Duke, age 60, is admitted to the hospital after complaining of right-sided weakness, slurring of speech, dysphagia, and some visual disturbances. She has a history of hypertension. The admitting diagnosis is a cerebrovascular accident.

18. What is the most probable cause of the admitting symptoms?

☐ 1. Transient ischemic attack (TIA).
☐ 2. Cerebral aneurysm.
☐ 3. Cerebral hemorrhage.
☐ 4. Meningitis.

19. The client has positive Babinski's reflex. This is indicated by which of the following?

☐ 1. Dorsiflexion of the great toe with plantar stimulation.
☐ 2. Tremor of the foot following brisk, forceful dorsiflexion.
☐ 3. Extension of the leg when the patellar tendon is struck.
☐ 4. Plantar flexion of the great toe with plantar stimulation.

20. Mrs. Duke is incontinent during the first few days of her hospitalization. What would be the most satisfactory means of handling this problem?

☐ 1. Insert an indwelling catheter.
☐ 2. Offer a bedpan q4h.
☐ 3. Offer a bedpan q2h.
☐ 4. Apply disposable diapers and restrict fluids.

21. While the nurse is bathing Mrs. Duke, she begins to mutter something unintelligible about the "plant," while pointing excitedly at a glass of water on the bedside stand. She indicates in pantomime that she wants a drink of water. This behavioral observation is most characteristic of which of the following types of aphasia?

☐ 1. Visual.
☐ 2. Hysterical.
☐ 3. Receptive.
☐ 4. Expressive.

22. This type of aphasia occurs when the injury is in the speech center. Where in the brain is the speech center located?

☐ 1. Medulla oblongata.
☐ 2. Around the central fissure (Broca's area).
☐ 3. Occipital lobe.
☐ 4. Parietal lobe.

23. What would be the most therapeutic nursing approach when Mrs. Duke's expressive aphasia is severe?

☐ 1. Anticipate her wishes so she will not need to talk.
☐ 2. Communicate by means of questions that can be answered by shaking her head.
☐ 3. Keep up a steady flow of talk to minimize her silence.
☐ 4. Encourage her to speak at every possible opportunity.

24. When Mrs. Duke is attempting to speak, she becomes frustrated. Her family asks how to deal with this problem. What is the best advice?

☐ 1. They should continue to encourage her.
☐ 2. They should realize it may be their frustration rather than Mrs. Duke's frustration.
☐ 3. They can help by anticipating her needs more.
☐ 4. Be patient with her, and do not expect too much progress at this time.

25. Mrs. Duke still has some dysphagia, but she is beginning to eat solid foods. What is the most important aspect when helping her to eat?

☐ 1. Use a bulb syringe when giving fluids.
☐ 2. Praise her consistently if she can feed herself.
☐ 3. Keep her positioned in semi-Fowler's position.
☐ 4. Allow her to attempt to feed herself.

26. Mr. Duke asks if his wife's right arm and leg will always be paralyzed. Which of the following is the nurse's answer primarily based upon?

☐ 1. Much of the initial paralysis is due to edema of brain tissue.
☐ 2. Strokes are characterized by functional, rather than organic, changes.
☐ 3. New neurons will be regenerated to replace the damaged ones.
☐ 4. Her future neurological status cannot be predicted this early.

27. When is the best time to begin an active rehabilitation program for Mrs. Duke?

☐ 1. When the physician orders it.
☐ 2. 24 hours after the critical phase of the illness.
☐ 3. When the client is medically stable.
☐ 4. When the entire health team can meet and decide on a comprehensive program.

28. Which one of the following would be considered most vital to success or failure of a rehabilitation program?

☐ 1. Physicians.
☐ 2. Nursing staff.
☐ 3. Significant others or family members.
☐ 4. Physical therapist.

29. Mrs. Duke has been taking anticoagulant medication. She will be discharged on a regimen of warfarin (Coumadin), 10 mg daily. What instructions would her family receive?

☐ 1. Ensure that weekly partial thromboplastin times (PTT) are done.

☐ 2. Eat foods that are high in vitamin K.

☐ 3. Check Mrs. Duke's skin daily.

☐ 4. Expect to see pink urine for several days.

Sally, age 2 years, has eczema.

30. In which age group is eczema most frequently seen?

☐ 1. Infancy.

☐ 2. Childhood.

☐ 3. Adolescence.

☐ 4. It is seen equally in all age groups.

31. The primary objective of nursing care of the infant or child with eczema is which of the following?

☐ 1. Treatment of pruritus.

☐ 2. Identification of the allergen.

☐ 3. Giving treated baths.

☐ 4. Education for diet regimen.

32. Sally's parents say she is irritable and does not sleep well. What is the most likely cause of Sally's irritability and lack of sleep?

☐ 1. Pruritus.

☐ 2. Pain.

☐ 3. Teething.

☐ 4. Hunger.

33. When planning to give Sally a bath, which of the following baths would the nurse recommend?

☐ 1. Warm water and soap.

☐ 2. Cool water and soap.

☐ 3. Tepid water only.

☐ 4. Warm water with lipid soap.

34. Which activity would be most appropriate for Sally?

☐ 1. Playing with clay.

☐ 2. Naming pictures in a book or magazine.

☐ 3. Building a column with plastic building blocks.

☐ 4. Drawing pictures of familiar objects with crayons.

35. When instructing Sally's parents about skin care at home, which of the following instructions is *not* appropriate?

☐ 1. Provide a cool, dry environment.

☐ 2. Wear wool clothing in the winter.

☐ 3. Rinse clothes twice during washing.

☐ 4. Keep nails short.

36. Which of the following responses indicates that Sally's parents do *not* fully understand how to prevent their daughter's scratching?

☐ 1. "Sally wears elbow restraints when we can't directly supervise her."

☐ 2. "Sometimes Sally wears cotton gloves so she won't irritate her rash."

☐ 3. "We've been dressing her in one-piece outfits."

☐ 4. "Sally wears close-fitting clothes."

37. To help Sally's parents promote her nutrition, which of the following observations indicates a need for teaching?

☐ 1. Sally is fed after her rest period.

☐ 2. She takes vitamin and mineral supplements.

☐ 3. Her parents occasionally allow her to have a favorite restricted food to encourage her eating.

☐ 4. Sally's parents allow her to feed herself.

38. Sally is placed on a hypoallergenic diet. Which of the following foods is *least* likely to be allowed?

☐ 1. Turkey.

☐ 2. Soy milk.

☐ 3. Pancakes.

☐ 4. Peaches.

Renata Jones is a 44-year-old woman whose divorce was final 2 months ago. She is having trouble sleeping, is unable to eat, and reports having very little energy. She has been having trouble taking care of her house.

39. The symptoms that Mrs. Jones describes are most likely a manifestation of which of the following?

☐ 1. Depression.

☐ 2. Anxiety.

☐ 3. Psychosis.

☐ 4. Paranoia.

40. Which of the following is the most appropriate goal for Mrs. Jones?

☐ 1. The client will be free of signs of suspicious behavior after 1 month.

☐ 2. The client will resume activities of daily living within 1 month.

☐ 3. The client will be able to distinguish between what is real and what is not real within 2 weeks.

☐ 4. The client will demonstrate more calm and rational behavior within 2 weeks.

41. Which of the following best explains Mrs. Jones' symptoms?

☐ 1. She has lost a sense of reality orientation.

☐ 2. Her symptoms result from stimulation of the sympathetic nervous system related to high stress levels.

☐ 3. She lacks a feeling of trust in people.

☐ 4. She is angry about the loss of her relationships and is internalizing the anger.

42. During an interview with the nurse, Mrs. Jones begins to cry. The appropriate nursing response is which of the following?

☐ 1. "Don't cry, Mrs. Jones. You'll feel better in a day or so."

☐ 2. Leave her alone, and check on her in 15 minutes.

☐ 3. "This sounds like a difficult time for you, Mrs. Jones."

☐ 4. Force her to talk and reveal her feelings.

43. Mrs. Jones appears to be feeling much better the next day when the nurse talks with her. Mrs. Jones asks to be discharged, stating, "I can handle it on my own now. You've helped me so much." The nurse knows that the appropriate response to such a request is to do which of the following?

☐ 1. Deny discharge, and consider the possibility that she has decided to attempt suicide.

☐ 2. Discharge her.

☐ 3. Permit her a 2-day pass to see how she gets along.

☐ 4. Permit her a 2-hour pass.

44. The next week, Mrs. Jones is irritable. She is criticizing the staff and their treatment of her. The nurse is most likely to evaluate this behavior as which of the following?

☐ 1. Regression.

☐ 2. Dangerous to the staff.

☐ 3. Improvement.

☐ 4. Suicidal.

45. Which of the following would the nurse consider when evaluating Mrs. Jones' progress?

☐ 1. Her ability to deal with stress.

☐ 2. Her reality orientation.

☐ 3. Her preoccupation with suspicious thoughts.

☐ 4. Her handling of activities of daily living.

Gladys Witt, age 70, is undergoing hemodialysis for acute renal failure following a hysterectomy. An arteriovenous (AV) shunt has been placed in her right forearm.

46. Which of the following is the *least* likely cause of prerenal azotemia, such as Miss Witt is most likely experiencing?

☐ 1. Hypovolemia.

☐ 2. Severe crush injuries.

☐ 3. Shock.

☐ 4. Poisons.

47. What is the most important indication for hemodialysis?

☐ 1. To prepare the client for renal transplant.

☐ 2. To control a high and rising serum potassium level.

☐ 3. To increase the life span of a client with chronic renal failure.

☐ 4. To avoid excessive diet and fluid restrictions.

48. Which of the following is *not* an aim of hemodialysis?

☐ 1. To restore fluid and electrolyte balance.

☐ 2. To correct acid-base imbalance.

☐ 3. To replace the endocrine functions of the kidneys.

☐ 4. To remove the nitrogenous by-products of protein metabolism.

49. Miss Witt says she's concerned about needing to be on the kidney machine. Which is the most appropriate response?

☐ 1. "Don't worry. I'm sure your insurance will cover the cost."

☐ 2. "We can teach you to do your own treatments at home."

☐ 3. "Do you have family who can learn to do your dialysis?"

☐ 4. "It's unlikely you'll need long-term dialysis, and we'll keep you informed about how your kidneys are recovering."

50. The nurse plans to observe Miss Witt carefully for symptoms of disequilibrium syndrome during dialysis and immediately following. Which is *not* a symptom of this complication?

☐ 1. Agitation.

☐ 2. Lethargy.

☐ 3. Muscle twitching.

☐ 4. Convulsions.

51. During hemodialysis, the nurse is most concerned about observing for which of the following?

☐ 1. Anuria.

☐ 2. Infection.

☐ 3. Uremic intoxication.

☐ 4. Hypovolemic shock.

52. Why is regional heparinization used during the dialysis procedure?

☐ 1. To retard clotting in the cannula.

☐ 2. To prevent clotting in the dialyzer.

☐ 3. To minimize intravascular thrombosis.

☐ 4. To decrease embolization of clots from the cannula.

53. Which action is *inappropriate* when caring for the arteriovenous shunt?

☐ 1. Palpate to assess blood flow.

☐ 2. Apply a tight dressing to prevent cannula dislodgment.

☐ 3. Avoid blood pressure readings in the affected limb.

☐ 4. Apply antibiotic ointment to the shunt site.

Baby Girl Ortiz, 39 weeks' gestation, has been admitted to the observation nursery. She weighs 7 pounds 1 ounce and had Apgar scores of 9 at 1 minute and 10 at 5 minutes.

54. The nurse admitting the infant to the nursery notes a temperature of 96.8° F (36° C) on admission. Which nursing action is most appropriate at this time?

☐ 1. Chart the temperature reading.

☐ 2. Call the pediatrician to check the infant.

☐ 3. Place the infant in a warmed incubator.

☐ 4. Administer oxygen by mask.

55. If the temperature remains at 96.8° F (36° C) after 5 hours, which condition would the infant be most prone to develop?

☐ 1. Metabolic acidosis.

☐ 2. Hypercalcemia.

☐ 3. Polycythemia.

☐ 4. Hyperglycemia.

56. The nurse does a complete assessment. All of the following are noted. Which requires immediate attention?

☐ 1. Cephalohematoma.
☐ 2. Milia.
☐ 3. Moro's reflex.
☐ 4. Expiratory grunting.

57. What is the major reason why an injection of vitamin K is given to newborns in the nursery?
☐ 1. It helps conjugate bilirubin in the infant.
☐ 2. It prevent Rh sensitization in the infant.
☐ 3. It reduces the possibility of hemorrhage in the infant.
☐ 4. It increases the infant's resistance to infection.

58. While performing a newborn assessment, the nurse observes the following: respiratory rate 44 and irregular, apical heart rate 148, and bluish hands and feet. How would the nurse interpret these data?
☐ 1. Possible cardiovascular problem. Call the physician.
☐ 2. Respiratory distress. Administer oxygen.
☐ 3. Normal newborn. Continue to observe.
☐ 4. Cold stress. Place infant in heated Isolette.

59. Which of the following observations is considered normal for a full-term neonate?
☐ 1. Heart rate of 90/min.
☐ 2. Jaundice in the first 24 hours.
☐ 3. Nasal flaring.
☐ 4. Uncoordinated eye movements.

60. Mrs. Ortiz is worried because her 2-day-old infant has lost 5 ounces since birth. How would the nurse respond?
☐ 1. "Try giving her formula more frequently."
☐ 2. "The nurse probably made a mistake while weighing your baby."
☐ 3. "The nurses will feed your baby for you for a few days."
☐ 4. "It is normal for an infant to lose up to 10% of her weight in the first few days."

61. The nurse observes signs of jaundice in Baby Ortiz on the third day of life. What is the most likely explanation?
☐ 1. Liver failure.
☐ 2. Physiological jaundice.
☐ 3. Erythroblastosis fetalis.
☐ 4. Sepsis.

Mike Lane, an acutely ill 10-year-old, is hospitalized with an upper respiratory infection and right otitis media. He is pale and lethargic and has a low-grade fever. Mike's condition is diagnosed as lymphoblastic leukemia.

62. Mike's initial pallor and lethargy are most likely the result of which of the following?
☐ 1. An accumulation of toxic wastes in body tissues caused by poor kidney functioning.
☐ 2. Body tissues being deprived of oxygen because of a decrease in the number of red blood cells.

☐ 3. Excessive needs for energy because of Mike's respiratory and ear infections.
☐ 4. A slower-than-normal blood flow to body tissues caused by a decreased heart rate.

63. The nurse notes that Mike has petechiae; bleeding from his gums, lips, and nose; and bruises on various parts of his body. Which one of the laboratory findings would the nurse expect to find?
☐ 1. Low serum calcium level.
☐ 2. Faulty thrombin production.
☐ 3. Decreased platelet count.
☐ 4. Elevated partial thromboplastin time.

64. Which of the following nursing measures is *contraindicated* for Mike?
☐ 1. Alternate medications between oral and intramuscular routes.
☐ 2. Handle his extremities with care while turning him.
☐ 3. Use stool softeners prn.
☐ 4. Provide frequent oral hygiene.

65. Which statement best indicates that Mike understands the use of chemotherapy for treatment?
☐ 1. "I must be getting worse because the drugs make me so sick."
☐ 2. "I won't be able to return to school until my disease-fighting cells increase."
☐ 3. "I can tolerate the nausea, because I know the drugs will kill all the cancer cells."
☐ 4. "I don't want a wig, because boys don't lose their hair."

66. Mike returns to the hospital 2 years later in a terminal stage. His parents decide to remain with him continuously. What is the most reasonable nursing plan?
☐ 1. Be available to the Lanes for emotional support while providing most of Mike's care.
☐ 2. Leave the Lanes alone with Mike to help them work through their grief.
☐ 3. Provide all meals and sleeping accommodations for the Lanes.
☐ 4. Teach the Lanes to give Mike most of the care he needs.

Jane Smith, a 35-year-old single parent, has been hospitalized as the result of a court order for psychiatric evaluation and treatment following continuing physical violence toward her 3-year-old daughter. Her history indicates that she has been fired three times from waitress positions for "refusing to do things that are beneath me, like clearing off the table for those fat slobs. I told them that they are pigs, and they could clear their own messy table." Miss Smith's mother states that the client has no friends, probably because "she tricks people so much and hurts their feelings." While being evaluated in the emergency room, the client screams that her back is hurting her and refuses to be admitted to the psychiatric unit. She is first

admitted to the orthopedic unit to assess her back problem.

67. While making rounds on nights, the nurse observes that Miss Smith has diaphoresis and mild tremors. At 8 AM the following day, the client complains of nervousness and is noted to be grossly disoriented and hyperactive. What substance has most likely been abused by Miss Smith?
☐ 1. Diazepam (Valium).
☐ 2. Alcohol.
☐ 3. Barbiturates.
☐ 4. Marijuana.

68. Miss Smith tells one of the primary nurses that another nurse, Miss Levy, "is a royal ass. I like you, because you're a good nurse. You're the only one who really understands me. Miss Levy isn't a good nurse." Which of the following does the client's remark best indicate?
☐ 1. Ability to detect staff weaknesses.
☐ 2. Thought disorder.
☐ 3. Rigid defense mechanism.
☐ 4. Attempted manipulation of the staff.

69. Which of the following characteristics is most likely to suggest a personality disorder?
☐ 1. Complies readily and passively with hospital rules and regulations.
☐ 2. Minimal insight and poor impulse control.
☐ 3. Demonstrates ego disintegration and impaired thought processes.
☐ 4. Delusional and acting-out behavior.

70. When dealing with clients with personality disorders, staff most often experience which of the following emotional states?
☐ 1. Anger and helplessness.
☐ 2. Apathy and boredom.
☐ 3. Confusion and mild irritability.
☐ 4. Curious absence of feelings.

71. In addition to psychiatric evaluation, one of the goals of Miss Smith's hospitalization is that she will recognize and abide by the limits set on her behavior in her interactions with other clients and with staff. Which of the following approaches is the most therapeutic way for staff to deal with her behavior?
☐ 1. Provide her with attention when she is not manipulating others.
☐ 2. Do not intervene in Miss Smith's interactions with other clients.
☐ 3. Make decisions as soon as possible after she makes a request.
☐ 4. Give detailed explanations about what she is expected to do.

Rena Klein is a 73-year-old retired telephone operator who had a hemorrhoidectomy this morning. She has just returned from the recovery room, has an IV infusing, and is alert and oriented.

72. What step would the nurse take after checking her vital signs?
☐ 1. Auscultate her chest.
☐ 2. Check the surgical site for excess bleeding.
☐ 3. Check her abdomen for distension.
☐ 4. Percuss her bladder.

73. Six hours after her surgery, Mrs. Klein has not voided. What is the most appropriate nursing action to take at this time?
☐ 1. Ask her if she feels the need to urinate.
☐ 2. Catheterize her.
☐ 3. Help her to the bathroom.
☐ 4. Run warm water over her fingers.

74. Mrs. Klein progresses well on her second postoperative day. What care is appropriate?
☐ 1. Encourage Mrs. Klein to lie on her back when in bed.
☐ 2. Encourage Mrs. Klein to sit up for as long as possible.
☐ 3. Have Mrs. Klein sit on a rubber ring when in a chair.
☐ 4. Take Mrs. Klein's temperature orally.

75. Mrs. Klein tells the nurse that she is worried about having her first bowel movement. What is the best response?
☐ 1. "All clients with hemorrhoids are concerned about that."
☐ 2. "What concerns you about it?"
☐ 3. "Are you afraid that it will be painful?"
☐ 4. "Don't worry. Your doctor has ordered medication to make it as painless as possible."

76. Which of the following instructions would be best to give Mrs. Klein in order to help avoid postoperative infection?
☐ 1. "Do perineal care with antiseptic solution after every stool, and take as many sitz baths as you need to clean the incision."
☐ 2. "Do perineal care every morning and every evening, and take sitz baths as necessary to clean the incision."
☐ 3. "Do perineal care with antiseptic solution every evening, and take three sitz baths every day."
☐ 4. "Do perineal care with plain soap and water after every stool, and take a sitz bath four times a day."

77. Which of the following is important to tell Mrs. Klein in preparation for discharge?
☐ 1. "Limit your fluid intake."
☐ 2. "Notify your doctor if you have increased pain when having a bowel movement."
☐ 3. "Notify your doctor when you have your first bowel movement."
☐ 4. "Stay with a low-residue, soft diet for 3 weeks."

Jimmy Baker, age 1½, is brought to the emergency room by his mother. He has a skull fracture and multiple body bruises. Child abuse is suspected.

78. Assessing the situation, the nurse would find what information most useful?
    - ☐ 1. The interaction between Jimmy and his mother.
    - ☐ 2. When the accident occurred.
    - ☐ 3. Presence of other children in the family.
    - ☐ 4. Age of Jimmy's mother.
79. Which of the following actions would be taken by hospital personnel when child abuse is suspected?
    - ☐ 1. Confront Jimmy's mother.
    - ☐ 2. Notify the family.
    - ☐ 3. Notify the child protective services.
    - ☐ 4. Do nothing until the diagnosis is certain.
80. Before an effective working relationship with Jimmy's mother can be established, which of the following is most important for the nurse to do first?
    - ☐ 1. Identify family support systems.
    - ☐ 2. Learn to identify and deal with negative feelings about abusive caregivers.
    - ☐ 3. Review the family history thoroughly.
    - ☐ 4. Identify referral sources for abusive caregivers.
81. A nursing goal for Mrs. Baker is that she will learn about parenting skills. Which of the following indicates that she has, at least partially, met this goal?
    - ☐ 1. She attends Parents Anonymous group meetings.
    - ☐ 2. She brings Jimmy presents in the hospital.
    - ☐ 3. She calls the hospital several times a day to check on Jimmy's progress.
    - ☐ 4. After discharge, she brings Jimmy to the clinic to visit.

Jack Silsbe is a 64-year-old client with a 30-year history of cigarette smoking. A chest x-ray, bronchoscopy, and biopsy confirm oat-cell carcinoma.

82. Mr. Silsbe's cancer is inoperable. External radiation is prescribed as a palliative measure. What side effect is Mr. Silsbe most likely to experience?
    - ☐ 1. Alopecia.
    - ☐ 2. Bone marrow suppression.
    - ☐ 3. Stomatitis.
    - ☐ 4. Dyspnea.
83. Nursing management of Mr. Silsbe's irradiated skin will *not* include which of the following?
    - ☐ 1. Applying A and D Ointment prn to relieve dry skin.
    - ☐ 2. Cleansing the skin with tepid water and a soft cloth.
    - ☐ 3. Avoiding direct exposure to the sun.
    - ☐ 4. Redrawing the skin markings if they are accidentally removed.
84. Mr. Silsbe tells you that he fears he is radioactive and a danger to his family and friends. How would the nurse dispel his fears?
    - ☐ 1. Inform him that radiation machines are risk free.
    - ☐ 2. Explain that once the machine is off, radiation is no longer emitted.

- ☐ 3. Avoid telling him that his fears are in fact true.
- ☐ 4. Instruct him to spend short periods of time with his family and friends.

85. Fatigue is part of a radiation syndrome not related to the site of therapy. How might the nurse best ensure that Mr. Silsbe receives adequate rest?
    - ☐ 1. Schedule all Mr. Silsbe's hospital activities early in the morning so that he has the remainder of the day to rest.
    - ☐ 2. Encourage Mr. Silsbe's family to carry out all his activities for him so that he will not overexert himself.
    - ☐ 3. Maintain Mr. Silsbe's bed rest with bathroom privileges only.
    - ☐ 4. Balance Mr. Silsbe's daily activities with frequent rest periods.

Jim Taylor, a 6-month-old infant, is admitted to the hospital with diarrhea for the past 2 days. The physician suspects the infant has eaten something contaminated by salmonella.

86. Which of the following foods or fluids are most likely to be contaminated by salmonella?
    - ☐ 1. Water and fruits.
    - ☐ 2. Eggs and poultry.
    - ☐ 3. Milk and vegetables.
    - ☐ 4. Beef and pork.
87. At Jim's age, what is the most critical clinical manifestation of the degree of dehydration?
    - ☐ 1. Sunken fontanel.
    - ☐ 2. Weight loss.
    - ☐ 3. Decreased urine output.
    - ☐ 4. Dry skin.
88. Jim develops hypokalemia, which would be manifested by which of the following?
    - ☐ 1. Muscle weakness.
    - ☐ 2. Hunger.
    - ☐ 3. Hyperreflexia.
    - ☐ 4. Apnea.
89. What is the primary cause of Jim's hypokalemia?
    - ☐ 1. Diarrhea.
    - ☐ 2. Salmonella.
    - ☐ 3. Oliguria.
    - ☐ 4. IV fluid without added potassium.

Cathy Lubbick, a 32-year-old woman, reports to her gynecologist for her yearly Pap test. She states she has been in good health but complains of a watery vaginal discharge. She is concerned because there is a family history of cancer.

90. Assessing Mrs. Lubbick, the nurse keeps in mind the signs of cancer. Which of the following are signs of cancer of the cervix?
    - ☐ 1. A dark, foul-smelling vaginal discharge.
    - ☐ 2. Pressure on the bladder or bowel, or both.

☐ 3. Pain and weight loss.

☐ 4. Vaginal discharge (leukorrhea).

91. While assessing Mrs. Lubbick, the nurse considers the possibility of endometrial cancer. Which of the following statements is *incorrect* concerning endometrial cancer?

☐ 1. Diagnosis is most frequently established by a dilatation and curettage (D&C).

☐ 2. Prolonged use of exogenous estrogen increases the occurrence.

☐ 3. The first and most important symptom is abnormal bleeding.

☐ 4. This malignancy tends to spread rapidly to other organs.

92. The Pap smear reveals that Mrs. Lubbick has cancer of the cervix. The mode of treatment is an abdominal hysterectomy. She voices concern about undergoing menopause. In counseling her, which of the following statements would be most appropriate?

☐ 1. A surgical menopause will occur, and treatment with estrogen therapy will be necessary.

☐ 2. The ovaries will continue to function and produce estrogen, thus preventing menopause.

☐ 3. Ovarian hormone secretion ceases, but the hypothalamus will continue to secrete FSH, preventing menopause.

☐ 4. The ovaries will cease functioning; thus it will be necessary to administer estrogen.

93. Estrogen therapy is often prescribed to suppress the symptoms experienced by the menopausal client. Which of the following symptoms would *not* be characteristic of menopause?

☐ 1. Anxiety and nervousness.

☐ 2. Vasomotor instability.

☐ 3. Osteoporosis resulting in backache.

☐ 4. Dysmenorrhea and mittelschmerz.

94. Following the hysterectomy, which of the following symptoms would most likely indicate that Mrs. Lubbick is experiencing a serious complication of a hysterectomy?

☐ 1. Gas pains and difficulty defecating.

☐ 2. Moderate amount of serosanguinous drainage on the perineal pad.

☐ 3. Low-back pain, decreased urinary output.

☐ 4. Incisional pain requiring narcotic administration for relief.

95. In providing postoperative discharge instructions for Mrs. Lubbick, the nurse would *not* include which of the following?

☐ 1. Return to the clinic in 10 days for the removal of the vaginal packing.

☐ 2. Carry out abdominal strengthening exercises.

☐ 3. Expect to experience periodic crying spells.

☐ 4. Avoid activities that increase pelvic congestion.

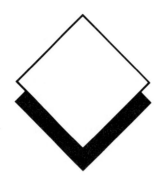

Test 2, Book III

ANSWERS WITH RATIONALES

KEY TO ABBREVIATIONS
Section of the Review Book

P = Psychosocial and Mental Health Problems
   T = Therapeutic Use of Self
   L = Loss and Death and Dying
   A = Anxious Behavior
   C = Confused Behavior
   E = Elated-Depressive Behavior
   SM = Socially Maladaptive Behavior
   SS = Suspicious Behavior
   W = Withdrawn Behavior
   SU = Substance Use Disorders
A = Adult
   H = Healthy Adult
   S = Surgery
   O = Oxygenation
   NM = Nutrition and Metabolism
   E = Elimination
   SP = Sensation and Perception
   M = Mobility
   CA = Cellular Aberration
CBF = Childbearing Family
   W = Women's Health Care
   A = Antepartal Care
   I = Intrapartal Care
   P = Postpartal Care
   N = Newborn Care
C = Child
   H = Healthy Child
   I = Ill and Hospitalized Child
   SPP = Sensation, Perception, and Protection
   O = Oxygenation
   NM = Nutrition and Metabolism
   E = Elimination
   M = Mobility
   CA = Cellular Aberration

Nursing Process Category

AS = Assessment
AN = Analysis
PL = Plan
IM = Implementation
EV = Evaluation

Client Need Category

E = Safe, Effective Care Environment
PS = Physiological Integrity
PC = Psychosocial Integrity
H = Health Promotion and Maintenance

1. no. 1. Latent phase (stage one) generally spans from 0 to 3 or 4 cm dilatation and is accompanied by minimal discomfort in most women. CBF/I, AN, PS

2. no. 1. Demerol should be given late enough in the labor that it doesn't slow the labor, yet not so late that it causes the newborn to be "sleepy" when delivered. The situation given describes the optimum time to administer the pain medication. CBF/I, IM, PS

3. no. 3.
$$\frac{100 \text{ mg}}{1 \text{ ml}} \times \frac{75 \text{ mg}}{X \text{ ml}} = 100 X = 0.75$$

OR

75/100 ml × 1 ml = 75/100 = 0.75 ml
CBF/I, IM, PS

4. no. 3. The effects of selected medications on the fetus are generally heightened by increasing the dosage, giving the drug intravenously, and administering the agent close to delivery. CBF/I, AN, PS

5. no. 3. Antacids may neutralize the highly acidic gastric juice and thereby prevent a fatal chemical pneumonitis if vomiting and aspiration occur during general anesthesia. CBF/I, AN, PS

6. no. 2. Occiput refers to vertex presentation; the

words right and posterior refer to those portions of the maternal pelvis. Option no. 1 is correct but does not answer the client very specifically; no. 3 and no. 4 are incorrect. CBF/I, IM, PS

7. no. 1. A major consequence of malpresentation is the lengthening of labor through decreased efficiency of contractions, longer time for the presenting part to descend, and weaker forces working on the cervix, all of which slow dilatation. Nursing actions should be designed to provide physical comfort and emotional support when labor is prolonged. CBF/I, IM, PS

8. no. 3. The client's symptoms are typical of severe anxiety panic. Mild anxiety does not produce the discomfort that this client is experiencing; it motivates growth and creativity. Moderate anxiety, which narrows the perceptual field, can be redirected with help, and clients can feel challenged to cope. The severely anxious person might have a greatly reduced perceptual field or develop a denial of existing feelings with selective inattention. Although problem solving is difficult, it is not impossible. P/A, AN, PC

9. no. 4. The highest priority is to reduce the client's anxiety. Priorities differ in the emergency room as opposed to other acute care settings. The focus is not immediately on relationship, although trust in relationships with helpers will occur. An immediate goal of gaining insight is impossible since she is now experiencing a level of anxiety where cognitive functioning is blocked. P/A, PL, E

10. no. 1. Persons in an acute anxiety state need to feel that someone understands their terror and that they will not be left alone. Reassurance negates the experience and discounts the terror of the present. Clients in panic must not be left alone because panic is experienced as dread and terror. Acting out and/or verbal expression of true feelings of anger and helplessness would be blocked. P/A, IM, PC

11. no. 2. Clients may not want medication but may come to recognize their need for it and therefore ready themselves. Respond to the anxiety, not to the content of the client's remark. The first remark is authoritarian and defensive. It makes an assumption that client cannot refuse ordered medication. Options no. 3 and no. 4 are patronizing and discount the client's fear of addiction. P/A, IM, PC

12. no. 3. Orient assessment toward finding out the factors that precipitated the client's present stage of anxiety. Be specific. Clients in a panic state need great assistance in staying focused. Option no. 1 is very generalized and assumes a high level of awareness on the part of the client. Option no. 2 assumes a connection between client's present situation and her anxiety with little input from client. If the client

knew how to be helped, she would not be in the emergency room. People seek assistance from health providers because they do not know how to help themselves. P/A, AS, PC

13. no. 3. Drowsiness, vertigo, and dizziness are the most common side effects of diazepam. Her level of anxiety (panic) does not manifest itself in faintness and dizziness. Allergic responses to diazepam are skin rash, urticaria, fever, angioneurotic edema, and bronchial spasms. There is no indication that she has been sleepless or experiencing exhaustion. P/A, AN, PS

14. no. 1. Removing the nipple frequently while feeding breaks the suction, causing the child to swallow more air. This also frustrates the child, and crying further aggravates the problem. Breastfeeding is permitted, but it is more difficult. C/NM, IM, E

15. no. 1. This child will swallow a lot of air because of the abnormal openings. The other answers are contraindicated. C/NM, PL, PS

16. no. 1. Most surgeons prefer to repair the palate before the child develops faulty speech patterns. By 12 to 18 months of age, palatal growth has progressed enough to allow surgery. Although some surgeons prefer to wait until 4 or 5 years of age to allow complete palatal development, by that age the child's speech will have been permanently affected by the deformity. C/NM, AN, PS

17. no. 4. Speech and hearing problems are common after this repair because of the necessary change in the palate arch and concomitant change in eustachian tubes. Contractures of the mandible are unrelated to this repair. C/NM, AN, H

18. no. 3. With her history of hypertension, cerebral hemorrhage is the most probable cause of the CVA. TIAs produce sudden neurological deficits; these usually disappear within minutes or hours. A cerebral aneurysm and meningitis do not result in these types of signs and symptoms. A/SP, AN, PS

19. no. 1. A positive Babinski reflex is extension or dorsiflexion of the great toe and the fanning of the other toes when a hard object is applied to the lateral surface of the sole, starting at the heel and going over the ball of the foot, ending beneath the great toe. The normal response to plantar stimulation is to plantar-flex the foot and flex all toes (called a negative Babinski reflex). A/SP, AS, PS

20. no. 3. Offering the bedpan q2h is the first step in initiating bladder training, which is part of rehabilitation. The 2-hour interval is gradually lengthened as control is gained. Catheters can cause bladder infections and should be avoided when possible. Wearing a diaper may cause embarrassment and skin breakdown. Restricting fluids would be inappropriate. A/SP, PL, PS

21. no. 4. There is no such thing as hysterical aphasia. In expressive aphasia, the client has difficulty in selecting, organizing, and initiating motor speech. Expressive aphasia is also termed motor, Broca's, or nonfluent aphasia. In contrast, the client with receptive (sensory, Wernicke's, or fluent) aphasia generally has impaired auditory comprehension and auditory feedback. A/SP, AN, PS

22. no. 2. The occipital lobe holds the visual center; the medulla deals with essential functions (e.g., temperature); the parietal lobe deals mainly with sensory function. A/SP, AN, PS

23. no. 4. Encourage her to speak at any possible opportunity. Although time consuming, it is more therapeutic for the client. Options no. 1, no. 2, and no. 3 actually discourage the rehabilitation of verbal communication. A/SP, IM, E

24. no. 1. Have the family continue to encourage Mrs. Duke's efforts. If the aphasia is expressive, she may be able to choose another word to communicate her needs. A/SP, IM, H

25. no. 3. Keeping Mrs. Duke positioned in semi-Fowler's position is important to prevent aspiration, a frequent complication after a CVA. Although the other options may be appropriate, client safety comes first. A/SP, PL, E

26. no. 1. Initial damage to any tissue creates edema and impairs functioning. As the cerebral edema decreases, muscle function begins to return and can improve for a period of up to 6 months. The most dramatic changes in functional gains generally occur within the first 3 months after the onset of the stroke. A/SP, AN, PS

27. no. 3. Rehabilitation attempts to reduce the impairments and disability in stroke and to restore and develop physical and psychological functioning. A/SP, PL. PS

28. no. 3. With the help of significant others or family, rehabilitation efforts are continued over the long term, resulting in a more optimal recovery. A/SP, AN, H

29. no. 3. Daily skin checks are done to note any potential bleeding. Pink urine may be from hematuria and must be reported immediately. Foods high in vitamin K will enhance the clotting mechanism and counteract the effects of the drug. Prothrombin levels, not partial thromboplastin times, are measured in clients receiving warfarin (Coumadin). A/SP, IM, PS

30. no. 1. Eczema is most often seen in infancy. The most frequent cause is cow's milk and egg albumin allergy. The infant is at highest risk for developing an allergic response because the immune system is still not fully mature. C/SPP, AS, PS

31. no. 2. Before treatment can be effective, the allergen that is causing the problem must be identified. C/SPP, PL, PS

32. no. 1. Pruritus is the most difficult symptom of eczema to control. It causes infants and children to be irritable and interferes with sleep. Eczema is not usually painful unless infection occurs. Although teething is common at age 2, it does not cause long periods of irritability and sleeplessness. Hunger is unrelated but may be manifested by a diet that is restrictive to the point that the child does not like any of the foods allowed. C/SPP, AN, PS

33. no. 3. Soaps are drying agents and are not used. Lipid lotions or agents are not good cleansing agents. Warm water increases itching; cool water promotes chilling and loss of body heat. Tepid baths soothe irritated skin and decrease itching. C/SPP, PL, PS

34. no. 2. This is an age-appropriate activity that would provide a distraction for Sally without giving her anything to scratch with. Working with clay requires more coordination than the average 2-year-old has; additionally, the clay may prove irritating to Sally's skin condition. Although building columns with blocks is age appropriate for Sally, she may use the blocks to scratch or irritate her eczema. Until her eczema clears, Sally should play with safe objects with rounded edges. Although the average 2-year-old is able to hold a crayon and make circular and linear lines, they do not typically associate these markings with specific objects. C/SPP, IM, H

35. no. 2. Wool is not used because it can irritate the skin. Synthetic materials are substituted for wool in coats, hats, gloves, etc. C/SPP, IM, H

36. no. 4. Close-fitting clothes cause irritation and perspiration and increased itching. These should be avoided. Loose-fitting, one-piece clothing prevents access for itching. C/SPP, EV, H

37. no. 3. Allowing restricted foods, even occasionally, can cause the exacerbation of eczema. Options no. 1, no. 2, and no. 4 encourage intake in a toddler. C/SPP, EV. H

38. no. 3. Pancakes are not included because they are usually made from wheat flour. Soy milk is used if there is an allergy to cow's milk. Turkey and chicken are permitted, as are bland fruits (e.g., apples, pears, peaches, and bananas). C/SPP, PL, PS

39. no. 1. Reactive depression is characterized by a loss, sleeping disorder, eating disorder, or decreased energy. She may be experiencing anxiety about being alone, but the symptoms indicate depression. Psychosis would include more severe symptoms such as a thought disorder. Paranoia would include symptoms of a rigid belief system and delusions of persecution. P/E, AN, PC

40. no. 2. One indication of increased well-being in the client is resumption of activities of daily living.

There is no evidence in the situation to suggest that the client is suspicious or has a thought disorder. When Mrs. Jones starts taking better care of herself, it will indicate that the immobility imposed by the depression is lifting. Options no. 1 and no. 3 reflect a person with a psychosis, and no. 4 reflects a goal for a person with anxiety. P/E, PL, E

41. no. 4. Reactive depression is characterized by an identifiable loss of some type. In Mrs. Jones' case, it is the loss of a relationship with her husband. The anger at the loss of her husband is not directly expressed externally or verbally. It is turned inward; she takes the anger out on herself and becomes depressed. Option no. 1 reflects a person with a psychosis, no. 2 reflects an anxiety disorder, and no. 3 reflects a person with paranoia. P/E, AN, PC

42. no. 3. This response is client centered and reflects the nurse's empathy. Option no. 1 gives false reassurance and ignores the client's feelings and situation. Option no. 2 may help the nurse feel better by getting him or her out of the situation, but it may not meet the client's need. The nurse can offer to help the client discharge feelings but should not force the client to talk. P/E, IM, PC

43. no. 1. Clients who are depressed and suddenly get better may have made the decision to commit suicide or may now be feeling better and have the energy to make a suicide attempt. Discharging her or giving her a pass as soon as she feels better is premature. P/E, AN, PC

44. no. 3. When Mrs. Jones becomes irritable, it is a sign that the anger is moving from being inwardly directed to being directed out. This is a sign that the depression is lifting. An indication of regression would be acting childish. Mrs. Jones is not threatening the staff, nor is she acting suicidal. P/E, EV, PC

45. no. 4. Improved mental well-being of a client is evidenced by an increased ability to carry out activities of daily living. When the depression is less incapacitating, the client has more energy to act. Option no. 1 reflects improvement from an anxiety disorder, no. 2 reflects improvement from psychosis, and no. 3 reflects improvement from paranoia. P/E, EV, PC

46. no. 4. Prerenal azotemia refers to causes outside the kidneys; poisons cause renal azotemia. A/E, AN, PC

47. no. 2. Hyperkalemia is an immediate and life-threatening problem associated with renal failure. Clients on hemodialysis have diet and fluid restrictions. Hemodialysis sustains a client until renal transplant is scheduled. A/E, PL, PS

48. no. 3. The hemodialysis machine works on the simple physical principles of filtration, osmosis, and diffusion. It cannot duplicate the complex endocrine functions of the kidneys (e.g., the production of erythropoietin). The other options reflect the purposes of hemodialysis. A/E, PL, PS

49. no. 4. Postoperative renal shutdown is usually reversible. A/E, IM, PC

50. no. 2. Lethargy is a symptom of a high BUN. Disequilibrium syndrome is caused by a rapid decline of electrolytes or wastes. A/E, AS, PS

51. no. 4. The shift of too much blood to the dialyzer produces symptoms of hypovolemic shock. Accidental disconnection of the tubing also results in rapid exsanguination and hypovolemic shock. A/E, PL, PS

52. no. 2. Regional heparinization prevents clotting in the hemodialyzer without subjecting the client to the risks of systemic anticoagulation. A/E, PL, PS

53. no. 2. Blood flow must be maintained in the cannula to prevent clotting. A tight dressing constricts flow. A/E, IM, PS

54. no. 3. The infant's temperature normally drops immediately after birth if the infant is not dried and well wrapped. The large body surface area and the difference in external temperature from the mother's internal temperature predispose the infant to chilling. The infant must be warmed immediately. The one way to do this is placement in a warmed incubator. CBF/NR, IM, PS

55. no. 1. Cold increases an infant's metabolic rate because of inability to shiver. This increases both oxygen and calorie consumption, necessitating the administration of more oxygen and calories. If they are unavailable, the infant develops metabolic acidosis, which is manifested by lowered blood pH. CBF/NR, AN, PS

56. no. 4. Grunting is an abnormal breathing pattern, usually indicative of respiratory distress. Cephalohematoma, a collection of blood between the bone and periosteum, is the result of pressure sustained at birth, usually requiring no treatment. Milia, resulting from blocked sebaceous glands, is a normal newborn characteristic, as is the Moro or startle reflex. CBF/NR. AS, PS

57. no. 3. Synthesis of vitamin K by *E. coli* bacteria occurs in the intestinal tract. Newborns have a sterile intestinal tract and lack the vitamin, which is essential in the formation of prothrombin and for normal blood clotting. CBF/NR, AN, PS

58. no. 3. Acrocyanosis is usually present in a normal neonate because of immature peripheral circulation. Average pulse rate is 100 to 160 and respirations are 30 to 60 and irregular. CBF/NR, AN, PS

59. no. 4. Uncoordinated eye movements are a normal finding in full-term neonates, because they have poor control of eye muscles. The normal heart rate is 100

to 160. Jaundice in the first 24 hours is considered pathological. Nasal flaring is a sign of respiratory distress. CBF/NR, AS, PS

60. no. 4. During the first few days after birth, the infant may lose 5% to 10% of her birth weight because of loss of excess fluid and minimal intake of nutrients. CBF/NR, IM, PS

61. no. 2. Approximately 50% of full-term newborns develop jaundice around the third day of life in the absence of disease or a specific cause. This is called physiological jaundice because of the rapid breakdown of fetal cells, resulting in an increase in bilirubin. This subsides approximately 5 to 7 days after birth. CBF/NR, AN, PS

62. no. 2. The immense metabolic needs of the proliferating leukemic cells cause bone marrow depression and reduce red blood cell production. C/CA, AN, PS

63. no. 3. Platelets are involved in clotting and coagulation and are decreased in number because of leukocytosis. C/CA, AS, PS

64. no. 1. Intramuscular injections can precipitate bleeding and are to be avoided. C/CA, PL, PS

65. no. 2. This indicates that he is aware that myelosuppression occurs and is temporary. C/CA, EV, E

66. no. 1. This is the most realistic because it is supportive to the family without overburdening them. Options no. 2, no. 3, and no. 4 place too much responsibility on the family and do not allow them a respite. C/CA, PL, H

67. no. 2. Alcohol withdrawal involves four stages. Signs and symptoms occurring in stage I (8 hours or more after cessation of drinking) include mild tremors and nervousness. In stage II, symptoms include hyperactivity and disorientation. Miss Smith was admitted on the previous day, and sufficient time had elapsed without alcohol ingestion, resulting in several signs of alcohol withdrawal. Signs of diazepam (Valium) withdrawal are tremors, abdominal and muscle cramps, and convulsions. Barbiturate withdrawal would include nausea, vomiting, diarrhea, sleep disturbance, diaphoresis, irritability, hostility, and agitation. Marijuana does not produce withdrawal symptoms. P/SU, AN, PS

68. no. 4. Clients with personality disorders "use" or manipulate other persons for their own motives. They have a tendency to ascribe their own motivations and behaviors to others. In psychiatric settings, these clients consistently try to split the staff by complaining about one staff member to another and by flattering some staff members. Miss Smith is describing her reaction to Miss Levy, not identifying her weaknesses. Manipulative behavior is well-thought-out and deliberate, not irrational as with a thought disorder or unconscious as with a defense mechanism. P/SM, AN, PC

69. no. 2. Clients with personality disorders have no impairment of thought, no ego disintegration, and no delusional behavior the way psychotic clients do. The client with a personality disorder has minimal insight and poor impulse control, which results in acting-out behavior. Compliance and passivity are seen in clients with low self-esteem who wish to please others to be liked. P/SM, AS, PC

70. no. 1. Clients with personality disorders consistently arouse uncomfortable feelings of anger, frustration, helplessness, and defensiveness in staff. The deliberate, manipulative behaviors are blatant enough that there is no confusion about what is happening. An absence of feelings is sometimes seen in response to schizophrenic clients, and boredom can be experienced with withdrawn, depressed clients. P/SM, AS, PC

71. no. 1. Because staff feel so angry and helpless with clients with personality disorders, these clients are rarely sought out. Reinforcing positive behavior is an effort to reward the client with attention. Options no. 2 through no. 4 tend to foster the client's chronic manipulative behavior. P/SM, IM, PC

72. no. 2. Checking for excess bleeding is the next priority, since hemorrhage is the priority complication in the immediate postoperative period. Urine retention is a more frequent complication in men. A/E, IM, PS

73. no. 1. Postoperative clients should void within 8 to 12 hours after surgery. At this time, it is most appropriate to assess the client's status by asking her if she feels the need to urinate. Catheterization is done as a last resort when other measures (e.g., no. 3 and no. 4) are ineffective. Further assessment of the client's need to void comes before interventions such as options no. 3 and no. 4. A/E, IM, PS

74. no. 4. Mrs. Klein's temperature should be taken orally, not rectally. Avoid the supine position, sitting for prolonged periods, and sitting on rubber rings, all of which increase venous stagnation in the rectal area. A/E, IM, PS

75. no. 2. This option gives Mrs. Klein the opportunity to voice her concerns. The other options assume the cause of the client's worry. A/E, IM, PS

76. no. 1. In order to avoid postoperative infection, Mrs. Klein should do perineal care after each stool, and she may have sitz baths as needed to clean the incision or to provide for comfort. A/E, IM, H

77. no. 2. Increased pain with bowel movements is a symptom of anal stricture, and Mrs. Klein should notify her physician. She should drink 2500 to 3000 ml of fluid daily and eat a low-residue, soft diet for the first postoperative week. Mrs. Klein will have had her first bowel movement before she is discharged. A/E, IM, H

78. no. 1. Observe the interaction between Jimmy and

his mother. Abusers frequently do not offer appropriate comfort or support to the distressed child. The abused child frequently appears wary of the caregivers or does not seek them out for comfort and affection. Options no. 2, no. 3, and no. 4 may prove useful, but no. 1 will provide the most important information to assess child abuse. P/SM, AS, PC

79. no. 3. All suspected cases of child abuse must be reported to the child welfare and protective services agency. Personnel cannot be prosecuted for defamation of character if their suspicions prove to be incorrect. Option no. 1 is not helpful at this time and would create further problems. The law requires the use of protective services rather than the police directly. If nothing is done, the child's life will continue to be endangered. P/SM, IM, E

80. no. 2. Although identification of support systems is important, the ability to deal with any negative feelings is imperative in establishing a working relationship. Family history does have value, but it has a lower priority and is more likely to be obtained after a relationship is established. Option no. 4 has a lower priority and does not necessarily facilitate an effective working relationship. P/SM, IM, PC

81. no. 1. Attendance at a parent-support group indicates that Mrs. Baker might be willing to invest her time and that there is at least a minimal level of motivation to change. Bringing gifts to Jimmy and calling the hospital do not necessarily indicate a commitment to furthering parenting skills. Attendance at the parents' group (which deals with feelings and needs of parents and children) demonstrates interest, motivation, and commitment. P/SM, EV, H

82. no. 4. The majority of side effects of external radiation are dependent on the specific site being radiated. Because the client's site is the lung, radiation will result in irritation of the lung mucosa, resulting in dyspnea. A/CA, AS, PS

83. no. 4. Skin markings must not be removed in any way. If they are inadvertently washed off, markings are redrawn only by the radiation technician. A/CA, PL, PS

84. no. 2. It is important to understand the difference between external and internal radiation so that the nurse can be accurate when correcting the client's misconceptions. He is not radioactive and does not need to limit contact with others. Options no. 1, no. 3, and no. 4 are incorrect. A/CA, IM, PC

85. no. 4. Encourage the client to participate in his own care as much as possible, but provide periods of uninterrupted rest in a quiet environment between periods of activity. A/CA, PL, PS

86. no. 2. The most common sources of salmonella infection are poultry and eggs. Other sources may be dogs, cats, hamsters, and pet turtles. C/NM, AN, PS

87. no. 2. The posterior fontanel is closed by 2 months, and the anterior closes at 12 to 18 months but is usually covered with hair. Although the anterior fontanel can be an indicator of dehydration at 6 months, the weight of the infant is a more reliable sign of fluid loss and dehydration. C/NM, AS, PS

88. no. 1. The infant with a potassium deficit has muscle weakness and hyporeflexia, is anorexic, and develops cardiac dysrhythmias, rather than apnea. C/NM, AS, PS

89. no. 3. Potassium is lost primarily from the gastrointestinal tract. Salmonella is indirectly a cause because it is the cause of the diarrhea. Diuresis, rather than oliguria, leads to hypokalemia. Because IV fluids were not ordered, option no. 4 is not applicable. C/NM, AN, E

90. no. 4. The two chief symptoms of cancer of the cervix are metrorrhagia (vaginal bleeding or spotting at irregular intervals and between periods) and a watery vaginal discharge. A/CA, AS, PS

91. no. 4. Cancer of the endometrium tends to be slow-spreading. Once it has spread to the cervix, invaded the myometrium, or spread outside the uterus, the prognosis is poor. A/CA, AN, PS

92. no. 2. Menstruation will cease following a hysterectomy, but as long as the ovaries are left in place, they will continue to function, and surgical menopause will not occur. A hysterectomy is removal of the uterus and usually cervix. A/CA, IM, PS

93. no. 4. Menstrual irregularities occur with menopause, but these do not include dysmenorrhea (menstrual cramps) and mittelschmerz. A/CA, AN, PS

94. no. 3. A serious complication of a hysterectomy is the accidental ligation of the ureter during surgery. These symptoms would be found if that had occurred. A/CA, AS, PS

95. no. 1. Vaginal packing is not used following an abdominal hysterectomy. Crying spells may be related to her change in body image. A/CA, IM, H

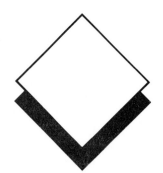

Test 2, Book IV

Questions

Mary Phillips, 28 years old, is admitted with the following complaints: urgency, frequency, dysuria, suprapubic pain, and hematuria. Her admitting diagnosis is cystitis.

1. What is the most likely cause of Miss Phillips' urgency?
   □ 1. Contracted bladder.
   □ 2. Inflamed bladder.
   □ 3. Enlarged bladder.
   □ 4. Increased vascularity in the bladder.

2. Fluids should be encouraged for this client, especially those that can aid in altering the urinary pH. Her nurse would advise her to take liberal quantities of which of the following?
   □ 1. Apple juice.
   □ 2. Tea and coffee.
   □ 3. Vitamin C.
   □ 4. Orange juice.

3. Miss Phillips will be given a drug that acts only on bacteria in the urine and is not absorbed systemically. This drug is which of the following?
   □ 1. Sulfisoxazole (Gantrisin).
   □ 2. Penicillin.
   □ 3. Ampicillin.
   □ 4. Tetracycline.

4. What organism is this drug most effective against?
   □ 1. *E. coli*.
   □ 2. *Pseudomonas*.
   □ 3. *Salmonella*.
   □ 4. *Klebsiella*.

Eight-year-old Randall, a third-grader, visits his pediatrician for an annual health checkup and a camp physical examination. The nurse begins a history and exam.

5. When obtaining a nursing history from Randall and his mother, the nurse questions Randall about his school activities and achievements. This is important because, according to Erikson's stages of development, Randall should be developing a sense of

□ 1. Initiative.
□ 2. Industry.
□ 3. Generativity.
□ 4. Identity.

6. Randall's weight is at the 95th percentile, and his height is at the 75th percentile. Based on this information, which of the following conclusions is most warranted?
   □ 1. Randall is overweight and should be referred to the dietitian for nutrition counseling.
   □ 2. Randall's weight is disproportionate to his height, and he should be counseled to reduce his caloric intake.
   □ 3. Randall's weight and height indicate he is growing normally.
   □ 4. Additional information should be collected before drawing conclusions.

7. The nurse screens Randall's vision using the Snellen alphabet chart. The results show Randall has 20/30 vision in his left eye and 20/40 vision in his right eye. Corneal light reflex and cover tests are normal. Which follow-up action is most indicated?
   □ 1. Rescreen Randall in 1 month.
   □ 2. Test Randall for color blindness.
   □ 3. Discuss with the physician a referral to an ophthalmologist or optometrist.
   □ 4. Counsel Randall's mother that the findings are normal.

8. Randall's camp administrator requires that his immunizations be up-to-date. Before today, Randall had received the full recommended series of childhood immunizations. Which of the following would be appropriate to administer to Randall?
   □ 1. No immunization.
   □ 2. A tetanus booster.
   □ 3. Diphtheria (adult type) and tetanus booster.
   □ 4. Measles and mumps vaccines.

9. The nurse takes this opportunity to discuss general safety with Randall's mother. Which of the following approaches to encourage safety is *not* appropriate?

- ☐ 1. Live safely to show the child how it is done.
- ☐ 2. Anticipate that fatigue and strong emotions may increase the danger of accidents.
- ☐ 3. Comply with local laws and support law enforcement in action and attitude.
- ☐ 4. Restrict the child from experience with fire, tools, and electrical appliances.

Jerry Hall is a handsome, bright young man who has just been admitted to the psychiatric unit after 1 week in the alcohol withdrawal unit. He has a history of several marriages in the last 5 years, two children he does not support, and a criminal record. On the unit, he has been observed to be charming and helpful; he says he is doing fine and hopes to be discharged soon. His diagnosis is borderline personality disorder.

10. Which of the following is most characteristic of the client with borderline personality disorder?
- ☐ 1. Poor impulse control because of inadequate internal control.
- ☐ 2. Realistic appraisal of others.
- ☐ 3. Ritualistic behavior.
- ☐ 4. Unfounded, morbid fear of a seemingly harmless object.

11. Which of the following statements most often applies to clients with borderline personality disorder?
- ☐ 1. Will be helped greatly by psychotropic drugs.
- ☐ 2. Will be given electroconvulsive therapy.
- ☐ 3. Will not be given psychotropic drugs.
- ☐ 4. Will be given antidepressants.

12. In the initial stages of the therapeutic relationship, the nurse would be aware that Mr. Hall may most likely do which of the following?
- ☐ 1. Ruminate.
- ☐ 2. Hallucinate.
- ☐ 3. Manipulate.
- ☐ 4. Lose contact with reality.

13. Which of the following nursing actions would be inappropriate?
- ☐ 1. Set limits on behavior.
- ☐ 2. Maintain a firm, consistent, and positive attitude.
- ☐ 3. Expect Mr. Hall to act in a realistic, mature way, with the nurse knowing that he will not always fulfill this expectation.
- ☐ 4. Encourage Mr. Hall to assist staff with some of the more withdrawn clients.

14. Which of the following would be the most effective approach to attain the goal "client will strengthen ability to relate to others in socially acceptable ways"?
- ☐ 1. Allow the client to set his own standards of behavior on the unit.
- ☐ 2. Accept the client's evaluation of social problem areas.
- ☐ 3. Include the client in a mixed-diagnosis group for group therapy so that he learns to get along with different kinds of people.
- ☐ 4. Set rules for the client's behavior on the unit, and treat infractions of rules with loss of privileges.

15. Mr. Hall attends the daily discussion group, focuses group work on other clients' problems, and states, "My problems are over; I just want to help others." The nurse would be aware that the client is probably demonstrating which of the following behaviors?
- ☐ 1. Learning social skills.
- ☐ 2. Impulse control.
- ☐ 3. Learning problem-solving skillls.
- ☐ 4. Avoiding working on his own problems.

16. Mr. Hall stays late in the exercise yard and states that he forgot his appointment to talk with his primary nurse. Which response would be the most effective at this time?
- ☐ 1. "If you don't talk with me, I'll call your doctor."
- ☐ 2. Accept his excuse, and ask to have the client assigned to another staff member.
- ☐ 3. Ignore the forgotten appointment, and act as if it never happened.
- ☐ 4. Go to the exercise yard and state, "You and I are scheduled to talk for awhile now."

17. Mr. Hall tells his primary nurse on the 3-to-11 PM shift that the only help he is getting is from her. He complains that the day staff are too task oriented and that the night staff ignore his requests and stay in the nurses' station drinking coffee and chatting. Which of the following would be the most appropriate response?
- ☐ 1. Confront the night shift with these complaints.
- ☐ 2. Report the night shift behaviors to the 11 PM-to-7 AM supervisor.
- ☐ 3. Collect data on staff behavior from other clients at the evening client-government group.
- ☐ 4. Bring this information to daily staff conference to discuss the situation and decide on an approach to the client.

18. Which of the following is *not* an effective action to cope with the client who attempts to split the staff?
- ☐ 1. Review requests made by the client with other staff before permission is granted.
- ☐ 2. Be flexible, and let the client make his own rules.
- ☐ 3. Hold daily staff conference to discuss the matter, set an approach, and inform all staff of approaches and limits with the client.
- ☐ 4. Use written care plans for consistent approach.

Betty Pohl, 35 years old, is admitted to the unit for diagnostic tests. She is 5 feet 2 inches tall and weighs 120 pounds. She appears acutely ill and complains of pain and stiffness of the joints in her hands, feet, and knees. She says she is becoming dependent on her

family for her activities of daily living. The tentative diagnosis is rheumatoid arthritis.

19. Which of the following is most characteristic of rheumatoid arthritis?
    - ☐ 1. It most often occurs in women between the ages of 40 and 80.
    - ☐ 2. Nonsystemic involvement is most common in rheumatoid arthritis.
    - ☐ 3. Joints are affected bilaterally and symmetrically.
    - ☐ 4. It first occurs in a joint following a traumatic injury.

20. Which one of the following lab values would most support the diagnosis of rheumatoid arthritis?
    - ☐ 1. Elevated sedimentation rate.
    - ☐ 2. Decreased WBC count in the synovial fluid.
    - ☐ 3. Normal hematocrit and hemoglobin.
    - ☐ 4. Absence of rheumatoid factor in the serum.

21. The nurse is about to take Mrs. Pohl's history. Which of the following assessment findings would *not* be typical?
    - ☐ 1. A recent weight loss and anorexia.
    - ☐ 2. Stiffness that becomes more pronounced later in the day.
    - ☐ 3. Tender, hot, and red joints.
    - ☐ 4. Low-grade fever.

22. Which of the following would be *inappropriate* to include in a plan of care for Mrs. Pohl?
    - ☐ 1. Schedule her activities to allow for at least 8 to 10 hours of sleep every night, plus naps during the day.
    - ☐ 2. Educate the client and family to avoid quackery.
    - ☐ 3. Put the head of the bed in high position when helping her out of bed.
    - ☐ 4. Help her to select a high-calorie, high-protein, and high-calcium diet.

23. Preventing deformities is a major goal for Mrs. Pohl. Which of the following nursing actions would be *inappropriate* to achieve this goal?
    - ☐ 1. Place pillows under the major joints.
    - ☐ 2. Encourage her to lie prone several times a day.
    - ☐ 3. Place a pillow between her legs when she is positioned on the side.
    - ☐ 4. Provide her with a small pillow for her head.

24. Another goal is to help Mrs. Pohl to be as pain free as possible. Which of the following is an *incorrect* method of relieving pain?
    - ☐ 1. Apply hot, moist packs to the affected joints.
    - ☐ 2. Apply cold packs to the affected joints.
    - ☐ 3. Give analgesics on a regular schedule every 3 to 4 hours.
    - ☐ 4. Massage the joints when they ache.

25. Exercise is an important treatment modality for clients with arthritis. Which of the following responses by Mrs. Pohl indicates the need for further teaching regarding physical exercise guidelines?

- ☐ 1. "Exercise only to the point of pain, never beyond."
- ☐ 2. "Refrain from exercising affected joints until pain and swelling subside."
- ☐ 3. "Isometric exercises can be done independently and without supervision."
- ☐ 4. "An ongoing regimen of exercise at all times for all joints is essential."

26. Phenylbutazone (Butazolidin) is prescribed for its antiinflammatory actions. What instructions would be given to Mrs. Pohl regarding this drug?
    - ☐ 1. Take the drug 2 hours before and 2 hours after eating.
    - ☐ 2. Take alternately with aspirin.
    - ☐ 3. Examine the stools and urine for blood.
    - ☐ 4. You may need to take the drug indefinitely.

27. Mrs. Pohl tells the nurse that the physician may prescribe a gold preparation if the present medications are not effective. What is a major *disadvantage* of gold preparations?
    - ☐ 1. They must be administered several months before benefits can be determined.
    - ☐ 2. They must be given intravenously.
    - ☐ 3. The urine will turn green.
    - ☐ 4. Serious adverse effects commonly occur during the first week.

Julie Carter, age 36, has just had her first pregnancy confirmed. She has been married 5 years and appears excited and nervous after hearing she is pregnant.

28. In performing an initial assessment of Mrs. Carter during the first trimester, what is most appropriate for the nurse to assess?
    - ☐ 1. Pattern of weight gain.
    - ☐ 2. Cervical dilatation.
    - ☐ 3. Plans for childbirth preparation.
    - ☐ 4. Past medical history.

29. When a nursing history is taken, Mrs. Carter asks the nurse, "How soon can I find out if I'm carrying a normal baby?" Which response by the nurse would be most appropriate?
    - ☐ 1. "A 24-hour estriol can be done now."
    - ☐ 2. "An amniocentesis can be done at 14 weeks."
    - ☐ 3. "An oxytocin challenge test can be done at 16 weeks."
    - ☐ 4. "A nonstress test can be done immediately."

30. Mrs. Carter's history reveals that she smokes a pack of cigarettes each day. Which of the following problems would the nurse discuss with her that might occur as a result of smoking?
    - ☐ 1. Small-for-gestational-age infant.
    - ☐ 2. Spontaneous abortion.
    - ☐ 3. Fetal limb anomalies.
    - ☐ 4. Increased maternal weight gain in pregnancy.

31. Mrs. Carter's blood work at this visit demonstrates the following results: blood type A, Rh negative, rubella titer 1:64, hemoglobin 14 g, hematocrit 37%, serology for syphilis: nonreactive. How would the nurse interpret these data?
    - ☐ 1. Rubella vaccine should be given.
    - ☐ 2. Iron supplements are needed.
    - ☐ 3. Mr. Carter should be checked for the Rh factor.
    - ☐ 4. Baby Carter could acquire congenital syphilis.

32. Prenatal teaching for Mrs. Carter includes recommendations about rest and exercise. Which of the following is *not* appropriate advice for the pregnant woman?
    - ☐ 1. Avoid standing or sitting for long periods of time.
    - ☐ 2. Prevent fatigue, as pregnant women tire more readily.
    - ☐ 3. Continue usual exercise regimen.
    - ☐ 4. Begin a new active exercise program, such as jogging.

33. Mrs. Carter has active genital herpes simplex type 2. What kind of a delivery would the nurse advise her to expect if she still has active lesions when she goes into labor?
    - ☐ 1. Low-segment cesarean section.
    - ☐ 2. Vaginal delivery with low forceps.
    - ☐ 3. Induction at 36 weeks' gestation.
    - ☐ 4. Method selected by client.

34. Early in the second trimester, Mrs. Carter is scheduled to have an amniocentesis. Which of the following would be a reason for having an amniocentesis at this time?
    - ☐ 1. To assess fetal lung maturity.
    - ☐ 2. To estimate the gestational age of the fetus.
    - ☐ 3. To determine alphafetoprotein levels.
    - ☐ 4. To evaluate placental functioning.

35. During a prenatal visit in the seventh month of pregnancy, Mrs. Carter complains of severe leg cramps, especially at night. When the nurse is instructing her on ways of alleviating this problem, which of the following is the most appropriate action to advise?
    - ☐ 1. Walk briskly around the room.
    - ☐ 2. Get up and drink a cup of tea.
    - ☐ 3. Straighten her leg, and dorsiflex her ankle.
    - ☐ 4. Rub her leg until the pain subsides.

36. The nurse teaches Mrs. Carter about varicose veins in pregnancy. Which of the following would indicate that Mrs. Carter understands how to obtain relief from the discomfort of the varicosities in her legs?
    - ☐ 1. She is currently sitting with her legs crossed at the knees.
    - ☐ 2. She is currently wearing knee-high hose with stretch bands.
    - ☐ 3. She states she frequently elevates her legs above her hips when lying down or sitting.
    - ☐ 4. She is still employed as a secretary and remains sedentary most of her work day.

37. At Mrs. Carter's next antepartal visit, the nurse notes that she has gained 3 pounds since her last visit 2 weeks ago and is complaining that her wedding ring is tight. Her urine shows 1+ proteinuria, and her blood pressure is markedly increased from baseline. What is the suspected cause?
    - ☐ 1. Normal fluid retention of pregnancy.
    - ☐ 2. Early cardiac decompensation.
    - ☐ 3. Pathological changes accompanying polyhydramnios.
    - ☐ 4. Pathological changes of mild preeclampsia.

Twenty-month-old Ryan Shore has a diagnosis of iron-deficiency anemia.

38. Which of the following is most likely to be the cause of iron-deficiency anemia in a toddler?
    - ☐ 1. Excessive milk intake, which decreases the intake of solid foods.
    - ☐ 2. Insufficient iron stores at birth.
    - ☐ 3. Refusal to eat iron-rich foods because of their unappealing taste.
    - ☐ 4. A normal physiological occurrence during the toddler years.

39. Which of the following signs and symptoms would the nurse expect her assessment of Ryan to reveal?
    - ☐ 1. Overweight, normal exercise tolerance, and flushed face.
    - ☐ 2. Pallor, fatigue, and irritability.
    - ☐ 3. Pallor, average muscle tone, and accelerated growth rate.
    - ☐ 4. Exercise tolerance, good muscle tone, and average growth rate.

40. Mrs. Shore has been taught how to administer Ryan's oral iron preparation at home. Which statement by Mrs. Shore indicates the need for clarification by the nurse?
    - ☐ 1. "I'll give Ryan his medicine between meals with fruit or juice."
    - ☐ 2. "I'll use a straw, syringe, or dropper placed to the back of Ryan's mouth when I give him his medicine."
    - ☐ 3. "I'll help Ryan brush his teeth after he takes the medicine to decrease the likelihood of staining his teeth."
    - ☐ 4. "I'll expect the color of Ryan's stool to change to a dark yellow."

41. One month after discharge, Mrs. Shore returns with Ryan for a blood count. Which test result indicates that teaching for Mrs. Shore has been successful?
    - ☐ 1. Hemoglobin: 14.2 g/dl.
    - ☐ 2. Hematocrit: 28%.
    - ☐ 3. Platelets: 100,000/mm³.
    - ☐ 4. White blood count: 10,000 cells/mm³.

Andrea Stuben is admitted to the psychiatric unit with a diagnosis of reactive depression. She is 26 years old. She was severely injured in an automobile accident 2 months ago. Her husband and 3-year-old daughter were killed in the same accident. Because of her injuries, she was unable to attend their funeral. She is in two full-leg casts, is thin, and apathetic.

42. Which is the best explanation for Mrs. Stuben's behavior?
   ☐ 1. She is in poor physical condition from the accident.
   ☐ 2. The inability to attend the funeral has probably affected the process of grieving.
   ☐ 3. The realization she will not see her daughter grow up was overwhelming.
   ☐ 4. She is experiencing unbearable loneliness.

43. Mrs. Stuben has had a 10-pound weight loss since the accident. Which would be the most helpful for her?
   ☐ 1. Have her eat with a client who is recovering from depression.
   ☐ 2. Serve a tray in her room so others will not observe her poor appetite.
   ☐ 3. Allow her to eat in the cafeteria so she can select food that appeals to her.
   ☐ 4. Have the dietitian prepare special trays to ensure the inclusion of all food groups.

44. Mrs. Stuben has difficulty falling asleep. It is most appropriate to do which of the following?
   ☐ 1. Allow her to exercise the upper part of her body 20 minutes every night at 9 PM.
   ☐ 2. Provide a cool sponge bath and a cup of tea at bedtime.
   ☐ 3. Allow her to watch TV every night until midnight.
   ☐ 4. Provide a warm sponge bath and a warm glass of milk at bedtime.

45. Since there are variations in energy level in depressed clients, at what time of day would it be best to schedule Mrs. Stuben's activities?
   ☐ 1. Morning.
   ☐ 2. Noon.
   ☐ 3. Afternoon.
   ☐ 4. Evening.

46. Which of the following behaviors will demonstrate to the nurse that Mrs. Stuben is progressing in the resolution of her grief?
   ☐ 1. She reduces the amount of time spent crying.
   ☐ 2. She begins to talk about both the positive and negative aspects of relationships with the deceased.
   ☐ 3. She begins to demonstrate increased self-control by becoming more detached.
   ☐ 4. She begins to notice hospital staff members and seeks them out to discuss her concerns.

Harlan King, age 68, sustained a left-sided cerebrovascular accident 4 weeks ago. He has been transferred to a rehabilitation unit. He is able to communicate by minimal verbal expression and gesturing that he intends to walk again and use his right arm. His wife expresses the same goals.

47. In making assessments and initiating a program for Mr. King, what must all rehabilitation team members consider?
   ☐ 1. Initial assessments will need to be modified throughout the first week or two, because the transfer to a new environment and the client's fatigue during this period will affect the accuracy of assessments.
   ☐ 2. Try to accomplish as much as possible with this client in the first 2 weeks; after that, motivation will generally decrease and gains made thereafter will be minimal.
   ☐ 3. Mrs. King will need to find something to do outside the rehabilitation setting. Mr. King needs to concentrate on his rehabilitation program at this point, and too much stimulation from family members will confuse him.
   ☐ 4. While making diagnostic assessments, give the client as many cues as possible so that he will perform optimally.

48. Safety precautions are an important part of Mr. King's care. His right arm and leg have decreased sensation, along with the paresis, and could easily be injured. Based on these data, the plan of care would be to do which of the following?
   ☐ 1. Protect these extremities with an arm sling and bivalved leg cast.
   ☐ 2. Instruct Mr. King to observe his affected arm and leg frequently for positioning and to become aware of any movements that might injure them.
   ☐ 3. Concentrate on the positives; do not talk about the paralyzed extremities and depress the client.
   ☐ 4. Place any equipment (food tray etc.) on Mr. King's right side so he can help himself safely and gain self-esteem through increasing independence.

49. Mr. King is having difficulty attaining sufficient nutritional intake. He has some trouble swallowing and has choked while eating. How can eating be facilitated?
   ☐ 1. Teach him to eat slowly, and place food in the paralyzed side of his mouth.
   ☐ 2. Instruct Mrs. King to feed her husband after ensuring that all food is cut into bite-sized pieces.
   ☐ 3. Help him to a sitting position, place food in the unparalyzed side of his mouth, and have him concentrate on chewing and swallowing.
   ☐ 4. Restrict his intake to liquids until his chewing and swallowing capacities are fully restored.

50. It is important to minimize deformities in clients who

have sustained brain damage. How is this best accomplished?

☐ 1. Set up a program with the client, and let him be responsible for doing range-of-motion exercises on his own.

☐ 2. Schedule daily visits to physical therapy while the client is in the rehabilitation setting.

☐ 3. Remind Mr. King that he has flaccid paralysis of his right side and needs to prevent subluxation of his right shoulder by exercise.

☐ 4. Establish a schedule to assist him to exercise his right side with his unaffected side.

51. Which behavior best typifies the client with right-sided hemiplegia?

☐ 1. Unaware of limitations; plunges into activities unaware of safety factors.

☐ 2. Anxious; approaches tasks in a halting, fearful way; may respond best to simple gestures.

☐ 3. Content with verbal directives; feels gestures and pantomime are demeaning.

☐ 4. Especially prone to spatial-perceptual problems.

52. Mr. King spends a lot of time sitting in a chair. Where do decubitus ulcers most often develop when clients spend most of their time sitting?

☐ 1. Over the sacrum.
☐ 2. Over the coccyx.
☐ 3. Over the ischial tuberosities.
☐ 4. Heels.

Twelve-year-old Zachary has newly diagnosed insulin-dependent diabetes. He is on the pediatric unit.

53. Which of the following would *not* be an expected finding in Zachary's nursing history?

☐ 1. Rapid weight gain.
☐ 2. Drinking large amounts of fluids.
☐ 3. Lethargic and tired.
☐ 4. Sudden return of bed-wetting.

54. Zachary is admitted with ketoacidosis. The physician orders an "insulin IV push." Which type of insulin would the nurse anticipate that the physician will order?

☐ 1. Lente.
☐ 2. Regular.
☐ 3. NPH.
☐ 4. PZI.

55. Zachary has an order for an 1800-calorie, diabetic exchange diet. The nurse explains to Zachary and his parents that this means that Zachary can do which of the following?

☐ 1. Can eat what he wants as long as he avoids concentrated sweets.

☐ 2. Can substitute items on one food list with other items from the same food list.

☐ 3. Can substitute any food item for any other as

long as his total daily calorie intake remains the same.

☐ 4. Must carefully weigh or measure all portions of his food intake.

56. When teaching Zachary and his parents about insulin shock, the nurse emphasizes which of the following signs as indicating impending insulin shock?

☐ 1. Acetone breath.
☐ 2. Slowed respirations.
☐ 3. Tremors.
☐ 4. Increased thirst.

57. It is also important to teach Zachary and his parents about situations that will increase Zachary's insulin requirements. Which of the following will *not*?

☐ 1. Increased exercise.
☐ 2. Increased food intake.
☐ 3. Infectious disease.
☐ 4. Changes associated with puberty.

58. While being taught to administer his own insulin, Zachary becomes frustrated, throws down the syringe, and says, "I wish I could just forget this stuff!" What is the best explanation for this behavior?

☐ 1. Zachary lacks confidence in himself.

☐ 2. Zachary is not emotionally mature enough to assume full responsibility for his own insulin administration.

☐ 3. Zachary is having difficulty coping with the knowledge and implications of having a chronic illness.

☐ 4. Zachary is angry with the nurse.

59. How would the nurse respond to Zachary's behavior?

☐ 1. Discuss this reaction with Zachary's parents and physician.

☐ 2. Ask a 13-year-old boy on the unit who also has insulin-dependent diabetes to talk with Zachary.

☐ 3. Refer Zachary to the staff psychologist.

☐ 4. Tell Zachary, "You'll get used to this eventually, and it won't seem difficult."

Theodore Eliasson, a 32-year-old advertising executive, has had surgery for the removal of a peptic ulcer. He states he has been under increasing stress in his employment and is very concerned about being able to continue in his position.

60. Which of the following statements most accurately describes Mr. Eliasson's condition?

☐ 1. The stress of his environment has contributed to a physical condition of known organic origin.

☐ 2. Although there is stress in his environment, it is not a direct contributing cause of his physical problem.

☐ 3. His basic personality is the most influential factor in the cause of his physical problem.

☐ 4. Hereditary factors are the most important cause of his physical problem.

61. The principal ego-defense mechanism used by Mr. Eliasson is which of the following?

☐ 1. Rationalization.

☐ 2. Reaction formation.

☐ 3. Regression.

☐ 4. Repression.

62. A condition such as Mr. Eliasson's differs from malingering in which of the following ways?

☐ 1. The malingerer cooperates more readily in the treatment plan.

☐ 2. The malingerer unconsciously develops symptoms to avoid an undesirable situation.

☐ 3. The malingerer consciously develops symptoms to avoid an undesirable situation.

☐ 4. The malingerer does not adapt as easily to illness.

63. The nurse will need to take into consideration Mr. Eliasson's diagnosis when developing a treatment plan. For this reason, the nurse will assess three of the following behavioral characteristics. Which characteristic will *not* be evident?

☐ 1. Dependency issues.

☐ 2. Difficulty with decision making.

☐ 3. Excessive controlling behavior.

☐ 4. Poor reality orientation.

64. In the assessment, the nurse finds that Mr. Eliasson has difficulty with decision making. One of the main goals of nursing care will be to have which of the following occur?

☐ 1. Mrs. Eliasson will assume more responsibility for her husband's meals.

☐ 2. Mr. Eliasson will follow the physician's orders more closely.

☐ 3. Mr. Eliasson will work with the nurse to plan his care.

☐ 4. Mr. Eliasson will suggest to his wife what to make for his meals.

65. Mr. Eliasson tells the nurse he will be unable to walk down the hall today because he has a headache. When the nurse states that it is necessary for him to do so for his recovery, he yells, "You're the only nurse who makes me do that. You are cruel and heartless, and I refuse to be pushed around by you anymore." The nurse is surprised by his outburst, since he had not done it before. Which of the following responses would best meet Mr. Eliasson's nursing needs at this point?

☐ 1. "All right, if no one else does, then I won't either."

☐ 2. "I don't care what everyone else does; when I take care of you, you'll walk in the hall."

☐ 3. "You seem very angry and I'm not sure what about."

☐ 4. "Don't yell at me. Talk to me in a civilized tone or don't talk at all."

66. After a few days, the nurse notices that Mr. Eliasson begins to have frequent violent outbursts at the staff when he does not want to do something. The nurse sees these outbursts as Mr. Eliasson's way of gaining control over his environment. The best nursing approach would be to do which of the following?

☐ 1. Explain to him that yelling is not appropriate and that staff members will leave the room when he yells instead of talking.

☐ 2. Allow him to yell since he needs to feel some control while in the hospital.

☐ 3. Take away his television until he has not yelled for an entire day.

☐ 4. Allow him to yell at the staff, because they really have no right to yell back at him.

67. The most important contribution to the improvement of Mr. Eliasson's health is likely to be which of the following?

☐ 1. Taking time for more leisure activities so that stress will be reduced.

☐ 2. Appropriately sharing concerns and feelings so that emotional tensions are rechanneled.

☐ 3. Getting back to work so there is less time to focus on physical symptoms.

☐ 4. Realizing that emotions affect physical conditions.

Bonnie Turner, age 28, is suffering from metrorrhagia.

68. Mrs. Turner would be encouraged to seek medical assistance primarily because of which of the following?

☐ 1. Excessive bleeding during menses may lead to anemia.

☐ 2. Bleeding between periods may be the only early sign of cancer.

☐ 3. This is often symptomatic of a serious psychosomatic problem.

☐ 4. This is the main cause of failure to begin menses by 18 years of age.

69. In counseling Mrs. Turner, the nurse tells her that a yearly Pap smear is essential for which of the following reasons?

☐ 1. When uterine abnormalities are identified early, surgical treatment can be avoided.

☐ 2. Cervical cancer is usually curable in the preinvasive stage.

☐ 3. The Pap test is very reliable in diagnosing endometrial cancer.

☐ 4. The death rate for uterine cancer has steadily increased in recent years.

70. Mrs. Turner has had a Pap smear. The results reveal a stage 0 carcinoma in situ. It is decided that a conization will be the only treatment necessary. What is the major advantage of this procedure?

☐ 1. The procedure can be carried out on an outpatient basis.

☐ 2. Surgery carries less risk than the use of radiation.

☐ 3. The client retains the capacity to reproduce.

☐ 4. Leaving the ovaries intact while removing the uterus will prevent surgical menopause.

Colleen Green is in her third postpartum day. She has two children at home, age 7 and 2. She is breastfeeding for the first time.

71. Mrs. Green was unsuccessful in breastfeeding her first baby. Which of the following actions would be most beneficial in helping her to achieve her goal to breastfeed her new baby?

☐ 1. Explore the reasons why she failed the first time.

☐ 2. Tell her that breastfeeding will be easier with this baby since she is used to handling infants now.

☐ 3. Stay with her and assist her with feeding the infant as needed.

☐ 4. Ask her to put the call light on if she needs help.

72. Mrs. Green's infant is having difficulty grasping the nipple because of engorgement. The best initial nursing action is to tell Mrs. Green to do which of the following?

☐ 1. Use a nipple shield.

☐ 2. Discontinue breastfeeding.

☐ 3. Express some milk manually before each feeding.

☐ 4. Breastfeed more frequently.

73. Fundal height is measured daily to monitor the involution of the uterus. When would an *inaccurate* measurement be obtained?

☐ 1. Just after Mrs. Green has nursed her baby.

☐ 2. If Mrs. Green has a full bladder.

☐ 3. If Mrs. Green takes methylergonovine (Methergine).

☐ 4. If the baby is large (over 10 pounds).

74. Mrs. Green is having severe afterpains. What is the most appropriate explanation to give her?

☐ 1. "It is very individual. One cannot predict what the nature of the pains might be."

☐ 2. "Afterpains increase with each pregnancy. Breastfeeding also increases the intensity of the pains."

☐ 3. "They are not usual. I will call your doctor."

☐ 4. "Afterpains are due to clots within the uterus. The uterus contracts and tries to expel them."

75. Mrs. Green does not like to drink milk and wonders whether she can continue to nurse her baby because of this. What is the most appropriate response the nurse can give?

☐ 1. "Breastfeeding will have to be discontinued; milk is essential in the diet to produce milk."

☐ 2. "When you don't like milk, it is very important

to eat dark green vegetables as a source of calcium."

☐ 3. "Fruit juices can be used instead of drinking milk."

☐ 4. "This will not be a problem because there is no real advantage to drinking milk when lactating."

76. Mrs. Green has learned about the let-down reflex. Which one of the following statements most enables the nurse to conclude that Mrs. Green understands the nature of the reflex?

☐ 1. "I have excess milk now, but the quantity will adjust itself depending on the baby's needs."

☐ 2. "If I use a bottle often, I will stop secreting adequate milk for the baby."

☐ 3. "When milk drips from my other breast, I know that my baby is getting milk."

☐ 4. "The more the baby sucks and stimulates my breast, the more I will produce."

77. Mrs. Green is concerned that her 2-year-old daughter will not like the new baby. She asks the nurse what she might do. The nurse would suggest which of the following?

☐ 1. "Explain to your daughter that the baby is a permanent part of your family now."

☐ 2. "Expect your daughter to demand more of your attention when you bring the new baby home."

☐ 3. "Place limits on regressive behavior such as thumbsucking."

☐ 4. "Let your husband focus attention on your daughter while you focus on the new baby."

Alex Frankl is a 23-month-old boy with tetralogy of Fallot. At this time, he is admitted to the hospital for further evaluation and possible surgery.

78. During the initial nursing assessment of Alex, the nurse would most likely expect to find which of the following signs and symptoms of tetralogy of Fallot?

☐ 1. Bradycardia, dependent edema, and slow weight gain.

☐ 2. Pale, scrawny appearance; machinery murmur; and feeding difficulties.

☐ 3. Higher blood pressure in the arms than in the legs, weak pedal pulses, and epistaxis.

☐ 4. Clubbing of the fingers and toes, tachycardia, and cyanosis.

79. A child with tetralogy of Fallot is prone to several complications. The nurse would be alert for which of the following?

☐ 1. Clotting dysfunction.

☐ 2. Bone marrow depression.

☐ 3. Cerebral emboli.

☐ 4. Sickling of hemoglobin.

80. Alex suddenly begins to choke and cough, and he turns cyanotic. What would the nurse do first?

☐ 1. Help Alex assume a squatting position.

☐ 2. Put a Venturi mask over Alex's nose and mouth.

☐ 3. Place Alex upside down and pat his back vigorously.

☐ 4. Determine if Alex is trying to use his condition to gain attention.

81. The physician orders 65 μg of digoxin for Alex at 8 AM and 8 PM. What would be the best method for giving Alex his medicine?

☐ 1. Mix the digoxin with milk.

☐ 2. Allow Alex to drink the digoxin himself from a plastic medicine cup.

☐ 3. Use the dropper from the bottle.

☐ 4. Offer Alex a reward if he takes his medicine without difficulty.

82. Alex has an order for a low-sodium diet. Which one of the following foods would be most *inappropriate* for his diet?

☐ 1. Eggs.

☐ 2. Fruited yogurt.

☐ 3. Cottage cheese.

☐ 4. Cheddar cheese.

Jane Johnson, 22 years old, is admitted to the hospital for a diagnostic workup. For the past 2 months, she has been irritable and argumentative with her boyfriend. At other times, she has been almost euphoric. She has been depressed about recent body changes. She has gained 15 pounds; her face is puffy and flushed. She has also noted numerous bruises over her body; and while her abdomen has begun to protrude, her legs have become thin. Miss Johnson is admitted with the tentative diagnosis of Cushing's syndrome.

83. Assessments that would commonly lead the nurse to suspect a client has Cushing's syndrome include which of the following?

☐ 1. Low blood glucose and tachycardia.

☐ 2. Thickening of the skin and bruising.

☐ 3. Weight loss and sodium retention.

☐ 4. Delayed wound healing and osteoporosis.

84. What test results are most indicative of Cushing's syndrome?

☐ 1. Increased serum sodium and plasma free-cortisol levels.

☐ 2. Decreased serum potassium and BUN.

☐ 3. Increased serum epinephrine and norepinephrine.

☐ 4. Decreased urinary 17-ketogenic steroids and 17-hydroxycorticoids.

85. Which of the following would *not* be the possible cause of Cushing's syndrome in this client?

☐ 1. Adrenal tumor.

☐ 2. Ectopic source of ACTH.

☐ 3. Pituitary tumor.

☐ 4. Adrenal atrophy.

86. When Miss Johnson has been admitted to the hospital, the immediate nursing priority is which of the following?

☐ 1. Decrease stress in the environment.

☐ 2. Encourage liberal amounts of fluids.

☐ 3. Explain tests and procedures.

☐ 4. Provide diversional activities.

87. Which of the following fluid and electrolyte problems is most likely to occur with Miss Johnson?

☐ 1. Hyperkalemia.

☐ 2. Increased output of dilute urine.

☐ 3. Sodium and H_2O retention.

☐ 4. Decreased serum calcium.

88. The physician has ordered a plasma cortisol test. A positive test in a client with Cushing's syndrome would indicate elevated cortisol levels at what time of day?

☐ 1. Morning.

☐ 2. Afternoon.

☐ 3. Evening.

☐ 4. Morning and evening.

89. Miss Johnson is constantly hungry and is quite concerned that she cannot stop eating. This is probably occurring for which of the following reasons?

☐ 1. She is stressed and is compensating by eating.

☐ 2. She is hypoglycemic, and the body compensates with hunger.

☐ 3. She has increased cortisol levels that accelerate gluconeogenesis.

☐ 4. She has had an increase in energy output and requires more calories.

90. Miss Johnson's diet needs to be modified. Which of the following would be a good choice for lunch?

☐ 1. Chicken, brown rice, and sliced oranges.

☐ 2. Tomato soup, tuna fish sandwich, and vanilla pudding.

☐ 3. Macaroni and cheese, tomato salad, and baked apple.

☐ 4. Broiled steak, green beans, and ice cream.

91. The diagnosis of Cushing's disease has been confirmed. A bilateral adrenalectomy is scheduled. Client teaching will include which of the following?

☐ 1. Lifelong replacement of corticosteroids will be required.

☐ 2. She will need to have weekly ACTH injections.

☐ 3. Cortisol will be required in stress situations.

☐ 4. No replacement therapy will be necessary.

92. Preoperatively, the client says to the nurse, "I want to have this operation so I will look like my old self again." What would be an appropriate response?

☐ 1. "It will take several months before the changes are reversed."

☐ 2. "I can see this is bothering you. Can you tell me what concerns you the most?"

☐ 3. "Adjusting to body changes is never easy to do."

☐ 4. "Have you discussed this with your boyfriend?"

93. The most important postoperative adrenalectomy assessment is which of the following?
- ☐ 1. Type of nasogastric drainage.
- ☐ 2. Presence of drainage on abdominal dressing.
- ☐ 3. Heart rate.
- ☐ 4. Blood pressure.

94. On her third postoperative day, Miss Johnson shows signs and symptoms of a mild addisonian crisis. Why is this considered a medical emergency?
- ☐ 1. The increased cortisol levels can result in a hyperosmolar coma.
- ☐ 2. Loss of sodium and increased potassium levels can cause life-threatening fluid and electrolyte imbalances.
- ☐ 3. Increased aldosterone levels can trigger cardiac failure.
- ☐ 4. The posterior pituitary gland cannot produce enough antidiuretic hormone (ADH).

95. Miss Johnson continues to convalesce without any further complications. What is the most important point to be included in her discharge teaching?
- ☐ 1. Meticulous skin care.
- ☐ 2. Relaxation techniques.
- ☐ 3. Diet teaching.
- ☐ 4. Medication administration.

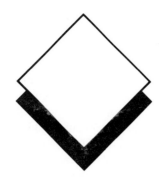

Test 2, Book IV

ANSWERS WITH RATIONALES

KEY TO ABBREVIATIONS
Section of the Review Book

P = Psychosocial and Mental Health Problems
   T = Therapeutic Use of Self
   L = Loss and Death and Dying
   A = Anxious Behavior
   C = Confused Behavior
   E = Elated-Depressive Behavior
   SM = Socially Maladaptive Behavior
   SS = Suspicious Behavior
   W = Withdrawn Behavior
   SU = Substance Use Disorders
A = Adult
   H = Healthy Adult
   S = Surgery
   O = Oxygenation
   NM = Nutrition and Metabolism
   E = Elimination
   SP = Sensation and Perception
   M = Mobility
   CA = Cellular Aberration
CBF = Childbearing Family
   W = Women's Health Care
   A = Antepartal Care
   I = Intrapartal Care
   P = Postpartal Care
   N = Newborn Care
C = Child
   H = Healthy Child
   I = Ill and Hospitalized Child
   SPP = Sensation, Perception, and Protection
   O = Oxygenation
   NM = Nutrition and Metabolism
   E = Elimination
   M = Mobility
   CA = Cellular Aberration

Nursing Process Category

AS = Assessment
AN = Analysis
PL = Plan
IM = Implementation
EV = Evaluation

Client Need Category

E = Safe, Effective Care Environment
PS = Physiological Integrity
PC = Psychosocial Integrity
H = Health Promotion and Maintenance

1. no. 2. The inflamed mucosa of the bladder is the most likely cause of the spasms that lead to symptoms of urgency. The other options are incorrect. A/E, AN, PS

2. no. 3. Vitamin C is the only choice given that will best acidify urine. Commercial juices may be too dilute to affect urine acidity. A/E, IM, PS

3. no. 1. Sulfisoxazole (Gantrisin) is excreted by the kidneys and not absorbed and is therefore more active in the urine than other antibiotics. The others listed are absorbed systemically. A/E, AN, PS

4. no. 1. *E. coli* is the most common cause of urinary tract infections and is very sensitive to sulfisoxazole (Gantrisin). *Pseudomonas* and *Klebsiella* infections are more commonly found in the respiratory system, and *Salmonella* infection is more commonly found in the gastrointestinal tract. A/E, AN, PS

5. no. 2. The school-age child is developing a sense of industry (doing, accomplishing, and achieving) to gain control through mastery and to build a positive self-concept. All the other options are too advanced for him. C/H, AN, H

6. no. 4. There is not enough information to make a judgment about Randall's growth. Information concerning his previous growth pattern, his dietary hab-

its and exercise patterns, and hereditary influences (growth of family members) is needed before conclusions can be drawn. C/H, AN, PS

7. no. 3. Results of visual-acuity testing are abnormal for Randall's age, and he should be referred for a more comprehensive evaluation at once. Option no. 4 is wrong; options no. 1 and no. 2 are inappropriate. C/H, PL, PS

8. no. 1. Since Randall has had the full recommended series, he will not need any additional immunizations until he is 14 to 16 years old. C/H, PL, PS

9. no. 4. Restricting a school-age child from experiences with fire, tools, and electrical appliances allows no opportunity to learn safety rules with these important objects. The child will remain unsafe. C/H, IM, E

10. no. 1. Such clients make unrealistic appraisals of others and usually do not demonstrate ritualistic or fearful behaviors. Most characteristic of a borderline personality is the poor impulse control because of inadequate internal control. Ritualistic behavior is seen in compulsive personalities. Morbid fear of a seemingly harmless object is true of a phobic client. P/SM, AS, PC

11. no. 3. Psychotropic drugs, electroconvulsive therapy, and antidepressants have not been found helpful in borderline personality disorder. Psychotropic drugs are used to treat psychotic disorders. Electroconvulsive therapy and antidepressants are used for clients with depression. P/SM, AN, PC

12. no. 3. Manipulation is characteristic behavior of clients like Mr. Hall. These clients seldom ruminate, lose contact with reality, or have ritualistic behavior. Rumination occurs mostly in depressed clients. Hallucinations occur in psychotic individuals and clients using street drugs (e.g., cocaine or PCP). Although depersonalization and splitting occur and are serious distortions of reality, actual psychosis is the exception rather than the rule. P/SM, AS, PC

13. no. 4. Since clients with borderline personality disorder have a tendency to manipulate and use others, they should not be asked to assist staff with other clients. Mr. Hall requires firm limits on his behavior since he has little inner control. A firm, consistent, and positive attitude will help strengthen the client's ego, which will help him deal with the emotional discomfort of psychotherapy. By expecting the client to act in a realistic, mature way, less regression should occur. P/SM, IM, PC

14. no. 4. Consistent limit setting is necessary in order to teach the client with borderline personality disorder to relate to others in socially acceptable ways. The client has little internal control and needs to learn control of impulsivity and acting-out behavior. Borderline clients often use flippancy and a light affect to minimize their desperation and pain. They often distort social problem areas and blame others for their problems. This client will antagonize others with critical and hostile complaints and verbal abuse. P/SM, IM, PC

15. no. 4. Clients with borderline personality disorder manipulate to avoid facing and working on their own problems. Genuine social skill development occurs very slowly. Impulse control is demonstrated when client shows restraint, not when focusing on other clients' problems. There is no evidence that the client is learning problem-solving skills. P/SM, EV, PC

16. no. 4. This approach is demonstrating consistent limit-setting in a matter-of-fact way. A firm and consistent approach is necessary so it is important not to ignore the incident. The nurse is responsible and accountable for meeting with the client. The nurse has been manipulated and is experiencing a common negative counter-transference reaction to the borderline client, that of aversion. This behavior by the nurse results in abandonment feelings in the client. P/SM, IM, PC

17. no. 4. Daily staff conferences must be held to discuss client behaviors and plan a consistent approach for all three shifts; clients with borderline personality disorder have an amazing ability to split the staff. Although clinical and managerial aspects of the matter must be explored by nursing management, better methods than that described in option no. 3 can be taken if staff behavior appears to be a problem. P/SM, IM, PC

18. no. 2. The client with borderline personality disorder needs limits and does not have the ability to adaptively set his own limits and rules. Reviewing requests, holding daily staff conferences, and using written care plans are very effective in decreasing manipulation and consequently staff anger as well as preventing splitting of staff. P/SM. IM, PC

19. no. 3. The other options are characteristic of osteoarthritis. Rheumatoid arthritis has familial tendencies and commonly occurs between the ages of 25 and 55 years. A/M, AS, PS

20. no. 1. The sedimentation rate is elevated and is the most consistent lab finding in rheumatoid arthritis. The serum white blood cell count is usually slightly elevated; the client is usually anemic; and protein antibodies and/or rheumatoid factor are present in 80% of clients. Synovial fluid is not tested in either type of arthritis. A/M, AS, PS

21. no. 2. Stiffness is more pronounced in the early morning; it diminishes with use of the joint in rheumatoid arthritis. A/M, AS, PS

22. no. 4. The client's weight is within normal limits. Increasing calories and weight would place extra stress on joints. Added calcium would cause serum

calcium to be high with increased risk of frozen joints. The client needs rest with spacing of activities to facilitate treatments for this systemic disease. Putting the head of the bed in high position prevents stress and strain on the joints when the client gets out of bed. A/M, PL, E

23. no. 1. Pillows under major joints contribute to the complication of flexion contractures. Options no. 2 and no. 4 prevent contractures. Option no. 3 maintains skin integrity. A/M, IM, E

24. no. 4. Massage tends to further traumatize swollen, inflamed, and painful joints. Cold packs produce an anesthetic effect. Heat or cold can both be used effectively in the treatment of arthritis to decrease muscle spasms. A/M, IM, PS

25. no. 4. Inflamed joints should not be exercised. All joints need not be exercised at all times. An appropriate exercise regimen must be flexible and adjustable. The other options are correct. A/M, EV, H

26. no. 3. Phenylbutazone (Butazolidin) causes bleeding; thus, stools and urine should be examined. Since acetylsalicylic acid (aspirin) also has ulcerogenic and anticoagulant effects, it should be avoided when taking phenylbutazone. A/M, IM, PS

27. no. 1. Several months of therapy are required before effectiveness can be determined. The drug is commonly given deep intramuscularly. Adverse effects most commonly occur late, often after treatment has been discontinued. A/M, AN, PS

28. no. 4. The client, by virtue of age, is a high-risk client. A medical history would be important to further assess for conditions affecting the course of pregnancy. Since this is the first prenatal visit, it would not be possible to determine a pattern of weight gain yet. Cervical dilatation determination would not be appropriate at this time. Plans for childbirth would be appropriate, but not as critical as the initial medical history. CBF/A, AS, PS

29. no. 2. Although a vast majority of birth defects will not be detected by amniocentesis as early as 14 weeks of gestation when adequate amniotic fluid can be obtained, this procedure can be used to assess specific disorders common in clients of advanced maternal age. The oxytocin challenge test, nonstress test, and urine estriols are carried out to determine fetal and placental functioning rather than chromosomal disorders. CBF/A, IM, PS

30. no. 1. Women who smoke give birth to small-for-gestational-age infants at a rate almost twice that of women who do not smoke. Smoking causes constriction in the vasculature of the mother as well as of the placenta. Fewer nutrients are thus delivered to the fetus. Smoking does not increase spontaneous abortion rates or maternal weight gain. CBF/A, AN, PS

31. no. 3. Maternal isoimmunization in the Rh-negative expectant mother may occur if the baby inherits the father's Rh factor; therefore it should be determined if Mr. Carter is Rh positive. All other data would require no action. CBF/A, AN, PS

32. no. 4. Strenuous new exercise should not be started during pregnancy. Current research indicates most fetuses can tolerate strenuous maternal exercise if the mother was previously conditioned to that level of activity. Jogging is also a controversial issue among physicians. CBF/A, IM, H

33. no. 1. The baby will contract the herpes through the birth canal if delivered vaginally. This virus has a devastating effect on newborns, and many will die if infected. CBF/A, IM, PS

34. no. 3. An increase in alphafetoprotein is indicative of neural defects in the fetus. Lung maturity is assessed in late pregnancy by determining the L/S ratio; a ratio of 2:1 indicates fetal lung maturity. Gestational age and fetal growth are more appropriately evaluated using serial ultrasonography. Placental functioning is not assessed by amniocentesis. CBF/A, AN, PS

35. no. 3. This is the only remedy known to eliminate the cramp quickly. The other methods listed do not work. CBF/A, IM, PS

36. no. 3. Swelling and discomfort from varicosities caused by impeded venous return can be decreased by lying down or sitting with the legs elevated. Relief measures are aimed at promoting venous return. Thus, increased periods of sitting (causing popliteal pressure) or constricting garments should be avoided. CBF/A, EV, PS

37. no. 4. Preeclampsia is the development of hypertension with proteinuria, edema, or both after the twentieth week of gestation. Normal fluid retention is reflected in lower extremity edema in late pregnancy. Blood pressure should remain within normal limits. Data do not support a diagnosis of cardiac decompensation or polyhydramnios. CBF/A, AN, PS

38. no. 1. Excessive milk intake limits ingestion of iron-rich foods. C/O, AS, PS

39. no. 2. Iron-deficiency anemia can cause symptoms including pallor, fatigue, irritability, decreased exercise tolerance, decreased growth rate, and poor muscle tone. C/O, AS, PS

40. no. 4. Stools, after administration of an oral iron preparation, will become a tarry-green color. C/O, EV, H

41. no. 1. A hemoglobin of 11 to 15.5 g/dl is within normal limits and is a valid measure of improvement in anemia. A hematocrit of 28% is abnormally low. Neither the platelets nor the WBC is affected by nutritional anemia. C/O, EV, PS

42. no. 2. Clients are often prevented from beginning resolution of their grief when they are unable to attend funerals of loved ones. Options no. 1, no. 3, and no. 4 are all possible explanations for why she is thin and apathetic, but she is having a delayed grief response because her physical condition prevented her from going through the normal funeral ritual. P/E, AN, PC

43. no. 3. Independence is encouraged by allowing her to select foods that appeal to her. Option no. 1 imposes another person upon her and places a burden on the other client. Option no. 2 causes isolation. Option no. 4 is a good second choice if she will not select her own foods. P/E, IM, PS

44. no. 4. These are appropriate nursing measures to promote sleep. Options no. 1, no. 2, and no. 3 are all stimulating actions that would increase arousal. P/E, IM, PS

45. no. 1. In reactive depression, the client usually feels best in the morning and worse as the day progresses. P/E, PL, E

46. no. 2. Resolution of grief is demonstrated by the ability to reminisce about both the positive and negative aspects of a relationship in a realistic manner. Crying is a normal response but will occur less often and for shorter periods. Detachment is a sign of abnormal grieving. Being able to talk about her concerns shows an ability to deal with the reality of the loss but does not show resolution; it shows the beginning of the working phase in dealing with the grief. P/E, EV, PC

47. no. 1. A change in environment affects concentration, but confusion is usually minimal unless the client is fatigued. The unfamiliar is overwhelming to a person with brain damage. The client's level of fatigue must be considered to obtain accurate assessment data. A/SP, AS, E

48. no. 2. Involve the client in his care with mutual goal setting and by promoting self-responsibility. These actions can enhance client compliance. Use arm sling and leg cast only during transport; these restrict range of motion if used continuously. Food trays and equipment should be positioned on the client's unaffected side. A/SP, PL, E

49. no. 3. This is the optimal way to facilitate eating. Feeding clients increases dependency. Chewing and swallowing may never be completely restored. Liquids are generally more difficult to handle than solids. A/SP, IM, PS

50. no. 4. A cerebrovascular accident is an upper motor neuron lesion; therefore spastic, not flaccid, paralysis is present. Clients should participate in exercises but cannot be expected to initiate and remember their own exercise program. A/SP, PL, E

51. no. 2. These behaviors are characteristic of left-brain lesions near the motor cortex. In contrast, right-brain lesions result in perceptual and spatial disabilities. A/SP, AS, PS

52. no. 3. Most pressure is on the ischial tuberosities when sitting. Any redness that does not resolve 20 minutes after the pressure is relieved is at risk for tissue breakdown. A/SP, AS, PS

53. no. 1. Weight loss is typical of diabetes in children. Since glucose is unable to enter the cells, the body quickly is in a state of starvation. C/NM, AS, PS

54. no. 2. Regular insulin is the only type given intravenously because it can act quickly to reduce the blood-glucose level. C/NM, AN, PS

55. no. 2. Zachary can exchange food items within each list (e.g., one vegetable for another vegetable from the same list), but he cannot exchange a vegetable for another food (e.g., meat or fruit). C/NM, PL, E

56. no. 3. Tremors or a shaky feeling indicate hypoglycemia and impending insulin shock. C/NM, AS, E

57. no. 1. Increased exercise will decrease Zachary's insulin requirements. C/NM, IM, H

58. no. 3. Zachary is expressing his frustration over his lack of control of the situation and the realization of the long-term nature of his illness. C/NM, AN, PC

59. no. 2. Peers are very important at this age, and talking with another boy with the same illness may help Zachary see things from a more positive perspective. C/NM, IM, PC

60. no. 1. The diagnosis of psychosomatic disorder is used when there is evidence of a relationship between the environment and its meaning to the client, and the initiation or exacerbation of a physical condition. The client is not always aware of the relationship. Personality and hereditary factors may have contributed to his physical problem, but the condition has been exacerbated by a stressful working environment. P/A, AN, PS

61. no. 4. The repression of emotional tension is unconsciously channeled through visceral organs. Rationalization is the falsification of experience by the construction of logically or socially approved explanations of behavior. Reaction formation is the development of conscious attitudes and behavior patterns that are opposite to what one really feels or would like to do. Regression is a retreat to earlier patterns of behavior. P/A, AN, PC

62. no. 3. The malingerer consciously produces symptoms so that some recognizable goal can be achieved. The malingerer does not cooperate with the treatment plan, fears getting well, and is more comfortable with the sick role. The malingerer is aware of his behavior and the environment and its effect. P/A, AN, PC

63. no. 4. Poor reality testing is a problem for clients

with a psychotic disorder; it is not a symptom of a psychosomatic disorder. Dependency issues, indecision, and excessive controlling behavior are all characteristic of clients with peptic ulcers. P/A, AS, PC

64. no. 3. Working cooperatively with another person, such as the nurse, is an effective way for a client to receive help in decision making. Taking an excessively assertive stand with clients is an ineffective way to teach them how to make decisions. Giving more responsibility to the client's wife will not help. A client is less likely to follow orders when he has not actively participated in their development. P/A, PL, E

65. no. 3. This response by the nurse encourages the client to express his feelings and redirects him from blaming her to discussing what is bothering him. This response does not blame or judge. To back down because of an angry outburst will encourage further use of that behavior in difficult situations. Option no. 2 introduces a power struggle between the client and the nurse. Option no. 4 is a parent-to-child communication and leaves the client feeling more frustrated. P/A, IM, PC

66. no. 1. This response by the nurse sets limits on the client's outbursts, protects the staff in their need not to be yelled at, and does not cause the client to feel judged or demeaned. Yelling is not a constructive method of communicating in any environment and does not enhance one's feeling of control. Removal of the television is a punitive measure and is not related to his yelling. Clients do not have the right to abuse staff members; the client needs to be taught how to successfully relate to others to have his needs met. P/A, IM, PC

67. no. 2. Participation in group or individual therapy and reevaluation of family relationships would help him understand his condition so that management of the environment can become more effective. Leisure activities may help to reduce the client's stress, but psychosomatic illnesses will recur if the client does not learn how to express his feelings and concerns constructively. Continued repression of emotional tension in a stressful environment will enhance the probability of a recurrence of his illness. Option no. 4 is a good first step, but the client needs to learn how to express his emotions. P/A, EV, H

68. no. 2. Metrorrhagia is bleeding between periods. It may be the first sign of cervical cancer. CBF/P, AN, PS

69. no. 2. When cervical cancer is diagnosed in the preinvasive stage, it carries a 95% to 100% cure rate. CBF/P, IM, H

70. no. 3. Conization may be the only type of therapy needed if an area of normal tissue surrounds the malignancy. Other treatments are hysterectomy and radiation, both of which result in infertility. Option no. 1 is an advantage, but not the primary one. CBF/P, AN, PS

71. no. 3. The fact that the first experience was unsatisfactory calls for supportive nursing action. CBF/P, IM, E

72. no. 3. Manual expression of breast milk before feeding will decrease engorgement and allow the baby to latch onto the nipple with greater ease. If this measure is unsuccessful, a nipple shield may be recommended. CBF/P, IM, PS

73. no. 2. The uterus is displaced by a full bladder. Both nursing the infant and the administration of methylergonovine (Methergine) will cause the uterus to contract; a large baby may result in decreased tone in the uterus. However, these factors will not result in an inaccurate assessment. CBF/P, AS, PS

74. no. 2. Afterbirth pains are uterine contractions that cause involution. The oxytocin released during breastfeeding intensifies the contractions. Afterbirth pains are more common in the multipara and breastfeeding mother. CBF/P, IM, PS

75. no. 2. Dark green vegetables are higher in calcium than most foods other than milk and milk products. CBF/P, IM, PS

76. no. 3. The let-down reflex causes milk to be pushed through the lacteal ducts. Oxytocin is released from the posterior pituitary for action on the myoepithelial cells of the mammary glands. As these cells contract, milk moves from the duct system to the lactiferous sinuses for ultimate delivery to the infant. The other options listed relate to milk secretion or production and not to the let-down reflex. CBF/P, EV, PS

77. no. 2. Regression and increased demands for attention are common occurrences in older siblings, and parents need to be alerted to expect this behavior. The 2-year-old requires the security and confidence that her mother as well as her father loves her in spite of the new baby. Option no. 1 is not developmentally appropriate for a 2-year-old. C/H, IM, E

78. no. 4. As one of the cyanotic heart defects, tetralogy of Fallot is characterized by cyanosis. Clubbing is due to chronic hypoxia, and tachycardia is an attempt by the heart to compensate for lack of oxygen. C/O, AS, H

79. no. 3. When a right-to-left shunt is present, the macrophage-filtering system of the lungs is bypassed. This gives bacteria and air access to the systemic circulation. Clients with congenital heart disease have areas of turbulent blood flow. These clients are more susceptible to the formation and deposit of clots or vegetative matter at these sites. The other options are not characteristic of tetralogy of Fallot. C/O, AN, PS

80. no. 1. Squatting alters the cardiovascular dynamics and improves pulmonary blood flow, thereby alleviating the symptoms of a choking spell. It is the position of choice often assumed spontaneously by these children. C/O, IM, PS

81. no. 3. Because the dose of digoxin must be measured so exactly, this is the recommended method of administration. C/O, IM, PS

82. no. 4. Because the child with heart disease is vulnerable to cardiac stress or failure, a restricted-sodium diet may be prescribed. Foods allowed in the cheese group on a low-sodium diet include unsalted cottage and low-sodium dietetic cheeses. Cheddar cheese contains a high amount of sodium and is contraindicated. C/O, IM, PS

83. no. 4. Cushing's syndrome is characterized by excessive amounts of cortisone. This delays wound healing (antiinflammatory) and interferes with calcium metabolism leading to osteoporosis. Other findings include easy bruising, sodium and water retention, potassium loss, hyperglycemia, and truncal obesity. A/NM, AS, PS

84. no. 1. Increased cortisone leads to sodium retention and higher levels of free cortisol. A/NM, AS, PS

85. no. 4. Adrenal atrophy results in hypocorticism (Addison's disease). A pituitary tumor might produce an increased ACTH that would stimulate the adrenal cortex to produce more cortisol and cortisone. An adrenal tumor might overproduce steroids. A/NM, AN, PS

86. no. 1. Because of increased cortisol levels, clients with Cushing's disease have a low tolerance for stress; in addition, the accuracy of diagnostic tests performed is dependent upon minimizing stress. Fluids may be given but usually not in liberal amounts. Explaining tests and procedures as well as providing diversional activities would be done; however, neither are the priority nursing concern. A/NM, PL, PS

87. no. 3. Increased amounts of glucocorticoids will cause increased sodium and water retention with loss of potassium in the urine. A/NM, AN, PS

88. no. 4. Normally, cortisol levels are highest between 6 AM and 8 AM and decrease during the evening hours, with a nadir around midnight. A client with Cushing's disease will have elevated levels regardless of wake pattern, sleep pattern, or time. A/NM, AS. PS

89. no. 3. Cushing's disease results in increased gluconeogenesis; hyperglycemia occurs, resulting in a diabetic state, and polyphagia is common. A/NM, AN, PS

90. no. 1. Diet should be high in protein, low in calories and sodium, and high in potassium. Complex carbohydrates should be included. A/NM, IM, PS

91. no. 1. Cortisone, the glucocorticoid of choice, will be taken on a daily basis for the rest of her life. When there is an increase in stress, the dosage may need to be temporarily increased. With total removal of a gland, replacement therapy is indicated. With partial removal, follow-up without replacement is possible. A/NM, IM, E

92. no. 2. Having the client verbalize the meaning of the body changes is essential before care can be planned. A/NM, IM, E

93. no. 4. Following the stress of surgery, addisonian crisis is a possibility if there has not been adequate steriod replacement. Change in blood pressure, a first indication of this problem, must be reported immediately. A/NM, AS, PS

94. no. 2. Decreased steroid production following an adrenalectomy can result in loss of sodium and water in copious amounts. In the absence of aldosterone, sodium is lost. Hypovolemic shock can occur quickly if the crisis is untreated. Also, potassium levels rise to dangerous levels, causing life-threatening dysrhythmias. A/NM, AN, PS

95. no. 4. Miss Johnson needs to know all the precautions about steroid therapy. Stress the importance of taking medications daily and informing a physician about the medication when ill or having surgery so that the dosage can be temporarily increased. A/NM, IM, H

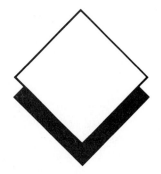

Appendix: Nursing Process and Client Need Categories

Editor's Note

There are two components of the NCLEX-RN test plan: Nursing Process and Client Needs. Nursing process is composed of five steps: assessment, analysis, planning, implementation, and evaluation. Four client needs have been identified: environmental safety, physiological integrity, psychosocial integrity, and health promotion. The practice of nursing requires knowledge in all these areas.

This appendix lists the categories of nursing process and client needs assigned to all the questions in this book.

Assignment of categories was made by item writers and nurse editors. Precise delineation of the categories is an evolving process and, as such, assignment of categories is also evolving.

The appendix is provided for you should you wish to use it. Remember that your test will be scored on your ability to answer a given question correctly and not on your ability to correctly assign a category to a given question.

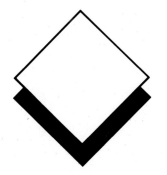

Nursing Process Categories

Section 2   Nursing Care of the Client with Psychosocial and Mental Health Problems

Assessment	11,	18,	19,	22,	28,	31,	33,	34,	38,
	45,	53,	54,	55,	70,	78,	81,	89,	96,
	99,	104,	110,	118,	119,	121,	147,	149,	152,
	153,	154,	159,	165,	166,	172,	173,	180,	189,
	208,	210,	222,	230					

Analysis	2,	5,	10,	15,	16,	26,	37,	42,	43,
	44,	58,	62,	71,	77,	82,	86,	95,	98,
	111,	113,	116,	122,	123,	124,	127,	130,	133,
	143,	144,	148,	156,	158,	168,	177,	178,	181,
	184,	187,	190,	191,	197,	198,	200,	221,	227,
	229,	235,	236,	247,	248,	249,	254		

Planning	8,	14,	30,	39,	46,	47,	48,	69,	87,
	92,	100,	105,	134,	163,	171,	174,	182,	194,
	203,	216,	217,	223,	244,	251			

Implementation	1,	3,	4,	6,	7,	9,	13,	17,	20,
	21,	23,	24,	25,	27,	29,	32,	35,	40,
	49,	50,	57,	59,	60,	61,	63,	64,	65,
	66,	67,	68,	72,	73,	74,	75,	76,	79,
	80,	83,	84,	85,	88,	90,	93,	94,	97,
	101,	102,	103,	106,	107,	108,	109,	112,	113,
	115,	117,	120,	125,	126,	128,	129,	131,	135,
	136,	137,	138,	139,	140,	141,	142,	145,	146,
	150,	155,	157,	160,	161,	162,	167,	169,	170,
	175,	176,	179,	183,	185,	186,	192,	193,	195,
	196,	199,	201,	202,	204,	205,	206,	209,	211,
	212,	213,	214,	215,	218,	219,	220,	224,	225,
	226,	228,	231,	232,	234,	237,	238,	239,	240,
	241,	242,	243,	245,	246,	250,	252,	253	

Evaluation	36,	41,	51,	52,	91,	151,	164,	188,	207,
	233								

Section 3   Nursing Care of the Adult

Assessment	5,	7,	10,	14,	31,	39,	44,	48,	49,
	51,	59,	63,	67,	68,	74,	76,	77,	78,
	79,	82,	86,	89,	93,	97,	100,	106,	108,
	109,	115,	132,	134,	135,	137,	139,	145,	150,

Section 3   Nursing Care of the Adult—cont'd

	156,	157,	170,	175,	179,	180,	182,	184,	188,
	190,	194,	199,	201,	202,	212,	215,	217,	220,
	224,	227,	228,	233,	235,	239,	243,	261,	262,
	265,	276,	280,	281,	282,	283,	287,	299,	306,
	312,	313,	327,	328,	332,	334,	341,	344,	354,
	355,	359,	364,	365,	368,	373,	374,	377,	379,
	384,	393,	394,	404,	406,	409,	421,	431,	436,
	441,	442,	444,	447,	459,	469,	479,	482,	495,
	496,	500,	507,	509,	519,	522			
Analysis	3,	6,	8,	9,	12,	13,	15,	16,	17,
	18,	19,	20,	21,	22,	25,	26,	28,	32,
	33,	34,	35,	36,	37,	38,	43,	46,	47,
	50,	53,	55,	61,	64,	66,	69,	70,	72,
	73,	75,	81,	83,	85,	87,	88,	90,	92,
	94,	95,	98,	99,	103,	104,	111,	114,	118,
	119,	120,	121,	122,	123,	124,	128,	129,	130,
	140,	144,	146,	148,	153,	158,	159,	163,	167,
	168,	171,	176,	181,	183,	186,	192,	195,	196,
	197,	198,	200,	226,	232,	236,	237,	240,	244,
	245,	246,	247,	248,	249,	256,	263,	264,	270,
	277,	278,	279,	284,	290,	292,	293,	294,	295,
	298,	300,	305,	307,	311,	314,	318,	321,	323,
	324,	325,	326,	329,	330,	333,	336,	338,	339,
	346,	347,	348,	349,	350,	351,	352,	357,	363,
	366,	371,	372,	375,	380,	381,	383,	385,	386,
	387,	389,	392,	395,	397,	399,	403,	405,	407,
	411,	412,	414,	422,	425,	426,	430,	435,	440,
	446,	448,	449,	450,	453,	454,	462,	475,	481,
	484,	486,	487,	488,	493,	494,	502,	508,	510,
	512,	518,	521,	523					
Planning	4,	42,	54,	60,	80,	96,	101,	110,	133,
	147,	151,	152,	154,	165,	172,	173,	178,	185,
	203,	213,	214,	242,	252,	262,	269,	271,	291,
	304,	309,	310,	315,	316,	331,	335,	343,	345,
	356,	360,	361,	362,	376,	378,	390,	391,	396,
	398,	401,	402,	408,	410,	415,	416,	418,	423,
	424,	429,	432,	451,	463,	464,	465,	467,	474,
	485,	489,	492,	511,	514				
Implementation	1,	2,	23,	24,	27,	29,	40,	41,	45,
	52,	56,	57,	58,	62,	65,	71,	84,	91,
	102,	105,	112,	113,	116,	117,	131,	138,	141,
	142,	143,	155,	160,	161,	162,	164,	166,	169,
	174,	177,	187,	189,	191,	193,	204,	206,	207,
	208,	209,	210,	211,	216,	218,	219,	223,	225,
	229,	230,	231,	234,	238,	241,	250,	251,	253,
	254,	255,	257,	261,	266,	267,	268,	272,	273,
	274,	275,	285,	286,	288,	296,	297,	301,	303,
	308,	317,	319,	320,	322,	337,	340,	342,	353,
	369,	370,	388,	400,	413,	417,	419,	420,	427,
	428,	433,	434,	437,	438,	439,	443,	445,	455,
	456,	457,	458,	460,	466,	468,	471,	472,	473,
	478,	480,	483,	490,	491,	497,	498,	499,	501,
	503,	504,	505,	506,	513,	515,	516,	517,	520
Evaluation	11,	30,	107,	136,	149,	221,	222,	258,	302,
	358,	367,	382,	461,	470,	476,	524		

Section 4   Nursing Care of the Childbearing Family

Assessment									
1,	7,	10,	13,	16,	17,	20,	23,	38,
39,	46,	47,	59,	64,	68,	71,	74,	77,
82,	84,	92,	95,	106,	109,	110,	111,	122,
132,	134,	136,	142,	149,	150,	152,	155,	156,
157,	158,	159,	160,	165,	166,	172,	173	

Analysis									
2,	3,	8,	11,	27,	33,	40,	41,	49,
50,	55,	57,	62,	66,	70,	72,	76,	79,
89,	90,	91,	94,	100,	107,	114,	117,	119,
124,	128,	133,	138,	139,	141,	145,	151,	167,
169,	176,	177,	178,	179				

Planning					
21,	54,	60,	61,	67,	147

Implementation									
4,	5,	6,	9,	12,	15,	18,	22,	24,
25,	26,	29,	30,	32,	34,	35,	36,	37,
42,	43,	44,	45,	48,	51,	52,	53,	56,
58,	63,	65,	69,	75,	78,	80,	83,	85,
87,	88,	93,	96,	97,	98,	99,	101,	102,
103,	104,	105,	108,	112,	113,	115,	116,	118,
120,	121,	123,	125,	126,	127,	129,	130,	135,
137,	140,	143,	144,	146,	148,	153,	154,	161,
163,	164,	168,	170,	171,	174,	180		

Evaluation							
14,	19,	28,	31,	73,	81,	86,	131

Section 5   Nursing Care of the Child

Assessment									
31,	43,	44,	62,	68,	79,	84,	92,	95,
101,	102,	104,	105,	111,	112,	118,	136,	143,
145,	149,	164,	174,	175,	177,	179,	187,	188,
190,	195,	196,	201,	205,	209,	210,	218	

Analysis									
3,	6,	14,	18,	19,	21,	26,	30,	36,
40,	49,	55,	66,	69,	80,	88,	90,	94,
98,	107,	109,	119,	120,	121,	126,	127,	128,
135,	137,	144,	147,	150,	161,	162,	163,	166,
167,	170,	171,	180,	197,	198,	200,	202,	211,
212,	214,	217						

Planning									
5,	12,	16,	17,	20,	23,	25,	28,	32,
33,	37,	41,	48,	52,	56,	59,	64,	70,
71,	74,	81,	82,	85,	86,	87,	98,	101,
106,	113,	123,	132,	138,	148,	153,	159,	165,
169,	178,	181,	183,	189,	201,	213,	220,	221

Implementation									
1,	4,	6,	7,	8,	9,	10,	11,	13,
15,	22,	24,	27,	34,	35,	38,	39,	40,
45,	46,	54,	58,	60,	61,	63,	65,	67,
76,	89,	91,	93,	96,	97,	100,	103,	108,
115,	116,	117,	122,	124,	125,	129,	130,	131,
134,	139,	140,	146,	149,	150,	151,	152,	154,
155,	160,	161,	176,	177,	182,	184,	185,	191,
193,	194,	199,	204,	206,	207,	208,	216,	219,
222								

Evaluation									
44,	50,	53,	72,	75,	78,	110,	114,	133,
141,	142,	186,	192,	203				

Section 6   Sample Tests

TEST 1, BOOK I

Assessment	1,	2,	6,	12,	24,	29,	30,	45,	48,
	49,	57,	61,	62,	77,	90			

Analysis	5,	8,	9,	15,	16,	23,	31,	34,	35,
	36,	37,	39,	43,	47,	52,	53,	66,	67,
	68,	69,	71,	75,	76,	86,	87,	91,	94,
	95								

Planning	4,	17,	19,	51,	59,	74,	81,	93

Implementation	3,	7,	13,	14,	18,	21,	22,	25,	26,
	27,	28,	32,	33,	38,	40,	41,	42,	44,
	46,	54,	56,	58,	60,	63,	64,	65,	72,
	73,	78,	79,	80,	84,	85,	88,	89,	92

Evaluation	10,	11,	50,	55,	70,	82

TEST 1, BOOK II

Assessment	5,	7,	11,	18,	20,	31,	36,	38,	39,
	40,	53,	58,	60,	63,	64,	69,	89	

Analysis	2,	4,	6,	8,	10,	13,	14,	15,	16,
	17,	21,	23,	25,	26,	28,	29,	32,	43,
	44,	54,	59,	62,	65,	74,	75,	76,	83,
	87,	91,	94,	95					

Planning	9,	22,	30,	34,	41,	42,	46,	47,	55,
	56,	68,	70,	71,	84,	90			

Implementation	1,	3,	12,	19,	27,	37,	45,	48,	49,
	50,	51,	57,	61,	67,	72,	73,	77,	78,
	79,	81,	82,	85,	88,	92,	93		

Evaluation	24,	33,	35,	52,	66,	80,	86

TEST 1, BOOK III

Assessment	2,	8,	13,	17,	19,	20,	21,	32,	33,
	34,	46,	53,	54,	61,	62,	63,	66,	68,
	74,	76,	79,	84,	88,	89			

Analysis	1,	6,	7,	9,	11,	25,	26,	35,	36,
	39,	40,	42,	43,	44,	45,	47,	48,	60,
	69,	71,	72,	75,	78,	86,	90,	91,	94,
	95								

Planning	3,	12,	15,	22,	23,	24,	50,	55,	64,
	93								

Implementation	4,	5,	10,	14,	16,	18,	27,	28,	29,
	30,	31,	37,	41,	49,	51,	56,	57,	58,
	59,	65,	70,	73,	77,	81,	82,	83,	87,
	92								

Evaluation	38,	67,	80,	85

TEST 1, BOOK IV

Assessment	3,	4,	5,	6,	8,	9,	12,	14,	15,
	16,	19,	23,	27,	31,	32,	41,	49,	50,
	61,	64,	69,	78,	79,	80,	86		

Section 6   Sample Tests—cont'd

Analysis	2, 37, 72,	7, 38, 73,	10, 39, 82	13, 44,	18, 47,	30, 56,	33, 62,	35, 65,	36, 67,
Planning	17, 74,	21, 81,	28, 83,	46, 89	48,	51,	53,	63,	71,
Implementation	1, 43, 70, 93,	11, 45, 75, 94,	20, 52, 76, 95	25, 54, 84,	26, 57, 87,	29, 58, 88,	34, 59, 90,	40, 66, 91,	42, 68, 92,
Evaluation	24,	77,	85						

TEST 2, BOOK I

Assessment	1, 35, 81,	7, 39, 84,	11, 44, 85	12, 52,	21, 58,	25, 66,	26, 73,	28, 74,	31, 80,
Analysis	5, 45, 63,	8, 46, 64,	10, 50, 78,	17, 53, 79,	20, 55, 87,	27, 56, 89,	36, 57, 93,	41, 59, 95	43, 62,
Planning	9, 90,	15, 92	23,	24,	37,	47,	51,	67,	69,
Implementation	2, 29, 61, 86,	3, 32, 65, 88,	4, 33, 68, 94	13, 38, 70,	14, 40, 72,	16, 48, 76,	18, 49, 77,	19, 54, 82,	22, 60, 83,
Evaluation	30,	34,	42,	71,	75,	91			

TEST 2, BOOK II

Assessment	9, 35, 82,	12, 44, 83,	15, 52, 91	17, 58,	19, 63,	25, 71,	27, 73,	30, 74,	34, 77,
Analysis	1, 45, 64,	4, 46, 65,	5, 47, 66,	6, 49, 69,	7, 55, 70,	10, 57, 72,	20, 59, 81,	32, 61, 88,	39, 62, 92
Planning	2, 68,	3, 78,	21, 86,	22, 93,	24, 94	42,	43,	56,	67,
Implementation	8, 31, 53, 87,	11, 36, 54, 89,	13, 37, 60, 90,	16, 38, 75, 95	18, 40, 76,	23, 41, 79,	26, 48, 80,	28, 50, 84,	29, 51, 85,
Evaluation	14,	33							

TEST 2, BOOK III

Assessment	12, 78,	19, 82,	30, 87,	50, 88,	56, 90,	59, 94	63,	69,	70,
Analysis	1, 22, 57, 93	4, 26, 58,	5, 28, 61,	8, 32, 62,	13, 39, 67,	16, 41, 68,	17, 43, 86,	18, 46, 89,	21, 55, 91,

Section 6   Sample Tests—cont'd

Planning	9, 47,	15, 48,	20, 51,	25, 52,	27, 64,	31, 66,	33, 83,	38, 85,	40,
Implementation	2, 29, 72, 92,	3, 34, 73, 95	6, 35, 74,	7, 42, 75,	10, 49, 76,	11, 53, 77,	14, 54, 79,	23, 60, 80,	24, 71, 84,
Evaluation	36,	37,	44,	45,	65,	81			

TEST 2, BOOK IV

Assessment	10, 51, 93	12, 52,	19, 53,	20, 56,	21, 63,	28, 73,	38, 78,	39, 83,	47, 88,
Analysis	1, 34, 70,	3, 37, 79,	4, 42, 85,	5, 54, 87,	6, 58, 89,	11, 60, 94	27, 61,	30, 62,	31, 68,
Planning	7,	8,	22,	45,	48,	50,	55,	64,	86
Implementation	2, 26, 59, 80,	9, 29, 65, 81,	13, 32, 66, 82,	14, 33, 69, 90,	16, 35, 71, 91,	17, 43, 72, 92,	18, 44, 74, 95	23, 49, 75,	24, 57, 77,
Evaluation	15,	25,	36,	40,	41,	46,	67,	76	

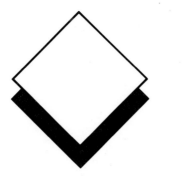

Client Needs
Categories

Section 2   Nursing Care of the Client with Psychosocial and Mental Health Problems

Environmental Safety									
	1,	2,	4,	8,	29,	30,	46,	47,	57,
	73,	79,	80,	83,	86,	87,	88,	93,	97,
	100,	105,	112,	117,	120,	130,	131,	133,	136,
	160,	162,	170,	172,	173,	174,	177,	178,	182,
	185,	188,	193,	194,	203,	212,	215,	217,	223,
	225,	241							

Physiological Integrity									
	15,	17,	28,	40,	56,	64,	74,	77,	85,
	89,	94,	101,	102,	119,	122,	123,	124,	132,
	137,	147,	148,	149,	157,	158,	159,	165,	168,
	169,	184,	187,	200,	201,	208,	210,	211,	226,
	228,	231,	234,	238,	240,	243,	247,	250,	254

Psychosocial Integrity									
	3,	5,	6,	7,	9,	10,	14,	20,	21,
	24,	26,	27,	31,	32,	33,	34,	35,	36,
	37,	38,	39,	41,	42,	43,	44,	45,	48,
	49,	50,	51,	52,	54,	55,	58,	59,	60,
	61,	62,	63,	66,	67,	70,	71,	78,	81,
	82,	84,	92,	95,	98,	99,	104,	106,	108,
	110,	111,	113,	115,	116,	118,	121,	126,	127,
	129,	135,	139,	141,	142,	143,	144,	145,	152,
	153,	154,	156,	161,	166,	167,	176,	180,	181,
	183,	189,	190,	195,	196,	197,	198,	199,	212,
	204,	205,	206,	209,	213,	214,	218,	219,	220,
	221,	222,	224,	227,	236,	237,	239,	242,	245,
	248,	249,	251,	252,	253				

Health Promotion									
	11,	12,	13,	16,	18,	19,	22,	25,	53,
	65,	68,	69,	75,	76,	91,	103,	107,	109,
	114,	125,	128,	138,	140,	150,	155,	163,	164,
	171,	175,	179,	191,	192,	207,	216,	232,	233,
	235,	244,	246						

Section 3   Nursing Care of the Adult

Environmental Safety									
	56,	65,	80,	84,	85,	105,	118,	131,	133,
	139,	142,	144,	151,	154,	155,	160,	161,	162,
	165,	173,	177,	181,	185,	189,	191,	193,	194,
	213,	214,	224,	225,	227,	238,	242,	253,	260,
	261,	265,	266,	268,	269,	272,	273,	274,	285,
	286,	288,	296,	315,	322,	334,	335,	340,	361,

Section 3   Nursing Care of the Adult—cont'd

362,	378,	390,	396,	400,	408,	413	417	423,
420,	429,	437,	438,	439,	445,	449,	451,	468,
470,	471,	473,	474,	485,	489,	490,	504,	506,
510,	511,	512,	514,	520				

Physiological Integrity

1,	2,	3,	4,	5,	6,	7,	8,	9,
10,	11,	12,	13,	14,	15,	16,	17,	18,
19,	20,	21,	22,	23,	24,	25,	26,	29,
30,	31,	32,	33,	34,	35,	36,	37,	38,
39,	40,	44,	46,	47,	48,	49,	50,	51,
52,	53,	54,	55,	56,	57,	61,	62,	63,
64,	66,	67,	68,	69,	70,	71,	72,	73,
74,	75,	76,	77,	78,	79,	81,	82,	83,
86,	87,	88,	89,	90,	92,	93,	94,	95,
96,	97,	98,	99,	100,	101,	102,	103,	104,
106,	107,	108,	109,	111,	113,	114,	115,	119,
120,	121,	122,	123,	124,	125,	126,	127,	128,
129,	130,	132,	134,	135,	137,	138,	140,	141,
143,	145,	146,	147,	148,	149,	150,	152,	153,
156,	157,	158,	159,	163,	164,	167,	168,	169,
170,	171,	172,	175,	176,	178,	179,	180,	182,
183,	184,	186,	188,	190,	192,	195,	196,	198,
199,	201,	202,	203,	205,	206,	208,	209,	212,
215,	217,	219,	220,	226,	228,	230,	231,	232,
233,	234,	235,	236,	237,	239,	240,	243,	244,
245,	246,	247,	248,	249,	250,	251,	252,	254,
255,	256,	259,	262,	263,	264,	267,	270,	275,
276,	277,	278,	279,	280,	281,	282,	283,	284,
287,	289,	292,	293,	294,	295,	297,	298,	299,
300,	301,	304,	305,	306,	307,	316,	317,	318,
319,	320,	321,	322,	323,	324,	325,	326,	327,
328,	329,	330,	332,	333,	336,	337,	338,	339,
341,	343,	344,	345,	346,	347,	348,	349,	350,
351,	354,	355,	356,	357,	358,	359,	360,	363,
364,	365,	366,	367,	368,	369,	371,	373,	374,
375,	376,	377,	379,	380,	381,	382,	383,	384,
385,	386,	387,	388,	389,	391,	392,	393,	394,
395,	396,	403,	404,	405,	406,	407,	409,	411,
412,	414,	418,	419,	421,	422,	424,	425,	427,
430,	433,	434,	435,	436,	440,	441,	442,	444,
446,	447,	450,	453,	454,	455,	456,	459,	461,
462,	463,	465,	466,	467,	469,	472,	481,	482,
484,	486,	488,	487,	488,	489,	492,	493,	494,
495,	496,	498,	500,	505,	507,	515,	518,	519,
521,	522,	523						

Psychosocial Integrity

28,	204,	207,	218,	229,	291,	303,	457,	458,
491,	497,	501,	503,	508,	509			

Health Promotion

27,	41,	42,	43,	45,	57,	58,	91,	110,
112,	116,	117,	136,	166,	174,	187,	197,	200,
210,	211,	216,	221,	222,	223,	241,	257,	258,
271,	290,	302,	308,	342,	352,	353,	369,	372,
397,	401,	402,	410,	415,	416,	420,	426,	431,
432,	443,	448,	452,	460,	464,	475,	476,	477,
478,	479,	480,	498,	506,	513,	516,	517,	524

Section 4   Nursing Care of the Childbearing Family

Environmental Safety								
16,	17,	24,	25,	31,	36,	43,	44,	48,
53,	54,	58,	60,	61,	67,	75,	87,	88,
89,	102,	103,	105,	106,	108,	112,	118,	125,
126,	144,	147,	168,	171				

Physiological Integrity								
1,	2,	3,	6,	7,	8,	9,	10,	11,
13,	20,	23,	28,	32,	33,	34,	37,	38,
39,	40,	41,	42,	46,	47,	49,	50,	51,
52,	55,	56,	57,	59,	62,	64,	65,	66,
70,	71,	72,	74,	77,	82,	83,	84,	85,
86,	90,	91,	92,	93,	94,	95,	96,	97,
98,	99,	100,	104,	107,	109,	110,	111,	114,
116,	117,	119,	122,	123,	124,	127,	128,	129,
132,	133,	134,	135,	136,	138,	140,	141,	142,
145,	149,	151,	152,	155,	156,	157,	158,	159,
160,	162,	165,	166,	167,	169,	172,	173,	175,
176,	177,	178,	179					

Psychosocial Integrity								
15,	22,	26,	27,	45,	68,	69,	76,	78,
79,	81,	113,	120,	121,	123,	139,	174,	180

Health Promotion								
4,	5,	12,	14,	18,	19,	21,	29,	30,
35,	63,	73,	80,	101,	115,	130,	131,	137,
143,	146,	148,	150,	153,	154,	161,	163,	164,
170								

Section 5   Nursing Care of the Child

Environmental Safety								
22,	24,	25,	27,	32,	56,	59,	61,	81,
99,	103,	137,	138,	139,	149,	153,	154,	160,
161,	165,	182,	191,	199,	206			

Physiological Integrity								
8,	12,	23,	28,	29,	30,	31,	33,	36,
37,	39,	40,	42,	44,	47,	48,	49,	50,
51,	52,	55,	62,	63,	64,	65,	66,	67,
68,	69,	70,	71,	73,	74,	79,	80,	82,
83,	87,	88,	89,	90,	91,	92,	94,	96,
98,	101,	102,	105,	106,	107,	108,	109,	112,
118,	120,	123,	124,	125,	126,	127,	128,	129,
130,	143,	145,	146,	147,	151,	152,	155,	159,
164,	166,	167,	168,	175,	177,	179,	180,	181,
183,	184,	185,	186,	187,	188,	189,	190,	192,
193,	194,	200,	201,	204,	205,	207,	208,	210,
211,	212,	213,	214,	215,	216,	218,	220	

Psychosocial Integrity								
10,	13,	18,	19,	20,	21,	57,	58,	76,
77,	106,	115,	116,	117,	129,	131,	134,	135,
144,	150,	162,	171,	197,	203			

Health Promotion								
1,	2,	3,	4,	5,	6,	7,	9,	11,
14,	15,	16,	34,	35,	38,	41,	43,	45,
46,	53,	54,	60,	72,	75,	84,	85,	86,
95,	100,	104,	110,	111,	112,	113,	114,	121,
132,	133,	136,	141,	142,	148,	169,	174,	176,
177,	178,	195,	197,	202,	209,	219,	221,	222

Section 6   Sample Tests

TEST 1, BOOK I

Environmental Safety

1,	3,	4,	7,	17,	19,	33,	51,	59,
62,	78,	88						

Physiological Integrity

2,	12,	13,	14,	15,	16,	18,	20,	21,
22,	23,	24,	26,	29,	30,	31,	32,	34,
35,	45,	46,	47,	48,	49,	50,	52,	53,
57,	60,	61,	65,	66,	67,	68,	69,	71,
72,	73,	74,	84,	85,	90,	91,	92,	93,
94,	95							

Psychosocial Integrity

5,	6,	8,	9,	10,	11,	36,	37,	38,
39,	40,	41,	42,	43,	44,	56,	75,	76,
77,	79,	80,	81,	82,	83,	86,	89	

Health Promotion

25,	27,	28,	54,	55,	58,	63,	64,	70

TEST 1, BOOK II

Environmental Safety

1,	22,	24,	30,	41,	46,	55,	61,	64,
67,	71,	84						

Physiological Integrity

2,	3,	4,	5,	6,	7,	10,	11,	12,
13,	14,	15,	16,	17,	18,	19,	20,	21,
23,	28,	29,	31,	32,	34,	36,	37,	38,
39,	40,	42,	54,	60,	62,	63,	65,	66,
68,	69,	70,	74,	75,	76,	82,	83,	85,
86,	87,	88,	89,	90,	91,	93,	94,	95

Psychosocial Integrity

9,	26,	25,	27,	44,	45,	47,	48,	49,
50,	51,	52,	57,	72,	73,	77,	78,	79,
80								

Health Promotion

8,	33,	35,	43,	53,	56,	58,	81,	92

TEST 1, BOOK III

Environmental Safety

3,	14,	16,	22,	23,	28,	30,	31,	50,
55,	64,	73,	77					

Physiological Integrity

1,	2,	11,	12,	13,	15,	17,	20,	21,
24,	25,	26,	32,	33,	34,	35,	36,	37,
39,	40,	41,	42,	43,	44,	45,	46,	49,
51,	60,	61,	62,	63,	65,	66,	68,	69,
70,	71,	72,	74,	75,	76,	78,	79,	80,
82,	83,	84,	85,	86,	87,	88,	89,	90,
91,	92,	93,	94,	95				

Psychosocial Integrity

4,	6,	7,	8,	9,	10,	18,	29,	47,
53,	54,	56,	57,	58,	59,	81		

Health Promotion

5,	19,	38,	48,	52,	67

TEST 1, BOOK IV

Environmental Safety

20,	28,	51,	54,	63,	75,	87,	89

Physiological Integrity

9,	10,	11,	14,	16,	17,	18,	19,	21,
22,	23,	25,	26,	27,	30,	32,	33,	34,
35,	36,	37,	38,	39,	40,	41,	44,	45,
47,	49,	50,	52,	53,	60,	61,	62,	63,
64,	65,	67,	68,	70,	71,	72,	73,	74,
78,	79,	80,	81,	83,	84,	85,	86,	88,
90,	91,	92,	93,	94				

Section 6   Sample Tests—cont'd

Psychosocial Integrity	1,	2,	3,	4,	5,	6,	7,	8,	12,
	13,	14,	55,	56,	57,	58,	59,	66,	82
Health Promotion	24,	26,	29,	31,	42,	43,	46,	48,	69,
	76,	77,	95						

TEST 2, BOOK I

Environmental Safety	22,	23,	36,	37,	38,	76,	86,	90,	94
Physiological Integrity	5,	6,	7,	8,	9,	10,	11,	12,	13,
	16,	17,	18,	19,	20,	21,	24,	25,	26,
	27,	28,	29,	35,	39,	40,	41,	42,	43,
	44,	45,	46,	58,	59,	60,	61,	62,	63,
	64,	65,	66,	67,	68,	70,	74,	77,	78,
	79,	80,	81,	83,	84,	85,	87,	89,	92,
	93,	95							
Psychosocial Integrity	2,	13,	15,	31,	32,	33,	48,	49,	50,
	51,	52,	53,	54,	55,	56,	73,	82	
Health Promotion	1,	3,	4,	30,	34,	47,	57,	69,	71,
	72,	75,	88,	91					

TEST 2, BOOK II

Environmental Safety	13,	21,	22,	43,	48,	57,	67,	84,	86,
	93								
Physiological Integrity	1,	2,	3,	4,	5,	6,	7,	8,	12,
	17,	19,	20,	23,	25,	27,	28,	32,	44,
	47,	49,	53,	63,	64,	65,	66,	69,	70,
	71,	72,	73,	74,	75,	76,	77,	80,	81,
	82,	85,	87,	91,	92,	94,	95		
Psychosocial Integrity	9,	10,	11,	15,	18,	26,	29,	34,	35,
	36,	37,	39,	40,	41,	50,	51,	58,	59,
	60,	61,	62,	78,	79				
Health Promotion	14,	16,	24,	30,	31,	33,	38,	52,	54,
	55,	56,	68,	83,	88,	89,	90		

TEST 2, BOOK III

Environmental Safety	9,	14,	23,	25,	40,	65,			
Physiological Integrity	1,	2,	3,	4,	5,	6,	7,	13,	15,
	16,	18,	19,	20,	21,	22,	26,	27,	29,
	30,	31,	32,	33,	38,	46,	47,	48,	50,
	51,	52,	53,	54,	55,	56,	57,	58,	59,
	60,	61,	62,	63,	64,	67,	72,	73,	74,
	75,	82,	83,	85,	86,	87,	88,	89,	90,
	91,	92,	93,	94					
Psychosocial Integrity	8,	10,	11,	12,	39,	41,	42,	43,	44,
	45,	49,	68,	69,	70,	71,	78,	80,	84
Health Promotion	17,	24,	28,	34,	35,	36,	37,	66,	76,
	77,	81,	95						

TEST 2, BOOK IV

Environmental Safety	9,	22,	23,	45,	47,	48,	50,	55,	56,
	64,	71,	76,	91,	92				

Section 6   Sample Tests—cont'd

Physiological Integrity	1,	2,	3,	4,	6,	7,	8,	19,	20,
	21,	24,	26,	27,	28,	29,	30,	31,	33,
	34,	35,	36,	37,	38,	39,	41,	43,	44,
	49,	51,	52,	53,	54,	60,	68,	70,	72,
	73,	74,	75,	78,	79,	80,	81,	82,	83,
	84,	85,	86,	87,	88,	89,	90,	93,	94
Psychosocial Integrity	10,	11,	12,	13,	14,	15,	16,	17,	18,
	42,	46,	58,	59,	61,	62,	63,	65,	66
Health Promotion	5,	25,	32,	40,	57,	67,	69,	77,	95

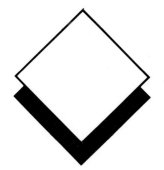

Index*

---

*The letters and numbers that follow each entry refer to the clinical section and the question number. For example: A301 following "Abdominoperineal resection" indicates question 301 in *Nursing Care of the Adult*. Consult the following key:

A = Adult C = Child CF = Childbearing Family P = Psychosocial
T1B1 = Test 1 Book 1 T1B2 = Test 1 Book 2 T1B3 = Test 1 Book 3
T1B4 = Test 1 Book 4 T2B1 = Test 2 Book 1 T2B2 = Test 2 Book 2
T2B3 = Test 2 Book 3 T2B4 = Test 2 Book 4.